D1568708

THORACIC
IMAGING
A Practical Approach

NOTICE

Medicine is an ever-changing science. As new research and clinical experience broaden our knowledge, changes in treatment and drug therapy are required. The editors and the publisher of this work have checked with sources believed to be reliable in their efforts to provide information that is complete and generally in accord with the standards accepted at the time of publication. However, in view of the possibility of human error or changes in medical sciences, neither the editors nor the publisher nor any other party who has been involved in the preparation or publication of this work warrants that the information contained herein is in every respect accurate or complete, and they are not responsible for any errors or omissions or for the results obtained from use of such information. Readers are encouraged to confirm the information contained herein with other sources. For example and in particular, readers are advised to check the product information sheet included in the package of each drug they plan to administer to be certain that the information contained in this book is accurate and that changes have not been made in the recommended dose or in the contraindications for administration. This recommendation is of particular importance in connection with new or infrequently used drugs.

THORACIC IMAGING
A Practical Approach

Richard M. Slone, M.D., F.C.C.P.

Assistant Professor of Radiology, Thoracic Imaging, and Body CT
Mallinckrodt Institute of Radiology
Washington University School of Medicine
St. Louis, Missouri

Fernando R. Gutierrez, M.D.

Associate Professor of Radiology, Thoracic Imaging, and Body CT
Director of Cardiac Radiology
Mallinckrodt Institute of Radiology
Washington University School of Medicine
St. Louis, Missouri

Andrew J. Fisher, M.D.

Director of Emergency and Trauma Radiology
Division of Musculoskeletal Radiology
Mallinckrodt Institute of Radiology
Washington University School of Medicine
St. Louis, Missouri

With contributions from

Matthew J. Fleishman, M.D.

Radiology Imaging Associates
Denver, Colorado

Robert Y. Kanterman, M.D.

St. Luke's Hospital
Chesterfield, Missouri

McGRAW-HILL
Health Professions Division

New York   St. Louis   San Francisco   Auckland   Bogotá   Caracas   Lisbon   London   Madrid
Mexico City   Milan   Montreal   New Delhi   San Juan   Singapore   Sydney   Tokyo   Toronto

A Division of The McGraw·Hill Companies

THORACIC IMAGING

Copyright © 1999 by *The McGraw-Hill Companies*, Inc. All rights reserved.
Printed in the United States of America. Except as permitted under the United
States Copyright Act of 1976, no part of this publication may be reproduced or
distributed in any form or by any means, or stored in a data base or retrieval
system, without prior written permission of the publisher.

1234567890 DOCDOC 998
ISBN: 0-07-058223-8

This book was set in Times Roman by V&M Graphics, Incorporated.
The editors were James Morgan III and Muza Navrozov.
The production supervisor was Helene G. Landers.
The cover was designed by Marsha Cohen/Parallelogram.
The index was prepared by Jerry Ralya.
R. R. Donnelley & Sons Company was printer and binder.

This book is printed on recycled, acid-free paper.

Library of Congress Cataloging-in-Publication Data
Slone, Richard M.
    Thoracic imaging : a practical approach / Richard M. Slone,
Fernando R. Gutierrez, Andrew J. Fisher.—1st ed.
        p. cm.
    Includes index.
    ISBN 0-07-058223-8
    1. Chest—Imaging. 2. Chest—Diseases—Diagnosis. 3. Diagnosis,
Differential. I. Gutierrez, Fernando R. II. Fisher, Andrew J.
III. Title.
    [DNLM: 1. Thoracic Diseases—diagnosis. 2. Diagnostic Imaging.
3. Radiology, Thoracic. 4. Thorax—radionuclide imaging.
5. Thorax—ultrasonography. 6. Lung Diseases—diagnosis.WF 975
S634t   1999]
RC941.S53   1999
617.5'40754—dc21
DNLM/DLC
for Library of Congress.

To my son Logan
—————
RMS

To my wife and best friend
—————
FRG

To Mom and Pop—my first and greatest teachers
—————
AJF

CONTENTS

PREFACE

Chest diseases encompass a broad spectrum of pathologies and affect a wide range of patients. Diagnostic imaging, including conventional chest radiography, computed tomography, and magnetic resonance imaging of the thorax, is an important means of detecting and diagnosing diseases of the heart, lungs, and chest wall. Interventional techniques play an important role in the diagnosis and treatment of some patients. Follow-up imaging studies are crucial in assessing the success of treatment and evaluating patients for new or recurrent disease following medical and surgical management of thoracic diseases.

This book is intended as a concise, yet complete, overview of thoracic imaging, diagnostic techniques, differential diagnosis, and diseases involving the thorax and is designed for radiologists, internists, and surgeons involved in the care of patients with chest disease. There are many excellent, comprehensive textbooks covering radiology and diseases of the chest which are generally well illustrated, large, and expensive. This book is not intended to replace those, but rather to serve a complementary role as a source for review and as a handy reference which is affordable, manageable in size, and easy to use.

Chapter 1 presents a review of pulmonary physiology, diagnostic imaging techniques, pulmonary function testing, bronchoscopy, and mediastinoscopy. Chapter 2 provides an extensive presentation of differential diagnoses based on specific radiographic findings. Chapters 3 through 8 present a reasonably comprehensive overview of specific thoracic diseases broken down by organ system, including etiology, diagnosis, management, treatment, and prognosis. Chapters 9 through 12 cover pediatric chest, trauma, postsurgical, portable and intensive care unit imaging, disease management, particularly thoracic surgical procedures, radiation therapy, chemotherapy, and thoracic implants, including prosthetic valves and pacemakers. Chapter 13 covers diseases of the upper abdomen involving the liver, spleen, stomach, kidneys, and adrenals. Chapter 14 covers interventional techniques, including percutaneous biopsy and pleural drainage procedures. The Appendix includes tables of the normal size of intrathoracic structures, common abbreviations, a comprehensive discussion of common syndromes, surgical eponyms, and current cancer staging criteria.

ACKNOWLEDGMENTS

We wish to thank the following individuals for their assistance in bringing this monograph to publication. Roger Yusen, M.D. from the Division of Pulmonary and Critical Care Medicine; Brian F. Meyers from the Division of Cardiovascular Surgery; Dennis Balfe, M.D. from the division of Abdominal Radiology; David Melson from the Electronic Radiology Laboratory, Michelle Thomas, Thomas Murry, and Norme Hente from Photograph for preparing all of the prints; Julie Larick and Vicki Friedman from Medical Illustration for preparing all of the drawings; Anna Langenberg and Debra Brouk for expert secretarial assistance, and the staff and residents at the Mallinckrodt Institute who contributed many of the teaching files used for illustrations.

THORACIC
IMAGING
A Practical Approach

Chapter 1

CHEST IMAGING
AND DIAGNOSTIC TESTING

Richard M. Slone

1.1 PULMONARY ANATOMY

- The right lung has three lobes, and the left lung has two. The **pleural fissures** are formed by the interface of the visceral pleura entering clefts separating the lobes (Fig. 1-1). The

major fissure separates the lower lobes from the remaining lung. The **minor fissure**, present only on the right, extends from the anterior chest wall to the major fissure posteriorly and separates the middle and right upper lobes. The fissures act as barriers to the spread of infection, creating a sharply marginated border to pneumonia or neoplasm. Air, infection, and neoplasia can spread between lobes when the fissures are incomplete.

- Pulmonary lobes are further divided into **bronchopulmonary segments** based on bronchial anatomy (Fig. 1-2). The right upper lobe has three segments—apical, posterior, and anterior. The middle lobe has two segments—medial and lateral. The right lower lobe has five segments, including the superior segment, which projects behind the middle lobe and hilum, and four basal segments—anterior, posterior, medial, and lateral. The left upper lobe has four segments—apicoposterior, anterior, superior lingular, and inferior lingular. The left lower lobe has four segments: superior and three basal segments—anteromedial, lateral, and posterior. In total, the right lung has ten segments, and the left, eight.

- The **airway** is a branching series of over 20 generations of progressively smaller tubes leading to the alveoli, the gas-exchanging units of the lung. The **trachea** is composed of 14 to 20 C-shaped hyaline cartilage rings and a posterior membrane. It extends from the cricoid cartilage to the carina at approximately T5, where it divides into the right and left main bronchi. The right main bronchus becomes the bronchus intermedius after the takeoff of the upper lobe bronchus. Further subdivisions into the bronchopulmonary segments are shown in Figure 1-2.

- The **conducting zone**, which has no direct communication with alveoli, begins with the trachea and continues

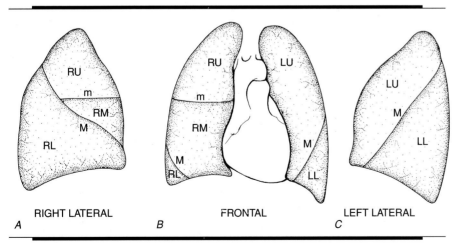

FIGURE 1-1 Pulmonary lobes and pleural fissures. Right lateral (*A*), frontal (*B*), and left lateral (*C*) views of the lungs, showing the major (M) and minor (m) fissures separating the right upper (RU), right middle (RM), right lower (RL), left upper (LU), and left lower (LL) lobes.

1

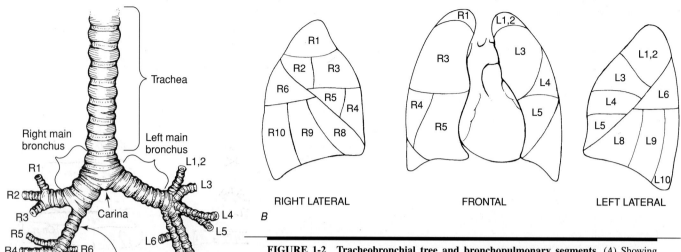

FIGURE 1-2 **Tracheobronchial tree and bronchopulmonary segments.** (A) Showing bifurcation of the trachea at the carina into the right and left main bronchus and subsequently into lobar and segmental bronchi. Apical (R1), posterior (R2), and anterior (R3) segments of the right upper lobe; lateral (R4) and medial (R5) segments of the right middle lobe; superior (R6), medial (R7), anterior (R8), lateral (R9), and posterior (R10) basal segments of the right lower lobe; apicoposterior (L1 and L2), anterior (L3), superior (L4), and inferior (L5) lingular segments of the left upper lobe; superior (L6), anteromedial (L8), lateral (L9), and posterior (L10) basal segments of the left lower lobe. (B) Illustrating the surface projection of each segment. The segments are numbered as in (A). (The right medial basal segment (R7) is obscured by the lateral basal segment.)

out to the sixteenth generation, the terminal bronchioles. The **respiratory zone** contains the airways distal to the terminal bronchiole, including the respiratory bronchioles, which have occasional alveoli arising from their walls and alveolar ducts, which are lined by alveoli terminating in collections of alveoli known as *alveolar sacs.*

- The **secondary pulmonary lobule** is the primary structural and functional unit of the lung and begins at the level of the respiratory zone (Fig. 1-3). It is a 2- to 3-cm regular polyhedron with thin, straight walls called *interlobular septa,* which

contain the pulmonary veins, lymphatics, and connective tissue. The pulmonary lobule is subdivided by *intralobular septa* into about 10 *acini* supplied by terminal bronchioles and pulmonary arterioles which travel together into the lobule center. Acini are further divided into *alveoli.* The lung contains about 300 million alveoli, each about 0.3 mm in diameter.

Type I pneumocytes are relatively large, thin cells providing most of the surface coverage of the alveoli. **Type II pneumocytes** are less prevalent, more cuboidal, and produce

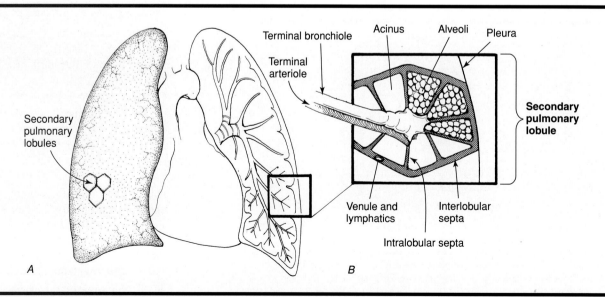

FIGURE 1-3 **Pulmonary architecture.** (A) Coronal section through the left lung and (B) enlarged view of a single secondary pulmonary lobule showing detailed anatomy of the respiratory zone.

surfactant. **Surfactant** is a fluid that lines the alveolar walls and lowers surface tension, increasing compliance and reducing the work required to expand the lung. The reduced surface tension also stabilizes alveoli, which are interdependent, and reduces movement of fluid into the alveoli.

- The **visceral pleura** covering the lung includes mesothelial cells lining the surface, underlying connective tissue, and a vascular layer. Blood is supplied by both pulmonary (98 percent) and bronchial (2 percent) arteries. The potential **pleural space** normally contains a small amount of pleural fluid (10 ml), primarily produced and resorbed by the parietal pleura, providing lubrication.

- The **parietal pleura** lines the thoracic cavity, mediastinum, and diaphragm. There is an overlying layer of connective tissue and extrapleural fat along the chest wall surface below the endothoracic fascia. The parietal pleural is innervated with sensory nerves, whereas the visceral pleura is not. Blood is supplied by systemic vessels.

- The **chest wall** includes the thoracic cage, muscle, fat, vessels, and lymphatics. The **thoracic cage** includes components of the axial skeleton (vertebral bodies, ribs, and sternum) and appendicular skeleton (clavicles and scapula). The **ribs** articulate with the vertebral bodies posteriorly and the sternum anteriorly. The costal cartilage of the first seven ribs articulates with the sternum directly, and the remainder combine to join inferiorly.

- The **diaphragm** is a thin, domed, musculotendinous structure that separates the thorax from the abdomen and is the primary muscle of respiration. The **muscular diaphragm** is composed of three groups: (1) the sternal portion arising from the xiphoid process, (2) the costal slips from the ribs, and (3) the crura from the upper three lumbar vertebrae. All three converge on the **central tendon**. There are three major openings in the diaphragm for the inferior vena cava, esophagus, and aorta, with accompanying thoracic duct, azygos, and hemiazygos veins.

- The **pulmonary arteries** receive the entire right heart output. The walls of the pulmonary arteries are thin and contain little smooth muscle. The arterioles travel alongside the bronchi and eventually branch into an extensive capillary network lining the alveolar walls, forming a sheet of blood for gas exchange. The **pulmonary veins** travel separately from the arteries and bronchi, converging into the right and left superior and inferior pulmonary veins which drain into the left atrium.

- The **bronchial arteries** arise from the aorta and supply blood to the bronchi out to the terminal bronchiole level. This blood returns to the left atrium via the pulmonary veins.

- The lung has an extensive **lymphatic network** within the peribronchovascular and subpleural connective tissue and interlobular septa. Drainage is to bronchopulmonary lymph nodes and subsequently to the ipsilateral hilar and then mediastinal lymph nodes. The American Thoracic Society mapping system is detailed in Fig. 5-4. In general, normal mediastinal lymph nodes are less than 1 cm in diameter.

Small intrapulmonary lymph nodes are occasionally identified on computed tomography (CT) as small (<4 mm), typically peripheral, oval nodules.

1.2 PULMONARY PHYSIOLOGY

- The **gas exchange** process involves ventilation, in which air is physically moved into and out of the lungs, diffusion of gases across lung tissue, pulmonary blood flow and ventilation-perfusion matching, gas transport within systemic vessels, and ultimate utilization of oxygen and production of carbon dioxide by mitochondria in cells.

- **Airway resistance** limits airflow and volume. Resistance is proportional to airway length and inversely proportional to the square of the radius, resulting in increased resistance and lower airflow speed in smaller airways. The higher resistance of small airways (<2 mm) is compensated for by their large number so that they account for less than one-quarter of total airway resistance. Thus, significant small-airways disease can be present before airflow limitation is clinically detected.

  Bronchi increase in size with inspiration, lowering inspiratory airflow resistance. Breathing at a high lung volume also reduces airway resistance, a technique unconsciously employed by patients with airflow limitations. Bronchial **smooth muscle tone** affects bronchial diameter and can be altered by the autonomic nervous system and drugs. Epinephrine, norepinephrine, and isoproterenol cause bronchodilatation, whereas acetylcholine, parasympathetic activity, and environmental irritants cause bronchoconstriction.

- **Compliance** of the lung is the volume change relative to the pressure change and depends on the volume at which it is measured. A stiff lung is less compliant, as seen with increased venous pressure, fibrosis, and alveolar edema. Compliance is increased with destruction of the elastic tissue due to emphysema or aging.

- **Inspiration** is an active process. In a normal breath, 500 ml of air is inhaled (tidal volume), but only 350 ml reaches the alveoli. The rest (150 ml) remains in the conducting airway as **anatomic dead space**. Approximately one-third of the respiratory cycle is spent in inspiration.

  Diaphragmatic contraction forces the abdominal contents downward, displacing the ribs upward and outward, thus increasing lung height and diameter. During normal breathing the diaphragm moves about 1 cm but may move 5 to 10 cm between deep inspiration and forced expiration. Contraction of the external intercostal muscles raises the ribs, increasing the thoracic diameter.

  Accessory muscles of inspiration may be recruited in severely dyspneic patients. They include the scalene muscles, which elevate the first two ribs, and the sternocleidomastoids, which raise the sternum.

- **Work of inspiration** is required to overcome the elastic forces of the lung as well as airway and tissue resistance. The **work of exhalation** must overcome airway and tissue resistance by passively using the energy stored in the expanded elastic structures. As the breathing rate increases, work increases because of airway resistance. Patients with airflow obstruction tend to breathe slowly, and patients with stiff lungs take rapid, shallow breaths to reduce the work of breathing.

Exhalation is normally a passive process. The lung has intrinsic recoil due to its elasticity and surface tension on the alveoli, enhanced by surfactant. This is balanced by the tendency of the chest wall to expand. These opposing forces keep the lung expanded and produce a negative intrapleural pressure. **Functional residual capacity** (end expiration) represents this equilibrium where the inward pull of the lung is matched by the outward pull of the thoracic wall at rest. A pneumothorax allows the lung to collapse and the thorax to expand outward.

Forced expiration involves contraction of the abdominal wall musculature, which increases intra-abdominal pressure and forces the diaphragm up, reducing lung volume. Contraction of the internal intercostal muscles pulls the ribs together, moving them downward, backward, and inward, decreasing the anteroposterior and transverse dimension of the chest.

Maximum flow is determined by the elastic recoil of the lung, airway resistance, lung volume, and effort. **Maximum expiratory flow rate** decreases with lung volume and is relatively independent of effort at low volumes. Elastic forces also provide outward radial traction on airways. This is reduced in emphysema, contributing to significant airflow limitation during expiration.

- **Ventilation** varies from apex to base, partly because of the weight of the lung and varying distending pressures throughout the lung. The lung is easier to inflate at low volumes; therefore the lower lobes, which have a lower resting volume due to the weight of the lung above it, expand more on inspiration. In the upright position, the lung bases receive three times the minute ventilation of the apices per unit volume (Fig. 1-4).

Perfusion plays a crucial role in the respiratory process and also varies as a gravity-induced pulmonary blood pressure gradient. In the upright position, blood flow to the lung bases is almost 20 times greater than to the lung apex. The peripheral lung receives less blood flow than the central areas. With exercise, blood flow becomes more evenly distributed in the upper and lower lobes as a result of recruitment and distention of capillaries.

Ventilation/perfusion (V/Q) ratios are highest in the lung apices and lowest in the lung bases in the resting upright patient. In the supine patient, the V/Q ratio is highest anteriorly and lowest posteriorly.

Oxygen and carbon dioxide concentrations also vary by region, primarily because of differences in the V/Q ratio. The upper lobes have a higher equilibrium oxygen concentration and a lower carbon dioxide concentration than the lower lobes. The lower carbon dioxide concentration in the upper lobes produces a relatively alkaline environment (Fig. 1-5).

- **Pulmonary vascular resistance** is about one-tenth that of the systemic circulation, allowing pulmonary perfusion at a mean pressure of only 15 mmHg. Pulmonary vascular resis-

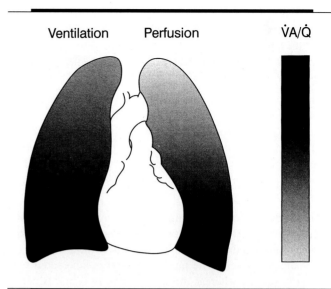

FIGURE 1-4   Pulmonary ventilation and perfusion distribution. Illustrating the relative distribution of ventilation, which ranges from 0.24 L/min in the apex to 0.82 L/min in the lung base (1:3). Perfusion ranges from 0.07 L/min in the apex to 1.29 L/min in the lung base (1:18). As a consequence, the ventilation/perfusion ratio is higher in the apex (3.3) than in the lung base (0.6).

tance increases as lung volumes decrease. Oxygen, acetylcholine, isoproterenol, and inhaled nitric oxide produce pulmonary vasodilatation. Serotonin, norepinephrine, and histamine cause smooth muscle contraction and increase pulmonary vascular resistance. Gas transfer between alveoli and blood is by passive diffusion from high to low partial

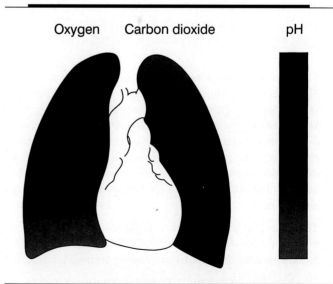

FIGURE 1-5   Oxygen and carbon dioxide gradients. Illustrating the higher alveolar oxygen concentration in the apex (130 mmHg) compared to the lung base (90 mmHg) and the lower alveolar carbon dioxide concentration in the apex (28 mmHg) compared to the lung base (42 mmHg). As a consequence of the carbon dioxide gradient, pH ranges from an alkaline environment of 7.51 in the apex to a normal systemic pH of 7.39 in the lung base.

pressures across the alveolar epithelium, interstitium, and capillary endothelium (blood-gas barrier). Although each red blood cell spends less than 1 sec in the capillary network, there is near complete equilibration of oxygen and carbon dioxide between the alveoli and blood. This mechanism is extremely efficient because of the very thin barrier (<0.5 μm) and the tremendous surface area of alveoli (almost 100 m^2).

The partial pressure of oxygen (P_{O_2}) in blood returning from the systemic circulation and entering the pulmonary capillaries is about 40 mmHg. The P_{O_2} of inspired air is about 150 mmHg and is reduced to 100 mmHg in the alveoli as equilibrium is reached with oxygenated blood. The partial pressure of carbon dioxide (P_{CO_2}) in blood entering the capillary bed is 45 mmHg. This value decreases to about 40 mmHg in the alveoli at equilibrium. Alveolar gas transfer is normally limited by blood flow rather than diffusion.

- **V/Q mismatch** or **inequality** may impair both oxygen and carbon dioxide transfer. In the setting of inadequate ventilation, gas exchange is impaired. Blood passing through areas of high ventilation relative to perfusion gains relatively little additional oxygen compared to areas with matched V/Q which have higher proportional blood flow.

   Similarly, if perfusion is inadequate relative to ventilation, alveolar oxygen levels increase and carbon dioxide levels decrease, approaching that of inspired air. Lung that is ventilated but not perfused does not contribute to gas exchange and is termed *alveolar dead space*.

   Although carbon dioxide would be expected to rise in V/Q mismatch, chemoreceptor response increases ventilation to maintain normal Pa_{CO_2}. This increased ventilation does not significantly improve Pa_{O_2} because of the difference in the shapes of the oxygen and carbon dioxide dissociation curves. Carbon dioxide has a much greater solubility than oxygen and diffuses about 20 times faster.

- **Hypoxemia** can result from (1) V/Q mismatch due to collapse, consolidation, or thrombosis, (2) hypoventilation due to drugs or paralysis, (3) impaired diffusion due to thickening of the blood-gas barrier by disease, (4) a shunt in which blood returns to the systemic circulation without passing through the ventilated lung, or (5) low inspired oxygen concentration.

   Hypoxic vasoconstriction occurs when pulmonary alveolar oxygenation decreases below 70 mmHg. This has a beneficial effect in shunting blood away from hypoxemic regions of the lung. This effect can be deleterious, however, in the setting of global hypoxemia (such as high altitudes) where global pulmonary vasoconstriction occurs and hypertension ensues. A low blood pH also leads to vasoconstriction.

- **Shunting** occurs when blood travels from the right to the left heart without being ventilated as a result of congenital heart disease, vascular malformations, collapsed lung, etc. Subsequent mixing of venous and arterial blood results in variable degrees of hypoxemia that cannot be completely corrected with supplemental oxygen. Similar to V/Q mismatch, shunting does not usually lead to hypercapnea because of increased respiratory drive.

- **Pulmonary interstitial fluid** results from an imbalance in the oncotic and hydrostatic forces that produces a net outward flow of fluid from the capillaries into the interstitium. This fluid travels in the peribronchovascular space where it is collected by lymphatics and transported to hilar lymph nodes. Increased production leads to interstitial edema. As production increases, fluid eventually crosses into the alveoli, leading to alveolar edema and interference with gas exchange. In contrast to cardiogenic or hydrostatic edema, damage to the capillary endothelium or alveolar epithelium in noncardiogenic edema or acute respiratory distress syndrome (ARDS) can cause fluid leakage in the absence of increased pressures.

- **Pulmonary clearance** is the combined result of filtration of inspired air by the nose which removes large particles, coughing, mucociliary clearance of material impacting on bronchial walls, phagocytosis by macrophages, and lymphatic drainage. **Coughing** serves to clear the lungs and is a protective maneuver against foreign materials. Diaphragmatic movement is a major contributor, resulting in more effective clearance in the lung bases (Fig. 1-6).

   The **mucociliary apparatus** plays an important role in pulmonary clearance. Most foreign particulate material entering the lung impacts on the airway walls and is subsequently moved proximally up the trachea and swallowed. There is little regional difference in the efficiency of this mechanism. Dust tends to settle in the region of the respiratory bronchioles.

   Foreign material reaching the alveoli is phagocytized by alveolar macrophages. **Pulmonary lymphatics**, beginning at the level of the terminal bronchiole, travel within the pulmonary interstitium toward regional lymph nodes. Complete clearance by lymphatics may take several weeks and

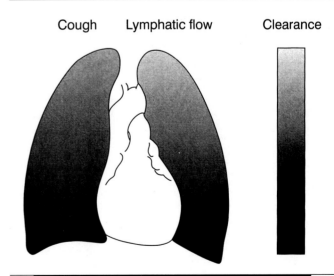

Cough   Lymphatic flow   Clearance

FIGURE 1-6 Pulmonary clearance. Cough, which is predominantly a diaphragmatic function, is much more efficient in the base than in the lung apex. Also, interstitial fluid production and lymphatic flow are approximately four times higher in the base than in the lung apex. As a consequence, overall pulmonary clearance is much better in the base than in the lung apices. There is no regional difference in mucociliary clearance within the lung.

is highest in the lung bases because of the greater relative hydrostatic pressure and interstitial fluid production.

- **Strain** is a result of the weight of the lung, which creates tension on the interconnected and interdependent supporting interstitium present throughout the lung. As a result, strain is greatest in the apex (Fig. 1-7).

- **Intrapleural pressure** is negative relative to the atmosphere because of the inward elastic recoil of the lung and outward recoil of the chest and further decreases on inspiration. The distribution of forces occuring in the lung and chest wall results in the intrapleural pressure being more negative in the apex than in the lung base.

- The pulmonary capillary bed serves to **filter** particulate material such as small thromboemboli before they reach the left heart and systemic circulation. The lung also serves an important **metabolic function** involving phospholipid and protein synthesis; carbohydrate metabolism; conversion of angiotensin I to angiotensin II; and partial inactivation of bradykinin, serotonin, norepinephrine, leukotrienes, and prostaglandins.

- In **summary**, relative to the lung apices, the lung bases have greater ventilation (3:1), higher perfusion (18:1), a lower ventilation/perfusion ratio, lower oxygen concentration, higher carbon dioxide concentration, lower pH, better clearance because of the cough mechanism and greater lymphatic flow, a less negative intrapleural pressure, and lower strain on the pulmonary interstitium.

- These regional physiologic differences can help explain some **patterns of disease** distribution. For example, the high ventilation/perfusion ratio in the lung apices results in a

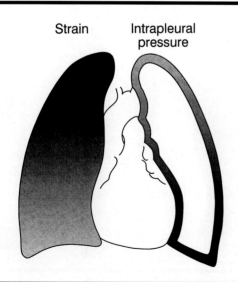

FIGURE 1-7 Strain and intrapleural pressure. Illustrating higher strain in the pulmonary parenchyma of the apex compared to the lung base because of the weight of the lung. Intrapleural pressure is negative because of the inward elastic recoil of the lung and outward elastic recoil of the chest wall. The weight of the lung creates a more negative intrapleural pressure in the apex than in the lung base.

relatively greater concentration of noxious gases and particulate matter compared to the lung base. Consequently damage, such as smoking related emphysema, is typically greatest in the lung apices. The lower carbon dioxide concentration, which leads to a relatively alkaline environment in the lung apex, accounts for the precipitation of calcium in patients with metastatic calcifications.

The greater efficiency of lower lobe clearance by coughing possibly contributes to the upper lobe predominance of infection and bronchiectasis in cystic fibrosis. Lower clearance may contribute to accumulation of particulate material such as silica dust in the apex accounting for the upper lobe predominance of silicosis. The higher apical oxygen concentration may contribute to the localization of tuberculosis to this region. Blebs, many probably associated with strain on the pulmonary architecture, are more common in the apex where forces are greatest.

1.3 CHEST RADIOGRAPHY AND FLUOROSCOPY

- **Chest imaging** includes standard and portable screen-film and digital radiography, various supplementary views, fluoroscopy, standard and high-resolution computed tomography (HRCT), magnetic resonance imaging (MR), nuclear medicine, and angiography. Each has specific indications, unique advantages, and limitations. The technique chosen depends on the clinical question, prior studies available, and the condition of the patient.

- **Chest radiography** is the principal imaging examination employed in the investigation of chest disease and is the most frequent examination performed in most radiology departments. A *standard examination* includes both erect posteroanterior (PA) and left lateral views of the chest. The PA provides substantial information, but the lateral provides a better view of the spine, posterior costophrenic angles, lung bases, and retrosternal region. A PA examination alone should be considered an incomplete study. If an examination is clinically indicated, a complete examination should be performed (Fig. 1-8).

A **PA radiograph** is obtained with the patient's chest against the cassette, chin lifted, back of the hands on the hips, and elbows rolled forward to rotate the scapula off the lungs. The x-ray source is positioned 6 ft behind the cassette so that the beam traverses the patient from back to front. A left **lateral examination** is obtained with the patient's left chest against the film cassette and arms above the head, usually grasping a bar. Both are obtained in deep inspiration.

Standard chest radiography is typically performed using a dedicated chest unit which automatically feeds the exposed film into a processor and reloads for the next examination. Development time, including fixing, washing, and drying, is 90 seconds. Proper processing is important and requires careful attention to quality control, including temperature and chemistry replenishment.

- The introduction of **high-kilovoltage techniques** (>110 kVp) to improve penetration of the highly attenuating medi-

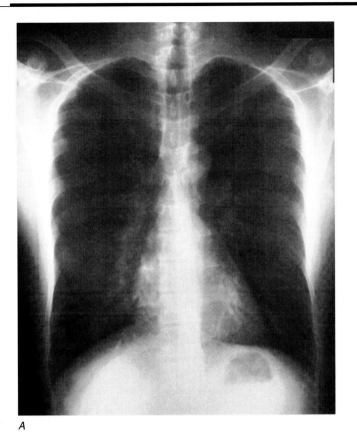
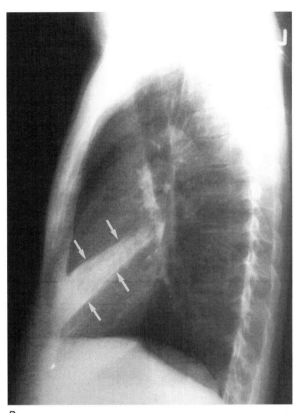

A   *B*

FIGURE 1-8   **Middle-lobe atelectasis.** (*A, B*) PA and lateral chest radiographs in a 35-year-old man. The lateral examination clearly demonstrates increased density and volume loss in the middle lobe (arrows) characteristic of atelectasis. This abnormality is not nearly as conspicuous on the PA examination where only a faint area of increased opacity is seen.

astinal and soft tissue structures and the use of wide-latitude (low-contrast) dual-screen film systems for chest imaging have greatly improved film quality in the past decade. Even so, the optimal exposure for visualizing the soft tissues of the chest wall and particularly the mediastinum would overexpose the lungs. Most chest radiographs are obtained primarily to evaluate pulmonary pathology, and exposure is generally optimized more for lung than soft tissue evaluation. (Fig. 1-9).

A high-kVp technique minimizes exposure time, and therefore cardiac and respiratory motion artifacts, but the low subject contrast limits evaluation of bone pathology and diminishes the conspicuity of calcification within pulmonary nodules.

The film is not actually exposed by the x-rays directly, rather the film, which has a light-sensitive emulsion layer on each side, is sandwiched between two image-intensification screens within a cassette. The screens absorb x-rays which are converted to light which subsequently exposes the film, reducing the total patient dose required compared to direct film exposure.

- An **antiscatter grid** is typically placed between the patient and the film to reduce the effect of Compton scatter, which predominates at high kVp. A grid is a series of very thin radiopaque strips sandwiched between radiolucent strips (typically 40 per centimeter) to absorb scattered x-rays approaching the film cassette at oblique angles. Much of the radiation that would contribute to film density but not information is eliminated, and so the patient dose increases about twofold to maintain film density.

- **Phototiming** is used to standardize film density by controlling the exposure time. A typical system employs a radiolucent ionization chamber which is integrated into the film changer between the patient and the film. It terminates the exposure once a predetermined number of x-ray interactions have occurred.

  The phototimer is typically positioned over the patient's right lung, or one over each lung for the PA examination and in the middle of the field for the lateral examination. If the patient is malpositioned, the duration of exposure is increased to try to achieve what would typically be lung density, and the resulting image will be too dark.

- Standard examinations should be obtained whenever feasible, but **portable radiography**, performed at the bedside, can provide valuable information when the patient cannot be transported. Portable radiographs are often obtained daily on patients in intensive care units, in part to monitor the location

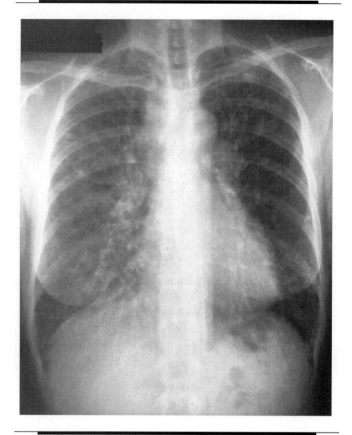

FIGURE 1-9 Metastatic renal cell carcinoma. Optimally exposed PA chest radiograph in a 62-year-old woman with metastatic carcinoma. There are pulmonary nodules, mediastinal adenopathy, and nodular interstitial infiltrates representing lymphangitic spread. Note adequate visualization of the upper abdominal soft tissues, spine, retrocardiac, and subdiaphragmatic regions without overpenetration of the lungs.

of multiple support lines and catheters and to identify associated complications. Portable examinations may constitute half of all chest examinations in a hospital setting.

Most are performed as anteroposterior (AP) examinations at a source-to-image distance of 40 inches, which accentuates the magnification of structures further from the film compared to PA radiography performed at 6 ft. The heart appears about 20 percent larger.

Because of equipment power limitations, a relatively low kVp of 80 to 100 is used, leading to relative underpenetration of the mediastinum and abdomen and longer exposure times which increase cardiac and respiratory motion artifacts. Patient positioning is difficult, and grids are not often used because of difficulty with alignment. Phototiming is not possible, and exposure is estimated by the technologist.

Proper positioning is often difficult, and examinations are often obtained with the patient in a semierect or nearly supine position. It is also difficult for patients to take a deep inspiration while sitting or reclining, and lung volumes are smaller, contributing to apparent cardiac enlargement.

Thus certain gravity-dependent pathologies such as pleural effusions are less conspicuous. In the supine position, fluid layers along the posterior chest, creating a hazy appearance but no air-fluid interface. The meniscus seen on erect films is absent. Portable films obtained with a slight lordotic orientation result in foreshortening of the lung and often obscuration of the left hemidiaphragm.

Also, blood flow distribution is altered in the supine patient. In the erect position, the more dependent lower lobe vessels are larger and the upper lobe vessels smaller. In the supine position, the vessels anterior in location are smaller and posterior vessels are larger, but since these overlap, vessels in the upper and lower lobes appear equal in size.

- **Additional radiographic examinations** may include oblique, apical lordotic, or decubitus examinations or films obtained with nipple markers, in expiration or dedicated examinations of the ribs. An esophogram or upper gastrointestinal examination with barium can be useful in the evaluation of suspected esophageal disease or hiatal hernia (Fig. 1-10).

- Metallic **skin markers** are sometimes placed on a mole or the nipples to help determine if a focal opacity is due to a skin lesion or to a true pulmonary nodule. They may be placed prospectively for examinations in oncology patients in which the principal indication is identification of pulmonary nodules.

- **Rib detail films** consist of coned-down and oblique projections of the chest wall obtained at a low kVp (60 to 80) to increase the subject contrast. This increases the conspicuity of bone relative to lung, allowing easier detection of destructive lesions or fractures (Fig. 1-11).

  Radiographs obtained with a **low-kVp** technique also increase the conspicuity of calcifications within nodules, helping to characterize a nodule.

- **Expiratory radiographs** can be helpful by demonstrating air trapping and increasing the conspicuity of a small pneumothorax. Bulla, blebs, and pleural and trapped air maintain the same volume and density, whereas the remainder of the lung decreases in size and increases in density, making these air collections more conspicuous.

- Radiographs obtained in an **oblique projection** can be helpful in evaluating a suspected nodule by separating superimposed structures. Oblique radiographs are also useful in visualizing pleural plaques which become more conspicuous when seen on edge.

- An **apical lordotic view** improves visualization of the lung apices by projecting the first rib and clavicles above the lung apex. They are obtained in an AP projection with the patient leaning back slightly against the cassette and the x-ray beam projected cranially rather than perpendicular to the patient. The lordotic view is most useful for evaluating suspected apical lesions.

- A **lateral decubitus view** is a frontal projection of the chest obtained with a horizontally directed x-ray beam and the

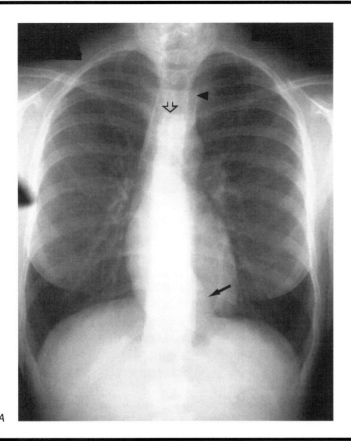
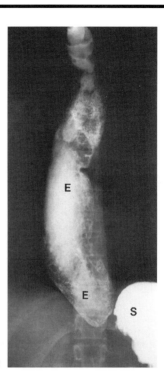

FIGURE 1-10   Achalasia. (*A*) PA chest radiograph showing an air-fluid level (open arrow) in the upper medi-astinum, a dilated air-filled upper esophagus (arrowhead), and retrocardiac opacity (arrow). (*B*) The esophogram confirms a dilated, atonic esophagus (E). There was no evidence of a distal esophageal lesion. S, Stomach.

patient lying on their side (right lateral decubitus or right-side-down decubitus; left lateral decubitus or left-side-down decubitus). They are useful in evaluating the presence or mobility of a suspected pleural effusion, particularly a sub-pulmonic effusion.

Both the dependent and nondependent sides of the chest can be evaluated, although the size of the pleural effusion on the nondependent side is not easily determined. The view is also useful in evaluating the otherwise obscured underlying lung and for demonstrating a pneumothorax in the non-dependent lung in patients who cannot be positioned upright.

- **Digital chest radiography** refers to the use of computers and media other than screen-film to capture images digitally. With conventional screen-film techniques, the film serves the roles of detection, display, and storage. Decoupling these three tasks allows performance to be optimized—detectors can be designed for wider latitude, image data can be manip-ulated to improve visualization, and data can be efficiently stored.

- **Computed radiography** (CR) utilizes standard radiographic equipment but replaces the screen-film cassette with a reusable photostimulable phosphor plate for image capture. When exposed to x-rays, the image is captured as electrons within the phosphor plate are stimulated to higher energy

levels. The CR reader scans the plate with a laser, causing light emission with an intensity proportional to the original exposure. Raw image data are typically captured at roughly 2000 lines with 2000 pixels per line with a 12-bit gray scale. Recently 4k detector systems have been developed. The phosphor plates are then initialized for reuse.

A major advantage of CR is the extremely wide latitude of the receptor, which in combination with image processing techniques allows diagnostically acceptable images with pre-determined density and contrast despite extremes of under- or overexposure. Image noise (quantum mottle) is, however, affected by the exposure, with underexposure resulting in a granular, photopenic image. CR has proven particularly effective for portable chest radiography.

- Once in the digital domain, image processing techniques can be used to optimize spatial frequency and contrast. "Edge enhancement" (unsharp masking) boosts the high-frequency components, resulting in improved visualization of lines and tubes or trabecular detail. Other algorithms are designed to enhance the gray scale characteristics.

- Digital images can be printed onto laser film for hard-copy display or displayed on a monitor for soft-copy viewing. Using networked workstations to form a picture archive and communication system (**PACS**) provides the opportunity for

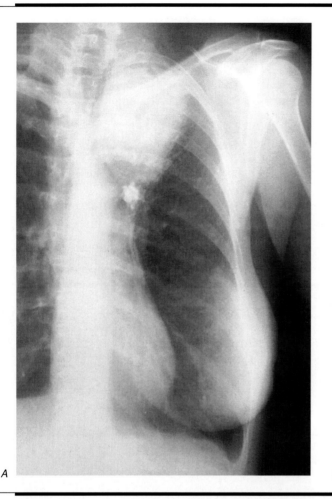

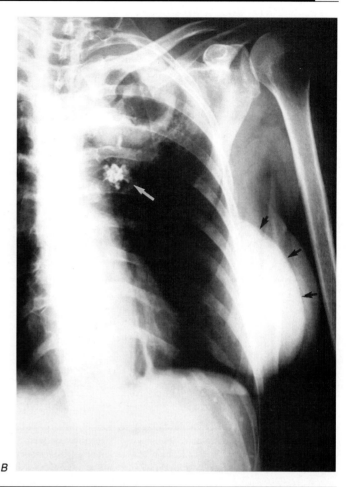

FIGURE 1-11   Comparison of standard chest and rib detail techniques. (*A*) PA chest radiograph obtained using a wide-latitude screen-film system and a high-kVp technique (115 kVp). (*B*) Film from a rib detail series obtained using a low-kVp technique (65 kVp). The lower kVp reduces Compton scatter and increases the contribution of the photoelectric effect, making high-atomic-weight materials like calcium more conspicious. Note better visualization of bone, the breast implant (black arrows), and the calcified nodule (white arrow) in this patient with an apical mass.

both remote viewing and availability to multiple sites and viewers simultaneously. Although 2k monitors are often advocated, 1k resolution is generally adequate for portable radiography. The raw or processed image data can be archived as a hard-copy image or as digital information on a hard drive, optical disk, or magnetic tape for short- and long-term storage.

- The intrinsic high-attenuation difference between the lung and mediastinum has led to attempts at equalizing exposure differences using filters or variations in the intensity of incident x-rays to deliver a higher dose over poorly penetrated regions and a lower dose over the lungs.

  More recently, selenium-based image detectors have been developed for large field-of-view imaging. Thoravision® (Philips Medical) is a dedicated selenium-based digital chest imaging system. Preliminary experience has demonstrated image quality superior to that of standard screen-film techniques.

- **Fluoroscopy** allows real time visualization of thoracic structures and is useful in evaluating suspected pulmonary nodules, assessing diaphragm movement, and guiding transthoracic needle biopsies. Fluoroscopy can be performed to determine if an opacity seen on radiography represents a true pulmonary nodule. Fluoroscopy allows direct control of the obliquity and observation of the opacity during respiration to determine the nature and location. Low-kVp spot films may demonstrate subtle calcifications not visible on a standard high-kVp chest radiograph, obviating the need for CT.

  Fluoroscopy can also be used to assess motion and coordination of the diaphragm. This technique is preferably performed with the patient erect but can be performed supine. A **sniff test** refers to fluoroscopic observation during rapid inhalation, which is nearly a pure diaphragmatic event. A paralyzed hemidiaphragm moves up in inspiration as a result of reduced intrathoracic pressure, in marked contrast to a normal hemidiaphragm which rapidly moves down. If the image-intensifying screen is small, the patient can be positioned in an oblique or lateral orientation to better visualize both hemidiaphragms simultaneously. Fluoroscopy is also used to evaluate mechanical prosthetic cardiac valve function, particularly leaflet excursion in patients with Björk-Shiley and St. Jude valves.

- **Patient radiation dose** from a chest radiograph is approximately 20 to 30 mrem per view. This is comparable to the background radiation individuals receive on a monthly basis in the United States from environmental radon and cosmic radiation. Chest radiography can safely be performed in pregnant women. Typically, a PA projection is obtained with careful attention to shielding the abdomen with a lead apron. On review of this single view, a lateral examination can be obtained as needed. Chest CT results in a patient dose of approximately 2000 mrem, 100 times that of a single-view chest radiograph.

1.4 COMPUTED TOMOGRAPHY AND HRCT

- **Conventional tomography**, previously invaluable in the assessment of pulmonary, mediastinal, and central airway abnormalities, has been completely replaced by CT. Similarly, **bronchography**, previously crucial in the evaluation of airway disease, particularly bronchiectasis, has been replaced by CT, specifically high resolution CT (HRCT).

- **CT** is the primary cross-sectional imaging technique for most chest conditions, with MR preferred in select situations such as assessing the chest wall. CT has better spatial resolution and depicts lung parenchyma and cortical bone better. Advantages of MR include direct multiplanar imaging, better soft tissue characterization, and demonstration of blood flow without intravenous (IV) contrast.

  The cross-sectional image orientation and high contrast sensitivity of CT are ideal for detecting, characterizing, and distinguishing among diseases of the lung, mediastinum, pleura, soft tissues, and bones of the thorax and upper abdomen (Figs. 1-12 to 1-16). Pleural and parenchymal processes difficult to distinguish on plain radiographs can be clearly displayed, and benign abnormalities that mimic pathology on plain films are clearly identified. The adrenal glands and liver, common sites of metastases, can be examined.

- **Conventional CT** acquires one image at a time. The patient table is stationary during data acquisition as the x-ray tube circles the patient. The radiation transmitted through the patient is collected by detectors, and an image is reconstructed from the projectional data. The patient table moves, and the process is repeated. **Collimation** refers to the width of the x-ray beam and determines section thickness.

  Typically, the patient breaths between scans, with imaging occurring during suspended inspiration. This may introduce respiratory misregistration if the depth of inspiration is inconsistent. As a result, portions of lung appear in more than one section, and others not at all. Small nodules can be missed or appear smaller.

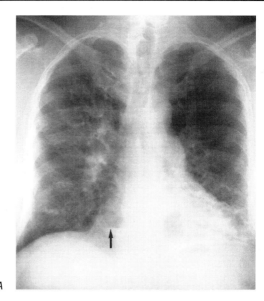

A

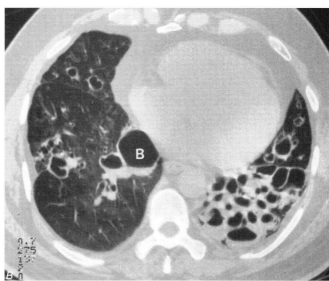

FIGURE 1-12 Bronchiectasis. (*A*) PA chest radiograph showing diffusely abnormal lung parenchyma and cystic lucencies, some with air-fluid levels (arrow). (*B*) CT clearly demonstrating the nature of the pulmonary abnormalities. There is extensive cystic bronchiectasis, some with air-fluid levels (B) but also intervening normal lung parenchyma.

- **Spiral CT** is a technique in which continuous rotation of the x-ray tube and data acquisition are coupled with continuous movement of the patient through the gantry. A large area, typically the entire thorax, can be imaged during a single 20- to 30-second breath hold. This eliminates respiratory misregistration.

- **Pitch** is the ratio of table speed to collimation. A table speed of 1 cm/s coupled with a collimation of 5 mm results in a pitch of 2. The greater the pitch, the larger the area covered for a given collimation, but as pitch increases there is associated image degradation due to slice profile broadening. A

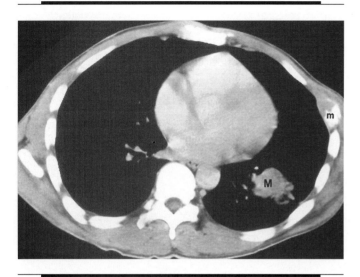

FIGURE 1-13   Stage IV bronchogenic carcinoma. CT showing
a left lower lung mass (M) representing bronchogenic carcinoma
and a destructive rib lesion with extraosseous soft tissue extension
representing a bone metastasis (m).

pitch of 1 should be used when possible, 1.5 is acceptable,
and 2 is the upper limit for chest imaging. Coverage = scan
time × collimation × pitch.

- **Reconstruction interval** is the spacing of images. Section
  thickness is always equal to the collimation used during data
  acquisition. Images can be reconstructed at any interval
  desired, including overlapping. For example, a useful technique when screening or following multiple small pulmonary

nodules <5 mm in diameter is to perform a spiral examination with 8-mm collimation and reconstruct the image data
set at 5-mm intervals, thus creating overlapping images
which increase sensitivity and measurement accuracy.

- The **field of view** should be small to maximize spatial resolution, and it should extend no further than the chest wall and
  axilla. Targeted imaging to include less than the entire thorax
  in the field of view is useful when coupled with narrow
  collimation for characterizing focal abnormalities such as
  indeterminate pulmonary nodules.

- **Follow-up** studies to characterize nodules should precisely
  replicate the original image using the same collimation, field
  of view, reconstruction technique, window settings, and
  image size. This facilitates subjective comparison and measurements.

- **Intravenous contrast** is frequently unnecessary for chest
  examinations, particularly for evaluating pulmonary nodules
  or interstitial lung disease. Contrast can help to distinguish
  lymph nodes from hilar vessels, identify the enhancing rim
  characteristic of empyemas (Fig. 1-17), demonstrate the
  vascular component of arterial venous malformations and
  sequestrations, and detect pulmonary emboli.

  IV contrast should be **avoided** in patients with a cre-
  atinine level above 2.0, in patients with multiple myeloma,
  and in those with a suspected pheochromocytoma. Nonionic contrast is preferred in patients with drug allergies, a
  history of asthma, or heart disease. Steroid pretreatment
  sometimes supplemented with antihistamine diminishes the
  risk of adverse reactions in patients with a history of prior
  mild contrast reactions such as hives.

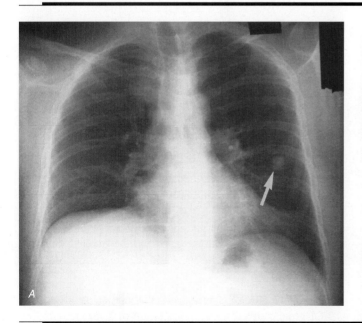

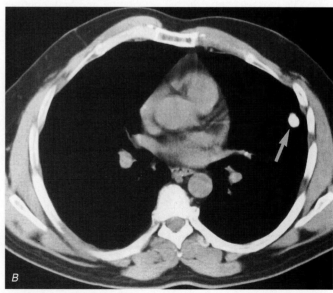

FIGURE 1-14   Calcified granuloma. (*A*) PA chest radiograph showing a pulmonary nodule (arrow). (*B*) CT
filmed for soft tissue detail demonstrating diffuse calcification (arrow) characteristic of a benign lesion, in this
case old healed granulomatous disease.

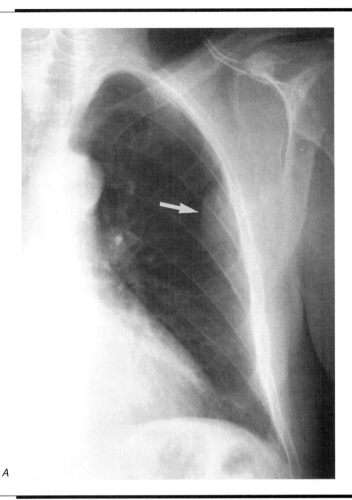

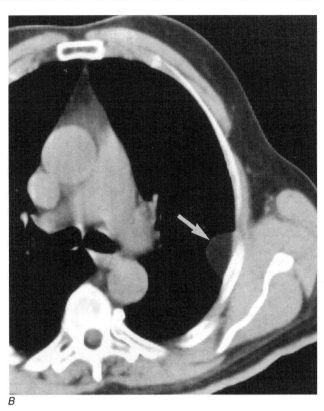

B

A

FIGURE 1-15 **Lipoma.** (*A*) PA chest radiograph showing a pleura-based mass (arrow). (*B*) CT demonstrates the fat density characteristic of a benign lipoma (arrow). (With permission from Slone RM, Gierada DS. Pleura, chest wall and diaphragm. In: Lee JKT, Sagel SS, Stanley RJ, Heiken JP, eds. *Computed Body Tomography with MRI Correlation.* 3rd ed. New York: Lippincott-Raven; 1998.)

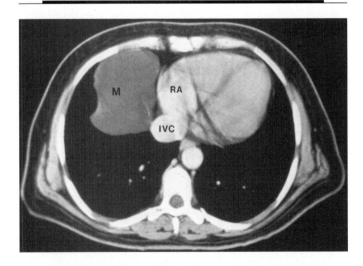

FIGURE 1-16 **Pericardial cyst.** CT in a 48-year-old woman with a right cardiophrenic angle mass on chest radiograph, showing a large fluid attenuation mass (M) adjacent to the right atrium (RA) and inferior vena cava (IVC) characteristic of a benign pericardial cyst.

Contrast should not be used despite pretreatment in patients with prior serious contrast reactions such as laryngeal edema or anaphalaxis.

A single 8-oz cup of **oral contrast** immediately before scanning or a few spoonfuls of barium paste can coat the esophagus in patients with suspected esophageal disease.

- **Quantitative CT (QCT)** refers to the analysis of CT image data to calculate lung volumes and to study lung morphology by evaluating lung density distribution.

- **High-resolution CT (HRCT)** involves obtaining representative sections with 1- to 2-mm collimation, a minimal field of view, and a high spatial frequency reconstruction algorithm to obtain detailed images comparable to gross tissue inspection. HRCT improves visualization of fissures and depicts bronchi out to the peripheral quarter of the lung and vessels as small as 0.5 mm. HRCT can detect disease at an earlier stage than radiography and enable characterization of vague lesions seen on CT. HRCT is valuable in detecting bronchiectasis, mild emphysema, and interstitial disease, particularly fibrosis and pneumoconiosis (Figs. 1-18 and 1-19).

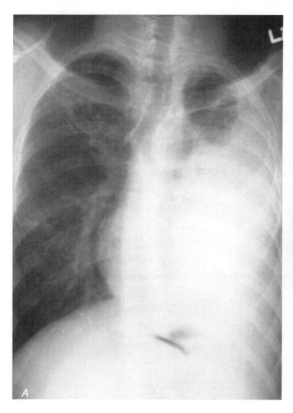

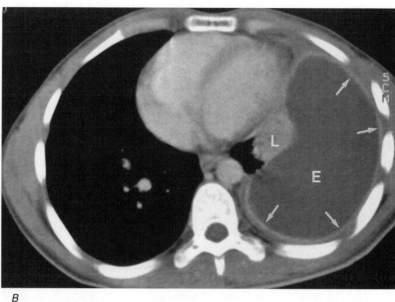

FIGURE 1-17   Empyema. (*A*) PA chest radiograph showing near-complete opacification of the left hemithorax. (*B*) Contrast-enhanced CT showing a large pleural effusion (E), collapsed left lung (L), and enhancing pleura (arrows) characteristic of an empyema.

The **section spacing** chosen depends on whether the study is intended to detect, exclude, or characterize disease. For example, pulmonary emphysema is generally diffuse, and sampling at 3- to 5-cm intervals is adequate to provide representative images; however, images at 1-cm intervals are required to confidently exclude subtle silicosis or bronchiectasis.

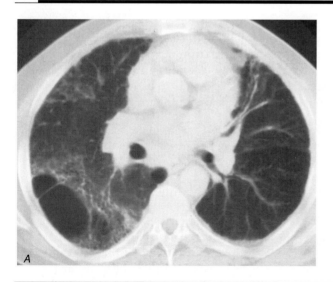

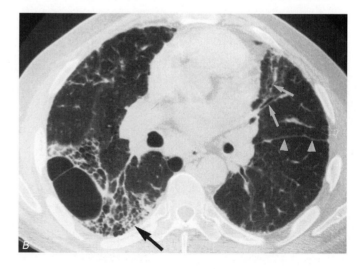

FIGURE 1-18   Fibrosis. (*A*) Conventional CT obtained using 10-mm collimation compared to the HRCT (*B*) obtained with 2-mm collimation showing improved demonstration of the fissures (arrowheads), fibrosis (black arrow), and traction bronchiectasis (white arrows) in a man with a history or prior massive acute silica dust exposure.

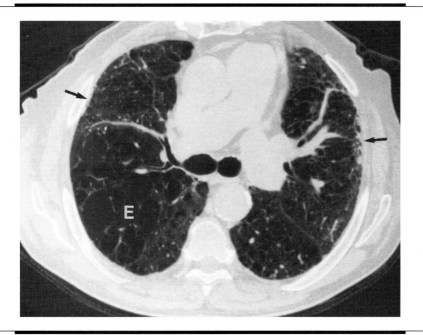

FIGURE 1-19   Fibrosis and emphysema. HRCT showing areas of lung destruction characteristic of pulmonary emphysema (E) as well as peripheral fibrosis (arrows) in a man with a history of asbestos exposure, smoking, and mixed restrictive and obstructive changes on pulmonary function testing. (With permission from Sagel SS, Slone RM. The lung. In: Lee JKT, Sagel SS, Stanley RJ, Heiken JP, eds. *Computed Body Tomography with MRI Correlation.* 3rd ed. New York: Lippincott-Raven; 1998.)

Supine positioning often results in gravity-induced "dependent atelectasis" which can be mistaken for pulmonary fibrosis. **Prone positioning** reverses this distribution of microatelectasis, and allows a distinction between gravity-related changes and inflammation or fibrosis.

Imaging at total lung capacity maximizes pulmonary aeration and minimizes dependent atelectasis, thus improving disease conspicuity. **Expiration** accentuates air trapping in emphysema and small-airways diseases such as bronchiolitis obliterans.

Proper **window center** and **width** are important in optimizing the display of normal and pathologic findings. Window width is analogous to contrast, and window center is analogous to brightness. Typical values are a width of 1500 to 1800 Hounsfield units (HU) and center of −500 to −600 HU for the lung and 400 to 500 HU, with a center of 10 to 50 HU, for soft tissues. Too narrow a window width for lung produces a blooming artifact, enlarging the apparent size of arteries, veins, and bronchial walls.

Although HRCT alone may be adequate for evaluating diffuse infiltrative lung disease, it is typically performed in conjunction with conventional CT to avoid underestimating or overlooking disease. Branching vessels can be mistaken for nodules, and pulmonary metastases can be missed. Conventional CT is superior for evaluating micronodules because of the increased number of nodules per section and better distinction from branching vessels.

1.5 MAGNETIC RESONANCE IMAGING, ULTRASOUND, NUCLEAR MEDICINE, AND ANGIOGRAPHY

- **Magnetic resonance imaging** has the unique ability to directly obtain multiplanar images and demonstrate blood flow without IV contrast. Fluid is easily identified, and tumor can better be distinguished from fibrosis. MR provides higher soft tissue contrast than CT and is preferred to CT for studying the central nervous, cardiac, and musculoskeletal systems but can also perform a problem-solving role in the chest in assessing mediastinal, central vascular, chest wall or diaphragm invasion by tumors. Primary indications include thoracic aortic aneurysms, aortic dissection in stable patients, superior sulcus tumors (Fig. 1-20), and brachial plexus and posterior mediastinal masses.

  There are no standard MR protocols for evaluating chest disease. Each examination must be tailored to the clinical problem with regard to pulse sequences, imaging planes, slice thickness, field of view, and coil used. If the area of interest is localized, a surface coil can be used to improve resolution and the signal-to-noise ratio. Phased-array surface coils simultaneously optimize coverage and tissue signals.

  MR scans of the chest are degraded by cardiac and respiratory motion. Cardiac gating minimizes cardiac motion artifact, and respiratory motion artifact can be minimized using respiratory compensation techniques without affecting imaging time. Spatial presaturation "bands" outside the area of interest can reduce motion artifacts. Positioning the patient with the area of interest down diminishes movement.

  T1-weighted spin-echo images are generally obtained in two orthogonal planes, followed by a multiple spin-echo T2-weighted pulse sequence in the plane best demonstrating the abnormality. Repetition times are constrained by the patient's heart rate if cardiac gating is used. Fast spin-echo techniques reduce the time needed for T2-weighted sequences and allow breath-hold images.

  Fast gradient-echo techniques can be used to assess vascular patency. Fat suppression, and short T1 inversion recovery (STIR) can be used to maximize lesion contrast. The minimum acceptable matrix size is 128 × 256. IV gadolinium enhancement is used selectively following review of the initial findings.

- **Ultrasound** is limited in the thorax because ultrasound waves are not propagated through air or bone. This technique

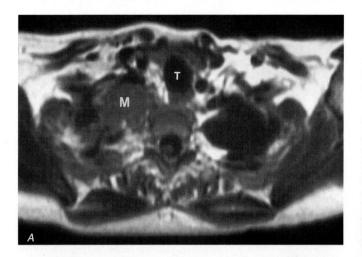 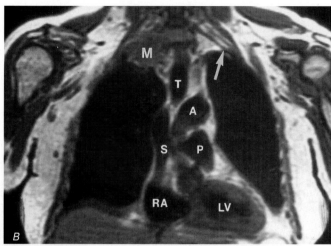

FIGURE 1-20   Superior sulcus tumor. (*A*) Axial and (*B*) coronal T1-weighted MR of the chest showing the extent of a soft tissue mass (M) which is invading the chest wall, displacing the subclavian vessels and involving the brachial plexus. Note normal brachial plexus on left (arrow). T, Trachea; A, aorta; S, superior vena cava; P, pulmonary trunk; RA, right atrium; LV, left ventricle. (Figure courtesy of DS Gierada, Mallinckrodt Institute of Radiology.)

can be used to evaluate cardiac, pleural, chest wall, diaphragmatic, and mediastinal lesions. Its principal role is in localizing pleural effusions and guiding thoracentesis, particularly with small or loculated effusions.

- **Nuclear medicine** imaging studies useful in the evaluation of chest disease include ventilation-perfusion scanning, gallium, indium, and bone scintigraphy, and positron emission tomography. **Ventilation perfusion** scanning allows noninvasive assessment of regional pulmonary blood flow and ventilation. It is most commonly performed to assist in the diagnosis of pulmonary embolism but can be used to assess the regional contribution of ventilation and perfusion in patients scheduled for surgical resection.

  Ventilation scanning can be performed with a radioactive gas or aerosolized particles such as technetium DTPA or Technigas®, a carbon-based particulate. Xenon-133 gas is most commonly used. An initial "breath-hold image" is followed by tidal breathing to demonstrate the "wash-in phase" during which the gas is distributed. Eventually an "equilibrium phase" occurs when radioactive gas equilibrates between the lung and spirometer. The "wash-out phase" recorded while the patient resumes breathing room air is the most sensitive for detecting ventilation abnormalities.

  Perfusion scanning is performed following the IV injection of approximately 300,000 technetium-labeled macroaggregated albumin particles which lodge in the pulmonary capillaries. Less than 1 percent of capillaries are occluded during this process, and the albumin disintegrates and is cleared within 8 hours.

  Perfusion studies are sensitive, and specificity is improved by making a comparison with the chest radiograph and ventilation images. Segmental or larger defects in the presence of a normal chest radiograph and ventilation study are characteristic of pulmonary arterial occlusion. In addition to thromboembolism, nonembolic disease such as Takayasu arteritis, fibrosing mediastinitis, or tumor invasion of the pulmonary arteries can cause perfusion defects.

- **Gallium 67** accumulates in metabolically active tissue, including neoplasm and inflammation. The most common thoracic application is to follow disease activity in patients with lymphoma. Both Hodgkin and non-Hodgkin lymphoma may be gallium-avid. If a particular tumor demonstrates activity, gallium scanning can be used to follow treatment response and tumor recurrence.

  Gallium may also accumulate in adenopathy from bronchogenic carcinoma, *Mycobacterium arium intracellularis* (MAI), or sarcoidosis. Pulmonary uptake occurs in patients with *Pneumocystis carinii* pneumonia (PCP), cytomegalovirus (CMV), cryptococcus, tuberculosis, and nonspecific interstitial pneumonitis associated with AIDS. Kaposi sarcoma does not accumulate gallium. **Indium**-labeled white blood cells can also be used in the evaluation of acute and subacute infection.

- **Positron emission tomography (PET)** is based on demonstrating uptake of radiolabeled fluorodeoxyglucose (FDG) by metabolically active cells. It has proven particularly useful in the evaluation of indeterminate pulmonary nodules. Intense uptake favors malignancy but can be seen in some infections. Mild activity suggests inflammatory disease. Absent or very mild activity reliably excludes malignancy although exceptions exist such as some forms of bronchoalveolar cell carcinoma.

  PET is valuable for the detection of distant metastases, particularly in candidates for surgical resection of esophageal cancer where it is more sensitive than CT. Limited spatial resolution reduces the value of PET in determining the T stage and detecting lymph nodes immediately adjacent to the primary.

- **Bone scintigraphy** is useful in detecting osteogenic metastases and is sometimes helpful in evaluating primary bone lesions and direct bone invasion by malignancy or infection.

- **Aortography**, previously crucial in the evaluation of aortic disease, has been replaced to a large extent by CT, MR, and transesophageal echocardiography for the evaluation of aneurysms, congenital anomalies such as coarctation, aortic dissection, and screening for traumatic transection. **Aortography, bronchial arteriography** including bronchial artery embolization in patients with bronchiectasis or mycetomas, and **pulmonary angiography** for evaluation of pulmonary emboli are discussed in Sections 14.1, 14.2, and 14.3, respectively.

1.6 BLOOD GAS ANALYSIS, PULMONARY FUNCTION, AND EXERCISE TESTING

- Routine **pulmonary function tests** include spirometry to measure airflow, plethysmography or gas dilution to measure lung volumes (Fig. 1-21) and diffusing capacity of carbon monoxide, and arterial blood gas analysis to assess gas exchange and acid-base disturbances. Airway resistance, work of breathing, respiratory muscle function, physiologic dead space, and shunt, lung, and chest wall compliance can also be assessed. Exercise tests can be used to evaluate work, ventilation, oxygen consumption, and other physiologic parameters.

- **Arterial blood gas** measurements are usually obtained from the radial artery. pH, arterial oxygen (Pa_{O_2}), and carbon dioxide tension (Pa_{CO_2}) are easily measured. Pa_{O_2} and Pa_{CO_2} should total less than 150 mm Hg in normal adult patients breathing room air. As a general rule, in normal individuals, Pa_{O_2} should be equal to 500 divided by the concentration of inspired oxygen (0.2 for room air).

  Causes of **hypoxemia** include hypoventilation, ventilation-perfusion imbalance, impaired diffusion, right-to-left shunt, and low concentration of inspired oxygen. Causes of **hypercapnea** include hypoventilation and sometimes ventilation-perfusion inequality, although a reflex increase in ventilatory drive often corrects the latter.

- **Spirometry** is performed by having the patient breathe through a tube connected to apparatus that determines the volume and rate of airflow. **Tidal volume** is the volume of air moved inward and outward during a normal respiratory cycle and is typically about 500 ml. **Vital capacity (VC)** refers to the amount of air that can be exhaled following maximal inspiration. **Forced vital capacity (FVC)** is the volume of air that can be forcefully expired after a maximum inspiration (Fig. 1-21).

  Forced expiratory volume (FEV) refers to the amount of air that can be forcefully exhaled following a maximal inspiration during a specified time, usually 1 second (FEV_1). FEV_1 is normally about 4 L at age 30, decreasing about 30 ml each year to about 3 L at age 65. FEV_1 is normally about 80% of the FVC. FEV_1 can be reduced by increased airway resistance or reduced elastic recoil (as in pulmonary emphysema), low lung volumes, or poor effort.

  Total lung capacity (TLC) refers to the total volume of air that can be contained in the lungs. **Residual volume (RV)** is the amount of gas remaining in the lungs after a maximal exhalation. **Functional residual capacity (FRC)** refers to the volume of air in the lungs after a tidal volume exhalation. Gas dilution or plethysmography is required to measure or calculate RV and TLC.

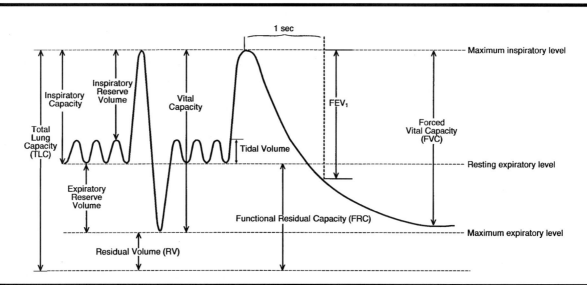

FIGURE 1-21 Pulmonary function testing. Composite diagram illustrating results of spirometry to measure flow rates and plethesmography to determine lung volumes.

- **Gas dilution techniques** are used to measure lung volumes. The patient breathes into a closed system containing a known concentration of a relatively insoluble gas such as helium that equilibrates with pulmonary air. The equilibrium concentration of these gases can be used to determine various lung volumes. Lung volumes can also be determined by measuring nitrogen gas concentration exhaled from a patient breathing 100% oxygen.

- A **plethysmograph** is an airtight box used to measure lung volumes. The patient sits in the box and breathes through a mouthpiece which may be occluded. During occlusion, the patient pants, taking small, quick breaths in and out, changing lung volumes and therefore pressure. By using pressure-volume relationships (Boyle's law), the **thoracic gas volume (TGV)** can be determined and the RV and TLC can be calculated. **Airway resistance** can also be measured using a body plethysmograph.

  A body plethysmograph measures the total volume of gas in the lung. Gas dilution techniques measure only the volume of gas that communicates freely with the upper airways. Although usually the same, in patients with significant air trapping, such as in emphysema, the gas methods underestimate lung volumes. The difference between the two methods of measuring TLC provides an indication of **trapped gas volume**, which is increased in patients with obstructive lung disease.

- Patients with **obstructive lung disease** such as chronic bronchitis and emphysema have very low flow rates relative to their large lung volumes and expiration is prolonged. There is a greater reduction in FEV_1 compared to FVC, and the FEV_1/FVC ratio is low. TLC, RV, and FRC are increased.

- Patients with **restrictive lung disease** such as pulmonary fibrosis typically have reduced flow rates and low lung volumes due to reduced compliance of the lung. Reduced compliance of the chest wall or weakness of the respiratory muscles may also produce a "restrictive" spirometry pattern. Typically both FEV_1 and FVC are reduced, but the FEV_1/FVC ratio is normal. TLC, RV, and FRC are also reduced.

- The **diffusing capacity** of the blood-gas barrier in the lung can be measured with a carbon monoxide (CO) gas mixture using either a single-breath technique ($D_L CO$) in which the inspired and expired CO concentrations are measured, or using a steady-state method. Diffusing capacity may be reduced in patients with lung destruction (emphysema), interstitial lung disease (sarcoidosis, diffuse interstitial fibrosis, etc.), or vascular disease such as pulmonary thromboembolism.

- **Maximum inspiratory pressure** is determined during a maximum inspiratory effort at RV or FRC against a closed system. This is a direct test of inspiratory muscle strength and therefore valuable in assessing patients with neuromuscular disease or thoracic cage abnormalities.

- **Exercise testing** on a bicycle or treadmill is useful in the assessment of patients with heart, lung or neuromuscular disease. Normal individuals have a tremendous pulmonary reserve, and maximal exercise is limited by cardiac output and muscle metabolism. In patients with pulmonary disease, exercise may be limited by ventilatory capacity and gas exchange.

- Heart and respiratory rate, ventilation, oxygen consumption, and expired gas concentrations can all be measured. Exercise testing can be used to determine supplemental oxygen requirements, support specific diagnoses, assess work capacity, identify factors limiting exercise tolerance, study the impact of therapy and rehabilitation in patients with COPD, evaluate changes from disease progression or therapeutic intervention, and help decide therapies.

1.7 INVASIVE MONITORING, BRONCHOSCOPY, AND MEDIASTINOSCOPY

- A **pulmonary artery** balloon-tipped (Swan-Ganz) catheter is a multilumen central access line used to (1) measure right atrial, pulmonary artery, and pulmonary capillary wedge pressures (PCWP), (2) calculate cardiac output using thermodilution techniques, (3) sample mixed venous blood for oxygenation measurement, and (4) obtain data used to calculate parameters such as systemic vascular resistance. These measurements are useful for determining volume status and oxygen delivery and for assessing therapy.

  Placement is often via a sheath in the subclavian, jugular, or femoral vein. Once the flow directed catheter with the balloon tip inflated is advanced through the heart, the catheter tip is positioned in a proximal pulmonary artery. Though kept deflated when not in use, an inflated balloon will occlude flow in a segmental branch of a pulmonary artery at which point "wedging" occurs. At that point, PCWP measurements are made.

  Placement should be proximal enough in the PA to allow blood flow around the catheter except when the balloon tip is inflated for PCWP measurement. **Complications** include pneumothorax during placement, hematoma or thrombosis due to vascular injury at the insertion site, line sepsis and pulmonary artery infarct, rupture, or pseudoaneurysm.

- **Thoracentesis** can be performed for diagnostic purposes to determine the contents of a pleural effusion and occasionally for therapeutic purposes in patients with a large effusion causing respiratory distress. Ultrasound guidance can facilitate aspiration of small or loculated effusions. Pleural drainage procedures are discussed in Section 14.5.

- **Fiberoptic bronchoscopy** allows direct visualization of the tracheobronchial tree and has widespread diagnostic and sometimes therapeutic applications. It has nearly replaced rigid bronchoscopy except for surgical procedures such as some foreign body removal, treatment of massive hemoptysis, stricture dilatation, stenting, and laser procedures. It can be performed without general anesthesia or endotracheal intubation. Bronchoscopes range from 3 to 6 mm in diameter and have one or more channels for irrigation, suctioning, and passing instruments.

Indications include evaluation of hemoptysis, nodules, stridor, cough, unresolved pneumonia, diffuse lung disease, atelectasis, or infection. The bronchoscope may be introduced orally, nasally, or by endotracheal tube. Supplemental oxygen and a topical anesthetic are administered and IV or intramuscular (IM) sedatives may be used as well. Pulse oximetry and vital sign monitoring is performed.

A **standard examination** includes evaluation of the nasal pharynx, larynx, vocal cords, and airways to the subsegmental level. The color, texture, position, size, and patency of the tracheobronchial tree can be assessed. Acute and chronic inflammation can be identified, and the nature and quantity of secretions determined.

Tissue sampling techniques include bronchial washings, brush biopsies, endobronchial and transbronchial forcep or needle biopsies, bronchoalveolar lavage, and transtracheal and transcarinal needle aspirates. The diagnostic yield approaches 95% in patients with an endoscopically visible neoplastic lesion. Random biopsies can often be diagnostic in the setting of diffuse lung disease, particularly in patients with sarcoid, lymphangitic carcinomatosis, or infection.

Bronchoalveolar lavage involves installation of liquid aliquots in a bronchial segment through a channel in the bronchoscope and recovery of the fluid through the bronchoscope suction channel. It is a valuable means of acquiring material for identification of infection, alveolar proteinosis, and alveolar hemorrhage carcinoma.

Therapeutic applications include removal of retained or impacted secretions causing atelectasis or pneumonia, removal of foreign bodies, dilatation of strictures, laser-assisted tracheobronchial procedures, and endobronchial balloon placement to manage hemorrhage.

Contraindications include respiratory distress and significant hypoxemia or coagulation disorders. **Complications** include pneumothorax, bleeding, pneumomediastinum and infection. Almost all patients develop some degree of hypoxemia which may last several hours, and transient fever is not uncommon, especially after lavage.

- **Mediastinoscopy** allows direct visualization and access to portions of the mediastinum to sample mediastinal lymph nodes, primarily for staging bronchogenic carcinoma and occasionally for biopsy of a mediastinal mass. Pneumothorax occurs in less than 1% of cases, and serious bleeding or damage to the esophagus, thoracic duct, vocal cord, trachea, or bronchus even less frequently.

Cervical mediastinoscopy is carried out through a suprasternal incision with dissection down to the trachea. A rigid metal mediastinoscope is inserted after blunt finger dissection, along the anterior tracheal wall down to the carina. Lymph nodes directly accessible include high and low paratracheal, azygos, and right tracheobronchial and anterior subcarial lymph nodes. Most lymph nodes in the hilum, AP window, subaortic region and anterior mediastinum are inaccessible and require thoracoscopy or anterior mediastinotomy for access.

Parasternal mediastinotomy, sometimes called a *Chamberlain procedure*, refers to an anterior mediastinal exploration through the second intracostal space or cartilage. It allows access to the anterior mediastinum and the aortic arch, including the AP window. It is primarily employed to biopsy lymph nodes in patients with left upper lobe carcinoma or to biopsy an anterior mediastinal mass which is not approachable through a standard cervicle mediastinoscopy.

1.8 RADIOGRAPH INTERPRETATION AND APPROACH TO UNKNOWN CASES

- The **standard chest radiograph** contains a wealth of information. Confident interpretation to extract relevant and important information can be difficult. Studies have shown that **errors** in interpretation are common but fortunately usually related to incidental and inconsequential findings. Misinterpretation of subtle but important findings can have a deleterious impact on diagnosis and treatment.

- Proper review of the chest radiograph begins with some elementary guidelines. Paramount is that the examination is of the patient in question and for the date of interest. Therefore, the patient **name** and **date** on the radiograph should always be checked.

- **Appropriate viewing conditions** are important. Unnecessary ambient light impacts the ability to detect subtle contrast differences. It is therefore crucial to turn off unnecessary viewbox lights and mask the film edges if necessary. Room lighting should also be minimized. A bright light (hot light) should be readily available to improve visualization of over-penetrated portions of the film.

- **Additional considerations** include evaluation of film quality, including patient positioning (rotation), level of inspiration, motion artifacts, and exposure. With conventional techniques, an optimally exposed chest radiograph is dark enough to allow visualization of pulmonary vessels through the left heart and diaphragm, and visualization of vertebral bodies and disk spaces through the mediastinal structures. This should be possible without producing a film so dark that lung parenchyma cannot be adequately evaluated without a hot light.

- **Prior radiographs** are often invaluable for comparison with the current study to determine the time course of a disease process, particularly to establish the chronicity, and therefore benign nature, of some lesions. Comparison with prior examinations also makes subtle abnormalities more conspicuous.

- Ideally the radiograph should be reviewed first without reviewing the **clinical information** or history to provide an unbiased objective evaluation. Prior to reporting the study, the clinical history and previous imaging reports should be sought to ensure a focused interpretation.

- **Interpreting** the radiograph begins with careful observation and description of the abnormalities. An initial gestalt of the film often reveals striking abnormalities, but the examination should be reviewed in a systematic fashion to avoid overlooking subtle abnormalities. One common pitfall is the phenomenon of *satisfaction of search* in which there is failure to evaluate the entire study after one abnormality is detected, such as failing to note a destructive rib metastases once a dominant pulmonary mass has been identified. It is often said that "an easy way to miss an abnormality is to have another abnormality present."

- **Clues to a pathologic process** may include alteration in tissue density (increased opacification or lucency), alteration of normal contour, and destruction or absence of normal anatomic structures. The order in which various tissues or areas on the radiograph are examined is less important than developing a comprehensive **systematic approach** that includes review of the soft tissue and bones of the chest wall, the upper abdomen, the mediastinum (including the central airway, heart, and central pulmonary vascular structures), and pulmonary parenchyma. The corners of the film should be specifically reviewed. Table 1.1 lists specific features of the chest radiograph that should be considered when reviewing an examination.

Once relevant observations including pertinent positive and negative ancillary findings are noted, a **differential diagnosis** can be considered. Categories of disease process provide a reliable general approach. These include inflammatory and infectious processes, neoplasm, congenital abnormalities, traumatic or iatrogenic injury, vascular, connective tissue disease, and metabolic disorders.

- **Errors in interpretation** include false-negative reports in which an abnormality is overlooked or discounted (noting but disregarding an abnormality). An additional type of error is a false-positive report in which a pathologic lesion is reported that is not present. There are more false-negative than false-positive readings.

TABLE 1.1. SYSTEMATIC REVIEW OF THE CHEST RADIOGRAPH

Item or Region	Specific Observation
Demographic data	Match paperwork and radiograph to ensure name and exam date are correct.
Technical quality	Exam type (portable or standard), patient positioning (AP or PA, rotation, supine or erect), right and left marked correctly, adequacy of exposure, depth of inspiration.
Comparison	Direct comparison with prior radiographs.
Appliances and potential complications	Catheters or chest tubes and potential pneumothorax, prosthetic valves or pacemaker, orthopedic instrumentation, abdominal catheters, complications in position, malfunction or damage.
Prior surgery	Thoracotomy, median sternotomy, hemoclips in chest or abdomen.
Lungs	Volume, symmetry, focal or diffuse infiltrates, atelectasis or nodules.
Pleura and fissures	Thickening, plaques, calcification, effusion size and location, accessory fissures.
Pulmonary vessels	Increased, decreased, or normal size or redistribution.
Hila	Size, shape, density, adenopathy or vascular enlargement.
Mediastinum	Adenopathy, mass, central airway.
Heart	Global or chamber enlargement, calcifications in valves, pericardium, myocardium or coronary artery distributions.
Aorta	Location, enlargement, tortuosity, calcification.
Diaphragm	Shape (eventration, hernia), location (hyperinflation), symmetry (paralysis).
Chest wall and bones	Anterior and posterior ribs, shoulder girdle, spine and sternum. Overall density and texture, acute or healed fractures, bone destruction, sclerotic or lytic areas, congenital deformity (cervical ribs, scoliosis).
Upper abdomen	Bowel gas pattern, free air, organ enlargement, abnormal calcifications.
Film edges and corners	Review film margins including structures obscured by demographic data or labels.
Clinical history and prior reports	Consider age, sex, and clinical information provided. Make inquiries as needed. Review prior report. Search should include targeted assessment of film to answer question at hand (e.g., rule out pneumothorax after bronchoscopy) and search for abnormalities overlooked related to the patient's underlying medical condition (e.g., if are there any sclerotic bone metastases in a patient with prostate cancer).
Report	Convey written results in concise, precise terms and by phone if indicated.

TABLE 1.2. SYSTEMATIC APPROACH TO UNKNOWN CASES

Description (20%)	Adequate detail for someone not seeing the films to "visualize" the findings.
Exam type	Portable or standard, supine or erect, PA or AP.
Sex and age	Obtain from film flasher or estimate from appearance.
Primary finding	Striking abnormality.
Size	Estimate dimensions in centimeters.
Location	Anatomic location, compartment and reason, e.g., chest wall, pleural, posterior mediastinum, pulmonary lobe.
Characteristics	Density, borders, cavitation, effect on adjacent structures (invasion or displacement).
Associated and ancillary observations	Enumerate pertinent positive and negative findings and avoid getting sidetracked on extraneous observations of unlikely relevance (see Table 1.1).
Summary	Summarize findings in one sentence.
Differential diagnosis (70%, 2–3 min)	Note additional observations of importance as necessary but try not to return to description. (Ideally everything pertinent already mentioned.)
Time course	Differentiate acute from chronic when possible by comparison with prior radiographs or history.
Category approach	Begin with most applicable category and most likely diagnoses. Mention disease, why specifically it is a consideration, and two or three potential distinguishing features or management issues.
Neoplasm	Primary and metastatic.
Infection	Specifics related to immune status.
Congenital	
Vascular	
Inflammatory or collagen vascular	Connective tissue, autoimmune, sarcoid.
Trauma	
Iatrogenic	Including drug reactions.
Metabolic or endocrine	
Summary (10%)	
Top differentials	Briefly summarize your reasoning and top differential choices in order of decreasing likelihood.
Definitive action indicated	Treatment, further history, testing or imaging that you would recommend, including follow-up or importance of seeking prior films.

- Failure to report a lesion may result from lesions being below the limit of visibility, typically 8 mm for a noncalcified pulmonary nodule. A double reading either by the same or different observers reduces error. Finally, of crucial importance, is accurate and concise **communication** of results to the patient's physician both by written report and verbally when indicated.

- Table 1.2 provides some guidelines for approaching an unknown case in a **teaching** or **board setting** where there is a known diagnosis and possibly other confirmatory imaging or clinical testing and the goal is to evaluate the discussant's observation skills and knowledge.

- **Be pragmatic** and limit discussion to realistic possibilities. In general this means 3 to 5 entities distributed in a few categories. Mention entities that generally might be considered but that are clearly not likely given a specific facet of the case and indicate why. For example, commenting that "although primary bronchogenic cancer is a common explanation for a solitary lung mass with associated adenopathy, it would be exceedingly rare and is not a reasonable consideration in this 20-year-old."

- Stress the importance of an unlikely diagnosis in differentials that remain important because of impact on management. For example, "Cancer must be excluded although infection is more likely," or "Tuberculosis must be excluded although bacterial pneumonia is more likely."

- Throughout the discussion, cite the value of specific historical information, laboratory data, or additional imaging studies that you would like to consider if available, including old films. Recommend history and physical examination before ordering expensive tests for further work-up.

  For example, given a cavitary lung mass, state that "absence of a fever would strongly favor neoplasm over abscess." The examiner or consultant may then provide you with this specific information. If not, you have indicated how that information would guide your thoughts were it available. *Do not* ask for "history," rather use your knowledge to ask for specific details, particularly in a testing situation. Always be able to defend your request, i.e., state exactly how information would be useful in a particular case.

- Stay with a current modality, such as recommending a lateral, lordotic, decubitus, or examination with nipple markers, before advancing to more sophisticated imaging studies. For example, given a PA film with blunting of the costophrenic angle, indicate that a lateral radiograph would be valuable for visualizing the posterior costophrenic angle to better determine whether this is scarring or fluid.

Bibliography

Aguv AMR. *Grant's Atlas of Anatomy*. 9th ed. Baltimore: Williams & Wilkins; 1991.

Armstrong P, Wilson AG, Dee P, Hamsell DM. *Imaging of Diseases of the Chest*. 2nd ed. St. Louis: Mosby-Year Book; 1995.

Fishman AP, Elias JA, Fishman JA, Grippi MA, Kaiser LR, Senior RM. *Fishman's Pulmonary Diseases and Disorders*. 3rd ed. New York: McGraw-Hill; 1998.

Fraser RG, Paré JAP, Paré PD, Fraser RS, Genereux GP. *Diagnosis of Diseases of the Chest*. Vol. 1, 3rd ed. Philadelphia: WB Saunders; 1988.

Freundlich IM, Bragg DG. *A Radiographic Approach to Diseases of the Chest*. 2nd ed. Baltimore: Williams & Wilkins, 1997.

Hasleton PS. *Spencer's Pathology of the Lung*. 5th ed. New York: McGraw-Hill; 1996.

West JB. *Physiological Basis of Medical Practice*. 12th ed. Baltimore: Williams & Wilkins; 1990.

West JB. *Respiratory Physiology*. 5th ed. Baltimore: Williams & Wilkins; 1995.

Chapter 2

DIFFERENTIAL DIAGNOSIS FOR THE CHEST

Richard M. Slone

Differential diagnosis lists serve several purposes. The most important is to provide a few practical diseases that represent the most likely etiologies for a radiologic observation. In this sense, the only practical differential is a short list from which a clinician can work to arrive at a diagnosis. An exhaustive list based solely on the radiologic observation is essentially useless. In this vein, we have provided within each differential list up to five items demarcated in **boldface** that represent the most common entities in a general clinical setting.

Another role for differential diagnosis lists is to help bring into consideration uncommon etiologies. Sometimes an unusual case is encountered in which a particular clinical presentation or information from other testing has eliminated the common entities and suggests that a "zebra" might explain the "hoofprints." In support of this, we have provided an exhaustive list of entities in each differential list, including rare etiologies or uncommon manifestations denoted in *italics*.

The following lists represent a composite of standard and "classic" radiology differentials (see Bibliography) balanced by our own practical experience. When patient symptoms, age, sex, immune status, and other relevant clinical history are considered in combination with the pattern and chronicity of the radiologic observation in a specific case, these differential lists can be reduced to a few likely entities.

Lung Volumes and Global Patterns

1. Increased Lung Volumes
2. Reduced Lung Volumes
3. Unilateral Small Lung
4. Unilateral Large Lung
5. Hyperlucent Hemithorax
6. Hyperlucent Lungs
7. Diffuse Lung Disease
8. Diffuse Unilateral Lung Disease
9. Unilateral Dense Hemithorax
10. Perihilar Lung Disease
11. Peripheral Lung Disease
12. Upper Lung Disease
13. Lower Lung Disease
14. Posterior Lung Disease

Pulmonary Nodules and Masses

15. Solitary Pulmonary Nodule (≤3 cm)
16. Solitary Pulmonary Mass (>3 cm)
17. Peripheral Pulmonary Mass
18. Pulmonary Nodules with Adenopathy
19. Well-Defined Pulmonary Nodules
20. Ill-Defined Pulmonary Nodules
21. Tiny Nodules (<5 mm, Micronodular, Miliary)
22. Calcified Pulmonary Nodules

Cavities and Lucent Lesions

23. Localized Pulmonary Lucency
24. Cystic Lesions with Lobar Enlargement
25. Multiple Lucent Lesions or Cysts
26. Cavitary Nodule or Mass
27. Multiple Cavitary Nodules

Airway Abnormalities, Atelectasis, and Collapse

28. Tracheal Wall Thickening
29. Tracheal Enlargement
30. Tracheal Narrowing
31. Tracheoesophageal Fistula
32. Tracheal Mass
33. Endobronchial Lesion
34. Atelectasis and Pulmonary Collapse
35. Bronchiectasis

Consolidation and Airspace Disease

36. Acute Diffuse or Patchy Pulmonary Consolidation
37. Chronic Diffuse Airspace Disease and Consolidation
38. Unilateral Airspace Disease
39. Pulmonary Hemorrhage
40. Localized Consolidation
41. Consolidation with Lobar Enlargement
42. Chronic Lobar Consolidation
43. Recurrent Pneumonia
44. Bronchopneumonia

Interstitial Lung Disease

45. Acute Diffuse Interstitial Lung Disease
46. Chronic Diffuse Interstitial Lung Disease (Not Nodular)
47. Chronic Nodular Interstitial Lung Disease
48. Diffuse Interstitial Lung Disease with Pleural Effusion
49. Diffuse Interstitial Lung Disease with Adenopathy
50. Diffuse Disease with Normal or Increased Lung Volumes
51. Peripheral Pulmonary Infiltrates
52. Pulmonary Edema
53. Unilateral Interstitial Lung Disease
54. Migratory Pulmonary Infiltrates
55. Focal Reticulonodular Pattern
56. Diffuse Reticulonodular Pattern
57. Peripheral Reticulnodular Pattern
58. Upper Lung Reticulonodular Pattern
59. Lower Lung Reticulonodular Pattern

High-Resolution CT Patterns

60. Ground Glass Opacities
61. Interlobular Septal Thickening (Kerley Lines)
62. Intralobular Septal Thickening
63. Peribronchovascular Interstitial Thickening
64. Honeycombing
65. Cystic Lesions
66. Interstitial Nodules
67. Small Perilymphatic Nodules
68. Small Randomly Distributed Nodules
69. Centrilobular Nodules

Pleural Abnormalities

70. Pneumothorax
71. Spontaneous Pneumothorax with Diffuse Lung Disease
72. Unilateral Pleural Effusion
73. Bilateral Pleural Effusion
74. Pleural Effusion with Cardiomegaly
75. Transudate
76. Exudate
77. Hemothorax
78. Chylothorax
79. Pleural Thickening
80. Pleural Mass
81. Multiple Pleural Masses
82. Pleural Calcifications

Diaphragm and Chest Wall Abnormalities

83. Flattened Hemidiaphragm
84. Elevated Hemidiaphragm
85. Bilateral Hemidiaphragm Elevation
86. Extrapleural Lesion
87. Soft Tissue Calcifications
88. Peripheral Pulmonary Disease and Chest Wall Mass
89. Chest Wall Mass
90. Vertebral Compression Fracture
91. Sclerotic Bone Lesion
92. Lytic Bone Lesion
93. Diffuse Bone Sclerosis

94. Inferior Rib Notching
95. Superior Rib Notching
96. Distal Clavicular Resorption

Mediastinal and Hilar Abnormalities

97. Unilateral Hilar Enlargement
98. Bilateral Hilar Enlargement
99. Calcified Lymph Nodes
100. Low Attenuation Lymph Nodes
101. Enhancing Lymph Nodes
102. Pneumomediastinum
103. Ipsilateral Mediastinal Shift
104. Contralateral Mediastinal Shift
105. Enlarged or Widened Mediastinum
106. Thoracic Inlet or Superior Mediastinal Mass
107. Anterior Mediastinal Mass
108. Middle Mediastinal Mass
109. Posterior Mediastinal Masses
110. Cardiophrenic Angle Mass
111. Low Attenuation Mediastinal Mass

Cardiac Abnormalities

112. Dextrocardia
113. Small Heart
114. Enlarged Cardiac Silhouette
115. Cardiac Mass
116. Pericardial Effusion
117. High-Output Heart Disease
118. Congestive Heart Failure in Neonates
119. Left Atrial Enlargement
120. Left Ventricular Enlargement
121. Right Atrial Enlargement
122. Right Ventricular Enlargement
123. Cardiac Calcifications
124. Aortic Insufficiency
125. Mitral Insufficiency
126. Tricuspid Insufficiency
127. Left-to-Right Shunt
128. Right-to-Left Shunt
129. Normal or Decreased Pulmonary Vascularity with Cyanosis
130. Congenital Heart Disease with Increased Pulmonary Vascularity

Vascular Abnormalities

131. Perfusion Defects on Lung Scan
132. Reversed Ventilation-Perfusion Mismatch on Lung Scan
133. Unilateral Decreased Perfusion on Lung Scan
134. Enlarged Ascending Aorta
135. Mirror Image Right-Sided Aortic Arch
136. Coronary Artery Aneurysms
137. Pulmonary Venous Hypertension (Edema)
138. Enlarged Pulmonary Arteries
139. Enlarged Superior Vena Cava
140. Enlarged Azygos Vein

Clinical Differential Diagnosis

LUNG VOLUMES AND GLOBAL PATTERNS

1. Increased Lung Volumes

- **Deep inspiratory effort** (more common in a young adult or child)
- **Emphysema** (increased lucency, attenuated vessels, lung destruction)
- Asthmatic attack (more common in a child)
- Cystic fibrosis (associated upper lobe-predominant bronchiectasis)
- *Eosinophilic granuloma (upper lobe predominant cysts or nodules, in a young woman)*
- *Lymphangioleiomyomatosis (innumerable pulmonary cysts, in a young woman)*

2. Reduced Lung Volumes

- **Poor inspiratory effort**
- Elevated diaphragm (obesity, hepatosplenomegaly, pregnancy, ascites, neuromuscular disease)
- Fibrosis (reticular interstitial pattern, IPF, connective tissue disease)
- Subpulmonic effusions (separation between gastric air and lung base)

3. Unilateral Small Lung

- **Lobar atelectasis** or **collapse** (obstruction with foreign body, endobronchial tumor, or mucus)
- **Prior partial pulmonary resection**
- **Paralysis of the phrenic nerve** (surgical, tumor, idiopathic)
- Hemidiaphragm displacement (distended stomach or colon, enlarged liver or spleen, subphrenic mass or fluid collection)
- Eventration of hemidiaphragm (broad based, most commonly right anterior portion)
- Subpulmonic effusions (separation between gastric air and lung base)
- Hernia
- Hypoplastic lung
- Swyer-James-Macleod's syndrome (bronchiolitis obliterans in childhood)
- *Unilateral transplant for pulmonary fibrosis*

4. Unilateral Large Lung

- Asymmetric emphysema
- Tension pneumothorax (hemidiaphragm and mediastinum displaced)
- Airway obstruction in a child (atelectasis more common in an adult)
- *Unilateral transplant for pulmonary emphysema*

5. Hyperlucent Hemithorax

- **Normal lung** (increased density of contralateral hemithorax from effusion, edema, etc.)
- **Patient rotation** (right lung more lucent in RPO position, left lung in LPO position)
- Asymmetric chest wall (**mastectomy**, Poland syndrome, scoliosis)
- Technical (grid cutoff, heal effect)
- Pneumothorax

5. Hyperlucent Hemithorax (*continued*)

- Increased aeration
    Asymmetric emphysema
    Compensatory hyperinflation (ipsilateral lobectomy, *contralateral lobar collapse*)
    Endobronchial obstruction* (mucus plug, bronchogenic carcinoma, broncholith, carcinoid, foreign body, endobronchial metastasis)
    Ipsilateral bronchiolitis obliterans with air trapping (Swyer-James-Macleod's syndrome)
    Congenital lobar emphysema (usually in first few weeks of life)
- Decreased vascularity
    Pulmonary thromboembolism (focal oligemia, Westermark sign)
    Pulmonary artery hypoplasia, agenesis, or stenosis
    Hypogenetic lung (scimitar syndrome)
- *Congenital bronchial atresia (left upper lobe most commonly)*
- *Unilateral lung transplant for emphysema*

*Postobstructive air trapping may be seen in a child, collapse is more common in an adult.

6. Hyperlucent Lungs

- **Overpenetrated film** (overexposure)
- **Emphysema** (hyperinflation, oligemia)
- Air trapping
    Multiple bullae or pneumatoceles
    Cystic fibrosis (hyperinflation, bronchiectasis)
    Asthmatic attack (hyperinflation, normal vascular markings)
    Bronchiolitis (hyperinflation, ill-defined opacities)
    Tracheal obstruction or compression (foreign body, relapsing polychondritis, tumor)
- Thin chest wall (**thin body habitus**, bilateral mastectomy)
- Decreased pulmonary vascularity
    Right-to-left pulmonary arterial shunt
    Pulmonary artery hypertension (central pulmonary artery enlargement)
    Pulmonary thromboembolism (massive)

7. Diffuse Lung Disease

- **Pulmonary edema** (cardiogenic, fluid overload, renal failure, and noncardiogenic)
- **Pneumonia**
    Pneumocystis carinii
    Mycoplasma
    Viral (cytomegalovirus, varicella)
    Fungus (*Aspergillus*, *Candida*, histoplasmosis)
    Mycobacterium (TB, MAI)
    Eosinophilic
- **ARDS**
- Pulmonary fibrosis (reduced lung volumes)
- Sarcoidosis
- Pneumoconiosis (silicosis)
- Bronchiectasis (cystic fibrosis, immotile cilia syndrome, idiopathic)
- Pulmonary hemorrhage (coagulopathy, Goodpasture syndrome)
- Aspiration
- Drug reaction or inhalation injury
- Bronchoalveolar cell carcinoma
- Metastatic disease

- Lymphangitic carcinomatosis
- *Fat emboli*

8. Diffuse Unilateral Lung Disease

- **Pneumonia** (bacterial, fungal, tuberculosis, aspiration, postobstructive)
- **Pleural effusion** (simulates diffuse lung disease in supine position)
- Bronchoalveolar cell carcinoma (can present as mass, nodules or consolidation)
- Unilateral pulmonary edema (lateral decubitus positioning, reexpansion after thoracentesis)
- Lymphangitic carcinomatosis
- Hemorrhage
- Pulmonary contusion (trauma)
- Lobar collapse
- Radiation pneumonitis or fibrosis
- *Bronchiectasis*
- *Recent bronchoalveolar lavage*

9. Unilateral Dense Hemithorax

- **Large pleural effusion** (usually with associated pulmonary collapse)
- **Pulmonary collapse** (volume loss, bronchogenic carcinoma, mucus plug, carcinoid, right mainstem intubation)
- **Prior pneumonectomy**
- Pneumonia (bacterial, fungal, mycobacterial)
- Pleural tumor (mesothelioma with circumferential pleural involvement, pleural metastasis)
- *Pulmonary agenesis or aplasia*
- *Ruptured ipsilateral hemidiaphragm*
- *Chest wall mass*

10. Perihilar Lung Disease

- **Pulmonary edema** (cardiogenic, renal failure, fluid overload)
- ***Pneumocystis carinii* pneumonia**
- Inhalation injury (smoke, toxic fumes)
- Vasculitis or pulmonary hemorrhage
- Aspiration pneumonia (superior segments of lower lobe)
- Sarcoidosis (peribronchovascular nodules)
- Bronchitis or bronchiectasis
- Viral pneumonia
- *Lymphangitic carcinomatosis (nodular interstitial thickening)*
- *Cystic fibrosis (predominantly upper lobe bronchiectasis, increased lung volumes)*
- *Alveolar proteinosis*
- *Drug reaction*

11. Peripheral Lung Disease

- **Pulmonary fibrosis** (idiopathic, scleroderma, rheumatoid, asbestosis)
- **Pulmonary metastases**
- Sarcoidosis (subpleural and septal nodules on HRCT)
- Eosinophilic pneumonia (airspace disease)
- Bronchiolitis obliterans with organizing pneumonia (BOOP, patchy peripheral consolidation)
- Hypersensitivity pneumonitis (alveolitis and ill-defined centrilobular nodules on HRCT)

12. Upper Lung Disease

- **Pneumonia** (bacterial, active granulomatous disease)
- **Cystic fibrosis** (bronchiectasis, hyperinflation, mucus plug)
- Sarcoidosis (nodules and fibrosis; may spare apex and base)
- Tuberculosis (consolidation, nodules, cavitation)
- Eosinophilic granuloma (small nodules and cysts)
- Silicosis and coal worker's pneumoconiosis (symmetric tiny nodules, often calcified, similar to talcosis)
- *Bronchiolitis*
- *Ankylosing spondylitis*

13. Lower Lung Disease

- **Pneumonia** (aspiration, lipoid from chronic oil aspiration)
- **Pulmonary fibrosis**
    Idiopathic (IPF, UIP, DIP)
    Collagen vascular disease (sclerodema, lupus, rhematoid arthritis, dermatomyositis)
    Asbestosis
    Drugs
- Pulmonary metastases (smooth, round nodules of various sizes)
- Bronchiectasis
- *Hypersensitivity pneumonitis (alveolitis, ill-defined nodules)*
- *Kaposi sarcoma*
- *Neurofibromatosis*

14. Posterior Lung Disease

- **Pulmonary fibrosis**
    Idiopathic (IPF, UIP, DIP)
    Collagen vascular disease (sclerodema, lupus, rhematoid arthritis, dermatomyositis)
    Asbestosis
    Drugs
- Silicosis (symmetric tiny nodules, often calcified)
- Pulmonary edema
- Dependent atelectasis (supine positioning)

PULMONARY NODULES AND MASSES

15. Solitary Pulmonary Nodule (≤3 cm)*

MIMICS
- **Nipple** (look for contralateral nipple on PA and skin location on lateral)
- **Confluence of shadows** (superimposed pleura, chest wall, or vascular structures)
- **Costochondral cartilage** (particularly the first rib end)
- Skin lesion (mole, wart, nevus, desmoid, neurofibroma)
- Artifact (button, ECG electrode)
- Rib or bone lesion (bone island, healed fracture)
- Pseudotumor (loculated fluid in a fissure)
- Pleural plaque (particularly calcified plaques seen en face)

INFLAMMATORY (HALF OF TRUE NODULES)
- **Granuloma** (tuberculoma or histoplasmoma; satellite lesions common, usually small, smooth, often calcified when healed)
- **Scar** (often linear and extending to pleura)
- Aspergilloma (in preexisting cavity)

- Organizing pneumonia (nocardia, actinomycosis)
- Lung abscess (bacterial—may be fluid-filled and appear solid, *amebic abscess*)
- Fungus (blastomycosis, coccidioidomycosis, cryptococcosis, histoplasmosis, aspergillosis)
- Septic emboli (usually multiple, may cavitate; *Staphylococcus* is common)
- *Round pneumonia (almost exclusively in children; Pneumococcus, Legionella, Nocardia)*
- *Echinococcal cyst*

NEOPLASM
- **Bronchogenic carcinoma** (adenocarcinoma, squamous, large cell, bronchoalveolar)
- **Solitary metastasis** (sarcoma, melanoma, colon, renal cell, testicular cancer)
- **Hamartoma** (smooth, 15 percent contain calcification and 50 percent fat)
- Bronchial adenoma (carcinoid, 80 percent are central)
- *Papilloma (usually multiple, cavitate)*
- *Fibrous tumor of pleura (may attach to visceral pleura in fissure simulating a pulmonary process)*
- *Lymphoma (particularly non-Hodgkin, usually multiple and rare without mediastinal adenopathy)*

VASCULAR
- **Prominent vessel** (seen on end)
- Pulmonary infarct (peripheral, wedge shaped)
- Arteriovenous malformation (half associated with Osler-Weber-Rendu)
- Hematoma (evidence of trauma, resolves over weeks)
- *Pulmonary artery pseudoaneurysm*
- *Pulmonary vein varix (near left atrium)*

OTHER CAUSES
- **Rounded atelectasis** (associated pleural disease)
- Bronchogenic cyst (15 percent are intrapulmonary)
- Intrapulmonary lymph node (benign, peripheral, 2 to 4 mm)
- Bronchocele/mucoid impaction (allergic bronchopulmonary aspergillosis, bronchial atresia, cystic fibrosis)
- Wegener granulomatosis (usually multiple)
- *Amyloidosis*
- *Rheumatoid nodules (usually multiple)*

*Rarely malignant before age 40

16. Solitary Pulmonary Mass (>3 cm)

NEOPLASM
- **Bronchogenic carcinoma** (adenocarcinoma, squamous, large cell, bronchoalveolar)
- Solitary metastasis (sarcoma, melanoma, colon, renal cell, testicular cancer)
- Pseudotumor (loculated fluid in fissure)
- **Hamartoma** (smooth, 15 percent contain calcification and 50 percent fat)
- *Pleural tumor (mesothelioma, fibrous tumor of the pleura)*
- *Lymphoma (particularly non-Hodgkin, usually multiple and rare without mediastinal adenopathy)*

INFLAMMATORY
- **Organized pneumonia** (*Nocardia, Actinomyces*)
- **Lung abscess** (thick irregular walls, may appear solid)
- **Round pneumonia** (almost exclusively in children; pneumococcus, *Legionella, Nocardia*)
- Granuloma (usually small, smooth, often calcified)
- Fungus (cryptococcosis, blastomycosis, coccidioidomycosis, histoplasmosis)
- *Echinococcal cyst*
- *Lipoid pneumonia (chronic oil aspiration, fat density on CT)*

OTHER
- **Rounded atelectasis** (associated pleural disease)
- Progressive massive fibrosis (complicated silicosis, coal worker's pneumoconiosis)
- Bronchogenic cyst (central lung, may cavitate with infection)

16. Solitary Pulmonary Mass (>3 cm) *(continued)*

- Hematoma (evidence of trauma, mass resolves over weeks)
- Wegener granulomatosis (usually multiple)
- *Pulmonary sequestration (interlobar may cavitate with infection, most common in LLL)*

17. Peripheral Pulmonary Mass

- **Bronchogenic carcinoma** (typically large cell or adenocarcinoma)
- **Rounded atelectasis** (in contact with associated pleural disease)
- **Organized pneumonia** (usually air bronchograms, may be associated with bronchiolitis obliterans)
- Fungus (blastomycosis, coccidioidomycosis)
- Loculated effusion
- Lymphoma
- Granuloma
- Hamartoma (15 percent contain calcification and 50 percent fat)
- Pulmonary infarct (wedge shaped, volume loss, effusion or enlarged PA)
- *Metastasis (usually smooth, peripheral and multiple)*
- *Pulmonary sequestration (interlobar may cavitate with infection, most common in LLL)*

18. Pulmonary Nodules with Adenopathy

- **Sarcoidosis**
- **Metastatic disease** (testicular, renal cell cancer)
- **Granulomatous infection**
- Non-Hodgkin lymphoma
- Silicosis

19. Well-Defined Pulmonary Nodules

- **Granulomatous disease** (tuberculosis, histoplasmosis, coccidioidomycosis, cryptococcosis, aspergillosis)

TUMOR
- **Metastases** (variable size, usually smooth and peripheral, lower lobe predominance)
  - Large: sarcoma, seminoma, renal cell, thyroid, colon cancer
  - Miliary: melanoma; thyroid, lung, breast, renal cell cancer
  - Calcified: osteosarcoma, chondrosarcoma, mucinous adenocarcinoma
  - Tumors most likely to metastasize to lung: choriocarcinoma, melanoma, sarcoma, renal cell, thyroid, breast, testicular cancer
  - Most likely origin of pulmonary metastases: breast, renal, head and neck, colon cancer
- Bronchoalveolar cell carcinoma (mass, nodules, or consolidation)
- *Papillomas (frequently cavitate)*
- *Non-Hodgkin lymphoma*

VASCULAR
- **Wegener granulomatosis** (frequently cavitates, may have renal and sinus disease)
- Arteriovenous malformations (half associated with Osler-Weber-Rendu)
- Pulmonary infarcts (peripheral, wedge-shaped)

OTHER CAUSES
- Silicosis (small, calcified upper lobe nodules)
- Eosinophilic granuloma (small upper lobe nodules and cysts, young women)
- Skin lesions (neurofibromas)
- Mucoid impaction (particularly allergic bronchopulmonary aspergillosis)
- *Sarcoidosis (rare manifestation)*

- *Amyloidosis*
- *Rheumatoid nodules (often multiple and cavitate)*

20. Multiple Ill-Defined Pulmonary Nodules

INFECTION
- **Granulomatous disease** (tuberculosis, histoplasmosis, aspergillosis, coccidioidomycosis, cryptococcosis)
- Bacterial pneumonia (bronchopneumonia, *Nocardia, actinomycosis, Legionella*)

TUMOR
- **Metastases** (renal cell, thyroid; cancer of colon, breast, stomach; choriocarcinoma, hemorrhagic—melanoma)
- Bronchoalveolar cell carcinoma (mass, nodules, or consolidation)
- Kaposi sarcoma

VASCULAR
- **Wegener granulomatosis** (frequently cavitate, may have renal and sinus disease)
- **Septic emboli** (peripheral, ill-defined; *S. aureus*, gram-negative organisms, anaerobes, streptococcus)
- Pulmonary infarcts (peripheral, wedge shaped)

OTHER CAUSES
- Eosinophilic granuloma (small upper lobe nodules and cysts, young women)
- Extrinsic allergic alveolitis
- *Sarcoidosis (rare manifestation)*
- *Non-Hodgkin lymphoma*
- *Progressive massive fibrosis (conglomerate masses, silicosis, coal worker's pneumoconiosis)*

21. Tiny Nodules (<5 mm, micronodular, miliary)

INFLAMMATORY
- **Granulomatous disease** (histoplasmosis, calcification and frequently calcified lymph nodes, blastomycosis, cryptococcosis, coccidioidomycosis)
- Miliary tuberculosis
- Viral pneumonia (varicella)
- *Extrinsic allergic alveolitis (hypersensitivity pneumonitis, farmer's lung)*
- *Nocardia*
- *Bronchiolitis*

MALIGNANCY
- **Pulmonary metastases** (thyroid, pancreas, renal cancer, breast cancer, choriocarcinoma, melanoma)
- Bronchoalveolar cell carcinoma
- Lymphangitic carcinomatosis (nodular interstitial pattern)
- *Lymphoma*

OTHER CAUSES
- **Silicosis** (small, calcified upper lobe nodules, also coal worker's pneumoconiosis)
- Sarcoidosis
- Eosinophilic granuloma
- *Other pneumoconiosis (siderosis, berylliosis, stannosis)*
- *Alveolar microlithiasis*
- *Amyloidosis*
- *Hemosiderosis (idiopathic, chronic venous hypertension, pulmonary hemorrhage)*

22. Calcified Pulmonary Nodules

- **Old, healed granulomatous disease** (frequently calcified lymph nodes, histoplasmosis, coccidioidomycosis, tuberculosis)
- **Silicosis** (small, calcified upper lobe nodules, often calcified lymph nodes)
- Varicella pneumonia (healed infection, lower lobe predominance)

---

22. Calcified Pulmonary Nodules (*continued*)

- *Hypercalcemia*
- *Mitral stenosis (left atrial enlargement, may have valve calcification, secondary hemosiderosis)*
- *Alveolar microlithiasis (diffuse, fine calcifications)*
- *Parasites*
- *Metastatic calcification (hyperparathyroidism)*
- *Amyloidosis (peripheral calcification)*
- *Calcified metastases (osteosarcoma, chondrosarcoma; cystosarcoma phyllodes; mucinous adenocarcinoma from breast, ovary, or colon; papillary adenocarcinoma from ovary or thyroid; radiation therapy of pulmonary metastases)*

CAVITIES AND LUCENT LESIONS

23. Localized Pulmonary Lucency

- **Bulla** or **bleb**
- **Pneumatocele**
    Infection (*S. aureus, H. influenzae, P. carinii, M. tuberculosis, Pneumococcus, E. coli, Klebsiella, Legionella*)
    Trauma (healed hematoma or laceration)
- Loculated pneumothorax
- Healed abscess cavity (tuberculosis)
- Lung abscess (usually thick-walled)
- Hernia containing bowel (hiatal, Bochdalek, Morgagni)
- Normal bronchus (seen on end)
- Cystic bronchiectasis
- *Necrotic or treated metastasis (usually thick-walled)*
- *Cystic adenomatoid malformation (fluid-filled at birth)*
- *Congenital lobar emphysema*
- *Pulmonary sequestration (intralobar, lower lobe)*
- *Bronchogenic cyst (15 percent parenchymal, air-filled after infection)*
- *Ecchinococcal cyst (hydatid)*

24. Cystic Lesions with Lobar Enlargement

- **Large bullae** emphysema
- Cystic adenomatoid malformation (multiloculated cysts, fluid filled at birth)
- Congenital lobar emphysema

25. Multiple Lucent Lesions or Cysts

- **Bullae** and **blebs, emphysema** (blebs arise in visceral pleura)
- Eosinophilic granuloma (may have nodules, cysts, or both)
- Pneumatoceles
    Infection (*S. aureus, H. influenzae*, gram-negative organisms, *P. carinii, M. tuberculosis, Pneumococcus, E. coli, Klebsiella, Legionella*)
    Trauma (healed hematoma or laceration)
- Cystic bronchiectasis
- Honeycombing (fibrosis)
- *Tracheobronchial papillomatosis*
- *Tuberous sclerosis*
- *Lymphangioleiomyomatosis (young woman)*

26. Cavitary Nodule or Mass

INFLAMMATORY
- **Lung abscess, necrotizing pneumonia** (thick, irregular wall, often aspiration-related)
  - Bacterial (*Staphylococcus, Pseudomonas, Klebsiella, E. coli*, gram-negative organisms, anaerobes, actinomycosis, *Nocardia, Streptococcus, Legionella*)
  - Fungal (blastomycosis, aspergillosis, histoplasmosis, coccidioidomycosis, cryptococcosis, mucormycosis)
  - *Amebic*
- Mycobacteria (particularly tuberculosis)
- *Chronic round pneumonia*
- *Echinococcal cyst*

TUMOR
- **Bronchogenic carcinoma** (classically squamous cell, also adenocarcinoma, bronchoalveolar)
- Carcinoid tumor
- Metastasis (usually multiple, smooth, peripheral; squamous cell, transitional cell, adenocarcinoma, sarcoma)
- *Lymphoma (Hodgkin)*

CONGENITAL
- Bronchogenic cyst (may cavitate following infection)
- *Cystic adenomatoid malformation*
- *Intralobar sequestration (may cavitate following infection, most common in LLL)*

VASCULAR
- Pulmonary infarct (peripheral, wedge-shaped)
- Septic embolus (usually multiple, ill-defined)
- Hematoma (trauma)
- Wegener granulomatosis (30 percent cavitate)

OTHER CAUSES
- **Hiatal hernia**
- Progressive massive fibrosis (usually bilateral and asymmetric, silicosis, coal worker's pneumoconiosis)
- *Amyloidosis*
- *Rheumatoid nodule*

27. Multiple Cavitary Nodules

INFLAMMATORY
- **Septic emboli** (peripheral, ill-defined, endocarditis, septic thrombophlebitis)
- Fungal infections (coccidioidomycosis, *Aspergillus*)
- *Tuberculosis*

TUMOR
- **Pulmonary metastases** (4 percent cavitate, squamous cell of head and neck or cervix, sarcoma, usually smooth and peripheral)
- *Lymphoma*
- *Tracheobronchial papillomatosis*

OTHER CAUSES
- Eosinophilic granuloma (upper lobe predominance of cysts, nodules, or both)
- Progressive massive fibrosis (silicosis or coal worker's pneumoconiosis)
- Wegener granulomatosis (30 percent cavitate)
- *Rheumatoid necrobiotic nodules*
- *Multiple pulmonary infarcts*
- *Amyloidosis*
- *Sarcoidosis*

AIRWAY ABNORMALITIES, ATELECTASIS, AND COLLAPSE

28. Tracheal Wall Thickening

- Amyloidosis
- Relapsing polychondritis
- Tracheopathia osteochondroplastica
- Sarcoidosis
- Wegener granulomatosis
- Inhalation injury
- Infection (tuberculosis, *Klebsiella rhinoscleroma*, fungus)

29. Tracheal Enlargement*

- **Tracheomalacia** (endotracheal cuff damage)
- **Tracheobronchomegaly** (Mounier-Kuhn syndrome)
- Cystic fibrosis
- Immunoglobulin deficiency
- Adjacent pulmonary fibrosis
- Relapsing polychondritis
- *Tracheocele*
- *Ehlers-Danlos complex*

*Wider than 26 mm in men and 23 mm in women.

30. Tracheal Narrowing

EXTRINSIC
- Thyroid mass (**goiter**)
- Mediastinal mass (esophageal cancer, bronchogenic cyst)
- Central bronchogenic carcinoma (small cell, squamous cell)
- Adenopathy (sarcoidosis, lymphoma, granulomatous disease, *metastases*)
- Radiation fibrosis
- Fibrosing mediastinitis (calcified adenopathy from histoplasmosis or tuberculosis)
- Saber sheath trachea (advanced emphysema)
- *Vascular ring*

INTRINSIC
- **Trauma** (burn or chemical aspiration)
- Cartilage deficiency (**tracheomalacia**, trauma, radiation therapy, intubation injury)
- **Tracheal thickening** (amyloidosis, relapsing polychondritis, tracheopathia osteochondroplastica, sarcoidosis, Wegener granulomatosis, infection)
- Prior tracheostomy
- Infection (tuberculosis, fungus, croup)
- Inflammation (epidermolysis bullosa)
- Bronchitis
- Carcinoma (squamous cell)
- *Congenital*

31. Tracheoesophageal Fistula

- **Congenital**
- **Esophageal cancer**
- Central bronchogenic carcinoma
- Tracheal cancer (squamous cell, adenoid cystic)
- Penetrating trauma (gunshot, endoscopy)

- Radiation therapy
- Infection (actinomycosis, tuberculosis)

32. Tracheal Mass

- **Squamous cell cancer**
- **Adenoid cystic carcinoma**
- **Metastasis** (breast, renal cell, colon cancer; melanoma)
- **Direct invasion** (esophageal, lung, thyroid cancer)
- Bronchial adenoma (carcinoid, mucoepidermoid, cylindroma = pleomorphic adenoma)
- Pseudotumor (mucus)
- Papilloma (most common laryngeal tumor in a child)
- Foreign body
- Benign tumor (hemangioma, chondroma, fibroma)

33. Endobronchial Lesion

- **Bronchogenic carcinoma**
- **Mucus plug** (asthma, allergic bronchopulmonary aspergillosis, *congenital bronchial atresia*)
- Bronchial adenoma (carcinoid, mucoepidermoid, cylindroma)
- Foreign body (may be radiolucent, cause hyperinflation in child)
- *Broncholith*
- *Endobronchial metastasis (renal cell, breast, colon cancer, melanoma, lymphoma, thyroid)*

34. Atelectasis and Pulmonary Collapse

- Obstructive or resorptive (endobronchial lesion, **bronchogenic carcinoma, mucus plug,** bronchial adenoma, foreign body, broncholith, endobronchial metastasis, benign stricture)
- Passive (**pleural effusion**, mass, pneumothorax, scoliosis)
- Cicatrizing (fibrosis)
    Granulomatous disease (tuberculosis, histoplasmosis)
    Connective tissue disease (scleroderma, lupus, rheumatoid arthritis)
    Fibrosing alveolitis (idiopathic pulmonary fibrosis)
    Sarcoidosis
    Radiation therapy
- Compressive (tumor, bullous emphysema)
- Adhesive (respiratory distress syndrome, pulmonary embolism)

35. Bronchiectasis*

- **Recurrent pneumonia** (particularly childhood infections; aspiration, obstructing tumor)
- **Fibrosis**, traction bronchiectasis (radiation therapy, infection)
- Congenital
    Cystic fibrosis (predominantly upper lobe cystic and cylindrical, increased lung volumes, mucus plugs)
    Chronic granulomatous infection (MAI)
    Cartilage deficiency (Williams-Campbell syndrome)
    Immune deficiency (agammaglobulinemia, variable immune deficiency)
    Immotile cilia syndrome (Kartagener syndrome)
- Artifact (respiratory or cardiac motion on CT)
- *Allergic bronchopulmonary aspergillosis (central bronchiectasis in patients with asthma)*
- *Tracheobronchomegaly (Mounier-Kuhn syndrome)*
- *Poststenotic (focal due to endobronchial lesion or extrinsic compression)*
- *Toxic fume inhalation*

*Focal cylindrical bronchiectasis may be transient following pneumonia in children.

CONSOLIDATION AND AIRSPACE DISEASE

36. Acute Diffuse or Patchy Pulmonary Consolidation

- **Pulmonary edema** (congestive failure, valvular disease, fluid overload, renal failure, drug reaction, neurogenic, high altitude)
- **Bronchopneumonia** (*Pseudomonas*, *S. aureus*, anaerobes, streptococcus, *Klebsiella*, *Mycoplasma*, *Legionella*, *Nocardia*, actinomycosis, histoplasmosis, tuberculosis, *P. carinii*, varicella)
- **Pulmonary hemorrhage** (DIC, bleeding diathesis, lupus, Goodpasture syndrome)
- **ARDS** (trauma, sepsis, shock, near drowning, oxygen toxicity, DIC, pancreatitis, burns, smoke inhalation, viral pneumonia, pulmonary contusions, multiple transfusions, sickle cell crisis)
- Massive aspiration (Mendelson syndrome)
- Drug overdose (cocaine, heroin, aspirin)
- *Gas inhalation (nitrogen dioxide, chlorine, hydrocarbon, phosgene)*
- *Pulmonary embolism (fat, amniotic fluid, septic, bland thrombus)*

37. Chronic Diffuse Airspace Disease and Consolidation

- **Pneumonia** (tuberculosis, virus, mycoplasma, eosinophilic, chemical; fungal, histoplasmosis, aspergillus, lipoid—chronic oil aspiration, *P. carinii*)
- **Pulmonary edema** (recurrent or chronic)
- **ARDS** (trauma, sepsis, shock, aspiration, fat embolism, near drowning, oxygen toxicity, DIC, pancreatitis, burns or smoke inhalation, viral pneumonia, drug overdose, amniotic fluid embolization, pulmonary contusions, multiple transfusions, sickle cell crisis)
- **Bronchoalveolar cell carcinoma** (can present as mass, nodules or consolidation)
- Bronchiolitis obliterans with organizing pneumonia (BOOP—typically peripheral)
- Vasculitis or hemorrhage (Wegener granulomatosis, Goodpasture syndrome, *hemosiderosis*)
- Eosinophilic pneumonia
- Lymphoma (mycosis fungoides)
- Radiation pneumonitis
- Alveolar proteinosis
- Sarcoidosis
- *Hemorrhagic metastases (irregular margins, choriocarcinoma, melanoma)*
- *Hypersensitivity pneumonitis*

38. Unilateral Airspace Disease

- **Pneumonia** (bacterial, tuberculosis, fungal)
  Aspiration (debilitated patients, posterior segment RUL, superior and posterior segments lower lobes)
  Obstruction (bronchogenic carcinoma, mucus plug, carcinoid, foreign body, broncholith, endobronchial metastasis)
  Lipoid pneumonia (chronic oil aspiration, fat density on CT)
- **Unilateral pulmonary edema**
  Lateral decubitus positioning
  Reexpansion edema (after thoracentesis)
  Mitral regurgitation (can have focal RUL edema from regurgitant jet)
  Contralateral arterial obstruction (thromboembolism or tumor with congestive failure)
  Ipsilateral venous obstruction (left atrial myxoma, fibrosing mediastinitis)
  Surgical systemic to pulmonary artery shunt
- Bronchoalveolar cell carcinoma
- Pulmonary contusion (trauma)
- Hemorrhage (bronchitis, bronchiectasis, PE, bronchogenic carcinoma, Goodpasture syndrome, Wegener granulomatosis, aspergilloma, anticoagulation, AVM, lupus, DIC)

- Recent bronchoalveolar lavage
- Radiation pneumonitis

39. Pulmonary Hemorrhage

- **Bronchitis**
- **Bronchiectasis**
- **Pulmonary contusion** (trauma)
- Impaired coagulation (**anticoagulation**, thrombocytopenia, drugs, DIC, *hemophilia, leukemia*)
- Bronchogenic carcinoma
- Pulmonary thromboembolism
- Vasculitis (Wegener granulomatosis, Goodpasture syndrome, lupus)
- Aspergilloma (fungus ball in preexisting cavity)
- AVM (smooth, often multiple, feeding artery and draining vein)
- *Mitral stenosis (LA enlargement, usually valve calcification)*
- *Idiopathic pulmonary hemosiderosis*

40. Localized Consolidation

INFECTION
- **Lobar pneumonia**
    Aspiration (anaerobes; gram-negative organisms)
    Postobstructive (mucus plug, bronchogenic carcinoma, foreign body)
    Bacterial (*Pneumococcus, Klebsiella, H. influenzae, Legionella, S. aureus*)
    Mycobacterium (tuberculosis)
    Fungus (cryptococcosis, histoplasmosis)
- Lung abscess
- *Eosinophilic pneumonia (Löffler syndrome, chronic eosinophilic pneumonia)*

OTHER CAUSES
- Atelectasis or collapse (obstructive, endobronchial lesion; cicatrizing, compressive)
- Hemorrhage (contusion, Goodpasture syndrome, Wegener granulomatosis)
- Pulmonary infarct (peripheral wedge shaped)
- Bronchoalveolar cell carcinoma (can present as mass, nodules, or consolidation)
- Radiation pneumonitis (follows radiation port margins)
- *Lipoid pneumonia (chronic oil aspiration, areas of fat density on CT)*
- *Lymphoma*
- *Sarcoidosis*
- *Progressive massive fibrosis (silicosis)*

41. Consolidation with Lobar Enlargement

- **Bacterial pneumonia**
    Postobstructive pneumonia (bronchogenic carcinoma)
    Pneumococcus
    Klebsiella (may cavitate, effusion common)
    Staphylococcus aureus (more commonly bronchopneumonia)
    Haemophilus influenzae
    Pseudomonas
- Primary tuberculosis
- Bronchogenic carcinoma (particularly bronchoalveolar cell)
- Lung abscess (*S. aureus, Klebsiella*, gram-negative organisms)
- *Pulmonary sequestration*

42. Chronic Lobar Consolidation

- **Bronchoalveolar cell carcinoma** (can present as mass, nodules, or consolidation)
- **Postobstructive pneumonia**, drown lung (bronchogenic carcinoma, foreign body, endobronchial metastasis)
- Fungal infection (histoplasmosis, aspergillus)
- Eosinophilic pneumonia
- BOOP
- Tuberculosis
- *Lipoid pneumonia (chronic oil aspiration, areas of fat density on CT)*
- *Pulmonary sequestration*
- *Lymphoma*
- *Sarcoidosis*

43. Recurrent Pneumonia

- **Bronchial narrowing or obstruction** (bronchogenic carcinoma, mucus plug, carcinoid, foreign body, broncholith, endobronchial metastasis)
- **Bronchiectasis**
- **Repeated aspiration**
    Alcoholism
    Debilitation
    Neurologic disorder (stroke)
    Esophageal disease (achalasia, stricture, tumor)
    Neuromuscular disease
    Tracheoesophageal fistula
- Cystic fibrosis (upper lobe predominance)
- *Pulmonary sequestration*

44. Bronchopneumonia (Lobular Pneumonia)

- ***Pseudomonas***
- ***Staphylococcus aureus***
- **Anaerobes** (oral flora)
- *Haemophilus influenzae*
- *Mycoplasma*
- *Streptococcus* (more often lobar, pleural effusion common)
- *Klebsiella* (more often lobar)
- *Bronchoalveolor cell carcinoma (mimics pneumonia)*
- *Lymphoma*
- *Legionella*
- *Nocardia*
- *Actinomycosis*

INTERSTITIAL LUNG DISEASE

45. Acute Diffuse Interstitial Lung Disease

- **Pulmonary edema**
    Congestive heart failure
    Valvular heart disease
    Fluid overload
    Renal failure

Noncardiogenic (neurogenic, drug reaction or overdose, chemical inhalation)
ARDS
- **Pneumonia**
  Pneumocystis carinii
  Mycoplasma
  Viral (mononucleosis, cytomegalovirus)
  Haemophilus influenzae
  Granulomatous disease (mycobacterial, fungal)
  Rocky Mountain spotted fever
- Extrinsic allergic alveolitis (hypersensitivity pneumonitis)

46. Chronic Diffuse Interstitial Lung Disease (Not Nodular)

- **Chronic edema** (ischemic heart disease, mitral stenosis, left atrial tumor, mediastinitis, pulmonary veno-occlusive disease)
- **Infection** (granulomatous disease—viral, mononucleosis—*Mycoplasma, P. carinii*)
- **Fibrosis** (chronic interstitial pneumonia, asbestosis, fibrosing alveolitis, IPF, UIP, DIP, collagen vascular disease)
- **Lymphangitic carcinomatosis** (nodular septal thickening)
- Lymphocytic interstitial pneumonia
- Lymphangiectasia (child)
- Leukemia and lymphoma
- Extrinsic allergic alveolitis
- Sarcoidosis (peribronchovascular distribution of nodular infiltrates)
- Eosinophilic granuloma (upper lobe predominance)
- *Lymphangioleiomyomatosis and tuberous sclerosis (multiple superimposed cysts mimicking interstitial disease)*
- *Hemosiderosis*
- *Amyloidosis*

47. Chronic Nodular Interstitial Lung Disease

- **Pulmonary fibrosis** (nodular thickening with architectural distortion)
- **Infection** (*Mycobacterium*, fungal, viral—mononucleosis—*Mycoplasma, P. carinii*)
- **Lymphangitic carcinomatosis** (nodular septal thickening)
- Pulmonary metastases (thyroid, melanoma)
- Lymphangiectasia
- Leukemia and lymphoma
- Extrinsic allergic alveolitis (hypersensitivity pneumonitis)
- Silicosis (upper lobe, tiny nodules, some calcified; berylliosis, siderosis)
- Sarcoidosis (peribronchovascular distribution of nodular infiltrates)
- Eosinophilic granuloma (upper lobe predominance)
- *Hemosiderosis*
- *Alveolar microlithiasis*
- *Amyloidosis*

48. Diffuse Interstitial Lung Disease with Pleural Effusion

- **Pulmonary edema** (CHF, renal failure)
- Collagen vascular disease (lupus, rheumatoid)
- Pneumonia
- Lymphangitic carcinomatosis
- *Lymphoma or leukemia*
- *Lymphangioleiomyomatosis*

49. Diffuse Interstitial Lung Disease with Adenopathy

- **Stage II sarcoidosis**
- **Lymphoma or leukemia**
- Infection (fungal, tuberculosis)
- Lymphangitic carcinomatosis
- Silicosis

50. Diffuse Disease with Normal or Increased Lung Volumes

- **Interstitial lung disease with superimposed emphysema**
- **Cystic fibrosis** (upper lobe predominance, bronchiectasis)
- Eosinophilic granuloma (upper lobe nodules)
- *Lymphangioleiomyomatosis (diffuse cysts in a young woman)*

51. Peripheral Pulmonary Infiltrates

- **Pneumonia**
  Bacterial
  BOOP (bronchiolitis obliterans with organizing pneumonia, typically airspace)
  Eosinophilic
- Pulmonary fibrosis (reduced lung volumes, IPF, connective tissue disease, asbestosis)
- *Lymphoma*
- *Pulmonary edema*
- *Sarcoidosis*
- *Hypersensitivity pneumonitis*

52. Pulmonary Edema

- Venous hypertension
  Congestive heart failure
  Valvular heart disease (aortic or mitral stenosis)
  Obstruction to venous return (pulmonary vein thrombosis, veno-occlusive disease, fibrosing mediastinitis, left atrial thrombosis or myxoma)
- **Fluid overload**
- **Renal failure**
- Hypoproteinemia (cirrhosis)
- Lymphatic obstruction (mediastinal tumor)
- Noncardiogenic edema and ARDS
  Sepsis, pancreatitis, viral pneumonia
  Aspiration (Mendelson syndrome)
  Trauma, shock, pulmonary contusion
  Burns, toxic inhalation (gas, smoke, dust, nitrogen dioxide, sulfur dioxide, phosgene, hydrocarbons, carbon monoxide)
  DIC, multiple transfusions
  Drug reaction or overdose (morphine, heroin, cocaine, aspirin, tricyclic antidepressants)
  Sickle cell crisis, uremia
  Neurogenic (head trauma, tumor, stroke)
  Other less common causes: high altitude, eclampsia, radiation pneumonitis, anaphylaxis, contrast reaction, upper airway obstruction, near drowning, oxygen toxicity, amniotic fluid or fat embolization, reexpansion edema (following thoracentesis or evacuation of a pneumothorax)

53. Unilateral Interstitial Lung Disease

- **Unilateral pulmonary edema**
  - Lateral decubitus positioning
  - Reexpansion edema (after thoracentesis)
  - *Mitral regurgitation (can have focal RUL edema from regurgitant jet)*
  - *Asymmetric emphysema or lobectomy*
  - *Bronchial obstruction (ipsilateral)*
  - *Swyer-James syndrome (contralateral)*
  - *Ipsilateral venous obstruction (left atrial myxoma, fibrosing mediastinitis)*
  - *Contralateral arterial obstruction (thromboembolism)*
  - *Surgical systemic to pulmonary artery shunt (Waterston, Blalock-Taussig, Potts)*
  - *Lymphatic obstruction (mediastinal tumor)*
- **Aspiration**
- **Pneumonia**
- Local lymphangitic spread of bronchogenic carcinoma
- *Pulmonary contusion*

54. Migratory Pulmonary Infiltrates

- **Pulmonary edema**
- Eosinophilic pneumonia

55. Focal Reticulonodular Pattern

- **Fibrosis**
  - Prior pneumonia
  - Radiation therapy
  - Chronic aspiration (lower lobes and posterior segments of upper lobes)
- Lymphangitic carcinomatosis (breast, pancreas, bronchogenic carcinoma, lymphoma, leukemia)

56. Diffuse Reticulonodular Pattern

PULMONARY FIBROSIS (HONEYCOMBING)
- **Idiopathic** (fibrosing alveolitis, IPF, UIP, DIP)
- **Drug-related** (bleomycin, amiodarone, nitrofurantoin, methysurgide, procainamide, busulfane, cyclophosphamide, BNCU)
- **Connective tissue disease** (usually peripheral and basilar, scleroderma, lupus, rheumatoid lung, *dermatomyositis*)
- **Sarcoidosis** (stage 4, may spare apex and base)
- **Granulomatous disease** (usually focal, histoplasmosis—associated calcification and frequently calcified mediastinal lymph nodes, tuberculosis)
- **ARDS** (trauma, sepsis, shock, aspiration, fat embolism, near drowning, oxygen toxicity, DIC, pancreatitis, burns or smoke inhalation, Mendelson syndrome, viral pneumonia, drug overdose, amniotic fluid embolization, pulmonary contusions, multiple transfusions, sickle cell crisis, noxious gas inhalation)
- Pneumoconiosis
  - Complicated silicosis (small, calcified upper lobe nodules)
  - Asbestosis (associated pleural plaques)
- Chronic aspiration (lower lobes)
- *Neurofibromatosis*
- *Ankylosing spondylitis (upper lobe, symmetric syndesmophytes and spine fusion)*

OTHER CAUSES
- **Lymphangitic carcinomatosis**
- Chronic pulmonary venous hypertension

56. Diffuse Reticulonodular Pattern (*continued*)

- Lymphoma
- Sjögren syndrome
- *Extrinsic allergic alveolitis (hypersensitivity pneumonitis)*
- *Eosinophilic granuloma (upper lobe predominance)*
- *Amyloidosis*

57. Peripheral Reticulonodular Pattern (Fibrosis)

- **Idiopathic**
- **Drug-related** (bleomycin, amiodarone, nitrofurantoin, methysurgide, procainamide, busulfane, cyclophosphamide, BNCU)
- Connective tissue disease
    Scleroderma (thickened soft tissues, esophageal dysmotility, basilar fibrosis)
    Lupus (often small pleural and pericardial effusions)
    Rheumatoid lung
    Dermatomyositis
- Asbestosis (associated pleural plaques)
- *Extrinsic allergic alveolitis* (hypersensitivity pneumonitis)

58. Upper Lung Reticulonodular Pattern

- **Granulomatous disease** (histoplasmosis—calcification and frequently calcified mediastinal lymph nodes)
- Sarcoidosis (stage IV)
- Post–primary tuberculosis
- Complicated silicosis (small, calcified upper lobe nodules)
- Eosinophilic granuloma
- *Ankylosing spondylitis (symmetric syndesmophytes and spinal fusion)*
- *Chronic hypersensitivity pneumonitis*

59. Lower Lung Reticulonodular Pattern

- **Idiopathic pulmonary fibrosis**
- **Connective tissue disease** (lupus, scleroderma, rheumatoid lung, dermatomyositis)
- Asbestosis (associated pleural plaques)
- Chronic aspiration
- *Amyloidosis*
- *Neurofibromatosis*

HIGH-RESOLUTION CT PATTERNS

60. Ground-Glass Opacities*

- **Pulmonary edema** (septal thickening)
- **Fibrosing alveolitis** (UIP, DIP—inflammatory phase of IPF)
- Pulmonary hemorrhage
- Connective tissue disease (lupus)
- *Eosinophilic granuloma (upper lobe nodules)*
- *Sarcoidosis*
- *Alveolar proteinosis*

Infection
- **Bacterial (alveolitis)**
- ***Pneumocystis carinii* pneumonia**
- Viral (cytomegalovirus)

- **Hypersensitivity pneumonitis**
- BOOP (typically peripheral, consolidation)
- *Mycoplasma*
- Mycobacterial (tuberculosis, MAI, centrilobular, tree-in-bud nodules)
- Bronchiolitis (centilobular nodules)
- Eosinophilic pneumonia (usually associated consolidation)
- *Lymphocytic interstitial pneumonia (children with AIDS)*

*Partial airspace filling or alveolar septal inflammation that does not obscure vessels.

61. Interlobular Septal Thickening (Kerley Lines)*

- **Pulmonary edema** (smooth, often associated areas of ground-glass opacity)
- **Lymphangitic carcinomatosis** (typically nodular)
- Sarcoidosis (often nodular)
- Lymphoma
- Pneumonia (*Mycoplasma*, viral, *P. carinii*)
- Lymphangiectasia (congenital)
- Pulmonary fibrosis (irregular, architectural distortion, cystic airspaces, and traction bronchiectasis)
- *Alveolar proteinosis*
- *Silicosis or coal worker's pneumoconiosis*
- *Hypersensitivity pneumonitis*

*Fluid or cellular infiltrates in interlobular septa.

62. Intralobular Septal Thickening *

- **Pulmonary fibrosis** (idiopathic, asbestosis; irregular, architectural distortion, cystic airspaces, and traction bronchiectasis)
- Hypersensitivity pneumonitis
- Sarcoidosis (typically nodular)
- Alveolar proteinosis (associated ground glass opacities)
- *Lymphangitic carcinomatosis (typically nodular)*
- *Pulmonary edema (smooth)*

*Fluid or cellular infiltrates in intralobular septa.

63. Peribronchovascular Interstitial Thickening

- **Pulmonary edema** (smooth)
- Lymphangitic carcinomatosis (nodular)
- Lymphoma (smooth or nodular)
- Sarcoidosis (irregular)
- Fibrosing alveolitis (UIP, DIP-associated traction bronchiectasis)
- *Silicosis*
- *Chronic hypersensitivity pneumonitis*

64. Honeycombing*

- **Idiopathic pulmonary fibrosis** (UIP, DIP)
- **Connective tissue disease** (lupus, scleroderma, rheumatoid)
- End-stage lung disease (eosinophilic granuloma, sarcoidosis, silicosis)
- Asbestosis
- Chronic hypersensitivity pneumonitis
- ARDS
- Drug-related
- Chronic aspiration
- Pneumoconiosis

*Interstitial thickening with bronchiolectasis and architectural distortion.

65. Cystic Lesions

- **Bullae and blebs, emphysema** (blebs arise in visceral pleura)
- **Bronchiectasis**
- Pneumatoceles
    - Trauma (hematoma or laceration)
    - Infection (*S. aureus*, *H. influenzae* and gram-negative organisms, *P. carinii*, *M. tuberculosis*)
- Pulmonary fibrosis (honeycombing)
- Eosinophilic granuloma (upper lobe, often nodules)
- *Tuberous sclerosis*
- *Lymphangioleiomyomatosis (young women)*

66. Interstitial Nodules

INFECTION
- **Bronchopneumonia**
- **Granulomatous disease** (often calcified when healed)
- **Bronchiolitis** (obliterans, Asian panbronchiolitis; areas of ground-glass opacity, associated air trapping)
- **Mycobacterial infection** (hematogenous spread of tuberculosis)
- Hypersensitivity pneumonitis
- Lymphocytic interstitial pneumonia (ill-defined, children with AIDS)
- Fungal infection

TUMOR
- **Pulmonary metastases** (typically peripheral)
- **Lymphangitic carcinomatosis**
- Bronchoalveolar cell carcinoma
- Lymphoma

OTHER CAUSES
- **Silicosis** and coal worker's pneumoconiosis
- **Sarcoidosis** (upper lobe predominance)
- Eosinophilic granuloma
- Amyloidosis

67. Small Perilymphatic Nodules

- **Sarcoidosis**
- **Lymphangitic carcinomatosis**
- **Silicosis** and coal worker's pneumoconiosis (symmetric upper lobe, slight posterior predominance; some calcify)
- Lymphoma (peribronchovascular, septal, and subpleural)
- Amyloidosis (subpleural, septal, and centrilobular)
- Lymphocytic interstitial pneumonia in AIDS (ill-defined)

68. Small Randomly Distributed Nodules

- **Old granulomatous disease** (often calcified)
- **Pulmonary metastases** (typically peripheral)
- Miliary tuberculosis
- Fungal infection

69. Centrilobular Nodules*

- **Bronchiolitis** (obliterans, Asian panbronchiolitis; areas of ground-glass opacity, associated air trapping)
- **Mycobacterial infection** (endobronchial spread of tuberculosis, tree-in-bud pattern)
- **Bronchopneumonia**

- Bronchoalveolar cell carcinoma
- Hypersensitivity pneumonitis (typically areas of ground-glass opacity also present)
- Eosinophilic granuloma

*Peribronchiolar inflammation.

PLEURAL ABNORMALITIES

70. Pneumothorax

- **Mimics** (extrinsic artifact—sheet, tubing, skin fold, scapula edge, companion shadow of rib or clavicle)
- **Iatrogenic** (thoracentesis, thoracic or abdominal surgery, lung or pleural biopsy, central line or pacemaker placement)
- **Positive-pressure ventilation,** "volotrauma" (often preceded by pneumomediastinum)
- **Trauma** (rib fracture, penetrating injury, tracheobronchial injury; closed chest trauma)
- **Ruptured cystic airspace**
    Bullae or blebs (classically tall, thin men)
    Obstructive lung disease (emphysema, asthma, cystic fibrosis)
    Cystic lung disease (*P. carinii*, eosinophilic granuloma, lymphangioleiomyomatosis)
    Pneumatocele
- Asthmatic attack (pneumomediastinum is more common)
- Barotrauma (scuba diving)
- Necrotizing pneumonia or ruptured abscess (*Staphylococcus, M. tuberculosis*)
- Bronchopleural fistula
- Pulmonary fibrosis (idiopathic, sarcoidosis)
- Esophageal rupture (endoscopy, cancer, spontaneous)
- Dissection from pneumoperitoneum or pneumomediastinum
- *Pulmonary metastases (osteosarcoma)*
- *Bronchogenic carcinoma*
- *Catamenial (endometriosis)*

71. Spontaneous Pneumothorax with Diffuse Lung Disease

- **Cystic fibrosis**
- *Pneumocystis carinii* **pneumonia**
- Emphysema
- *Lymphangioleiomyomatosis*
- *Eosinophilic granuloma*
- *Pulmonary fibrosis*

72. Unilateral Pleural Effusion

CARDIOVASCULAR
- **Congestive heart failure** (right greater than left)
- **Pulmonary thromboembolic disease**
- Recent chest surgery
- Pericarditis
- Dressler syndrome (left greater than right, myocardial infarction, cardiac surgery)

INFLAMMATORY
- **Parapneumonic effusion** (associated lung disease)
    Bacteria (*Staphylococcus, Streptococcus, Klebsiella*)
    Mycobacterium (may lack associated lung disease with tuberculosis)
    Mycoplasma, fungus, viral, parasitic, protozoa

72. Unilateral Pleural Effusion (*continued*)

- Pericarditis
- Subphrenic abscess
- Pancreatitis (left greater than right)
- Pyelonephritis
- Radiation therapy (serous fluid)

MALIGNANCY
- **Pleural metastases** (lung, breast, lymphoma, stomach, pancreas)
- Bronchogenic carcinoma (direct extension to pleura)
- Mesothelioma (may see plaques from asbestos exposure)
- Lymphoma or leukemia

TRAUMATIC
- Vascular injury (catheter placement; hemothorax)
- Pulmonary contusion or laceration (blunt or penetrating; hemothorax)
- Esophageal rupture or fistula (cancer, dilatation, endoscopy)
- Thoracic duct rupture (low—right effusion; high—left effusion; chylothorax)

73. Bilateral Pleural Effusion

- **Congestive heart failure**
- **Pleural metastases** (breast, stomach, lymphoma, pancreas, lung)
- **Collagen vascular disease** (usually small, often associated lung disease; lupus, rheumatoid)
- Leukemia or lymphoma
- Recent chest surgery
- *Wegener granulomatosis*
- *Myxedema*
- *Drugs (nitrofurantoin, methysergide, methotrexate)*
- Asbestos exposure (usually small; often see pleural plaques)
- *Pericarditis*
- *Dressler syndrome (left greater than right)*

ABDOMINAL DISEASE
- **Renal failure** (uremia, often with edema)
- Pancreatitis (left greater than right)
- Nephrotic syndrome (diffuse body wall edema)
- Cirrhosis
- Ascites (peritoneal dialysis)
- *Meig syndrome (benign effusion with ovarian neoplasm)*

74. Pleural Effusion with Cardiomegaly

- **Congestive heart failure**
- Pericarditis
- Pulmonary embolism

ASSOCIATED PERICARDIAL EFFUSION
- Lupus
- Dressler syndrome
- Metastases
- Lymphoma and leukemia

75. Transudate*

- **Congestive heart failure**
- **Renal failure** (uremia, often with edema)
- Nephrotic syndrome (diffuse body wall edema)
- Cirrhosis
- Ascites (peritoneal dialysis)
- *SVC obstruction*
- *Myxedema*
- *Constrictive pericarditis*

  *Protein < 3 g/dl.

76. Exudate*

- **Parapneumonic effusion** (bacteria, tuberculosis)
- **Malignant effusion** (pleural metastases, bronchogenic carcinoma, lymphoma, leukemia, mesothelioma)
- Collagen vascular disease
- Pulmonary thromboembolic disease
- Subphrenic abscess
- Dressler syndrome
- *Drug-induced*
- *Pericardial disease*
- *Postpartum*
- *Meig syndrome*

  *Protein > 3 g/dl.

77. Hemothorax

- **Open or closed chest trauma** (torn intercostal vessel; may see rib fracture or contusion)
- **Malignancy** (bronchogenic carcinoma, pleural metastases, mesothelioma)
- Torn pleural adhesion (most common spontaneous cause)
- Coagulopathy (anticoagulation, hemophilia)
- *Dissecting aortic aneurysm*
- *Catamenial (endometriosis)*
- *Extramedullary hematopoiesis*

78. Chylothorax*

- **Traumatic injury to thoracic duct** (cardiothoracic surgery, penetrating and closed injuries; may take months to develop, low injury—right effusion; high injury—left effusion)
- Lymphangioleiomyomatosis (diffuse pulmonary cysts in young women)
- Lymphoma
- Metastatic disease
- *Lymphangioma and lymphangectasia*
- *Mediastinal fibrosis*
- *Central venous obstruction*
- *Tumor invasion*
- *Filariasis*

  *High lipid content.

79. Pleural Thickening

- **Extrapleural fat deposition** (symmetric)
- **Asbestos exposure** (often calcified)
- Artifact (skin fold, arm; can typically trace beyond the pleural edge)
- Prior empyema (particularly tuberculosis)
- Pulmonary fibrosis (when advanced)
- Organized pleural effusion (prior surgery, hemorrhage)
- Metastatic disease (nodular; adenocarcinoma—lung, breast, stomach, pancreas, ovary)
- Mesothelioma (may be focal or diffuse; typically lobulated)

80. Pleural Calcifications

- **Asbestos exposure** (bilateral, symmetric; parietal pleura)
- **Prior empyema** (unilateral, thick calcifications from tuberculosis; visceral pleura)
- Prior hemothorax (unilateral; visceral pleura)
- Pleurodesis
- *Chronic pancreatitis*
- *Chronic hemodialysis*
- *Talcosis (also mica, zeolites, minerals)*

81. Pleural Mass

- **Pleural plaques** (particularly from asbestos exposure)
- **Loculated effusion**
- **Rounded atelectasis** (adjacent pleural thickening)
- Pleural thickening (prior infection, hemorrhage, or surgery)
- Pulmonary infarct
- Empyema (split pleura sign, follows pleural contour, displaces lung; *S. aureus, Pneumococcus, E. coli, Klebsiella, Pseudomonas,* anaerobic)
- *Actinomycosis*
- *Thoracic splenosis (prior splenic and diaphragmatic trauma)*

NEOPLASM
- **Extraosseous extension of a rib tumor** (metastasis, multiple myeloma, chondrosarcoma, Ewing)
- **Peripheral lung cancer** (superior sulcus tumor)
- Pleural metastases (enhancing nodules, often associated effusion, breast, lung, adenocarcinoma)
- Invasive thymoma
- Lymphoma
- Extrapleural tumor (lipoma, neural—schwannoma, neurofibroma)
- Mesothelioma
- Fibrous tumor

82. Multiple Pleural Masses

- **Loculated effusions**
- **Pleural plaques** (asbestos—usually bilateral, often calcified)
- **Pleural metastases**
- Invasive thymoma
- Fibrous tumor of the pleura
- Mesothelioma
- *Endometriosis*
- *Thoracic splenosis*

DIAPHRAGM AND CHEST WALL ABNORMALITIES

83. Flattened Hemidiaphragm

BILATERAL
- **Emphysema**
- **Deep inspiration** (young, thin)
- Asthmatic attack (particularly children)
- Cystic fibrosis (upper lobe bronchiectasis)
- *Eosinophilic granuloma*
- *Lymphangioleiomyomatosis*

UNILATERAL (OFTEN CONTRATERAL MEDIASTINAL SHIFT)
- Pneumothorax
- Airway obstruction (foreign body, atelectasis in an adult, hyperinflation in a child)
- *Unilateral lung transplant (emphysema in native lung)*

84. Elevated Hemidiaphragm

- **Paralysis of the phrenic nerve** (surgical, tumor, idiopathic)
- **Distended stomach or colon**
- **Enlarged liver or spleen**
- **Volume loss** (atelectasis, collapse, hypoplastic lung, partial pulmonary resection)
- Pulmonary hypoplasia
- Splinting (rib fracture, pleurisy, pneumonia, pulmonary embolism)
- Subphrenic mass or fluid collection
- Eventration (broad based, most common right anterior portion)
- Mimics (subpulmonic effusion or large pleural tumor, diaphragm rupture—left more frequent than right, Morgagni or Bochdalek hernia—left more frequent than right)
- *Unilateral lung transplant for pulmonary fibrosis (fibrotic native ipsilateral lung)*

85. Bilateral Hemidiaphragm Elevation

- **Poor inspiratory effort**
- **Obesity**
- **Ascites**
- Hepatosplenomegaly
- Pregnancy
- Fibrosis (reticular interstitial pattern)
- Neuromuscular disease (multiple sclerosis)
- Subpulmonic effusions (simulates elevation of diaphragm)
- *Bilateral phrenic nerve paralysis (surgical, traumatic, thermal, idiopathic, tumor)*

86. Extrapleural Lesion

- **Lipoma** (characteristic fat density on CT)
- Hematoma (rib fracture, surgery, catheter placement)
- Rib metastasis or multiple myeloma (bone destruction with extraoseous soft tissue extension)
- Chest wall infection
- *Primary bone tumor*

87. Soft Tissue Calcifications

- **Injection granulomas**
- **Hemangioma** (small, round calcifications—phleboliths)

87. Soft Tissue Calcifications (*continued*)

- Scleroderma
- CREST syndrome
- Dermatomyositis
- Myositis ossificans
- Calcified lymph nodes
- Parasites (cysticerci, guinea worm, armillifer)
- Vascular (diabetes, hyperparathyroidism)
- Degenerating fibroadenoma (breast)
- Old hematoma (rim calcification)

88. Peripheral Pulmonary Disease and Chest Wall Mass

TUMOR
- **Bronchogenic carcinoma**
- Invasive breast cancer
- Lymphoma

INFECTION
- **Actinomycosis**
- Mucormycosis
- *Nocardia*

89. Chest Wall Mass

- **Sebaceous cyst**
- **Hematoma**
- Malignant tumor
    Bronchogenic carcinoma with chest wall invasion
    Bone (multiple myeloma, metastases, chondrosarcoma, Ewing sarcoma)
    Soft tissue (lymphoma, melanoma, *sarcoma—MFH, fibrosarcoma, rhabdosarcoma or liposarcoma*)
- Benign tumor (lipoma, fibroma, hemangioma—phleboliths and tortuous vessels, desmoid, neurofibroma,
    schwannoma, dermoid, exostosis)
- Infection
    Bacteria (actinomycosis, *Nocardia*, *Staphylococcus*)
    Fungus (blastomycosis, aspergillosis)
    Tuberculosis

90. Vertebral Compression Fracture

- **Osteopenia** (osteoporosis)
- Metastasis
- Multiple myeloma or plasmacytoma
- Trauma
- *Primary bone tumor*

91. Sclerotic Bone Lesion

- **Bone island** (focal, smooth, round)
- **Metastasis** (breast or prostate cancer, lymphoma)
- Osteochondroma (exostosis—most commonly primary benign bone tumor)
- Osteonecrosis (humoral heads)
- Paget disease (bone expansion)

92. Lytic Bone Lesions

MALIGNANCY
- **Metastasis** (renal cell, thyroid, lung cancer)
- **Multiple myeloma** or plasmacytoma
- Direct extension of primary tumor (lung)
- Primary bone tumor (Ewing sarcoma, chondrosarcoma, fibrosarcoma)

OTHER
- Benign cortical defect
- Osteomyelitis (*S. aureus*, *M. tuberculosis*, *Actinomyces*, *Nocardia*)
- Benign tumor
    Fibrous dysplasia (bone expansion without cortical disruption)
    Aneurysmal bone cyst
    Enchondroma
    Eosinophilic granuloma
- Fracture

93. Diffuse Bone Sclerosis

- **Widespread metastases** (breast and prostate cancer most commonly)
- **Sickle cell disease**
- **Renal osteodystrophy**
- Mastocytosis
- Osteopetrosis
- Lymphoma

94. Inferior Rib Notching

- **Arterial collaterals (aortic coarctation** or obstruction, pulmonary atresia, Blalock-Taussig shunt—unilateral notching)
- **Neurofibromatosis**
- Nerve sheath tumor (neuroma)
- Venous collaterals (SVC obstruction)
- Unilateral pulmonary obstruction
- Idiopathic
- *Arteriovenous malformation (involving an intercostal artery)*
- *Hyperparathyroidism*
- *Takayasu arteritis*

95. Superior Rib Notching

- **Neurofibromatosis**
- **Connective tissue disease** (rheumatoid arthritis, lupus)
- Paralysis
- Hyperparathyroidism
- Idiopathic

96. Distal Clavicular Resorption

UNILATERAL
- Posttraumatic osteolysis
- Infection

96. Distal Clavicular Resorption (*continued*)

BILATERAL
- Rheumatoid arthritis
- Hyperparathyroidism

MEDIASTINUM AND HILAR ABNORMALITIES

97. Unilateral Hilar Enlargement

- **Central bronchogenic carcinoma** (squamous cell, small cell)
- Primary mediastinal tumor
- Pneumonia in superior segment of lower lobe (hilar overlay sign)
- Bronchogenic cyst

ADENOPATHY
- **Metastases** (bronchogenic, head and neck, renal cell, testicular cancer)
- **Granulomatous infection** (tuberculosis, histoplasmosis, coccidiomycosis)
- Bacterial pneumonia or lung abscess
- AIDS
- *Mycoplasma*
- *Viral (mononucleosis)*
- *Sarcoidosis (usually bilateral)*
- *Castleman disease*
- *Lymphoma (usually bilateral)*

PULMONARY ARTERY ENLARGEMENT
- Pulmonary stenosis (left pulmonary artery enlargement)
- Massive pulmonary embolism
- Prior surgical systemic to pulmonary shunt (*Blalock-Taussig, Waterson-Cooley, Potts-Smith*)
- *Pulmonary artery aneurysm*

98. Bilateral Hilar Enlargement

VASCULAR
- **Pulmonary artery hypertension** (fibrosis, interstitial disease, emphysema, pulmonary emboli, idiopathic, left-to-right shunt)
- Normal variant (idiopathic dilatation in a young adult)
- Venous enlargement (mitral stenosis, mitral insufficiency, congestive heart failure)
- *Left-to-right shunt (patent ductus arteriosus, ASD, VSD)*
- *High-output heart disease (anemia, thyrotoxicosis)*

ADENOPATHY
- **Sarcoidosis**
- **Granulomatous infection** (tuberculosis, histoplasmosis, coccidiomycosis)
- **Metastases** (bronchogenic, head and neck, renal cell, testicular cancer)
- Lymphoma or leukemia (often asymmetric)
- Bacterial pneumonia or lung abscess
- *Viral (mononucleosis)*
- AIDS
- *Cystic fibrosis*
- *Silicosis (lung disease invariably present)*
- *Castleman disease*

99. Calcified Lymph Nodes

- **Old, healed granulomatous disease** (histoplasmosis, tuberculosis)
- Disseminated *P. carinii* (AIDS patient)
- Amyloidosis (may be very dense)
- Metastatic cancer (mucinous adenocarcinoma, osteosarcoma, *thyroid, bronchogenic*)

EGGSHELL CALCIFICATION
- Silicosis (associated small, calcified upper lobe nodules)
- Sarcoidosis
- Treated lymphoma

100. Low-Attenuation Lymph Nodes

- **Tuberculosis**
- **Metastases** (bronchogenic carcinoma, testicular, ovarian cancer)
- Pyogenic infection
- Fungal infections
- *Radiated lymphoma*
- *Lymphangioleiomyomatosis*

101. Enhancing Lymph Nodes

- Castleman disease
- Vascular metastases (renal cell, melanoma, thyroid, small cell, Kaposi sarcoma)
- HIV-related adenopathy
- Paraganglioma

102. Pneumomediastinum

- **Recent surgery** (tracheostomy, sternotomy)
- **Extension from neck or abdomen** (pneumoperitoneum or subcutaneous emphysema)
- **Volotrauma, barotrauma** (ventilated patient, stiff lungs—fibrosis)
- **Tracheobronchial injury** (intubation, bronchoscopy, chest trauma)
- **Esophageal tear** (endoscopy, dilatation, cancer, Boerhaave syndrome)
- Penetrating injury (neck or face)
- Asthmatic attack
- Pneumothorax
- Spontaneous (cough, vomiting)
- *Tracheal or esophageal fistula (tumor, infection)*

103. Ipsilateral Mediastinal Shift

- **Atelectasis or collapse**
- **Prior lobectomy** or partial pulmonary resection
- Unilateral fibrosis
- *Scimitar syndrome*

104. Contralateral Mediastinal Shift

- **Large effusion**
- Tension pneumothorax
- Asymmetric emphysema
- Scoliosis

105. Enlarged or Widened Mediastinum

- **Projectional** (anteroposterior or lordotic projection, scoliosis)
- **Lipomatosis** (fat deposition seen with obesity and steroid use)
- **Reduced lung volumes** (obesity, poor inspiratory effort)
- **Vascular** (tortuous or aneurysmal aorta or brachiocephalic vessels, enlarged azygos vein or SVC, left superior vena cava)
- **Adenopathy** (granulomatous, sarcoidosis, silicosis, lymphoma, Castleman disease, metastases, amyloidosis, bronchogenic carcinoma, reactive)
- **Tumor** (small cell, lymphoma, thymic, germ cell, lipoma, neurogenic, cystic hygroma, dermoid, hemangioma, central bronchogenic, bone tumor involving spine, posterior ribs, or sternum)
- Gastrointestinal (acholasia, esophageal tumor or diverticulum, hiatal or Bochdalek hernia)
- Hemorrhage (ruptured aneurysm, traumatic venous bleeding)
- Fluid collection (postoperative or perforated central venous catheter)
- Inflammation (median sternotomy, mediastinitis, fibrosing granulomatous mediastinitis)
- Duplication cysts (bronchogenic and esophageal)
- Pericardial cyst
- Loculated effusion
- Pleural thickening
- *Paraspinal abscess (discitis)*
- *Extramedullary hematopoiesis (anemia, often bilateral)*

106. Thoracic Inlet or Superior Mediastinal Mass

- **Thyroid mass** (**goiter**, adenoma, carcinoma, may compress trachea or esophagus)
- **Lymphoma** or leukemia (particularly CLL)
- Adenopathy (reactive, head and neck or bronchogenic cancer)
- Tortuous brachiocephalic vessels
- Thymic mass (thymoma, thymolipoma, thymic carcinoma, rebound hyperplasia, thymic cyst)
- *Cervical aorta (very high aortic arch)*
- *Parathyroid mass*
- *Cystic hygroma (cystic mass in children)*

107. Anterior Mediastinal Mass*

- **Thyroid mass** (goiter, adenoma, carcinoma, may compress trachea or esophagus)
- **Lymphoma** (particularly Hodgkin)
- Thymic mass
    - **Thymoma** (30% have myasthenia gravis; invasive and encapsulated forms)
    - Thymolipoma (contains fat)
    - Rebound hyperplasia
    - Thymic cyst (fluid density)
    - *Thymic carcinoma*
- **Fat deposition** (obesity, steroids)
- Vascular
    - **Ascending aortic aneurysm**
    - Enlarged superior vena cava (elevated central venous pressure or obstruction)
    - Tortuous brachiocephalic vessels
- **Germ cell neoplasm**
    - Mature teratoma (often contain fat or bone; cystic usually benign; solid usually malignant)
    - Seminoma
    - Embryonal cell carcinoma
    - Choriocarcinoma
- Morgagni hernia
- Fluid collection (postoperative or perforated central venous catheter)

- Hemangioma
- Lipoma
- Inflammation (median sternotomy, acute mediastinitis, fibrosing mediastinitis)
- Sarcoma (angiosarcoma, liposarcoma)
- Sternal mass (metastasis, multiple myeloma, Ewing sarcoma)
- Hematoma (posttraumatic)
- Pericardial cyst (most common in right cardiophrenic angle)
- *Parathyroid mass (adenoma, carcinoma, usually small)*
- *Cystic hygroma (children)*

*Bounded anteriorly by the sternum and posteriorly by the brachiocephalic vessels, aorta, and anterior pericardium.

108. Middle Mediastinal Mass*

VASCULAR
- **Ascending aortic aneurysm** (poststenotic dilatation in aortic stenosis, Marfan syndrome)
- Tortuous brachiocephalic vessels
- Pulmonary artery enlargement
- Right-sided or double aortic arch
- Left superior vena cava
- Enlarged azygos vein (CHF, vena cava obstruction, azygos continuation of IVC)
- Aberrant subclavian artery

LYMPHADENOPATHY
- **Lymphoma** or leukemia (CLL)
- **Bronchogenic carcinoma**
- Extrathoracic malignancy (renal cell, testicular, ovarian, head and neck, thyroid, breast, melanoma)
- Sarcoidosis
- Reactive (lung abscess, tuberculosis, histoplasmosis, coccidioidomycosis, cystic fibrosis, mononucleosis)
- Silicosis (invariable presence of small pulmonary nodules)
- *Castleman disease (hyperdense on contrast CT)*

PRIMARY TUMOR
- Central bronchogenic cancer (small cell or squamous)
- Tracheal tumors (squamous cell, adenoid cystic, metastases)
- Esophageal tumor (leiomyoma, squamous cell, adenocarcinoma)
- Parathyroid tumor
- *Cardiac tumors*

OTHER CAUSES
- **Duplication cyst** (bronchogenic or esophageal)
- Lipomatosis
- Morgagni hernia
- Pancreatic pseudocyst
- Pericardial cyst
- Thyroid mass (large goiter, often with calcification)
- Hematoma (trauma, surgery)
- Fluid collection (postoperative or perforated central venous catheter)
- Inflammation (median sternotomy, mediastinitis, fibrosing mediastinitis)

*Contains heart, ascending and transverse aorta, superior and inferior vena cava, brachiocephalic vessels, trachea and main bronchi, and central pulmonary arteries and veins.

109. Posterior Mediastinal Mass*

SPINAL MASS
- **Neurogenic tumors**
  Autonomic (schwannoma—neurilemoma, neurofibroma, neurofibrosarcoma, malignant schwannoma)
  Sympathetic (ganglioneuroma, neuroblastoma, ganglioneuroblastoma)
  Paragangliomas (chemodectoma, pheochromocytoma)

109. Posterior Mediastinal Mass* (continued)

- Paraspinal abscess (discitis, tuberculosis, Staphylococcus)
- Degenerative disease (exuberant osteophytes)
- *Compression fracture with hematoma*
- *Extramedullary hematopoiesis (anemia, often bilateral paraspinal mass)*
- *Bone tumor involving spine or posterior ribs (primary or metastases—renal cell, breast cancer)*
- *Neurenteric cyst*
- *Meningocele (often see spine or rib anomaly)*

GASTROINTESTINAL
- **Hiatal hernia**
- **Enlarged esophagus** (achalasia, scleroderma, obstructing stricture or tumor)
- Esophogeal duplication cyst or diverticulum
- Esophageal tumor (leiomyoma, squamous cell, adenocarcinoma)
- Bochdalek hernia (usually posterolateral left-sided)
- Pancreatic pseudocyst

VASCULAR
- **Descending thoracic aortic aneurysm**
- Enlarged azygos vein (right-sided, azygos continuation)
- Paraesophagel varices
- Hemangioma

PULMONARY OR PLEURAL (MIMICS POSTERIOR MEDIASTINAL MASS)
- Pleural thickening or loculated effusion
- Lipoma
- Lymphoma
- Rounded atelectasis (associated pleural thickening)
- *Extralobar sequestration*

*Bounded by the posterior pericardium anteriorly, the paravertebral gutters posteriorly, and the mediastinal pleura laterally. Contains esophagus.

110. Cardiophrenic Angle Mass

MEDIASTINAL
- **Enlarged cardiophrenic angle fat pad**
- **Pericardial cyst** (right more common than left)
- **Enlarged right atrium** (ASD, VSD, PDA, right ventricular failure, tricuspid stenosis or insufficiency, endocardial cushion defect, anomalous pulmonary venous return, Ebstein anomaly)
- Mediastinal tumor (thymoma)
- Pericardial effusion
- Left ventricular aneurysm
- Lymphadenopathy (pericardial, anterior diaphragmatic)
- *Large IVC*
- *Paraspinal abscess*

PULMONARY
- Peripheral lung mass (bronchogenic carcinoma, sequestration)
- Pneumonia
- *Scimitar syndrome*

PLEURAL
- **Pleural mass** (fibrous tumor, mesothelioma)
- Loculated effusion

ABDOMINAL
- **Morgagni hernia**
- Large hiatal hernia
- *Ruptured hemidiaphragm*

111. Low Attenuation Mediastinal Mass

FAT DENSITY
- **Fat deposition** (obesity, steroids)
- Lipoma
- Liposarcoma
- Thymolipoma
- Mature teratoma (often contain fat or bone; cystic usually benign, solid usually malignant)

FLUID DENSITY
- **Duplication cyst** (bronchogenic or esophageal)
- **Fluid collection** (seroma from trauma or surgery, perforated central venous catheter)
- **Pericardial cyst** (most common in right cardiophrenic angle)
- Germ cell tumors
- Loculated pleural effusion
- Pancreatic pseudocyst
- Paraspinal abscess (discitis, tuberculosis, *Staphylococcus*)
- Thymic cyst (fluid density)
- Cystic thymoma
- *Meningocele (often see spine or rib anomaly)*
- *Neuroenteric cyst*
- *Cystic hygroma (children)*

GASTROINTESTINAL
- **Hiatal hernia**
- Enlarged esophagus (achalasia, scleroderma, obstruction from stricture or tumor, diverticulum)
- Morgagni hernia
- Bochdalek hernia (usually posterolateral)

CARDIAC ABNORMALITIES

112. Dextrocardia

- **Kartagener syndrome** (a form of immotile cilia syndrome)
- Situs inversus totalis
- Dextroversion of heart in situs solitus (usually cyanotic patients)

113. Small Heart

- **Emphysema** (heart small relative to large lungs, vertical due to flattened diaphragm)
- Addison disease
- Dehydration
- Shock
- Malnutrition (anorexia)
- Constrictive pericarditis
- Normal variant

114. Enlarged Cardiac Silhouette

- **Congestive heart failure** (edema and effusion common)
- **Pericardial effusion** (idiopathic, infectious pericarditis, collagen vascular disease, cardiac surgery, Dressler syndrome, uremia, CHF, metastases, RT, trauma, coagulopathy, tumor)
- **Cardiomyopathy** (viral, ischemic, amyloidosis, hypothyroidism, drugs—Adriamycin, glycogen storage disease, Cushing disease, postpartum, idiopathic)
- Valvular heart disease (usually regurgitant lesions)
- Congenital heart disease (ASD, Ebstein anomaly)

115. Cardiac Mass

- **Bland thrombus**
- **Primary benign tumor**
  Myxoma (often pedunculated, attached to atrial septum, LA>>RA>RV location)
  Atrial septal lipoma
  Rhabdomyoma (patient with tuberous sclerosis)
  Fibroma
  Fibromyxoma
  Hamartoma
- **Tumor emboli** (renal cell, hepatoma)
- Direct invasion (lymphoma, lung, esophagus, thymoma
- Metastases (carcinoid, breast, melanoma, lymphoma, lung, osteosarcoma, chondrosarcoma)
- Primary malignant tumor
  Sarcoma (angiosarcoma, RA most common cardiac site)
- *Valve vegetation (endocarditis)*

116. Pericardial Effusion

- **Idiopathic** (one-third of all cases)
- **Infectious pericarditis** (tuberculosis, viral—coxsackie)
- Collagen vascular disease (particularly lupus—often chronic, small, pleural effusions)
- Recent cardiac surgery
- Dressler syndrome (effusion in 70 percent, fever, chest pain, pleural effusion or infiltrate)
- Uremia (renal failure)
- Congestive heart failure (often associated with pleural effusions)
- Tumor
  Metastases (lymphoma, breast cancer, melanoma)
  Direct invasion (lung, lymphoma)
  Primary tumor (angiosarcoma)
- *Radiation therapy*
- *Hemopericardium*
  Aortic dissection
  Trauma
  Coagulopathy

117. High-Output Heart Disease

- **Anemia** (sickle cell disease)
- **Fluid overload**
- Arterial venous malformations (extrapulmonary, vein of Galen aneurysm)
- Polycythemia vera (elevated hematocrit, splenomegaly)
- Pregnancy
- *Thyrotoxicosis*
- *Vitamin B_1 deficiency (beriberi)*

118. Congestive Heart Failure in Neonates

- **Coarctation**
- **Hypoplastic left heart syndrome**
- Overhydration
- Interruption of the aortic arch
- Cardiomyopathy
- Asphyxia
- Anomalous venous return

- Endocardial fibroelastosis
- Arterial venous malformations (extrapulmonary, vein of Galen aneurysm)
- Critical aortic stenosis
- Anomalous coronary artery origin (usually left coronary off pulmonary artery)

119. Left Atrial Enlargement

- **Mitral stenosis** (valve calcification, right ventricular enlargement, pulmonary vascular engorgement)
- Mitral insufficiency (left ventricular enlargement, usually due to myocardial ischemia or rheumatic heart disease)
- Left to right shunts (VSD, patent ductus arteriosus)
- *Left atrial myxoma (occasionally calcify)*

120. Left Ventricular Enlargement

- **Congestive heart failure** (effusions and edema common)
- **Ischemic heart disease** (may see coronary artery calcifications)
- **High-output heart disease** (anemia, sickle cell disease, fluid overload, arteriovenous fistulas, polycythemia vera, pregnancy, hyperthyroidism-thyrotoxicosis)
- Valvular heart disease
    Aortic insufficiency
    Aortic stenosis (poststenotic dilatation of the aorta in late stage of LV failure)
    Mitral insufficiency
- Acute myocardial infarction (variable degree of pulmonary edema)
- Coarctation of the aorta
- Hypertension (may have only left ventricular hypertrophy, not enlargement)
- Congenital heart disease (truncus arteriosus)
- Cardiomyopathy

121. Right Atrial Enlargement

- **Atrial septal defect**
- **Right ventricular failure**
- Endocardial cushion defect
- Anomalous pulmonary venous return
- Tricuspid stenosis or insufficiency (carcinoid syndrome, lupus, endomyocardial fibrosis, rheumatic heart disease)
- *Ebstein anomaly (box-shaped heart)*
- *Tumor (RA myxoma, angiosarcoma)*

122. Right Ventricular Enlargement

- **Cor pulmonale** (pulmonary artery hypertension and enlarged pulmonary artery; severe lung disease, pulmonary emboli, idiopathic)
- **Atrial septal defect**
- Valvular heart disease (pulmonary or tricuspid insufficiency)
- Partial anomalous pulmonary venous return

123. Cardiac Calcifications

- **Aortic valve** (bicuspid, rheumatoid, endocarditis, atherosclerosis)
- **Coronary arteries**
- **Pericardium** (prior viral or tuberculosis pericarditis—often spares apex; pyogenic, uremia, rheumatoid, syphilis, asbestos plaques)
- **Mitral annulus** (clinically insignificant)
- Mitral valve (rheumatic heart disease)

123. Cardiac Calcifications (*continued*)

- Left atrium (severe mitral stenosis)
- Myocardial (commonly involves cardiac apex; aneurysm, old MI)
- Ductus arteriosus
- Left atrial myxoma
- Left ventricular thrombus
- Ascending aorta
  - Atherosclerosis
  - Hyperlipoproteinemia (homozygous type II)
  - Diabetes
  - Syphilis (dense calcification, dilated)

124. Aortic Insufficiency

- **Bicuspid aortic valve**
- **Rheumatic heart disease**
- **Bacterial endocarditis** (acute AI)
- Cystic medial necrosis (Marfan syndrome)
- Dissecting aneurysm (acute AI)
- *Trauma*
- *Reiter syndrome*
- *Syphilitic aortitis*

125. Mitral Insufficiency

- **Rheumatic heart disease**
- **Mitral annulus dilatation** (left ventricular dilatation; cardiomyopathy)
- **Papillary muscle dysfunction**
- Bacterial endocarditis
- Rupture of chorda tendinea
- Mitral valve prolapse
- *Marfan syndrome*
- *Endocardial cushion defect*
- *Left atrial myxoma*

126. Tricuspid Insufficiency

- **Endocarditis** (IV drug abuse)
- Rheumatic heart disease
- Right ventricular dilatation
- Pulmonary hypertension
- *Endomyocardial fibrosis*
- *Endocardial cushion defect*
- *Ebstein anomaly*
- *Carcinoid heart disease—endocardial fibroelastosis*

127. Left-to-Right Shunt

- **Atrial septal defect** (enlarged PA, RA, RV, normal LA)
- **Ventricular septal defect** (increased pulmonary vascularity, enlarged LA, PA)
- **Patent ductus arteriosus** (enlarged LA, LV, PA)
- Endocardial cushion defect (frequently associated with Down syndrome)
- Anomalous pulmonary venous return (partial is often asymptomatic)

128. Right-to-Left Shunt

- **Tetralogy of Fallot**
- Pulmonary atresia with intact ventricular septum (right-to-left shunt usually through ASD)
- Tricuspid atresia
- Total anomalous pulmonary venous return

129. Normal or Decreased Pulmonary Vascularity with Cyanosis

- Tetralogy of Fallot
- Tricuspid atresia (unless large VSD)
- Pulmonary atresia with intact ventricular septum
- Ebstein anomaly (usually big heart)

130. Congenital Heart Disease with Increased Pulmonary Vascularity

WITH CYANOSIS
- **Total anomalous pulmonary venous return**
- Truncus arteriosus
- Transposition of the great vessels
- Tricuspid atresia (with large VSD)
- Single ventricle

WITHOUT CYANOSIS
- **Atrial septal defect** (normal sized LA)
- **Ventricular septal defect** (enlarged LA)
- **Patent ductus arteriosus** (enlarged LA)
- Other left to right shunts (endocardial cushion defect, PAPVR, aortopulmonary window)

VASCULAR ABNORMALITIES

131. Perfusion Defect on Lung Scan

- **Pulmonary thromboembolism**
- **Emphysema or cystic airspace** (bulla, bleb, pneumatocele)
- **Pleural effusion**
- Pneumonia
- Atelectasis
- Pulmonary mass
- Vasculitis
- *Lymphangitic carcinomatosis*
- *Radiation therapy*
- *Pulmonary fibrosis*

132. Reversed Ventilation-Perfusion Mismatch on Lung Scan

- **Pneumonia**
- **Pulmonary collapse**
- **COPD and asthma**
- Pleural effusion
- Partial bronchial obstruction
- *Cardiomegaly*
- *Bronchiectasis*

133. Unilateral Decreased Perfusion on Lung Scan

- Unilateral obstruction to arterial blood flow
  Pulmonary artery stenosis
  Pulmonary artery invasion by tumor (bronchogenic carcinoma)
  Swyer-James-Macleod's
  Compressed right pulmonary artery (mediastinal mass, aortic aneurysm)
  Massive pulmonary embolism
- Injection through pulmonary artery catheter
- Large pleural effusion or pneumothorax
- Pneumonectomy
- *Venous to pulmonary artery shunt (Glenn, Blalock-Taussig, Waterston)*
- *Unilateral obstructed venous return (fibrosing medistinitis, left atrial myxoma)*

134. Enlarged Ascending Aorta

- **Hypertension**
- **Aortic aneurysm** (atherosclerotic, mycotic, Marfan syndrome)
- **Aortic stenosis**
- Aortic insufficiency
- Syphilitic aortitis
- Coarctation
- Patent ductus arteriosus

135. Mirror-Image Right-Sided Aortic Arch*

- **Tetralogy of Fallot** (present in 25 percent)
- Persistent truncus arteriosus (present in 30 percent)
- Transposition of the great vessels (present in 10 percent)
- *Tricuspid atresia (present in 5 percent)*
- *Double outlet right ventricle (present in 15 percent)*

  *>95 percent have congenital heart disease

136. Coronary Artery Aneurysms

- **Atherosclerosis**
- Congenital
- Kawasaki disease (mucocutaneous lymph node syndrome)
- Postsurgical

137. Pulmonary Venous Hypertension (Edema)

- **Congestive heart failure** (LV failure, ischemic heart disease, cardiomyopathy)
- **Fluid overload**
- **Renal failure**
- Left atrial obstruction
  Atrial myxoma
  Mediastinal fibrosis
  Pulmonary veno-occlusive disease
  Mitral stenosis (LA and RV enlargement)
- *Constrictive pericarditis*
- *Mitral insufficiency (LA and LV enlargement)*
- *Anomalous pulmonary venous return*
- *Cortriatrium (pulmonary vein stenosis at LA)*

138. Enlarged Pulmonary Arteries

- **Pulmonary artery hypertension** (may have decreased peripheral vessel caliber)
  Severe lung disease (interstitial disease, fibrosis, emphysema, pneumoconiosis, sarcoidosis)
  Pulmonary vasculitis (polyarteritis nodosa)
  Pulmonary emboli (blood, tumor, fat)
  Primary (idiopathic in a young woman)
  Eisenmenger syndrome
- **Left-to-right shunt** (ASD, VSD, patent ductus arteriosus, endocardial cushion defect, anomalous pulmonary venous return)
- **Pulmonary venous hypertension** (mild PA enlargement; CHF, fluid overload, renal failure, LA obstruction, *constrictive pericarditis, mitral insufficiency or stenosis,* venoocclusive disease)
- High-output heart disease (anemia, sickle cell disease, arteriovenous fistulas, polycythemia vera, pregnancy, thyrotoxicosis)
- *Pulmonary valve stenosis (enlarged left PA, poststenotic dilitation)*
- *Behçet disease*
- *Idiopathic dilatation (may be normal in young adult)*
- *Hypoventilation (venoconstictive hypertension; high altitude, neuromuscular disorder, obesity, tracheal obstruction, sleep apnea)*

139. Enlarged Superior Vena Cava

- **Congestive heart failure**
- Anomalous pulmonary venous return
- Idiopathic
- Azygos continuation of inferior vena cava
- *Cardiac tamponade*
- Obstruction
  Central bronchogenic carcinoma (small cell, squamous cell)
  Fibrosing mediastinitis
  Radiation therapy-induced fibrosis

140. Enlarged Azygos Vein

- **Elevated central venous pressures** (congestive heart failure, fluid overload, renal failure, pregnancy)
- **Superior vena cava obstruction** (tumor, fibrosis)
- Portal hypertension
- Azygos continuation of inferior vena cava
- Pregnancy
- *Pulmonary sequestration*
- *Pulmonary vein obstruction*
- *IVC obstruction (Budd-Chiari syndrome)*

CLINICAL DIFFERENTIAL DIAGNOSIS

141. Chest Pain (with Radiographic Abnormalities)

- **Ischemic heart disease** (myocardial infarction can present with cardiogenic edema)
- **Pneumothorax**
- **Gastroesophageal reflux** (may see hiatal hernia)
- **Pneumonia**
- **Rib fracture**
- Aortic dissection (often with associated aneurysm)
- Pulmonary embolism (atelectasis, pleural effusion, focal oligemia—Westermark sign)

141. Chest Pain (with Radiographic Abnormalities) (continued)

- Costochondritis (Tietze syndrome)
- Esophageal tear (pneumomediastinum, pleural effusion)
- Thoracic compression fracture
- Pneumomediastinum
- Bronchitis (often radiographically occult)
- *Pleural tumor*
- *Pericardial disease*

142. Shortness of Breath (with Radiographic Abnormalities)

- **Pulmonary edema**
- **Pneumonia**
- Pneumothorax
- Pulmonary embolism (atelectasis, pleural effusion, focal oligemia—Westermark sign)

143. Complications following Cardiac Resuscitation (with Radiographic Abnormalities)

- **Rib fractures** (typically anterior)
- **Aspiration pneumonia**
- **Pulmonary edema** (fluid overload)
- Pulmonary contusion
- Pneumothorax
- *Pneumomediastinum*
- *Hemothorax*
- *Hemopericardium*

144. Hemoptysis

- **Bronchitis or bronchiectasis**
- **Pulmonary thromboembolism**
- **Bronchogenic carcinoma**
- **Vasculitis** (Wegener granulomatosis, Goodpasture syndrome, lupus)
- Aspergilloma (fungus ball in preexisting cavity)
- Pulmonary contusion (trauma)
- Impaired coagulation (anticoagulation, thrombocytopenia, DIC, drugs, hemophilia, *leukemia*)
- AVM (smooth, often multiple, may see feeding artery and draining vein)
- *Mitral stenosis (LA enlargement, may see valve calcification)*
- *Idiopathic pulmonary hemosiderosis*

145. Pulmonary Infections

- Gram-positive bacteria (*Pneumococcus*, *S. aureus*, *Actinomyces* and *Nocardia*—both previously classified as *fungi*)
- Gram-negative bacteria (*Klebsiella*, *Pseudomonas*, *Legionella*, *H. influenza*, *E. coli*)
- Anaerobic bacteria (oral flora—*Bacteroides*, *Fusobacterium*, *Peptococcus*)
- Fungus (histoplasmosis, blastomycosis, aspergillosis, coccidioidomycosis, *cryptococcus, candidiasis, mucormycosis*
- Parasites (*P. carinii, amebiasis, toxoplasmosis, ascariasis, strongyloidiasis, paragonimiasis*)
- Mycoplasma
- Viral (mononucleosis, varicella—skin rash invariably present, cytomegalovirus, *Rickettsia*, coxsackie, rubeola, RSV, adenovirus, influenza, parainfluenza)
- *Mycobacterium* (tuberculosis, avium intracellular complex—MAI, MAC)
- *Chlamydia*

146. Opportunistic Pulmonary Infections

- *Pneumocystis carinii*
- Virus (cytomegalovirus, varicella-zoster, herpes simplex)
- Tuberculosis
- Toxoplasmosis
- Bacteria (*S. aureus, Pseudomonas, Legionella, Nocardia*)
- Fungus (*Aspergillus, Candida, Cryptococcus,* mucormycosis)

Bibliography

Brant WE, Helms CA. *Fundamentals of Diagnostic Radiology.* Baltimore: Williams & Wilkins, 1994.

Burgener FA, Kormano M. *Differential Diagnosis in Conventional Radiology.* New York: Thieme Medical Publishers; 1991.

Chapman S, Nakielny R. *Aids to Radiological Differential Diagnosis.* 3rd ed. Philadelphia: WB Saunders; 1995.

Eisenberg RL. *Clinical Imaging: An Atlas of Differential Diagnosis.* 3rd ed. Philadelphia: Lippincott; 1997.

Fraser RG, Paré JAP, Paré PD, Fraser RS, Genereux GP. *Diagnosis of Diseases of the Chest.* 3rd ed. Philadelphia: WB Saunders; 1991, vol. 4.

Fraser RS, Paré JAP, Fraser RG, Paré PD. *Synopsis of Diseases of the Chest.* 2nd ed. Philadelphia: WB Saunders; 1994.

Freundlich IM, Bragg DG. *A Radiologic Approach to Diseases of the Chest.* 2nd ed. Baltimore: Williams & Wilkins, 1997.

Kreel L, Thornton A. *Outline of Medical Imaging.* Jordan Hill, Oxford: Butterworth-Heinemann, 1992.

Lange S, Walsh G. *Radiology of Chest Diseases.* 2nd ed. New York: Thieme Medical Publishers; 1998.

Lange S, Stark P. *Teaching Atlas of Thoracic Radiology.* New York: Georg Thieme Verlag, 1993.

Mettler FA, Guiberteau MJ. *Essentials of Nuclear Medicine Imaging.* 3rd ed. Philadelphia: WB Saunders; 1991.

Reed JC. *Chest Radiology.* 4th ed. St Louis; Mosby–Year Book; 1997.

Reeder MM, Bradley WM. *Reeder and Felson's Gamuts in Radiology.* 3rd ed. New York: Springer-Verlag; 1993.

Reeders JWAJ, Mathieson JR. *AIDS Imaging—A Practical Clinical Approach.* Philadelphia: WB Saunders; 1998.

Resnick D. *Bone and Joint Imaging.* Philadelphia: WB Saunders; 1989.

Scott J, William W, Scott PP, Trerotola SO. *Radiology of the Thoracic Skeleton.* Philadelphia: BC Decker; 1991.

Silverman FN, Kuhn JP. *Essentials of Caffey's Pediatric X-ray Diagnosis.* Chicago: Year Book Medical Publishers; 1990.

Sperber M. *Radiologic Diagnosis of Chest Disease.* New York: Springer-Verlag; 1990.

Stern EJ, Swensen SJ. *High-Resolution CT of the Chest: Comprehensive Atlas.* Philadelphia: Lippincott-Raven; 1996.

Sutton D, Young JWR. *A Short Textbook of Clinical Imaging.* New York: Springer-Verlag; 1990.

Webb WR, Müller NL, Naidich DP. *High-Resolution CT of the Lung.* 2nd ed. Philadelphia: Lippincott-Raven; 1996.

Weissleder R, Rieumont MJ, Wittenberg J. *Primer of Diagnostic Imaging.* 2nd ed. St Louis: Mosby; 1997.

Chapter 3

FOCAL LUNG DISEASE

Fernando R. Gutierrez

3.1 EVALUATING FOCAL LUNG DISEASE

- There are many causes of focal, discrete abnormalities affecting the lung parenchyma, including bronchogenic carcinoma, infection, vascular abnormalities, and atelectasis. Often the primary question is whether an abnormality represents a benign or a malignant condition.

- **Chest radiography** remains the primary imaging technique for evaluating focal lung disease because it is widely available, simple to obtain, and relatively inexpensive. Nonspecific or equivocal findings may require further diagnostic investigation. It cannot be overemphasized, however, that comparison with prior radiographs (perhaps located at another hospital) is extremely important in order to determine the chronicity of the abnormality in question. Occasionally, a patient undergoes an extensive diagnostic evaluation for a pulmonary nodule only to learn later that the same finding was present on a radiograph taken several years prior.

- **Computed tomography (CT)**, with its cross-sectional imaging format, allows better characterization and localization of lesions identified on chest radiographs. For example, a single pulmonary nodule not definitely calcified on a chest radiograph may be effectively evaluated for the presence of calcium. Ideally, spiral or thin-section (2 to 3 mm thick) CT should be obtained over the area of lung being interrogated. In addition, CT can detect smaller lesions not seen on plain films. In selected cases, intravenous (IV) contrast material may help determine the vascular nature of the lesion or its relationship to adjacent vascular structures.

- **Magnetic resonance imaging (MR)** plays a very limited role in the evaluation of focal lung disease. Only in selected patients with a suspected vascular lesion, for those who have had a previous adverse reaction to contrast material, or for those in whom chest wall or brachial plexus invasion by tumor is a consideration, is MR a practical diagnostic option. In most cases, MR is not more specific than CT in distinguishing between benign and malignant processes. One major limitation of MR is its inability to identify calcification, information often crucial for a definitive diagnosis.

- More recently, **positron emission tomography (PET)**, based on increased uptake of ^{18}F-fluorodeoxyglucose (FDG) in metabolically active tissues, has proven of value in determining the malignant potential of pulmonary nodules otherwise deemed indeterminate by other imaging modalities as well as for detecting distant metastasis, such as from esophageal cancer, not seen on conventional imaging. Further investigation is needed to determine the usefulness of PET in other disease states.

3.2 SOLITARY PULMONARY NODULE

- It has traditionally been established that a **pulmonary nodule** is a well-circumscribed opacity <3 cm in diameter. Anything larger is considered a mass, although the terms are sometimes used interchangeably (**Differential 15***).

  The first determination to be made is whether the opacity seen on a plain radiograph is in fact a true intrapulmonary nodule. Superimposition of bone islands, nipple shadows, and other nodular densities outside the lung may mimic an intrapulmonary location. CT can readily discern the exact location of the "nodule" in question. In addition, as previously stated, comparison with prior chest radiographs must be made before the diagnostic search is started so that interval change can be properly assessed.

- The **detection** of single pulmonary nodules (SPNs) is a challenging problem for radiologists. It has been estimated that

---

*Please refer to Chapter 2, in which the differential diagnoses are discussed in numerical order.

up to one-third of SPNs are not detected on the initial chest radiograph. Nodules less than 8 to 10 mm are usually not seen on radiographs. Sharply marginated pulmonary nodules are detected more readily than nodules with irregular borders, a fact that tends to reduce the early detectability of primary bronchogenic carcinoma. About 80 percent of SPNs are either granuloma or bronchogenic carcinoma.

- The **margins** of a SPN can be an important feature during radiographic surveillance. Rounded, spiculated, lobulated, or other morphologic characteristics may be identified in the nodule being investigated (Fig. 3-1). In general, spiculated or ill-defined nodules have a higher incidence of malignancy than well-defined rounded nodules. Lobulation of the nodule usually implies different rates of growth in different areas of the nodule. This pattern is frequently seen in malignant lesions.

- Hematogenous **pulmonary metastases** tend to be round and well defined since they are usually not locally invasive. Because of more abundant blood flow in the lower lobes, hematogenous metastases tend to be more numerous in these portions of the lung. Steps must be taken to exclude opportunistic infection in immunocompromised patients receiving

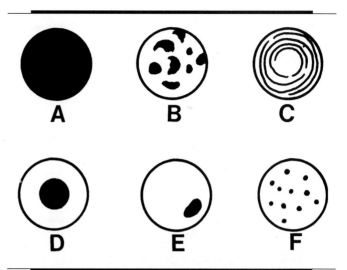

FIGURE 3-2   Patterns of calcifications in pulmonary nodules. (A) Diffuse, (B) popcorn, (C) laminar, and (D) central patterns all characteristic of benign lesions. (E) Eccentric and (F) stippled patterns can be seen with either benign or malignant lesions.

chemotherapy in which radiographic findings may be very similar (**Differentials 19, 20, 21, and 22**).

- **Calcification** of a single pulmonary nodule can be a very helpful diagnostic feature in differentiating between malignant and benign nodules. CT may be necessary to determine the presence and pattern of calcification. There are several patterns of calcification (Fig. 3-2).

  A pattern of **central** or **complete calcification** virtually excludes malignancy. The calcification pattern must be symmetric (diffuse, laminated, or central). When investigating multiple pulmonary nodules, the presence of calcium in one is meaningless with regard to the others. The most common cause of calcified pulmonary nodules is old, healed granulomatous disease, particularly histoplasmosis, coccidiomycosis, or tuberculosis, although granulomas often are not calcified (**Differentials 15 and 22**).

  Eccentric calcifications should be further investigated since a tumor may arise near a calcified granuloma and engulf it. Moreover, calcific metastatic nodules may be seen in tumors such as osteosarcoma, chondrosarcoma, and mucinous adenocarcinoma (Fig. 3-3) (**Differential 22**). The calcification in malignant tumors may be intrinsic or dystrophic from tumor necrosis.

  Other benign patterns of calcification include **ring patterns** seen in granulomas and **popcorn** calcifications seen in hamartomas. **Diffuse, stippled calcifications** can be seen in hamartomatous tumors, and are rarely seen in malignancy.

- The **rate of growth** of a pulmonary nodule is a helpful way to characterize it in a conservative fashion. Nodules that enlarge slowly are more likely to be benign, although low-grade adenocarcinomas and even metastases such as those from renal cell carcinoma may exhibit slow growth. Any nodule with documented size stability over a 2-year

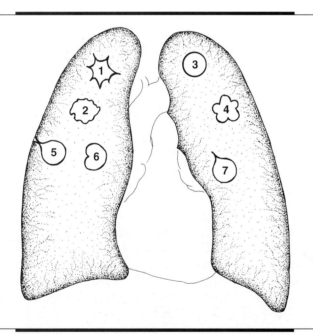

FIGURE 3-1   Variation in the contours of pulmonary nodules. (1) Spiculated nodule, worrisome for primary bronchogenic carcinoma. (2) Irregular, poorly defined margins suggestive of malignancy. (3) Rounded, well-defined nodule that can be seen in benign conditions as well as in metastatic disease. (4) Multilobulated lesion implying areas with different growth rates; also associated with malignancy. (5) "Pleural tail" is a strand of tissue extending to the adjacent pleura and can be seen in inflammatory and in neoplastic conditions. (6) Rigler's notch describes an indentation as a vessel enters a nodule; suggestive but not diagnostic of malignancy. (7) Rounded nodular density associated with parenchymal stranding or "tail sign" that can be seen both in neoplastic and in inflammatory conditions.

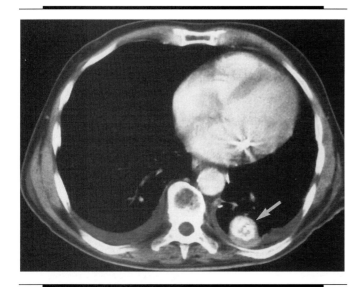

FIGURE 3-3 **Metastatic osteosarcoma.** CT of a single calcified pulmonary nodule (arrow) representing a metastatic focus.

period can be considered benign, and no further follow-up is usually needed.

Solitary pulmonary nodules should be followed with serial chest radiographs. A 25 percent increase in diameter is equivalent to a doubling of volume. Most bronchial carcinomas double their volume in 1 to 18 months with adenocarcinomas growing at the slower rates. Any SPN larger than 3 cm in diameter, unless it clearly shows a benign calcification pattern, is related to rounded atelectasis, or is a congenital malformation, should be aggressively investigated for its malignant potential.

- Besides the appearance, the **patient's age** can be very helpful in predicting the nature of the nodule. In a patient less than 30 years of age with no history of prior smoking, a rounded calcified nodule is almost certainly a benign lesion (granuloma). Any patient older than 30 years with a prior history of smoking, with an extrathoracic malignancy, or with an irregular, spiculated nodule requires a further diagnostic workup to exclude malignancy.

- The presence of **air bronchograms** within an SPN makes the diagnosis of malignancy unlikely with the exception of bronchioloalveolar cell carcinoma and lymphoma. With high-resolution CT (HRCT), air bronchograms are seen more frequently in primary bronchogenic carcinoma.

- **Cavitation** can be seen both in benign and in malignant nodules (Fig. 3-4) and is therefore not a very helpful diagnostic feature (**Differential 26**). The only information derived from a cavitated nodule is that it indicates an active disease process. The morphologic appearance of the cavities can also vary significantly. They may be uniloculated or multiloculated, have thin or thick outer walls, or contain air-fluid levels (Fig. 3-5).

- A **hamartoma** is a benign pulmonary tumor, with clefts lined by bronchial epithelium, which can contain cartilage and may also contain fat. They tend to be solitary and have slow growth, usually appearing in middle age. They are rare in children. Pathologically, they arise within the bronchial lumen, in a peripheral location of the lung, although more central tumors can occur. Symptoms are usually related to bronchial obstruction with atelectasis or hemoptysis.

Plain radiographs usually demonstrate a well-circumscribed peripheral tumor that may be rounded or lobulated. Calcification, particularly in larger tumors, is seen in about

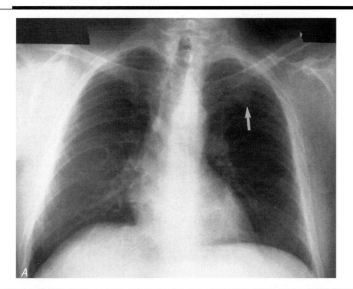
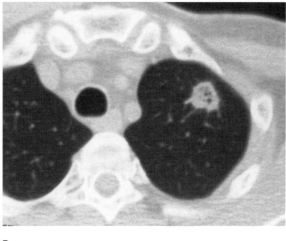

FIGURE 3-4 **Adenocarcinoma.** (*A*) PA chest radiograph showing a left upper lobe pulmonary nodule (arrow) in a 54-year-old smoker. (*B*) CT at the same level demonstrating multiple small areas of cavitation. Fine-needle aspiration demonstrated adenocarcinoma.

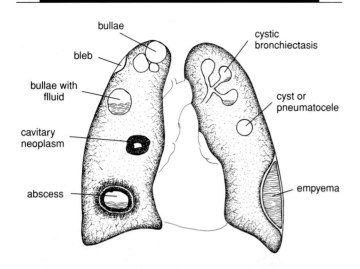

FIGURE 3-5   Cystic and cavitary lung lesions. Bullae are areas of lung destruction with displacement of pulmonary parenchyma. Blebs occur within the pleural surface. Pneumatoceles develop following infection, likely representing postobstructive dilatation of acini. Bulla and pneumatoceles can become fluid-filled, and the fluid may be sterile or infected. Squamous cell bronchogenic carcinoma and other lung masses can cavitate. Lung abscesses typically have poorly defined margins and surrounding pulmonary consolidation. Cystic bronchiectasis can appear as a collection of multiple pulmonary cysts, often with air-fluid levels. An empyema, in contrast to a lung abscess, is usually oblong, adjacent to the pleural surface, and displaces rather than destroys adjacent lung.

20 percent of cases. The pattern of calcification is usually of the "popcorn" variety (Fig. 3-6). The presence of fat within the tumor is a specific finding in about 50 percent seen better on thin-section CT. Absence of fat or even calcium by no means excludes the diagnosis.

3.3   PULMONARY MALIGNANCY

- Like tumors in other organs, pulmonary neoplasms can be divided into benign and malignant, the latter group being primary or metastatic.

- **Bronchial carcinoid** tumors arise from neuroendocrine cells (Kulchitsky cells) of the bronchial or gastrointestinal mucosa. 5 percent occur in the lung, where they arise in the bronchi near the hilum. They are very slow growing tumors that invade locally and have a low incidence of metastases. They can be seen at different ages.

    Typical carcinoid refers to a form of tumor that rarely metastasizes and is usually located centrally in the lung. **Atypical carcinoid**, on the other hand, has cytologic features resembling those of small-cell carcinoma, behaves in a more aggressive fashion, more frequently metastasizes, and tends to arise more peripherally in the lung.

    Because of their vascular nature, hemoptysis is frequent, and their central location within the bronchial tree makes

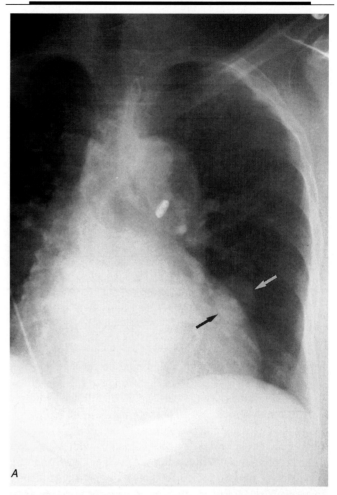

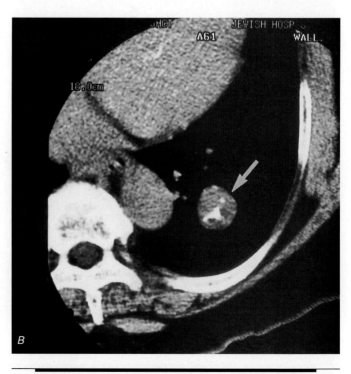

FIGURE 3-6   Hamartoma. (*A*) Chest radiographs showing a left lower lobe nodule partially projecting behind the heart (arrows). (*B*) Thin section CT windowed for soft tissue detail demonstrating calcium and fat (arrow).

wheezing, cough, and obstructive pneumonias frequent clinical manifestations. In addition, these tumors, even when of very small size, may secrete adrenocorticotrophic hormone (ACTH), causing Cushing syndrome. **Carcinoid syndrome** can sometimes be seen in patients with liver metastases.

Plain chest radiographs may show the tumor or evidence of obstructive changes from bronchial occlusion, usually atelectasis. Additionally, a slow growing tumor within a central bronchus may cause obstruction and mucus retention in the distal bronchus.

CT is the imaging modality of choice, particularly for smaller tumors that may not be readily apparent on a chest radiograph. Frequently, carcinoid tumors demonstrate different patterns of tumoral calcification which may involve a significant portion of the mass.

Octreotide radionucleide scanning has been used with some success in diagnosing carcinoid tumors because of their somatostatin receptors, however, the specificity of the test is rather low. Although percutaneous biopsy can provide the diagnosis, particularly for larger tumors, bronchoscopy is usually preferred.

- **Bronchogenic carcinoma** is the leading cause of cancer death in the United States, accounting for approximately 140,000 deaths annually. The incidence of lung cancer has increased significantly since 1950, and rates are usually related to smoking habits in different countries. The male:female ratio has dropped from 7:1 in 1960 to 2:1 at present, and lung cancer has overtaken breast cancer as the leading cause of cancer death in women. Twenty-five percent of patients have no symptoms at the time of diagnosis. Cough, hemoptysis, wheezing, and paraneoplastic syndromes are usual forms of clinical presentation.

  Etiology. Heavy cigarette smoking (over 40 cigarettes a day) produces a 20-fold increase in bronchogenic carcinoma compared to nonsmoking. Approximately 10 percent of heavy smokers will develop lung cancer. The risk falls to that of a nonsmoker after 10 years of not smoking. Cigarette smoking is most commonly associated with squamous cancer, small cell cancer and, to a lesser degree, adenocarcinoma. Other carcinogens include radon gas, asbestos, heavy metals, radiation, and urban pollutants. Sputum cytology and chest radiography are presently considered the preferred screening methods.

  Radiographically, a peripheral nodule is the most common manifestation (Fig. 3-7), particularly for adenocarcinoma and large-cell tumors. Squamous cell carcinomas can attain a large size and frequently cavitate, although a common manifestation is lung collapse and consolidation distal to the central bronchial obstruction (Fig. 3-8). Small cell carcinoma typically presents with mediastinal adenopathy.

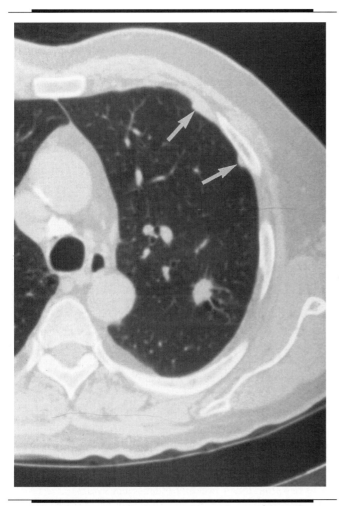

FIGURE 3-7 Bronchogenic cancer. CT showing a spiculated left upper lobe nodule in a 64-year-old man with asbestos-related pleural disease (arrows).

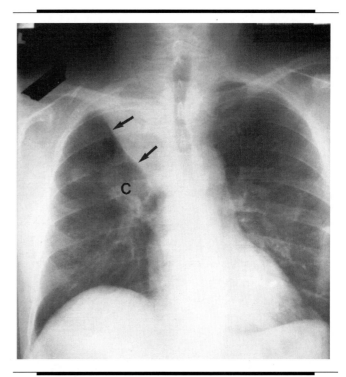

FIGURE 3-8 "S sign of Golden." PA chest radiograph in a 48-year-old man with hemoptysis, showing a hilar mass (C) and a collapsed right upper lobe marginated by displaced minor fissure (arrows) as a result of bronchogenic carcinoma.

- The **classification** of lung cancer consists of four major histologic types:

  Squamous (epidermoid) carcinoma arises in metaplastic squamous epithelium of the central bronchi and tends to remain localized more frequently than other histologic types. Rapid growth and cavitation are common. There is a strong predominance among males, usually those who are heavy smokers. Its incidence is decreasing (presently about 35 percent).

  Adenocarcinoma represents about 35 percent of the total number of lung cancer cases, and the incidence is rising, particularly in females. It is subdivided into well, moderately, and poorly differentiated forms, as is the case with other types. This tumor is characterized by the formation of glands or secretion of mucus by the tumor cells. It is commonly peripheral and is the most common cell type in nonsmokers.

  Bronchioloalveolar carcinoma is a variant of adenocarcinoma that arises from type II pneumocytes in alveoli. It can be localized and appear as a mass or focal consolidation simulating pneumonia. It can also be multifocal, having a poor prognosis (Fig. 3-9). Adenopathy, effusion, and cavitation are uncommon.

  Small cell (oat cell) carcinoma is believed to arise from neuroendocrine cells of the bronchial mucosa. It is highly malignant, and blood-borne metastases are common. It is more common in males. It usually occurs in central bronchi, with associated mediastinal and hilar adenopathy being a common presentation at the time of diagnosis (Fig. 3-10). Frequently, the primary tumor may be small and difficult to identify even with CT. Small cell carcinomas do not cavitate.

  Large cell undifferentiated carcinoma comprises about 10 to 15 percent of lung cancer cases. It is composed of large cells that show no squamous or glandular differentiation, although by electron microscopy many do show adenocarcinoma or squamous features.

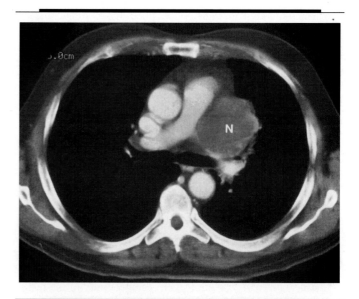

FIGURE 3-10　Small cell carcinoma. Chest CT demonstrating bulky mediastinal adenopathy (N).

- **Other primary lung neoplasms** are rare. **Mucoepidermoid carcinoma** and **adenoid cystic carcinoma** usually arise in the trachea or central bronchi, infiltrate locally, grow slowly, and have a very low incidence of metastasis. They seem to arise from the bronchial mucous glands and resemble the corresponding tumors in the salivary glands.

  Mixed types of tumors have also been described (e.g., adenosquamous carcinoma), probably arising from primitive cells that have the ability to differentiate in several directions.

- Lung carcinoma can **spread** in several ways. **Lymphatic metastases** can occur in all types of this disease, but particularly early in small cell types and less frequently in well-differentiated squamous types. Hilar and mediastinal node involvement is found in 50 percent of patients at the time of diagnosis (Fig. 3-11). Late in the disease, interstitial and retrograde lymphatic involvement referred to as "lymphangitic spread" can be seen with a typical reticular interstitial pattern on chest radiography and often pleural carcinomatosis.

  Local invasion by endobronchial or transbronchial growth is frequent. It can spread into mediastinal structures or the chest wall, a phenomenon that can be readily demonstrated with cross-sectional imaging (Fig. 3-12). Local spread and organ invasion are related to the proximity of the primary tumor to adjacent structures.

  Hematogenous spread is common in small cell carcinoma and less frequent in the other types. Common sites are adrenal gland, brain, bone, and liver.

  Pancoast tumor was originally described as a bronchogenic carcinoma of the superior sulcus invading the upper ribs or spine, lower brachial plexus, and sympathetic chain, causing Horner syndrome and arm pain. These lung tumors may be of any cell type, but squamous cell is most common. Asymmetric apical pleural thickening is an early radio-

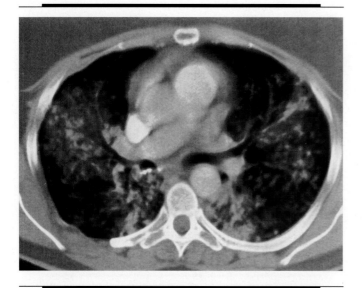

FIGURE 3-9　Multifocal bronchoalveolar cell carcinoma (BAC). CT showing multiple patchy areas of consolidation present throughout both lungs.

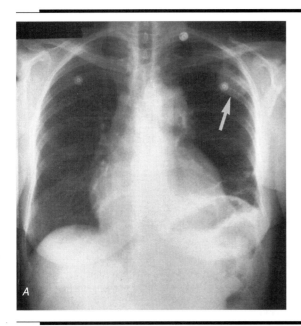
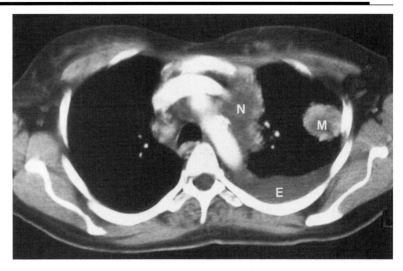

FIGURE 3-11 Metastatic adenocarcinoma. (A) Chest radiograph showing a left upper lobe mass (arrow), mediastinal fullness, and elevation of the left hemidiaphragm. (B) CT demonstrating the mass (M), mediastinal adenopathy (N) involving the left phrenic nerve and causing paralysis, and a pleural effusion (E) shown to be malignant.

graphic sign and should be monitored closely. MR is helpful in determining the extent of brachial plexus and spinal involvement.

- **Hypertrophic osteoarthropathy** refers to a syndrome consisting of arthralgias as well as swelling and stiffness of the joints (particularly the ankles, knees, fingers, and wrists) that is associated with periosteal thickening of the bones adjacent to the involved joints. This condition is most commonly found in patients with an intrathoracic malignancy, although benign tumors, particularly fibrous tumors of the pleura, infections, and other thoracic conditions can also be the cause.

- **Staging of lung cancer** (see Section 15.6) follows the tumor-node-metastases (TNM) system, dividing tumors into one of four stages. Staging is performed with CT, bronchoscopy, and mediastinoscopy to sample mediastinal nodes because of the lack of specificity of CT in determining nodal involvement. MR has not demonstrated an advantage over CT in staging lung cancer, with the exception of chest wall and brachial plexus involvement. Determination of mediastinal lymph node involvement should be based on the American Thoracic Society classification (Fig. 5-4).

Stage I includes T1 and T2 lesions without positive lymph nodes (N0) or metastasis (M0). They are usually resectable and have the best prognosis (65 percent 5-year survival following resection).

Stage II tumors represent T1 or T2 lesions with ipsilateral hilar or peribronchial lymph node involvement (N1) but no distant metastases (M0). Although these tumors are resectable, the prognosis is worse than for stage I (40 percent 5-year survival following resection).

Stage III tumors are subdivided into IIIA, which have limited and potentially resectable invasion of the chest wall or adjacent organs (T3) or subcarinal or ipsilateral mediastinal lymph node involvement (N2), and IIIB, which are nonresectable tumors that invade vital organs such as the heart, great vessels, or spine (T4) or have supraclavicular, scalene, or contralateral hilar lymph node involvement (N3) but no distant metastases (M0). They may be treated with radiation therapy.

Stage IV includes any tumor with distant metastases (M1).

- **Lymphomas** are divided into Hodgkin, which is characterized histologically by the Sternberg-Reed giant cell, and the more fatal non-Hodgkin lymphoma. **Hodgkin** disease is categorized into four subtypes: nodular sclerosing (50 percent of cases), lymphocyte predominance (10 percent), mixed cell (30 percent), and lymphocyte depletion (10 percent) with the worst prognosis. **Non-Hodgkin lymphomas** are classified into three grades corresponding to prognosis: low, intermediate, and high (Section 15.7).

  Parenchymal **lung involvement** at initial presentation is rare in lymphomas, although as the disease progresses it can become more common, particularly when the hila and mediastinum have been irradiated. Parenchymal lung involvement, when present, is more common in the Hodgkin variety and is almost universally accompanied by visible intrathoracic adenopathy. Isolated parenchymal involvement, however, can be seen in non-Hodgkin. Pleural and pericardial effusions can be associated with this condition and are probably related to lymphatic obstruction from enlarged nodes as well as mesothelial spread.

  Several radiographic patterns can be seen with lymphomatous involvement of the lung. Nodules may be dis-

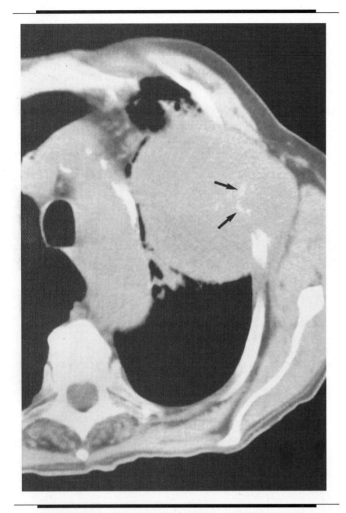

FIGURE 3-12   **Bronchogenic carcinoma.** CT showing a large soft tissue mass with associated rib destruction and chest wall invasion in a 79-year-old man. Note the focal fragments of bone in the periphery of the mass due to bone destruction (arrows), the most reliable feature of chest wall invasion in bronchogenic carcinoma.

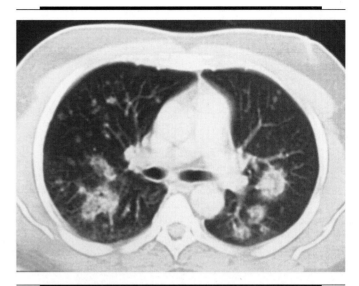

FIGURE 3-13   **Pulmonary lymphoma.** Multiple pulmonary nodules with air bronchograms.

• **Mycosis fungoides** is a T-cell non-Hodgkin lymphoma which may secondarily affect the lung. The lesion usually starts as a cutaneous T-cell lymphoma which disseminates to lymph nodes and other organs late in the disease. **Sèzary cells** are seen in the peripheral blood.

crete and multiple (**Differential 15**) or may be ill-defined and occasionally cavitate (Fig. 3-13). Areas of patchy consolidation with air bronchograms, particularly around the perihilar regions, may also occur. Less commonly, a diffuse reticulonodular form may be seen, which may be difficult to distinguish from other causes of diffuse lung disease (**Differential 49**).

Mucosa-associated lymphoid tissue (MALT) and **bronchus-associated lymphoid tissue (BALT)** refer to other forms of non-Hodgkin lymphoma which can involve the pulmonary parenchyma in the form of multiple nodules or masses.

• **Pseudolymphoma** refers to a condition once thought to represent a precursor of pulmonary lymphoma. Although it is histologically identical to well-differentiated small lymphocytic lymphoma, it can be differentiated using immunofluorescence techniques. Radiographically, it can present with pulmonary nodules or areas of consolidation with air bronchograms. It has a better prognosis than lymphoma.

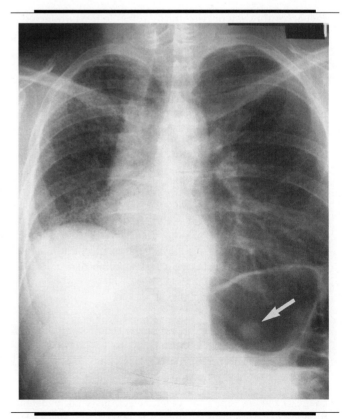

FIGURE 3-14   **PTLD.** Chest radiograph in a 40-year-old patient diagnosed with idiopathic pulmonary fibrosis, who had undergone left lung transplantation. Note the single pulmonary nodule in the left lower lobe projecting behind the gas-filled stomach (arrow).

- **Posttransplant lymphoproliferative disorder (PTLD)** is seen in about 3 percent of organ transplant recipients and is related to immunosuppression and the Epstein-Barr virus. It responds to reduction of immunosuppression and antiviral agents. The most common radiographic appearance is multiple pulmonary nodules (Fig. 3-14), with adenopathy and pleural effusions seen less frequently. Patchy pulmonary infiltrates may also be seen.

3.4 PULMONARY INFECTIONS (BACTERIAL AND VIRAL)

- **Pulmonary infections** can result from a large number of offending organisms. Although plain radiographs are insensitive in determining the exact cause of the pneumonia, several distinguishing features can help narrow the differential diagnosis and help direct the clinician toward a definitive diagnosis and appropriate therapy. Chest radiographs are also extremely useful in following response to treatment and in detecting complications.

    CT can be crucial not only in demonstrating characteristic features of an infection but also can provide a road map for the pulmonologist in planning bronchoscopy. Bacterial infections are generally divided into several types depending on their etiology: **community-acquired** or **nosocomial.**

- The radiographic pattern of pneumonia is quite variable depending on the offending organism. It is important to bear in mind that a specific organism can produce different radiographic patterns which may overlap within the same disease. Pneumonias can be grouped into several general radiographic patterns which include bronchopneumonias and lobar, rounded, and interstitial pneumonias.

    Bronchopneumonias are characterized by the absence of air bronchograms, a patchy distribution, and volume loss. This is one of the most common patterns (**Differential 44**).

    Lobar pneumonia is characterized by homogeneous consolidation of a segment or lobe but may also be multifocal (Fig. 3-15). Air bronchograms are present, and usually there is no volume loss. They are usually related to a bacterial organism such as *Streptococcus, Klebsiella,* or *Mycobacterium tuberculosis* or to a postobstructive infection (**Differential 40**).

    Rounded pneumonia represents an infection process that does not have a lobar pattern but rather presents as a rounded density that does not follow anatomic landmarks. Rounded or nodular forms of pneumonia are usually due to pneumococcal, *Legionella,* or fungal infections. This pattern is more common in children (Fig. 9-21).

    Interstitial pneumonia reveals a radiographic pattern in which the inflammatory process can be either localized or present with more extensive peribronchial thickening. Associated subsegmental and discoid atelectasis is frequently encountered. This pattern may be difficult to differentiate from other causes of interstitial lung disease such as interstitial pulmonary edema (**Differential 45**). This differentiation can be one of the biggest challenges to a radiologist inter-

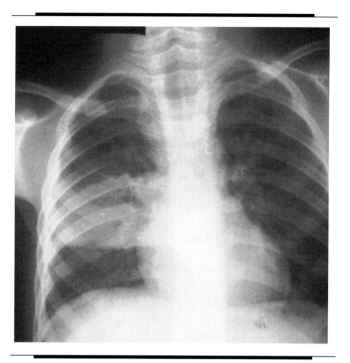

FIGURE 3-15   Lobar pneumonia. Chest radiograph in a 5-year-old boy showing opacification and air bronchograms in the superior segment of the right lower lobe characteristic of consolidation due to bacterial pneumonia. *Pneumococcus* was identified.

preting intensive care unit radiographs. Clues suggesting edema include cardiomegaly, bilateral pleural effusion, and vascular engorgement.

    A **milliary pattern** (see Section 5.10) is an unusual manifestation of infection that can be seen in cases of *M. tuberculosis* disease and histoplasmosis. The nodules are usually 2 to 4 mm in diameter (**Differential 21**).

    Cavitation, if present, is usually indicative of a bacterial (*Staphylococcus aureus*, gram-negative, and anaerobic) or mycobacterial infection (**Differentials 23–27**).

- Besides the radiographic pattern (e.g., viral and mycoplasma pneumonia usually appear as interstitial forms, whereas *Klebsiella* pneumonia is usually lobar), factors such as the patient's age, clinical symptoms, and predisposing conditions must be taken into account in the differential diagnosis. Other radiographic information can be particularly useful in narrowing the differential diagnosis.

Bacterial Pneumonia

- **Staphylococcal pneumonia** is frequently seen in older or debilitated patients, not infrequently occurring as a complication of influenza. The disease is commonly bilateral, starting as a patchy infiltrate with several lobes becoming involved rather rapidly. Volume loss in the affected segments or lobes and concomitant pleural effusions are frequent. Pneumatoceles are observed, particularly in children, and abscess formation can be seen at any age (**Differentials 23–25**).

- **Streptococcal (pneumococcal) pneumonia** is the most common community-acquired bacterial pneumonia and is frequently seen in debilitated patients. Lobar consolidation with air bronchograms is the classic radiographic presentation (Fig. 3-16). It can spread across segmental boundaries and can also be observed as patchy interstitial infiltrates. Frequently, concomitant pleural effusions are present. These parapneumonic effusions can become infected, leading to an empyema (see Section 7.5.)

- **Gram-negative pneumonias** due to organisms such as *Klebsiella, Enterobacter, Escherichia coli,* and *Haemophilus influenzae* are frequently hospital-acquired, occurring in patients with predisposing or debilitated conditions. Cavitation is a common feature. Pulmonary infiltrates can be variable. Patchy consolidation, segmental or lobar involvement, and ill-defined nodules can be seen alone or in combination. Pleural effusions and empyema are also frequent features.

- **Legionnaire disease** is an infection due to *Legionella pneumophila,* an organism frequently found in cooling water towers and humidifiers. Severe systemic symptoms are frequently associated with radiographic findings of rapidly developing peripheral consolidation, often bilateral, which resolves slowly. Pleural effusions and empyema are common. The diagnosis, which can be suspected by outbreaks, is usually confirmed serologically.

- **Actinomycosis** is the result of infection due to *Actinomyces israelis,* a filamentous bacteria formerly thought to represent a fungus. These bacteria represent part of the normal flora of the mouth, throat, and vagina of healthy individuals and have the capacity to proliferate and invade injured tissues. The dis-

ease can invade the chest either by aspiration of infected material or by direct extension of a cervicofacial infection (Fig. 8-15). Pulmonary infections are usually associated with fever, chills, chest pain, and weight loss.

The chest radiograph usually shows focal areas of pulmonary consolidation which may eventually cavitate, extending to adjacent pleural surfaces (Fig. 3-17) and even into the chest wall. Pleural effusions, empyema, and hilar and mediastinal adenopathy are common associated findings. The organism is difficult to culture, and the diagnosis usually rests with histologic identification after surgical resection. In hematoxylin- and eosin-stained tissues sections, the classic description is that of "sulfur granules." High-dose penicillin is the treatment of choice, and drainage of the affected areas of the lung and chest wall may be required.

- **Aspiration pneumonias** usually result from the aspiration of infected material from the oropharynx and esophagus into the respiratory tract. They are usually seen in debilitated or unconscious patients, alcoholics and patients with abundant gastroesophageal reflux. The dependent portions of the lungs are usually the most commonly affected areas (posterior segment of the right upper lobe and superior segment of lower lobes). Anaerobic bacteria are found in about 90 percent of cases, and the infections are usually polymicrobial.

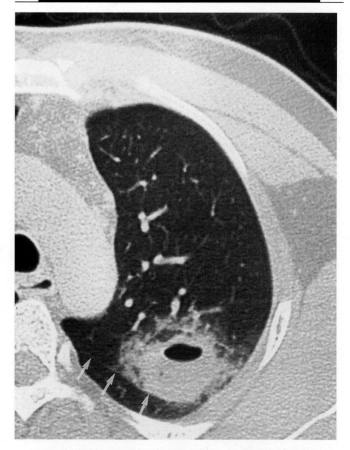

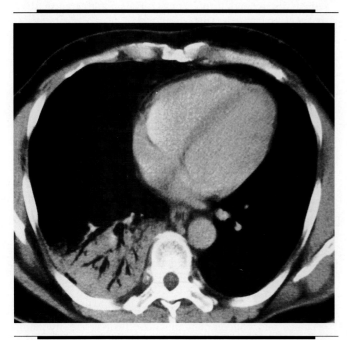

FIGURE 3-16   Right lower lobe bacterial pneumonia. CT showing nonspecific pattern of pulmonary consolidation with air bronchograms.

FIGURE 3-17   Actinomycosis. Thin-section CT of a cavitated left upper lobe mass that abuts the oblique fissure (arrows).

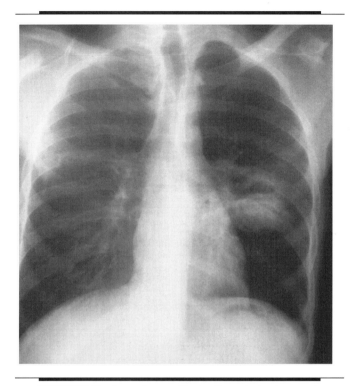

FIGURE 3-18 Lung abscess. Chest radiograph showing a cavitary mass with ill-defined margins and an air-fluid level in the superior segment of the left lower lobe. The abscess developed as a complication of a necrotizing pneumonia.

Necrotizing pneumonia and abscess formation are frequent (Fig. 3-18).

Viral Pneumonia

- **Viral infections** are among the most common diseases affecting humans, particularly children. Most begin within the respiratory tract, where over 100 types of rhinovirus can produce the common cold. However, only a limited number of viruses can infect the respiratory tract below the larynx. Serious viral respiratory tract infections are more common in infants, children, and immunocompromised adults.

- In children under 2 years of age, **respiratory syncytial virus (RSV)**, **parainfluenza 3**, and **adenovirus** are the most common causes of bronchiolitis and pneumonia. **Parainfluenza virus 1** and **2** are important etiologic factors in older children, in whom they can cause laryngotracheobronchitis (croup).

- **Adenovirus** infections can produce air trapping and lobar collapse as a result

of bronchial and peribronchial inflammation, with bronchiolitis obliterans, bronchiectasis, and **Swyer-James** syndrome as sequelae. Infection can also be seen in young adults, particularly military recruits.

- The **influenza virus** is a common cause of respiratory infections in children and adults. Influenza virus A and B are responsible for about one-third of cases, the others being attributable to a variety of viruses. Pneumonia is more serious in infants, the elderly, and ill patients. Headache, malaise, fever, prostration, and sore throat are usually followed by cough and lower respiratory tract symptoms. Associated bacterial infections, particularly those caused by *S. aureus*, *Pneumococcus*, and *H. influenzae*, are common.

  Radiographically, viral infections usually begin as a patchy interstitial infiltrate as necrotizing bronchitis and bronchiolitis develop. As infiltration of inflammatory cells and exudate develops, more confluent infiltrates may become evident, particularly in a bibasilar distribution and usually in a multifocal fashion (Fig. 3-19). Viral pneumonic infiltrates are difficult to differentiate from superimposed bacterial infections. Pleural effusions and cavitation are not common features of viral pneumonias.

  Respiratory tract infections may also occur as a complication of dissemination of a virus that primarily affects the skin.

- **Varicella zoster** virus can rarely produce pneumonia, particularly in immunocompromised patients. The usual radi-

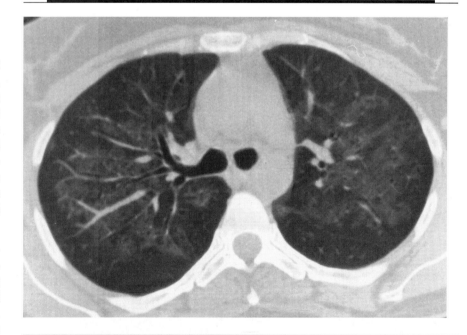

FIGURE 3-19 Viral pneumonia. HRCT demonstrating symmetric perihilar ground-glass opacities likely representing interstitial inflammation in a patient with an upper respiratory tract infection. (With permission from Sagel SS, Slone RM. The lung. In: Lee JKT, Sagel SS, Stanley RJ, Heiken JP, eds. *Computed Body Tomography with MRI Correlation*, 3rd ed. Lippincott-Raven; 1998.)

ographic pattern is one of multiple small, ill-defined pulmonary nodules that develop several days after the skin rash. These nodular densities can disappear within a few days, persist for months, or even calcify.

- **Rubeola** (measles) infection can result in lung infection secondary to the skin lesions. A widespread reticular infiltrate with lobar atelectasis, sometimes associated with hilar adenopathy, can be observed. Bacterial superinfections may occur. Radiographic findings may clear slowly.

- *Mycoplasma pneumoniae,* the smallest free-living organism, is a frequent cause of pulmonary infection that can resemble the common flu clinically and occur in outbreaks in healthy subjects. The radiographic findings are somewhat non-specific, with bibasilar interstitial infiltrates that can become confluent, resembling bacterial pneumonia. Pleural effusions are rare.

3.5 FUNGAL INFECTIONS

- **Fungal infections** of the lungs usually result from the inhalation of yeasts and molds growing in nature, although some fungi such as *Candida*, which are part of the normal flora, are opportunistic and can become respiratory pathogens. The ability to produce damage depends on the particular virulence of the pathogen, infecting dose, and host immune status.

    Once fungi reach the lungs, they can remain localized or disseminate via bronchial, hematogenous, or lymphatic routes, producing severe and often fatal disease. There has been a progressive rise in opportunistic fungal infections over the few decades resulting from the use of broad-spectrum antibiotic therapy, immunosupressive treatment for allograft rejection, chemotherapy, and acquired immunodeficiency syndrome (AIDS).

- **Aspergillosis** of the lung is the result of infestation with *Aspergillus fumigatus* which is usually present in soil and water. This organism has been isolated in sputum cultures of a large percentage of patients with bronchial asthma and other chronic forms of pulmonary disease. It can produce a wide spectrum of disease ranging from simple colonization to life-threatening invasive aspergillosis. Nodules of aspergillosis infection are often associated with surrounding areas of increased parenchymal density due to hemorrhage or edema (Fig. 3-20). This phenomenon has been described as a "halo sign" and can be seen in other focal pulmonary conditions.

    Fungus ball, mycetoma, and **aspergilloma** are terms reserved for a condition in which a preexisting lung cavity is colonized by a conglomerate of

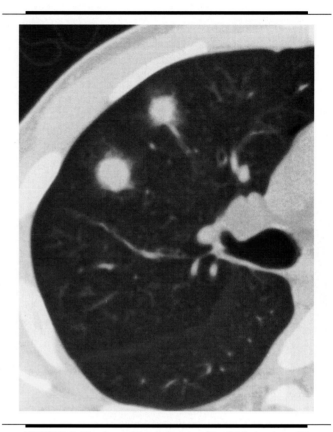

FIGURE 3-20 *Aspergillus* **infection with CT halo sign.** CT demonstrating two separate pulmonary nodules in the right upper lobe. Both have a surrounding zone of edema or hemorrhage referred to as a "halo" sign. This feature can be seen with infection or neoplasm.

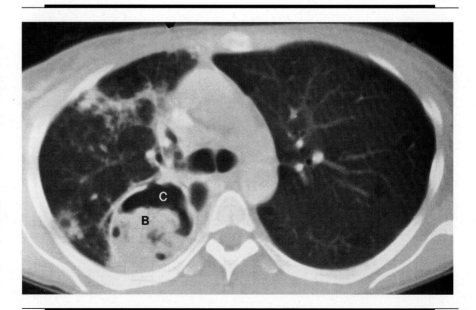

FIGURE 3-21   Aspergilloma. CT in a 35-year-old woman with necrotizing pneumonia showing a fungus ball (B) within a pulmonary cavity (C).

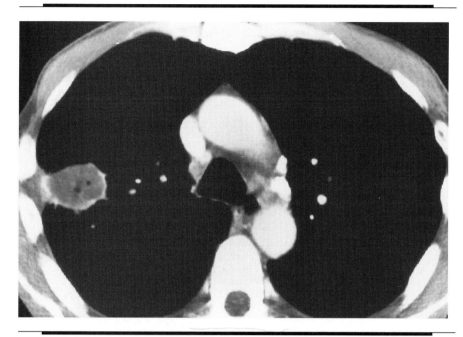

FIGURE 3-22 Mucormycosis. CT in a 56-year-old diabetic patient showing a cavitary area of consolidation in the right upper lobe with central necrosis and associated pleural thickening.

Infections rarely occur in patients without an underlying systemic disease (see Section 3.7).

- **Histoplasmosis** is caused by *Histoplasma capsulatum*, a fungus usually found in the soil as well as in excreta of chickens, pigeons, and bats. Humans are infected (frequently after cleaning bird cages) when they inhale the spores which subsequently convert to the yeast form. The disease is endemic to the Mississippi and Ohio river valleys and adjacent states and to Mexico, Venezuela, and Guatemala.

Millions of people in endemic areas become infected with the fungus, usually in the **asymptomatic form**. It is estimated that approximately 90 percent of patients develop this benign, self-limited form of the disease. A focal area of pulmonary infiltrate may develop, with eventual complete clearing or, commonly, leaving a focus of calcification. These focal areas are frequently associated with calcified lymph nodes in the hila and mediastinum as a result of accompanying inflammatory changes and subsequent necrosis in these structures (Fig. 3-23).

Symptomatic histoplasmosis comprises a variety of forms depending on the severity of symptoms, varying from mild to severe, usually resembling flu symptoms. The sever-

mycelial hyphae. Hemoptysis, which at times may be severe and uncontrollable, is a frequent clinical presentation (**Differential 145**). Sputum cultures are helpful in only about half of affected patients.

Radiographically, a filling defect may be seen within the preexisting cavity, usually in an upper lobe, frequently demonstrating air between the mass and the wall of the cavity (air meniscus sign) (Fig. 3-21). Changing the position of the patient may demonstrate the mobility of the fungus ball within the cavity. The diagnosis of aspergilloma rests on the triad of hemoptysis, intracavitary mass, and positive serology. Aspergillus may produce a more invasive infection in immunocompromised patients (see Section 3.7).

Allergic bronchopulmonary aspergillosis refers to aspergillus colonization in the proximal bronchi (usually upper lobe), a phenomenon usually seen in asthmatic patients who develop sensitivity to the fungus. Mucus impaction in affected bronchi results in branching pulmonary densities classically described as "gloved finger." Recurrence can lead to scarring, bronchiectasis, and upper lobe fibrosis.

- **Mucormycosis** refers to a variety of infections due to *Phycomycetes* usually occurring in patients with diabetes, leukemia, or lymphoma. (Fig. 3-22).

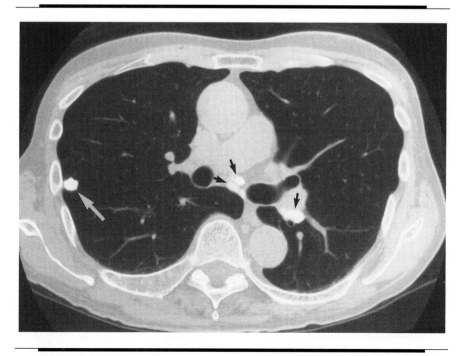

FIGURE 3-23 Healed histoplasmosis. CT showing a calcified granuloma in the right lung (white arrow), and calcified lymph nodes in the left hilum, and subcarinal region (black arrows) in a 78-year-old asymptomatic man.

ity of the disease is thought to be related to the extent of exposure, and it usually runs a limited course with no treatment. The chest radiograph is usually nonspecific, demonstrating patchy consolidation and adenopathy.

On rare occasions and following extremely heavy exposures (as in cave exploration), more severe forms may be encountered in which high fever, respiratory failure, and hepatosplenomegaly may be present. **Disseminated histoplasmosis** is a rare form of the disease usually seen in infants or immunosuppressed hosts such as AIDS and lymphoma patients (see Section 3.7).

Histoplasmoma refers to one or multiple rather well-defined, frequently calcified pulmonary nodules (granuloma) that may represent a necrotic focus of infection surrounded by an inflammatory reaction. They may grow slowly over years, making differentiation from a slow-growing bronchogenic carcinoma (particularly adenocarcinoma) difficult. Growth of a histoplasmoma does not represent general dissemination of the disease.

- **North American blastomycosis** is the result of infection with *Blastomyces dermatitidis*, an organism usually present in the soil, colonizing humans after inhalation. Once the organism has infected the lung, it can spread to other parts of the body such as the gastrointestinal tract, skin, and skeletal system. The chest radiograph may demonstrated nonspecific consolidation involving one or more segments, with a predilection for the upper lungs. These areas may cavitate and mimic tuberculosis.

These infiltrates may appear as small nodular lesions that can coalesce into areas of confluent infiltrate appearing rounded and masslike (Fig. 3-24). At times they may locally

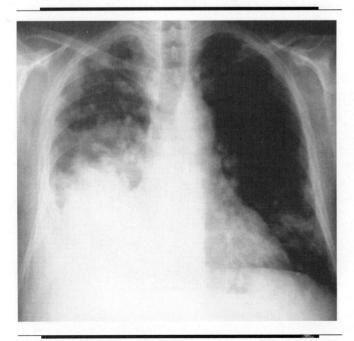

FIGURE 3-24 Pulmonary blastomycosis. Chest radiograph demonstrating multiple bilateral rounded densities which are confluent in the right lung base.

destroy adjacent bones in a fashion similar to an aggressive neoplastic process. Pleural effusions or thickening may be associated. Rarely, associated hilar or mediastinal adenopathy may be seen. The disease can spread in a hematogenous fashion and propagate to the rest of the lungs and other organs. Definitive diagnosis is usually based on identifying the organisms on microscopic examination or by culture.

- **Cryptococcosis** or European blastomycosis is caused by the inhalation of *Cryptococcus neoformans* spores usually found in pigeon droppings. The organism is a facultative intracellular yeast which can rarely cause pulmonary disease in healthy individuals and more commonly in immunocompromised hosts.

Once in the lungs, the organisms can produce local inflammation and caseation in healthy individuals or may spread to other areas of the body. The latter situation is particularly important in immunodeficiency states such as AIDS, diabetes mellitus, and lymphoma. The organism is very neurotropic, and systemic dissemination can lead to meningeal spread, meningitis, and meningoencephalitis.

The radiographic findings can vary from patchy interstitial infiltrates to nodules or rounded masslike infiltrates which may show cavitation. Pleural effusions and adenopathy may be associated, particularly in immunocompromised individuals who tend to develop more extensive forms of the disease. It may be difficult to differentiate from bronchogenic carcinoma, not only because of the rather striking radiographic similarities in both entities, but because they frequently coincide in the same hosts with chronic lung disease. Biopsy is often the only method of definitive diagnosis.

- **Coccidioidomycosis** is a pulmonary mycosis caused by the organism *Coccidioides immitis*, a fungus found in the soil of semiarid climates with short intense rainy seasons. The disease is endemic in southwestern North America, northern and central Mexico, and Argentina, Paraguay, Venezuela, and Guatemala. Most patients are asymptomatic, and after a short incubation period the rest develop flulike symptoms usually lasting about 2 to 3 weeks. Most individuals attain full recovery. However, a small percentage may have persistent clinical symptoms and radiographic findings, a condition referred to as **persistent coccidioidomycosis**. In immunocompromised patients, systemic dissemination may occur, particularly to the skin, bone, lymph nodes, and urinary tract.

The radiographic findings of coccidioidomycosis are variable and, for the most part, related to the severity of disease. During early stages, patchy infiltrates may be accompanied by hilar or mediastinal adenopathy and less frequently by pleural effusions. In cases of persistent disease, the infiltrates may persist and even enlarge, frequently demonstrating focal areas of confluence which are usually peripheral and can frequently cavitate with an upper lobe distribution somewhat similar to the findings in pulmonary tuberculosis. The infiltrates may acquire a more nodular appearance and be multiple and bilateral or be milliary in cases of hematogenous spread.

3.6 MYCOBACTERIAL INFECTIONS

- Mycobacterial lung infections are usually the result of *M. tuberculosis* or atypical mycobacteria including *M. kansasii* and *M. avium-intracellulare*, among others.

- *Mycobacterium tuberculosis* is the cause of pulmonary tuberculosis in humans and is usually transmitted by bacilli in aerosolized sputum from coughing. The disease has been well controlled in developed nations but is widespread in underdeveloped countries with poor sanitary conditions. There has been a rise in the incidence of this disease in the United States, particularly with the advent of AIDS and the increasing immigrant population.

   The **diagnosis** of tuberculosis usually requires demonstration of tubercle bacilli in smears of sputum or in tissue sections, but more accurately by culture of the slowly growing organism. **Imaging features** are variable and must be included in the differential diagnosis of many pulmonary conditions. **Tuberculin conversion** refers to a hypersensitivity reaction of the infected individual when injected intradermally with purified protein derivative (PPD) of the tubercle bacilli. Once infected, the test remains positive, presumably because of the presence of residual dormant organisms stimulating antibody formation.

- **Primary** or **childhood tuberculosis** results from initial contact with the tuberculous bacilli of a child who has had no prior exposure. Recently, primary tuberculosis has been increasingly seen in adult patients. Once the organism is inhaled, it enters the alveoli where it forms a **primary** or **Ghon complex** consisting of focal parenchymal inflammation accompanied by an enlarged hilar lymph node. Clinically, the patient may be asymptomatic or have mild flu-like symptoms. In the majority of cases, immunity inhibits progression of the disease and fibrosis occurs. If the individual is malnourished or immunodeficient, the disease can rapidly progress to caseation, bronchopneumonia, and even milliary tuberculosis.

   The chest radiograph may be normal in some cases of primary infections even if the individual undergoes PPD conversion or has positive sputum cultures. Small apical lesions may not be readily noticeable because of overlapping bony structures. However, in most cases of primary infection, particularly in children, a focal peripheral infiltrate associated with adenopathy can be identified (**Differential 100**). The peripheral infiltrate varies from patchy to segmental or lobar consolidation and may cavitate in a small percentage of cases (Fig. 3-25). These are slow to clear, leaving a scar or focal calcification in the parenchyma. Corresponding hilar or mediastinal lymph node cal-

cifications are common and may be rather bulky despite scanty parenchymal findings (**Differential 99**). Pleural effusions often are associated with the parenchymal infiltrates in primary tuberculosis and in rare cases can be the sole manifestation.

- **Adult** or **secondary tuberculosis** is the result of reinfection or, more commonly, reactivation of the dormant bacilli in an adult patient, usually as the result of a breakdown in the individual's immunity or of immunossuppressive therapy. Although reactivation of the tuberculous bacilli may occur at any site in the lung, the apical regions are most commonly affected since the higher oxygen concentration allows the aerobic bacilli to proliferate. As the organisms multiply, fibrocaseous granulomatous inflammation (tuberculoma) may cavitate and rupture into the bronchial lumen. Subsequent coughing can spread the bacilli and infect other individuals. Late in the disease or in very debilitated individuals, the bacilli can gain access to the bloodstream, resulting in systemic dissemination.

   The radiographic manifestations of **reactivation tuberculosis** may be variable and unilateral, bilateral, or multilobar. The anterior or posterior segments of the upper lobes and the superior segment of the lower lobes are frequently involved. Areas of parenchymal involvement often show cavitation, a sign of activity and potential infectious threat to other individuals (Fig. 3-26). Frequently, areas of fibrosis and calcification are seen surrounding or adjacent to the parenchymal infiltrates or cavities. Air-fluid levels may be seen within the cavitated areas of lung. Cavities may have thick or thin walls and be single or multiple. More confluent areas of consolidation are seen in cases of tuberculous bronchopneumonia.

- A **tuberculoma** represents a well-defined chronic granulomatous lesion which may mimic a pulmonary neoplasm except when calcification is present. Chronic infections can also lead to pulmonary scarring and parenchymal distortion

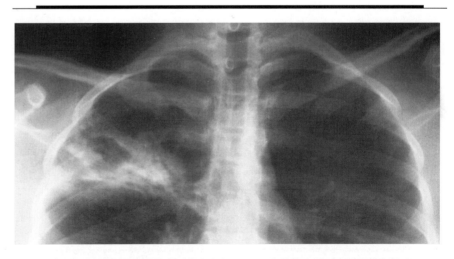

FIGURE 3-25 Tuberculosis. Chest radiograph in a 17-year-old woman showing a focal area of consolidation in the right upper lobe with evidence of cavitation.

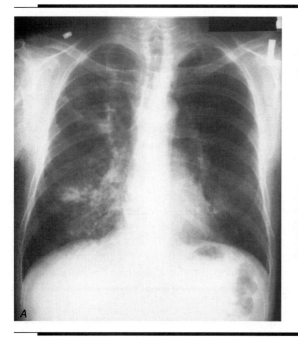
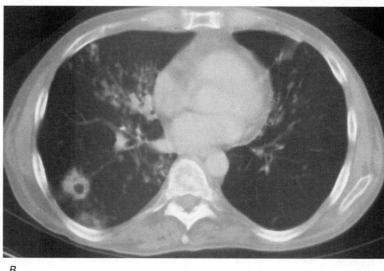

FIGURE 3-26   **Tuberculosis.** (*A*) Chest radiograph in a 52-year-old man showing a nodular infiltrate in the right lung. (*B*) CT showing cavitation in some of the larger nodules and subtle evidence of disease in the left lung.

with traction bronchiectasis and bronchial stenosis. Calcified tuberculous nodes may erode into the lumen of a bronchus, producing broncholithiasis. In addition, extrinsic bronchial compression may cause lobar or segmental collapse which

may be recurrent. The right middle lobe is the most common location for this condition (Fig. 3-27).

- **Atypical mycobacterial infections** result from *M. kansasii* and *M. avium-intracellulare*, among others. These organisms

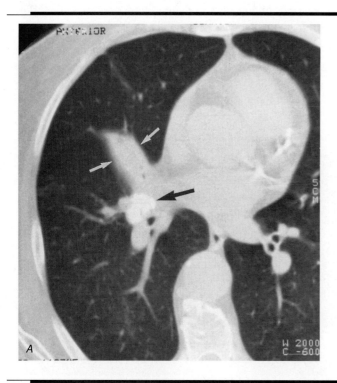
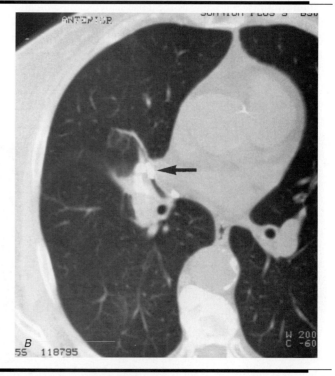

FIGURE 3-27   **Right middle lobe syndrome.** (*A*) CT demonstrating collapse of the middle lobe (white arrows). (*B*) Note calcified lymph nodes seen to obstruct the middle lobe bronchus (black arrow). Tuberculosis and histoplasmosis are the usual causes. (With permission from Sagel SS, Slone RM. The lung. In: Lee JKT, Sagel SS, Stanley RJ, Heiken JP, eds. *Computed Body Tomography with MRI Correlation*, 3rd ed. Lippincott-Raven; 1998.)

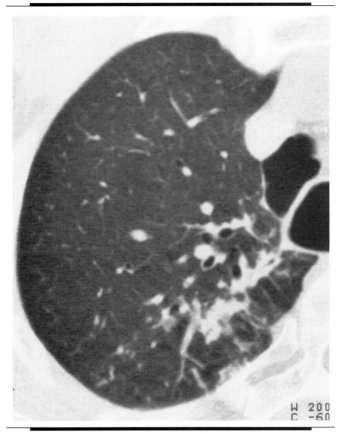

FIGURE 3-28 Atypical mycobacterium. Thin-section CT demonstrating a nodular infiltrate in the right upper lobe. Specimens sent for culture grew out *Mycobacterium kansasii*. (With permission from Sagel SS, Slone RM. The lung. In: Lee JKT, Sagel SS, Stanley RJ, Heiken JP, eds. *Computed Body Tomography with MRI Correlation*, 3rd ed. Lippincott-Raven; 1998.)

Most pulmonary nontuberculous mycobacterial infections can be classified into one of several categories. The **classical** form mimics tuberculosis radiographically and is predominantly seen in white male patients with underlying chronic lung disease. The **nonclassical** form is seen in elderly women without underlying chronic illness. Radiographically, this form is characterized by nodular infiltrates and bronchiectasis in a sporadic distribution (**Differential 35**).

Another nonspecific manifestation is asymptomatic nodules. Immunocompromised individuals are frequently asymptomatic and may have a wide variety of radiographic forms including disseminated infections. Patients with achalasia and repeated pulmonary aspiration are predisposed to mycobacterial infections, and the radiographic findings often resemble those for aspiration pneumonia.

3.7 IMMUNOCOMPROMISED PATIENTS

- The immune status of the individual determines the type, severity, and susceptibility to infection. Needless to say, patients with decreased immunity have an increased incidence of opportunistic infections. There has been a dramatic increase in the number of immunocompromised patients over the past two decades for many reasons.

  The number of **AIDS patients** and human immunodeficiency virus (HIV)-positive individuals has increased dramatically since the disease was first diagnosed in the early 1980s. In addition, there has been a tremendous increase in the number of allograft transplants performed and cancer patients being treated with immunosuppressive drugs. In the

are usually found in the soil and tend to be less pathogenic to humans. These infections are particularly problematic in individuals with chronic lung disease (Fig. 3-28), general debilitation, or an altered immune system.

The characteristic radiographic finding is a propensity for cavitation which is usually associated with fibrotic changes (fibrocavitary). Reticulonodular infiltrates are also a common radiographic feature. The disease may have a protracted course, not infrequently extending over several years. It may be difficult to distinguish atypical mycobacterial infections from tuberculosis since the areas of involvement (upper lobes, superior segments of lower lobes) are similar (Fig. 3-29). Distinguishing features are the low incidence of associated pleural effusions and adenopathy and poor response to traditional antituberculous therapy.

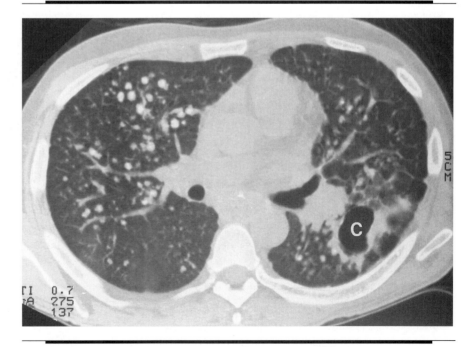

FIGURE 3-29 Atypical mycobacterial infection. 40-year-old man with sarcoidosis and occupational exposure to silica dust. CT illustrating multiple bilateral pulmonary nodules and a cavity in the left upper lobe. *Mycobacterium goldonae* was cultured.

7200: TB,Ehruhonic

previous sections, we described the different infectious agents, their particular epidemiology, and their radiologic presentation. In this section we will summarize the peculiarities of some of these infections, particularly in AIDS patients.

- Pulmonary infections and tumors in the **AIDS population** have a variable clinical and radiographic presentation. Correlation with the **CD4 T-lymphocyte** count can help narrow the differential diagnosis.

The major diagnostic consideration in patients with cavitary or noncavitary consolidation and a CD4 lymphocyte count above 200 cells/mm^3 is bacterial pneumonia and *M. tuberculosis*. The most common bacterial organisms are *Streptococcus pneumoniae, H. influenzae, Staphylococcus aureus,* and *Legionella* and *Mycoplasma* species.

The most likely diagnosis in patients with CD4 counts below 200 cells/mm^3 is *Pneumocystis carinii* pneumonia (PCP), which usually shows a ground-glass or reticular interstitial pattern. This organism is thought to represent a primitive fungus or unicellular protozoan and is so prevalent among AIDS patients that chemoprophylaxis is routine.

At CD4 lymphocyte counts between 50 and 200 cells/mm^3, disseminated fungal infections (Fig. 3-30) and Kaposi sarcoma also become prevalent.

At CD4 lymphocyte counts below 50 cells/mm^3, a reticular or nodular pattern on a chest radiograph may indicate AIDS-

related lymphoma, cytomegalovirus, or *M. avium-intracellulare* infections.

- The spread of AIDS has led to an increase in the number of **Tuberculosis** (TB) cases worldwide, particularly in intravenous drug users and ethnic minorities. Early in HIV, the radiographic findings are those of reactivation TB with cavitary infiltrates in the upper lobes and superior segments of the lower lobes. In more advanced cases of HIV infection, diffuse reticulonodular or airspace infiltrates or even a miliary pattern may be seen. Lymphadenopathy, even without concomitant pulmonary infiltrates, may be seen in up to 80 percent of cases. The enlarged nodes may exhibit low attenuation centers as well as peripheral enhancement. This pattern may also be seen with atypical mycobacterial infections. Although tuberculous infections are usually treatable, new drug-resistant strains have been described, particularly among drug users, and the mortality rate in this group is high.

- *Mycobacterium avium intracellulare* (MAI) is more common in cases of advanced HIV disease when the CD4 cell count falls below 50/mm^3. Besides the lungs, many other organs can be involved by this organism. Although the chest radiograph may be normal in patients infected with MAI, the most common patterns include bilateral reticulonodular infiltrates, focal alveolar infiltrates, or multiple pulmonary nodules. Cavitation and a miliary pattern are less common.

- Viral pulmonary infections can also be seen. **Cytomegalovirus (CMV)** infections are an infrequent cause of pneumonia (Fig. 3-31). The Epstein-Barr virus has been postulated as a cause of the **lymphoprolipherative disorder** in patients with AIDS.

*<200: PCP/KS/Fung·l   <50, LhA)
                              (CrV)
                              rAI*

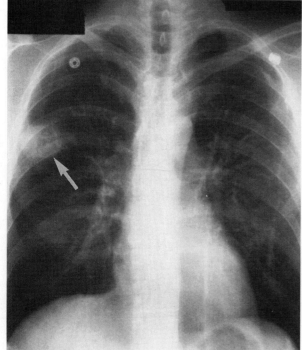

FIGURE 3-30 *Aspergillus.* Chest radiograph in a 42-year-old AIDS patient being treated with steroids for CMV encephalitis. Note the cavitary right upper lobe mass (arrow) shown to be aspergillus by aspiration lung biopsy.

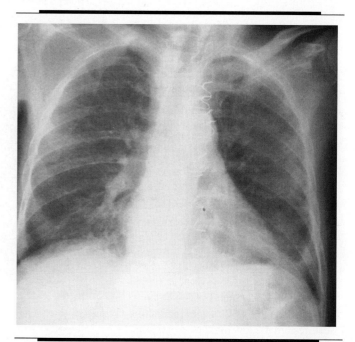

FIGURE 3-31 **CMV infection.** AP chest radiograph in a patient following heart transplantation, showing bilateral interstitial infiltrates.

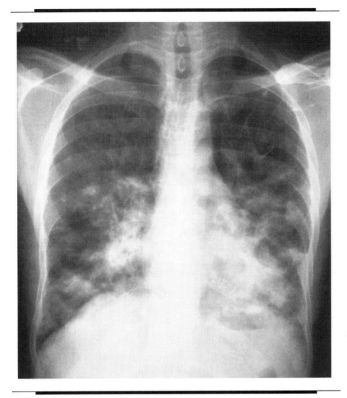

FIGURE 3-32   Pulmonary Kaposi sarcoma. Chest radiograph in a 35-year-old man with AIDS and mucocutaneous Kaposi sarcomas. Note the characteristic nodular lower lobe bronchovascular distribution.

tumor in HIV-positive children and the second most common thoracic neoplasm in HIV-positive adults. Most non-Hodgkin lymphomas are B cell. They are typically aggressive and patients often present with advanced disease, including extranodal involvement of the central nervous system, gastrointestinal tract, liver, spleen, and bone marrow. Thoracic disease is present in 20 percent of patients, with pulmonary nodules and pleural mass or effusion being more common than adenopathy. Peribronchovascular patterns that mimic Kaposi sarcoma also can occur.

- **Hodgkin disease** is not an AIDS-defining tumor, but AIDS patients often have atypical presentations, including pulmonary nodules and masses with or without pleural involvement or adenopathy and disease involving the central nervous system, skin, gastrointestinal tract, bone marrow, and oral pharynx. Treatment response is often poor and, pathologically, the disease has aggressive histologic features.

- **Lung carcinoma** has been reported with an increased incidence in HIV-positive patients. The imaging findings are similar to those in the general population, including a pulmonary mass with adenopathy and sometimes effusions. Disease is often advanced at diagnosis and prognosis is poor.

- Although the chest radiograph is nonspecific, certain radiographic patterns of disease may help suggest the etiology. A fine, bilateral interstitial infiltrate or ground-glass appearance is suggestive of PCP (Fig. 3-33). On rare occasions, calcified hilar and mediastinal nodes may be seen with PCP. Sponta-

- **Kaposi sarcoma** is the most frequent thoracic neoplasm in HIV-infected patients. Kaposi sarcoma is usually present on the skin when pulmonary involvement is seen. The most common presentation is focal parenchymal infiltrates with a bronchovascular distribution (Fig. 3-32). Adenopathy and pleural effusions are seen in about one-third of patients. While Kaposi shows a very low uptake of gallium, lymphoma shows avid uptake of both thalium and gallium.

- **Lymphocytic interstitial pneumonitis** (LIP) is an AIDS-defining condition in children but is uncommon in adults. Lymphocytic proliferation within the interstitium and adjacent to bronchioles produces a lower lobe–predominant reticulonodular pattern on imaging studies. Fibrosis may develop. LIP responds to steroid treatment. Progression to lymphoma is rare.

- **Non-Hodgkin lymphoma** is an AIDS-defining tumor. It is the most common

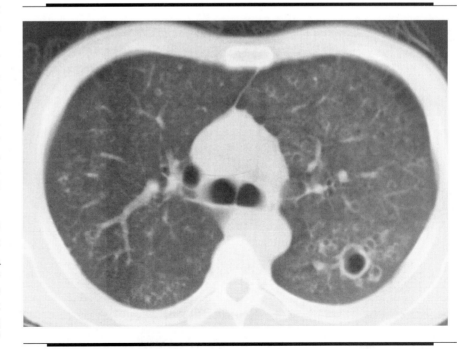

FIGURE 3-33   *Pneumocystis carinii pneumoniae.* CT in a 36-year-old man with AIDS, cough, and fever, showing diffuse interstitial infiltrates and cysts representing acute and chronic disease. (With permission from Sagel SS, Slone RM. The lung. In: Lee JKT, Sagel SS, Stanley RJ, Heiken JP, eds. *Computed Body Tomography with MRI Correlation*, 3rd ed. Lippincott-Raven; 1998.)

neous pneumothorax can be seen as a complication of AIDS-related PCP (Fig. 3-34). Although PCP can appear as lobar consolidation, this is unusual and consideration should then be given to bacterial infections. Effusions are rare.

In patients with pulmonary infection and a normal chest radiograph, gallium lung scanning may be helpful. Gallium scanning is highly sensitive for pulmonary infections, particularly PCP in patients with normal radiographs, although the specificity is low. A thallium-gallium mismatch pattern in immunodeficient patients is specific for mycobacterial infection. The presence of pleural effusion or mediastinal adenopathy also suggests an etiology other than PCP. Mycobacterial infections, Kaposi sarcoma, or lymphoma should be considered.

- Aside from AIDS, other causes of immune compromise, including immunosuppressive chemotherapy, can lead to opportunistic infections.

- **Invasive pulmonary aspergillosis** may produce infiltrates and lung consolidation and is difficult to differentiate from other pneumonias radiographically. This more aggressive form of infection seen in immunocompromised patients can invade the chest wall and be fatal (**Differential 89**). This devastating form of the disease is seen in debilitated patients with concurrent infections or on steroid therapy. Less than 30 percent of patients survive the infection. Amphotericin B is the chemotherapeutic agent of choice.

- **Mucormycosis** refers to a variety of infections due to **Phycomycetes**, usually occurring in patients with diabetes, leukemia, or lymphoma. Infections rarely occur in patients without an underlying systemic disease. These organisms can

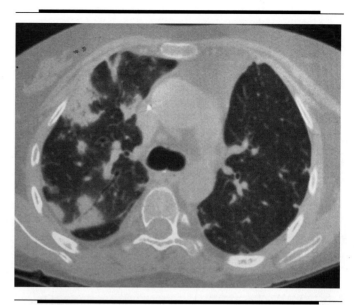

FIGURE 3-35   *Nocardia* **infection following renal transplantation.** CT demonstrating a nonspecific bronchopneumonia with multifocal areas of consolidation and air bronchograms. (With permission from Sagel SS, Slone RM. The lung. In: Lee JKT, Sagel SS, Stanley RJ, Heiken JP, eds. *Computed Body Tomography with MRI Correlation*, 3rd ed. Lippincott-Raven; 1998.)

erode through the bronchial wall, invading adjacent vessels, particularly arteries, and cause lung infarction. Infarcted areas tend to be rounded centrally and more wedge-shaped peripherally.

Foci of consolidation may spread rapidly, although the disease tends not to cross fissural boundaries. Cavitation is a common associated feature. The mortality rate is high even with aggressive treatment. Definitive diagnosis is difficult and usually depends on the identification of *mucoraceous hyphae* organisms in the respiratory tract.

- **Disseminated histoplasmosis** is a rare form of the disease usually seen in infants or immunosuppressed hosts such as AIDS and lymphoma patients. In these individuals, the disease may spread throughout the lungs, as well as other organ systems. The radiographic appearance varies from normal (particularly in infants) to various degrees of bilateral pulmonary infiltrates. Another characteristic form is that of diffuse bilateral milliary nodules similar to those of milliary tuberculosis.

- *Nocardia* species are a common cause of infection in immunocompromised patients. The radiographic findings are similar to those of tuberculosis (Fig. 3-35). Nodules may cavitate, and infiltrates and pleural effusions may be present. Patients with lymphoma, alveolar proteinosis, and leukemia have an increased incidence of *Nocardia* infections.

3.8 VASCULAR PULMONARY LESIONS

- **Pulmonary thromboembolism (PE)** is one of the most common causes of death in the United States, resulting in 50,000 to 100,000 fatalities each year. Most pulmonary

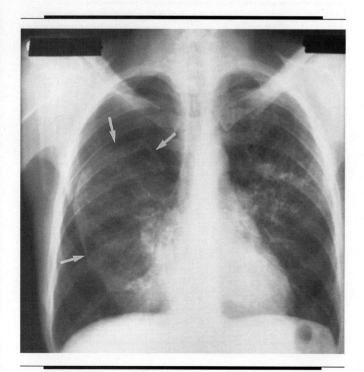

FIGURE 3-34   Spontaneous pneumothorax. Chest radiograph showing bilateral interstitial infiltrates and a large right pneumothorax (arrows) in a 42-year-old man with AIDS-related PCP.

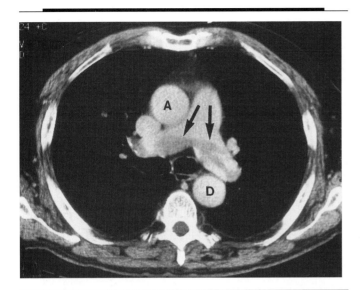

FIGURE 3-36 Pulmonary embolism. Chest CT with IV contrast performed in a 69-year-old man with chest pain to rule out dissection. There are large central filling defects representing pulmonary emboli (arrows) in the right and left main pulmonary arteries. Note the normal ascending (A) and descending (D) thoracic aortae.

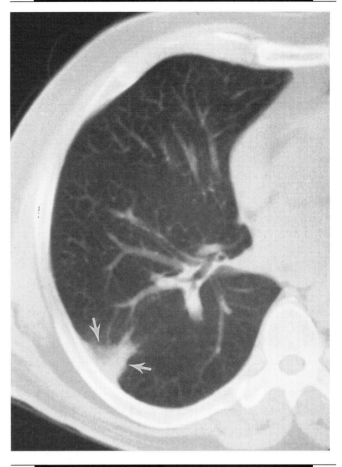

FIGURE 3-37 Pulmonary infarct. CT demonstrating a pleura-based triangular density (arrows) resulting from pulmonary infarct.

emboli are the result of deep venous thrombosis of the lower extremities. PEs most commonly occur in gravity-dependent portions of the lungs where blood flow is greatest.

The **diagnosis** of pulmonary embolism rests on a combination of clinical findings as well as chest radiography, ventilation-perfusion scintigraphy, and pulmonary angiography when necessary (see Figs. 14-1 and 14-2). Cross-sectional imaging, particularly spiral CT, is evolving as an important mean of diagnosis in some patients (Fig. 3-36). A current primary limitation is in the identification of small emboli in subsegmental artery branches; the clinical significance of these small emboli is not well known.

In most cases the chest radiograph is normal, although certain nonspecific findings such as atelectasis, pleural effusions, and infrequently peripheral wedge-shaped pleural-based densities may be identified. Often chest radiography plays an important role in suggesting a clear alternative diagnosis such a pneumothorax, rib fracture, pneumonia, or pulmonary edema in a patient with acute pleuritic chest pain or dyspnea. **Westermark sign** refers to a lobar or segmental area of oligemia seen on a chest radiograph. This results from mechanical obstruction or vasoconstriction. Although it is the most specific sign, it is rarely identified prospectively.

With extensive acute PE and occlusion of at least 70 percent of the vascular pulmonary bed, pulmonary arterial hypertension and enlargement of the central pulmonary arteries may occur. Recurrent episodes of PE may eventually lead to pulmonary arterial hypertension and cor pulmonale. Progressive dyspnea is one of the principal symptoms of the disease.

PE with infarction is seen in approximately 10 to 20 percent of surviving patients and more often in individuals succumbing to the disease. Peripheral areas of consolidation (Fig. 3-37), which may appear rounded medially (Hampton

hump), cavitations, and pleural effusions are characteristic radiographic findings. Cavitation within an area of infarction is a rare finding.

- **Septic emboli** are usually the result of infected vegetations of the endocardium or intravenous drug usage or infected grafts (Fig. 3-38). Areas of cavitation are frequently present (**Differential 27**).

- **Fat emboli** are usually due to traumatic fractures of long bones, with the incidence usually being related to the number and extent of the fractures. As a result of severed veins at the fracture site, fat droplets gain access to the central circulation and eventually lodge in the lung parenchyma where they act as chemical irritants. The usual radiographic presentation is that of air space disease occurring 24 to 48 hours after the traumatic event.

- **Congenital pulmonary arteriovenous malformations (AVM)** of the lung represent a direct communication between the pulmonary arteries and veins, bypassing the capillary bed and causing cyanosis as a result of right-to-left shunt. Dyspnea and hemoptysis are common clinical presentations. About 50 percent of pulmonary AVMs are associated with Osler-

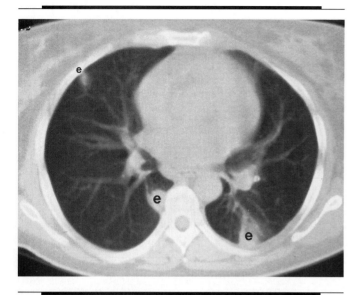

FIGURE 3-38   Septic emboli. CT in a 47-year-old patient with end-stage renal disease and an infected shunt graft resulting in staphylococcal sepsis. Note multiple peripheral pleura-based densities representing septic emboli.

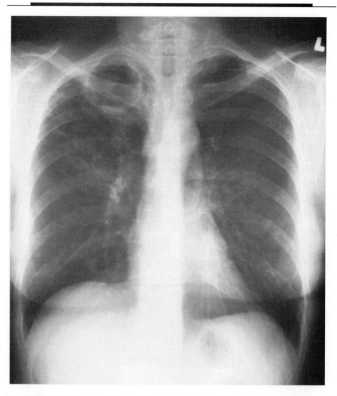

FIGURE 3-39   Cavitary Wegener granulomatosis. Chest radiograph showing a predominantly right perihilar and upper lobe infiltrate and a large air-filled cavity in the right apex in a 57-year-old woman.

Weber-Randu (hereditary hemorrhagic telangectasia). A pulmonary lobulated density associated with feeding vessels is the characteristic radiographic finding. Occlusion by means of coils or detachable balloons is the preferred form of therapy when symptomatic. (See Section 14.1 and Fig. 14-4.)

• **Pulmonary venous varices** are rare lesions, with less than 50 cases reported in the literature. In general, they present as pulmonary nodules in patients with no symptoms. They can also be seen in patients with elevated venous pressure, usually the result of mitral valve disease. Sudden formation of a venous varix in a patient with mitral stenosis may reflect acute elevation of left atrial pressures. Although they are benign in nature, death has been reported from bleeding.

• **Goodpasture syndrome** is an autoimmune disease affecting primarily young men. Antibodies against glomerular and alveolar basement membranes produce glomerulonephritis and pulmonary hemorrhage, which leads to hemosiderin deposition and eventually pulmonary fibrosis. Patients may have hepatosplenomegaly, anemia, hypertension, and hematuria.

Pulmonary involvement produces hemoptysis, cough, and dyspnea. Imaging studies show patchy consolidation with perihilar and lower lobe predominance, similar to pulmonary edema. Adenopathy may be present. Renal biopsy shows glomerulonephritis with characteristic IgG deposits. Death occurs as a result of renal failure.

• **Wegener granulomatosis**, an autoimmune disease, is a necrotizing vasculitis characterized by granulomatous involvement of small and medium-sized pulmonary vessels, upper respiratory tract ulcerations, and glomerulonephritis. Symptoms include cough and dyspnea. Most patients are middle-aged. Isolated thoracic involvement is uncommon.

Peripheral or pleural-based pulmonary nodules and cavities are the most common pulmonary manifestation (Figs. 3-39 and 3-40) (**Differential 27**). They often resolve and new nodules develop. A solitary mass is not uncommon. Prominent vessels are common next to the nodules, and they may be thrombosed. Ischemia is suspected as the etiology for cavitation. Pathologic examination demonstrates central necrosis

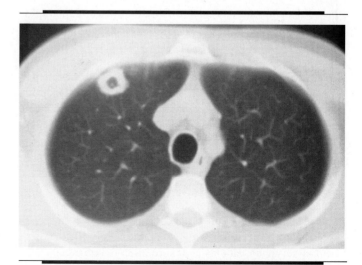

FIGURE 3-40   Wegener granulomatosis. CT showing a cavitary nodule in the right upper lobe in a 50-year-old man.

and granulomatous reaction. Endobronchial granulomas can cause obstruction. Focal or diffuse pulmonary hemorrhage can occur.

Other less common vasculitites affecting the lung include polyarteritis nodosa, Churg-Strauss disease, allergic angiitis, and lymphoid granulomatosis.

3.9 ATELECTASIS AND PULMONARY COLLAPSE

- **Pulmonary atelectasis** or **collapse** findings on chest radiographs have been well described and are generally well known. The two terms will be used interchangeably, with *collapse* referring to a larger degree of atelectasis. On certain occasions the radiographic appearance may be rather bizarre because of associated congenital variants, or more commonly because of fibrous adhesions between the lung and adjacent pleura. One of the most reliable signs of pulmonary collapse is displacement of the pulmonary fissures and mediastinum. CT not only helps clarify the extent of the collapse but also helps determine the etiology (**Differential 34**). Bronchoscopy can be extremely helpful in determining the histologic nature of the obstructing lesion.

- Several types of atelectasis are described depending on the etiology: **Obstructive atelectasis**, the most common form, is seen as a result of endobronchial tumors, foreign bodies, and mucus plugging. **Compressive atelectasis** is the result of adjacent masses that compress normal lung (Fig. 7-10). **Passive atelectasis**, usually occurring as a result of pleural effusions, is the result of insufficent space for the lung to completely expand on inspiration (See Fig. 7-12). **Adhesive atelectasis** is most frequently seen in newborns with hyaline membrane disease and in adults with pulmonary embolism. **Cicatrizing atelectasis** is the result of pulmonary fibrosis and is commonly seen following radiation therapy.

- **Rounded atelectasis** is thought to represent a sequelae of a previous exudative pleural effusion that "traps" the lung as it reabsorbs and forms pleural adhesions. Many causes have been postulated, particularly asbestos. Radiographically, a pseudotumor can be seen, particularly in the dorsal portions of the pulmonary bases. A swirling of the pulmonary vessels and bronchi occurs, producing a "comet tail" adjacent to the medial aspect of the atelectatic parenchyma with thickening of the adjacent pleura (Fig. 3-41). Although the CT findings are usually characteristic, requiring no further imaging, bronchogenic carcinoma may at times mimic the findings of rounded atelectasis (Fig. 3-42).

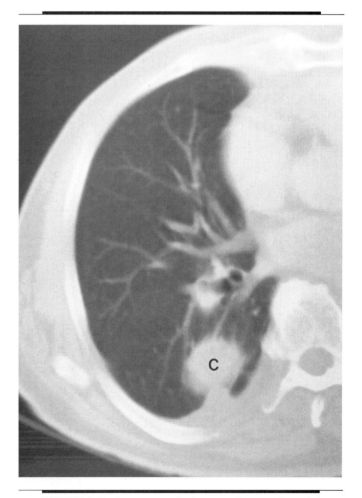

FIGURE 3-41 Rounded atelectasis. CT showing a rounded mass (R) in the right lobe with immediately adjacent pleural thickening (black arrow). Note associated areas of linear atelectasis and deviation of adjacent vessels. There is left-sided pleural thickening with calcification (white arrow) characteristic of prior asbestos exposure.

FIGURE 3-42 Lung cancer sharing some features of rounded atelectasis. CT in an 85-year-old man with an enhancing right lower lobe mass (C) and adjacent pleural thickening. Biopsy revealed primary bronchogenic carcinoma. Note vessels leading directly into mass rather than curving around periphery. (With permission from Sagel SS, Slone RM. The lung. In: Lee JKT, Sagel SS, Stanley RJ, Heiken J, eds. *Computed Body Tomography with MRI Correlation*, 3rd ed. Lippincott-Raven; 1998.)

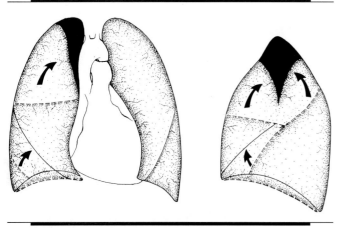
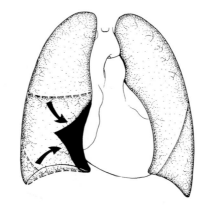
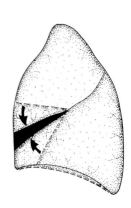

FIGURE 3-43   Right upper lobe collapse. The major and minor fissures (arrows) are displaced superoanteriorly.

FIGURE 3-44   Right middle lobe collapse. Note triangular density with base of triangle against right heart border and anterior chest wall. Major and minor fissures (arrows) move closer together.

- **Right upper lobe collapse** (Fig. 3-8) results in the right upper lobe collapsing superiority and medially. This produces a sharply defined triangular density bordered by the minor fissure laterally and the major fissure posteriorly, with elevation of the right hilum and hyperexpansion of the middle and lower lobes. The minor and upper portion of the major fissure move closer together. On the lateral view, a retrosternal area of increased density is seen anterior to the trachea. The right hemidiaphragm is slightly elevated as a result of volume loss (Fig. 3-43).

- **Right middle lobe collapse** may involve one or both segments. When the medial segment is involved, the frontal radiograph shows an opacity partially obliterating the right atrial border. As the lobe collapses, the minor and major fissures approximate each other. The lateral radiograph shows a triangular density with the base of the triangle against the anterior chest wall (Figs. 3-44 and 3-45). CT can often readily demonstrate the cause of collapse (Fig. 3-27).

- **The right lower lobe collapses** posteromedially, retracting the major and minor fissures inferoposteriorly, displacing the

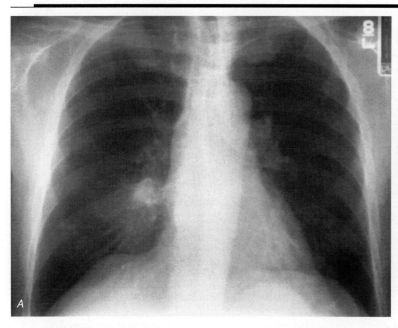
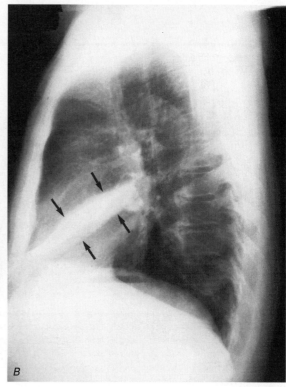

FIGURE 3-45   Right middle lobe collapse. (*A*) PA chest radiograph showing an ill-defined opacity adjacent to the right heart boarder. (*B*) The lateral radiograph shows the collapsed middle lobe sharply marginated by the minor and major fissures (arrows).

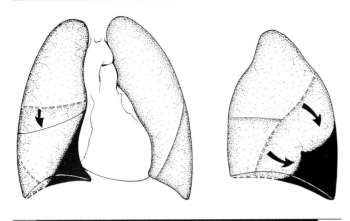
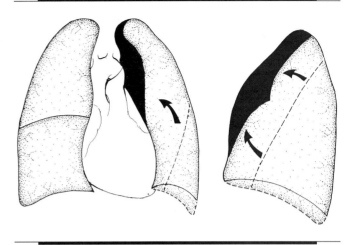

FIGURE 3-46   Right lower lobe collapse. The minor and major fissures (arrows) move inferoposteriorly.

FIGURE 3-47   Left upper lobe collapse. The oblique fissure (arrows) moves superoanteriorly.

right hilum inferiorly, and elevating the right hemidiaphragm (Fig. 3-46). A right paraspinal density is present on the frontal radiograph that silhouettes the right hemidiaphragm.

- The **left upper lobe collapses** in an anterosuperior direction. This causes a density in the left paramediastinal region on the frontal radiograph and in the retrosteral area on the lateral radiograph as the oblique fissure moves anterosuperiorly (Fig. 3-47). Compensatory hyperexpansion of the superior segment of the left lower lobe may cause an area of lucency

in the region of the aortic knob termed the "Luftsichel" sign. (Fig. 3-48).

- **Left lower lobe collapse** causes downward displacement of the left hilum and a left paraspinal density behind or adjacent to the left heart border parallel to the descending aorta (Fig. 3-49). This lobe collapses in a posteromedial direction and displaces the oblique fissure posteriorly (Fig. 3-50). The hyperexpanded left upper lobe appears hyperlucent, whereas the ipsilateral ribs may be approximated due to the volume loss.

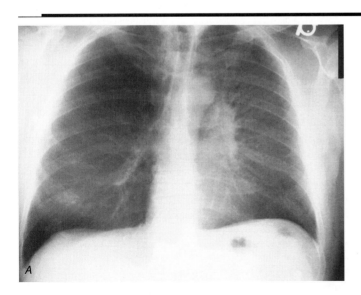
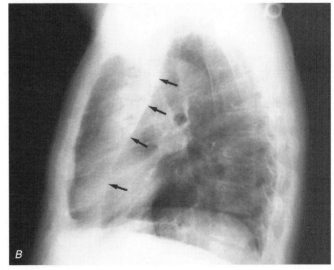

FIGURE 3-48   Left upper lobe collapse due to bronchogenic carcinoma. (A) PA chest radiograph showing an ill-defined density around the left hilum. The left apical lucency represents an hyperexpanded lower lobe. (B) Lateral radiograph showing an anteriorly displaced fissure (arrows).

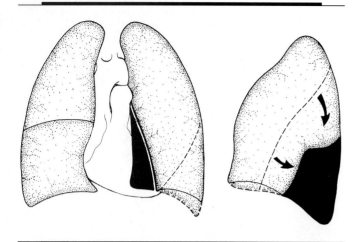

FIGURE 3-49   Left lower lobe collapse. The oblique fissure (arrows) moves in a posteromedial direction.

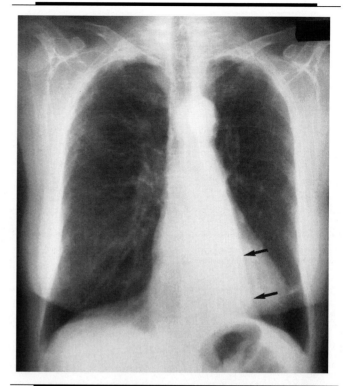

FIGURE 3-50   Left lower lobe collapse. PA chest radiograph in a 75-year-old man with asthma. Bronchoscopy identified a mucus plug as the cause of obstruction. Note the characteristic triangular retrocardiac opacity with a sharp lateral margin (arrows) formed by the major fissure.

Bibliography

Armstrong P, Wilson AG, Dee P, Hansell DM. *Imaging of Diseases of the Chest.* 2nd ed. St. Louis: Mosby-Year Book; 1995.

Chandrasoma P. *Concise Pathology.* 2nd ed. Norwalk, CN: Appleton & Lange;1995.

Dewan NA, Shehan CJ, Reeb SD, Gobar LS, Scott WJ, Ryschon K. Likelihood of malignancy in a solitary pulmonary nodule: Comparison of Bayesian analysis and results of FDG-PET scan. *Chest.* 1997;112(2):416–421.

Eagar G, Royal HD, Deyoe LA, Gutierrez FR. *Radiology of Pulmonary Embolism: RSNA Categorical Course in Diagnostic Radiology—Nuclear Medicine* 1996;79–95. Radiological Society of N.A., Oak Brooks, Illinois.

Fishman AP, Elias JA, Fishman JA, Grippi MA, Kaiser LR, Senior RM. *Fishman's Pulmonary Diseases And Disorders.* 3rd ed. New York: McGraw-Hill; 1998.

Fraser RG, Paré JA, Paré PD, Fraser RS, Genereux GP. *Diagnosis of Diseases of the Chest.* 3rd ed. Philadelphia: WB Saunders; 1989.

Goodman PC, Daley C, Minayi H. Spontaneous pneumothorax in AIDS patients with *Pneumocystis carinii* pneumonia. *Am J Roentgenol.* 1986;147:29–31.

Groskin SA, Massi AF, Randall PA. Calcified hilar and mediastinal lymph nodes in an AIDS patient with *Pneumocystis carinii* infection. *Radiology.* 1990;175(2):345–346.

Keiper MD, Beumont M, Elshami A, Langlotz CP, Miller WT Jr. CD4 T lymphocyte count and the radiographic presentation of pulmonary tuberculosis:

A study of the relationship between these factors in patients with human immunodeficiency virus infection. *Chest.* 1995;107(1):74–80.

Lange S, Walsh G. *Radiology of Chest Diseases.* 2nd ed. Stuttgart: Thieme;1998.

Lee VW, Cooley TP, Fuller JD, Ward RJ, Farber HW. Pulmonary mycobacterial infections in AIDS: Characteristic pattern of thallium and gallium scan mismatch. *Radiology.* 1994;193(2):389–392.

Miller WT Jr. Spectrum of pulmonary nontuberculous mycobacterial infection. *Radiology.* 1994;191(2):343–350.

Nathan MH. Management of solitary pulmonary nodules. *JAMA.* 1974; 227:1141–1144.

Proto AV, Tocino I. Radiographic manifestations of lobar collapse. *Sem Roentgenol.* 1980;15:117–173.

Reed JC. *Chest Radiology: Plain Film Patterns and Differential Diagnosis.* 4th ed. St. Louis: Mosby-Year Book, 1997.

Reeders JWAJ, Mathieson JR. *AIDS Imaging—A Practical Clinical Approach.* Philadelphia: WB Saunders; 1998.

Sha RM, Kaji AV, Ostrum BJ, Friedman AC. Interpretation of chest radiographs in AIDS patients: Usefulness of CD4 lymphocyte counts. *Radiographics.* 1997;17(1):47–58.

Swensen SJ. *Radiology of Thoracic Diseases: A Teaching File.* St. Louis: Mosby-Year Book; 1993.

Winn WC, Walker DH. *Viral Infections in Pulmonary Pathology.* Dail DH, Hammar SP, eds. 2nd ed. New York: Springer-Verlag.

Chapter 4

DIFFUSE LUNG DISEASE

Richard M. Slone

4.1 EVALUATING DIFFUSE LUNG DISEASE

- There are over 100 causes of diffuse infiltrative, airspace, and airway disease, but less than 20 are routinely encountered. Imaging in conjunction with clinical data, including pulmonary function testing, is the standard approach for evaluation. **Chest radiography** is the primary imaging technique but is insensitive for detecting mild infiltrative lung disease, bronchiectasis, and emphysema.

- **Computed tomography (CT)** allows earlier detection and better characterization, especially when performed using high-resolution techniques. Specific diagnosis may require transbronchial or open lung biopsy for pathologic evaluation. Imaging can help guide the location for these procedures. Currently, **magnetic resonance (MR) imaging** has no role in evaluating diffuse lung disease.

- **High-resolution CT (HRCT)** with representative 1- to 2-mm-thick sections at 1- to 5-cm increments, a minimal field of view, and high spatial frequency reconstruction enhances spatial resolution, providing detailed images comparable to gross tissue inspection. HRCT is sensitive for detecting, characterizing, and establishing the extent of disease, and for following response to treatment (Fig. 1-18). (See Section 1.4 for more details on HRCT technique.)

   When HRCT alone is performed, small vessels can be mistaken as pathologic nodules and true nodules can be missed. Depending on the clinical history, HRCT should be performed in conjunction with conventional CT using 5- to 10-mm-thick contiguous sections.

   Conventional CT is actually superior for evaluating micronodular patterns since more nodules are included in each section and there is better demonstration of branching vessels and bronchi; however, low-density micronodules may be obscured because of volume averaging.

   Scans obtained supine often have an area of gravity-induced increased density, termed **dependent atelectasis**, adjacent to the posterior chest wall that can be mistaken for pulmonary infiltrate or fibrosis. Scanning in the prone position reverses the distribution of this microatelectasis, and obtaining one exam supine and one prone allows confident distinction between gravity-related changes and pulmonary fibrosis.

- **Expiratory HRCT** may accentuate differences between normal and abnormal lung parenchyma in patients with air trapping in comparison with standard CT. Expiratory HRCT may be more sensitive than spirometry for detecting subtle air trapping in patients with emphysema and can be abnormal in patients with normal inspiratory scans having small-airways disease, such as bronchiolitis obliterans.

- **The secondary pulmonary lobule** is the primary structural and functional unit of the lung, visible on HRCT as a 2- to 3-cm regular polyhedron with thin, straight walls (Fig. 1-3). It is composed of *interlobular septa* which contain the pulmonary veins, lymphatics, and connective tissue, and about ten acini supplied by three to five terminal bronchioles separated by *intralobular septa*, which are visible only if thickened. Small dots or Y-shaped structures within the center represent the terminal airways and pulmonary arterioles (Fig. 4-1).

4.2 PATTERNS OF DISEASE

- **Diffuse lung disease** encompasses a broad array of patterns and etiologies. In general, diffuse disease can be divided into processes involving primarily the airspace, interstitium, or airways. Interstitial disease is the most common. Interstitial and airspace disease often coexist. Pure airspace disease is the least common pattern of parenchymal lung disease.

Diffuse
Dz. č Avol : LAM
CF
EG
Emphysema

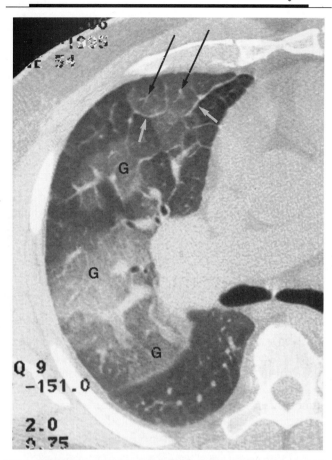

FIGURE 4-1   Septal thickening and ground-glass attenuation.
HRCT in a patient with congestive heart failure, showing areas of
ground-glass attenuation (G). Accumulation of fluid in the interstitium thickens the interlobular septa (white arrows) outlining the secondary pulmonary lobule. The central opacity (black arrows)
represents the terminal arteriole and bronchiole. (With permission
from Sagel SS, Slone RM. The lung. In: Lee JKT, Sagel SS, Stanley
RJ, Heiken JP, eds. In: *Computed Body Tomography with MRI Correlation.* 3rd ed. New York: Lippincott-Raven, 1998.)

Once established, a differential diagnosis can be refined
based on lung volumes, chronicity, global and regional distribution, associated findings such as pleural disease or adenopathy, and clinical symptoms.

- Most interstitial lung disease results in reduced **lung volumes** and a restrictive pattern of pulmonary function;
however, normal or increased lung volumes can be seen
in patients with eosinophilic granulomatosis, lymphangio-
myomatosis, cystic fibrosis, and concomitant emphysema
(Fig. 1-19) or asthma (**Differential 50***) (Fig. 4-2).

- Some diseases favor particular patterns of distribution, which
is helpful in narrowing the differential. Silicosis and cystic
fibrosis have predominantly upper lung involvement, sarcoid
often has midlung involvement, and pulmonary fibrosis typi-

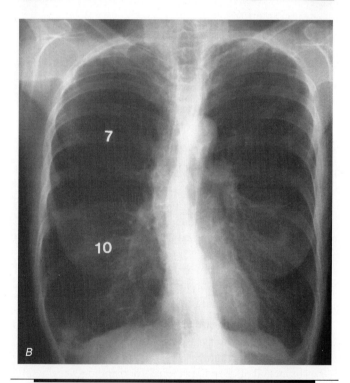

FIGURE 4-2   Lung volumes. (*A*) Chest radiograph in a 61-year-
old woman with idiopathic pulmonary fibrosis demonstrating
markedly reduced lung volumes and predominantly peripheral and
basilar honeycombing. (*B*) Chest radiograph in a 57-year-old
woman with advanced emphysema, demonstrating hyperlucent
lungs with parenchymal destruction, thoracic distention, and
downward displacement of the diaphragm. Note the position of the
seventh (7) and tenth (10) posterior ribs.

cally has a lower lung distribution. Kaposi sarcoma and sarcoidosis are characterized by a bronchovascular distribution
(**Differentials 10–14**).

- **Interstitial lung disease** involves the supporting structures
that surround the airspaces, including the bronchovascular
bundles, fissures, and interlobular and intralobular septa and

---

*Please refer to Chapter 2, in which the differential diagnoses are
discussed in numerical order.

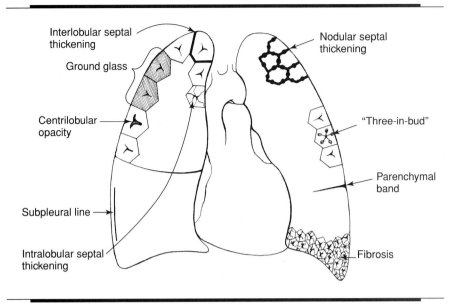

FIGURE 4-3   HRCT patterns. Illustrating the relative appearance of various patterns of diffuse lung disease.

may present as thickened septa, areas of reticulation, or nodules. HRCT is particularly well suited for evaluating interstitial lung disease (Fig. 4-3). The most common and earliest sign is indistinct bronchovascular margins and irregular thickening of the visceral pleura and fissures.

- **Smooth septal thickening** is the result of fluid or cellular infiltrates within the interlobular septa, most commonly pulmonary edema (Fig. 4-1). There is often a dependent distribution, associated cardiac enlargement, and pleural effusions (**Differentials 45, 46, 61, and 62**).

- **Irregular septal thickening** without architectural distortion, sometimes referred to as the "beaded septum sign," may be seen with lymphangitic carcinomatosis, sarcoidosis, and coal worker pneumoconiosis (**Differential 47**).

- **Honeycombing** refers to irreversible fibrosis, with coarse interstitial thickening and associated architectural distortion, typically as a result of end-stage lung disease. Traction on the pulmonary parenchyma produces cystic airspaces and bronchiectasis (**Differentials 56–59 and 64**).

- **Parenchymal bands** are elongated fibrotic opacities, several millimeters in width and up to 5 cm in length, extending to the pleura, which may be thickened or retracted.

- **Subpleural lines** are curvilinear opacities, only a few millimeters in thickness, which are parallel and usually less than 1 cm from the pleura. They result from atelectasis, edema, fibrosis, or inflammation.

- **Ground glass**, a pattern simulating frosted window glass, refers to a nonspecific pattern of increased parenchymal attenuation with preservation of bronchial and vascular margins as a result of alveolar septal inflammation or edema; partial filling of airspaces by macrophages, histiocytes, or other material; alveolar atelectasis; or rarely fibrosis below the resolution of CT. HRCT may reveal subtle areas of inflammation not evident on radiography or conventional CT. The most common cause is pneumonitis, alveolitis, or edema (**Differential 60**) (Fig. 4-4).

- **Airspace disease** may be diffuse or focal but, in general, spares the peripheral lung where interstitial processes are most prominent. In its earliest form, airspace disease may appear as an area of ground-glass attenuation or involve only the acinus where fluid-filled alveoli appear as small, ill-defined nodules. These nodules become confluent, resulting in lobular, subsegmental, or lobar areas of consolidation (Fig. 4-5).

- **Pulmonary consolidation** refers to homogeneous increased parenchymal attenuation that obscures vessels and airway walls, often producing air bronchograms. The most common cause is pneumonia (**Differentials 36–44**) (Fig. 4-6).

- **Cystic lung disease** refers to abnormal air-containing spaces within the lung, including dilated bronchi, pneumatoceles, cavities, blebs, and bullae resulting from inflammation, obstruction, necrosis, congenital abnormalities, neoplasm, lung retraction due to fibrosis, or areas of destruction caused by emphysema (**Differentials 23–25 and 65**).

- **Bullae** are round, air-containing spaces, larger than 1 cm, generally representing emphysema. **Blebs** occur within the pleural layers. A **cyst** is a round space with a well-defined wall lined by epithelium or fibrous tissue usually containing air, but without emphysema.

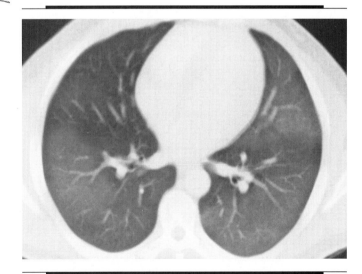

FIGURE 4-4   Noncardiogenic pulmonary edema. HRCT showing diffuse ground-glass attenuation following cocaine overdose. (With permission from Sagel SS, Slone RM. The lung. In: Lee JKT, Sagel SS, Stanley RJ, Heiken JP, eds. In: *Computed Body Tomography with MRI Correlation.* 3rd ed. New York: Lippincott-Raven, 1998.)

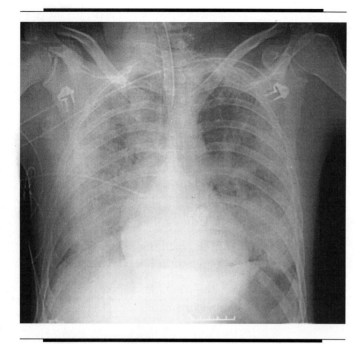

FIGURE 4-5   Pulmonary hemorrhage in Wegener granulomatosis. Portable chest radiograph showing diffuse predominantly airspace disease in a 19-year-old with alveolar hemorrhage confirmed at bronchoscopy.

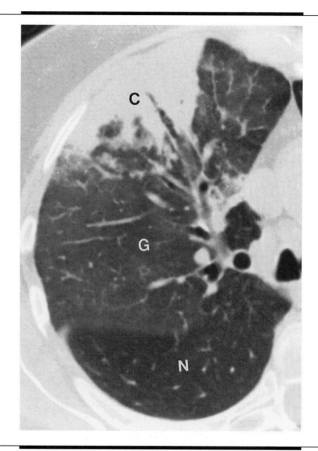

FIGURE 4-6   Pneumonia. HRCT demonstrating normal lung parenchyma posteriorly (N), ground-glass attenuation (G) that does not obliterate vessels, and consolidation (C) anteriorly where the vessels are obliterated and air bronchograms are seen. (With permission from Sagel SS, Slone RM. The lung. In: Lee JKT, Sagel SS, Stanley RJ, Heiken JP, eds. In: *Computed Body Tomography with MRI Correlation.* 3rd ed. New York: Lippincott-Raven, 1998.)

- **Honeycomb cyst** refers to focal airspaces, typically less than 1 cm, formed as a result of lung retraction by pulmonary fibrosis. They are typically subpleural and largest in the upper lobes. Honeycomb cysts and bronchiolectasis decrease in size on expiration as a result of free communication with the airway, whereas bullae do not (**Differentials 64 and 65**).

- **Air trapping** can be the result of fixed bronchial narrowing or reactive airway disease due to bronchial spasms. It is a characteristic finding in asthma, COPD, and bronchiolitis obliterans where it is caused by narrowing and occlusion of noncartilaginous bronchioles by granulation tissue. **Expiratory HRCT** is sensitive for demonstrating the differential attenuation between areas of air trapping and normal lung.

- **Mosaic perfusion**, or **mosaic oligemia**, refers to a lobular or multilobular patchwork pattern of varied attenuation specifically due to regional differences in perfusion. A more lucent, oligemic lung has a decreased number and size of pulmonary vessels compared to normal lung. Causes include thromboembolic disease, cystic fibrosis, bronchiolitis obliterans, infection, and hemorrhage.

  A pattern of **mosaic attenuation** can also be caused by infiltrative or inflammatory lung disease producing areas of high attenuation. The size and number of vessels do not differ between the two regions of lung. Patients with small-airways disease, such as asthma or bronchiolitis obliterans, may have a pattern of mosaic attenuation seen only on expiration, with lucent areas of air trapping adjacent to normal lung parenchyma.

- **Interstitial nodules** can be seen with sarcoidosis, histiocytosis-X, pneumoconioses, tuberculosis, hypersensitivity pneumonitis, pulmonary metastases, and amyloidosis. Nodular lesions in close proximity to blood vessels suggest a hematogenous process such as metastases, pulmonary infarcts, or septic emboli (**Differentials 19–21 and 66**).

- **Centrilobular nodules** may be seen on HRCT as a result of inflammation of the terminal briochioles (**Differential 69**). The *tree-in-bud* sign refers to nodular dilatation of the centrilobular branching structures.

- The **CT halo sign** (Fig. 3-20), originally described in association with invasive pulmonary aspergillus, refers to a rim of ground-glass attenuation due to edema and hemorrhage surrounding infectious and noninfectious nodules (**Differential 20**).

- Areas of high attenuation in the lung may be caused by **calcification**, iodine, barium, or radiopaque foreign bodies. Multiple parenchymal calcifications are most commonly the result of prior granulomatous infections but can be seen with other infections and pneumoconioses (**Differential 22**).

Metastases from osteogenic sarcoma, mucin-producing adenocarcinomas, and treated metastases may also calcify.

- **Pulmonary ossification** is an exceedingly rare condition consisting of mature bone formation within lung. It most commonly occurs in association with chronic cardiopulmonary disease, particularly mitral stenosis, but may be idiopathic or associated with pulmonary fibrosis due to chemotherapy, asbestos exposure, hemodialysis, acromegaly, or metastatic cancer.

4.3 PULMONARY EDEMA AND ACUTE RESPIRATORY DISTRESS SYNDROME

- **Pulmonary edema** is the most common cause of pulmonary infiltrates and is typically diagnosed based on radiographic and clinical information. Edema may be the result of increased pulmonary venous pressure (hydrostatic edema) due to congestive heart failure (CHF) or volume overload, reduced intravascular oncotic pressure, lymphatic obstruction, or increased vascular permeability due to capillary damage (noncardiogenic edema). Radiologic findings of hydrostatic edema can precede clinical manifestations which include dyspnea and peripheral edema, and when advanced, hypoxemia and mildly hemorrhagic sputum, and also may persist radiographically after clinical recovery.

- **Hydrostatic edema** is usually associated with cardiomegaly, but the heart size may be normal in cases of acute myocardial infarction or acute valve dysfunction. Impaired pulmonary venous return, most commonly a result of left ventricular failure, fluid overload, renal failure, or mitral valve disease leads to an increased pulmonary blood volume. Enlargement of pulmonary vessels allows smaller vessels not typically visualized to be seen, contributing to a "crowded" or "congested" appearance.

    Cephalization of pulmonary blood flow, termed *redistribution,* is one of the earliest findings and refers to relative enlargement of the upper lobe pulmonary vessels which are normally about half the size of lower lobe vessels. This is a combined effect of constriction and reduced compliance of lower lobe vessels which are surrounded by small amounts of interstitial fluid and decreased lower lobe ventilation leading to hypoxic vasoconstriction. The gradient changes to anteroposterior in supine patients. Redistribution is first seen when pulmonary capillary wedge pressures exceed 16 mmHg.

    As pulmonary venous pressures increase above about 20 mmHg, fluid leaks into the interstitium and the capacity of the lymphatic drainage is exceeded. Smooth septal and peribronchial thickening, fissural thickening due to subpleural edema, and pleural effusions develop (**Differentials 45 and 52**). Vessel margins become indistinct as a result of perivascular **interstitial edema.**

    Edema is usually greater in the perihilar regions and lung bases because of the higher hydrostatic pressure. **Kerley B lines** are thin, smooth peripheral septal lines representing interlobular septal fluid. **Kerley A lines** are central, are longer, and radiate from the hila; they are the result of fluid in the central bronchovascular interstitium.

    Diffuse, patchy, occasionally asymmetric **airspace edema** develops as the pulmonary capillary wedge pressure exceeds about 25 mmHg and fluid begins to enter the alveoli (Fig. 4-7). This impairs gas exchange, leading to hypoxemia and hypercapnea. Reduced compliance contributes to reduced lung volumes. The presence and patterns of edema can change rapidly. Chronic congestive failure can lead to fibrosis and hemosiderin-laden macrophages.

    Marked asymmetry can be seen as a consequence of lateral decubitus positioning, thromboembolism, tumor invasion of the pulmonary vessels, or underlying lung disease (**Differential 53**). Predominantly right upper lobe edema can rarely be seen with mitral regurgitation, presumably related to the direction of the regurgitant jet. Emphysema and fibrosis can alter the normal pattern of edema, leading to atypical patterns that mimic pneumonia. Superimposed pulmonary edema can make diagnosis of concomitant disease such as pneumonia difficult.

- **Noncardiogenic pulmonary edema** is the result of increased capillary permeability with leakage of fluid primarily into the airspaces (**Differential 52**). Vessel size and pressures are normal, and there are usually no pleural effusions or cardiomegaly.

    Acute upper airway obstruction from strangulation or laryngospasm can occasionally cause pulmonary edema, likely a combined effect of hypoxia, negative intrathoracic pressure, and neurologic factors. **Neurogenic edema** is the result of systemic vasoconstriction and increased capillary permeability associated with brain trauma, hemorrhage, or tumor. **Near-drowning** has a similar appearance (Fig. 4-8).

    High-altitude edema can occur following ascents over 9000 ft. Symptoms include dyspnea and cough. Patchy edema develops over 1 to 2 days and is usually activity-related. Cardiac size and pulmonary pressures are normal. The edema clears with oxygen therapy and return to normal altitude.

    Reexpansion pulmonary edema occurs following rapid drainage of a large pneumothorax or pleural effusion in which there was chronic pulmonary collapse or extraction of a large pulmonary embolism (reperfusion edema). It develops within a few hours and is likely a combined result of surfactant depletion and increased capillary permeability. It may progress over 1 to 2 days and usually resolves within a week.

- **Acute respiratory distress syndrome (ARDS)**, sometimes called "shock lung," refers to a constellation of severe respiratory distress, marked dyspnea, hypoxemia, and diffuse airspace consolidation as a result of severe medical or traumatic insult, causing diffuse alveolar damage. Common causes include septic or hemorrhagic shock, massive trauma, burns, acute pancreatitis, aspiration, drug intoxication, severe pneumonia, fat or amniotic fluid embolism, near-drowning, inhalation injury, and anaphylaxis (**Differential 52**).

    ARDS may develop rapidly or take days to develop, but often there is up to a 12-hour delay between onset of clinical symptoms and the appearance of radiographic abnormalities.

In contrast, radiographic abnormalities may appear prior to clinical symptoms in hydrostatic edema. Interstitial edema and diffuse, patchy ill-defined opacities develop in the first

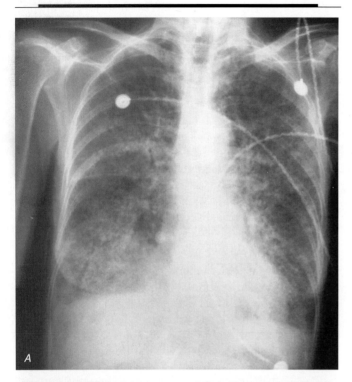

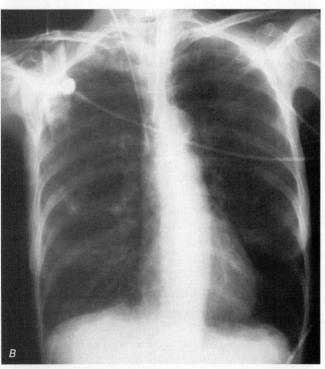

FIGURE 4-7   Flash pulmonary edema. (*A*) Portable chest radiograph showing severe diffuse interstitial and alveolar infiltrates and small pleural effusions in a 71-year-old woman with significant mitral regurgitation and coronary artery disease. Pulmonary edema was associated with a sudden ischemic episode. (*B*) Portable chest radiograph 17 hours later following intubation and placement of a central venous catheter showing resolution of the pulmonary edema.

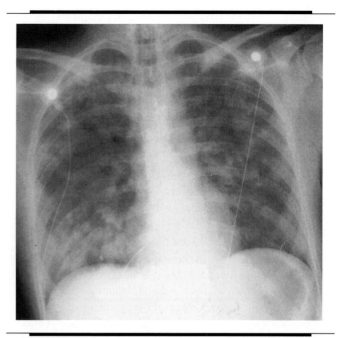

FIGURE 4-8   Near-drowning. Portable chest radiograph in a 34-year-old man following near-drowning. There are symmetric, predominantly airspace infiltrates diffusely distributed throughout both lungs characteristic of alveolar edema.

24 hours. This condition progresses to diffuse airspace consolidation with hemorrhagic alveolar edema and microatelectasis by 48 hours.

There is usually no cardiomegaly or pleural effusion, although patients with concomitant CHF may have these symptoms. Lung volumes decrease as a result of reduced compliance. The pulmonary disease may resolve, but fibrosis often develops, sometimes as early as 7 days. Treatment includes positive pressure ventilation and is primarily supportive to maintain cerebral and renal perfusion, prevent infection, and minimize barotrauma. Mortality, usually from multisystem failure, is common. Pneumothoracies, pneumomediastinum, and pneumonia are frequent complications.

4.4 LARGE-AIRWAYS DISEASE AND BRONCHIECTASIS

- **Bronchiectasis** refers to irreversible bronchial dilatation with bronchial wall thickening. It is the result of an inflammatory process, most commonly prior bacterial infections, but can also result from obstruction or congenital abnormalities such as cystic fibrosis, dysmotile cilia (Kartagener) syndrome, hypogammaglobulinemia, allergic bronchopulmonary aspergillosis (ABPA), impaired mucocilliary clearance, or other immunodeficiencies (**Differential 35**) (Fig. 4-9).

Symptoms include chronic cough, frequent recurrent infections, and sometimes hemoptysis. Medical management with antibiotics and respiratory therapy is the mainstay, but surgical resection of advanced localized disease may be

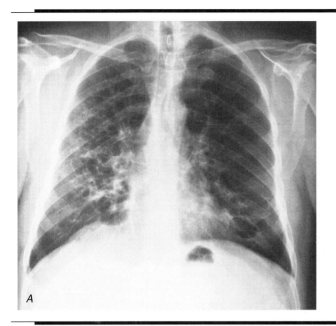 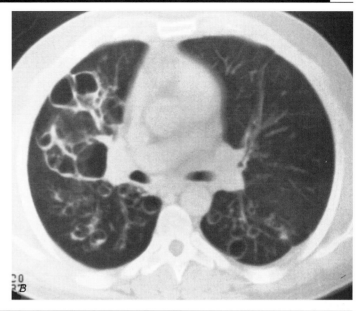

FIGURE 4-9   Bronchiectasis. (*A*) Chest radiograph showing cystic lucencies throughout the right lung and left base. (*B*) CT confirms cystic bronchiectasis.

warranted. Life-threatening bronchial artery hemorrhage may require emergency embolization.

   Idiopathic bronchiectasis is the most common etiology. It is often focal and most common in the lower lobes. Focal bronchiectasis can also result from bronchial stenosis or occlusion by benign or malignant endobronchial lesions with resultant mucoid impaction.

   The distribution and morphology of bronchiectasis generally differs depending on the cause, but there is considerable overlap between idiopathic and known causes. Impaired mucocilliary clearance and hypogammaglobulinemia have a lower lobe predominance. Cystic fibrosis has an upper lobe predominance. Bronchiectasis associated with ABPA is often central.

* **Bronchial wall thickening** or stenosis without dilatation is most commonly the result of bronchitis but can be seen with sarcoidosis, Wegener granulomatosis, amyloid deposition, and other inflammatory conditions. Normally the bronchial wall thickness is no more than 10 percent of the bronchial diameter. **Diseases of the trachea** are covered in Section 5.6.

* **Chronic bronchitis** is a clinical diagnosis based on excessive sputum production. Although imaging studies are usually normal, bronchial wall thickening without enlargement can be seen (Fig. 4-10).

* Although bronchography was previously required in many cases for the accurate diagnosis of bronchiectasis (Fig. 4-11), CT, specifically **HRCT,** has emerged as the imaging modality of choice for evaluating bronchiectasis. Radiography is relatively insensitive, and mild bronchiectasis can be overlooked on conventional CT. Abnormal findings include lack of tapering of bronchi, bronchial dilatation, wall thickening,

and mucus filling. The most striking abnormality is often visualization of bronchi further in the periphery of the lung than typically seen. Bronchi in the peripheral third of the lung on conventional CT or within a few centimeters of the pleura on HRCT suggests bronchiectasis.

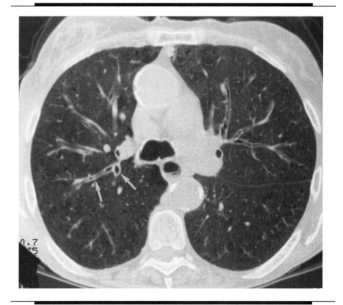

FIGURE 4-10 Bronchial wall thickening. HRCT showing bronchial wall thickening (arrows) due to chronic bronchitis. Note also small focal lucent areas of lung destruction characteristic of centrilobular emphysema. (With permission from Sagel SS, Slone RM. The lung. In: Lee JKT, Sagel SS, Stanley RJ, Heiken JP, eds. In: *Computed Body Tomography with MRI Correlation.* 3rd ed. New York: Lippincott-Raven, 1998.)

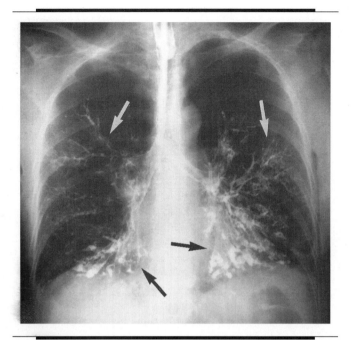

FIGURE 4-11 Bronchogram. Bronchography, now only of historical interest, was previously the modality of choice for imaging bronchiectasis. This examination shows contrast coating nearly the complete tracheobronchial tree with areas of cylindrical and saccular bronchiectasis, predominantly in the lower lobes (black arrows). There are normal bronchi in the upper lobes (white arrows).

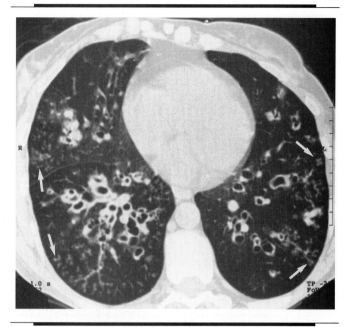

FIGURE 4-12 Bronchiectasis and bronchiolitis. HRCT showing central bronchiectasis and peripheral nodular opacities (arrows), termed tree-in-bud pattern, representing inflamed terminal bronchioles in a centrilobular distribution. (With permission from Sagel SS, Slone RM. The lung. In: Lee JKT, Sagel SS, Stanley RJ, Heiken JP, eds. *Computed Body Tomography with MRI Correlation.* 3rd ed. New York: Lippincott-Raven, 1998.)

The appearance of ectatic bronchi varies depending on their orientation. (Fig. 4-12). Bronchi in cross section appear as thickened rings, and bronchi in the plane of section as parallel thickened lines called "tram lines." In general, bronchi should be no larger than 1.2 times the diameter of the accompanying pulmonary artery. "Signet ring sign" refers to the relative enlargement of the bronchi in cross section as compared to the pulmonary artery, resulting in the artery forming the "stone" and the ectatic bronchi forming the "band" of the ring.

- **Bronchiectasis** is often classified as cylindrical, varicose, or saccular (cystic), although mixed patterns are common and distinction has little clinical impact (Fig. 4-13).

    Cylindrical or tubular bronchiectasis, referring to uniform fusiform dilatation of bronchi with loss of normal tapering and abrupt termination, is the most common type. It appears as thickened parallel lines when seen longitudinally, and thickened rings when viewed in cross section. It is seen in idiopathic, hypogammaglobulinemia, and impaired mucocilliary clearance syndromes. When confined to the central lung in asthmatics, ABPA is often the cause.

Varicose bronchiectasis presents as a "beaded" appearance caused by alternating areas of dilatation and bronchial constriction and is often seen in cystic fibrosis.

Cystic or saccular bronchiectasis is manifested by marked bronchial dilatation with peripheral ballooning producing cystic cavities, often with thick walls and air-fluid

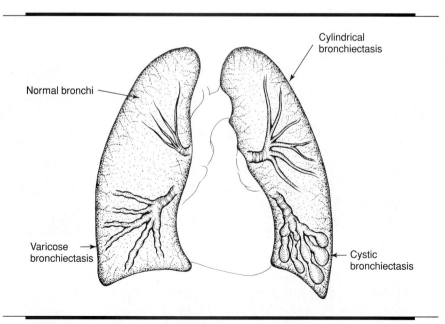

FIGURE 4-13 Patterns of bronchiectasis. Illustrating three common patterns of bronchiectasis.

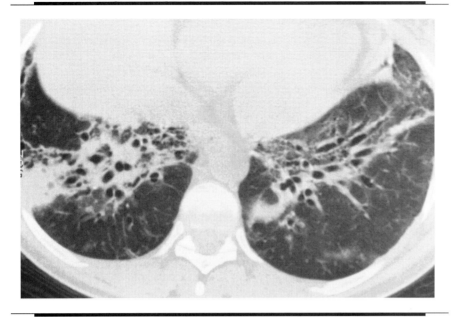

FIGURE 4-14 Traction bronchiolectasis. HRCT in stage IV sarcoidosis showing traction bronchiolectasis as a consequence of fibrosis rather than intrinsic airway disease. (With permission from Sagel SS, Slone RM. The lung. In: Lee JKT, Sagel SS, Stanley RJ, Heiken JP, eds. *Computed Body Tomography with MRI Correlation.* 3rd ed. New York: Lippincott-Raven, 1998.)

levels due to retained secretions (Fig. 1-12). It is often associated with bronchial stenosis.

- **Traction bronchiectasis** is a result of fibrotic distortion of the lung parenchyma caused by infection, radiation therapy, or end-stage lung disease rather than intrinsic airway disease. Traction bronchiectasis is common in the lung periphery of patients with fibrosis and contributes to the appearance of honeycombing (Fig. 4-14).

- **Mucoid impaction** in dilated bronchi is common. It may be seen as an isolated entity or in association with cystic fibrosis, ABPA, bronchial atresia, pulmonary sequestration, or as a result of bronchial obstruction by intrinsic or extrinsic lesions. The branching tubular opacities do not enhance following intravenous (IV) contrast, allowing distinction from vascular structures. Dilated mucus-filled bronchi may simulate pulmonary nodules.

- **Reversible bronchiectasis** refers to transient cylindrical bronchial dilatation seen primarily in children as a result of bronchial inflammation from bacterial pneumonia. The bronchial dilatation may persist for several months after resolution of the pneumonia, but follow-up studies show a return to normal diameter. Care should be taken in diagnosing bronchiectasis in the presence of acute infection.

- **Pseudobronchiectasis** is produced as a result of motion artifacts on CT. In particular, blurring of the fissures and vessels can simulate dilated bronchi seen in longitudinal section. Inspection of the section above and below almost always confirms the true nature of the finding. Inappropriate window settings can also produce a misleading appearance. Thickening of the bronchial walls can be simulated on thick-

section CT when bronchi take an oblique course through the imaging plane.

Some cystic pulmonary lesions may superficially mimic bronchiectasis such as histiocytosis-X, cystic *Pneumocystis carinii* pneumonia (PCP), cavitary metastases, or tracheopapillomatosis. These lesions are round rather than tubular and are not associated with pulmonary vessels as are dilated bronchi.

- **Allergic bronchopulmonary aspergillosis,** which represents a hypersensitivity to *Aspergillus*, presents as central, upper lobe predominant bronchiectasis with mucus plugging in patients with asthma (Fig. 4-15). Peripheral bronchi are normal. Atelectasis and transient or fixed postobstructive pneumonitis can be seen, and patients may develop pulmonary fibrosis. Patients have blood eosinophilia, positive skin reactions and elevated serum IgE.

- **Dysmotile cilia syndrome**, called Kartagener syndrome (Fig. 9-16) when situs inversus is present, is a deficiency in the dynein arms of the cilia resulting in abnormal mucocilliary function. This dysfunction causes sinusitis, bronchiectasis, deafness, and infertility. Imaging studies show hyperinflation, bronchiaectasis, and situs inversus in one-half of patients (see Section 9.2).

- **Cystic fibrosis**, also called fibrocystic disease and mucoviscidosis, is an autosomal recessive disease characterized by exocrine gland dysfunction and viscous secretions. It is the most common congenital disorder, affecting 1 in 1600 live births. One in 20 individuals is a heterozygous carrier. The highest incidence is in Caucasians. There are several associated genes and mutations resulting in variable severity, but all are associated with defective cell transport of salt and water.

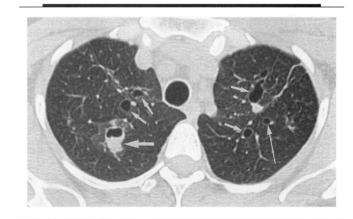

FIGURE 4-15 ABPA. HRCT showing central bronchiectasis (small arrows) and mucus plugging (large arrow) in a 29-year-old asthmatic. Note the "signet ring" appearance of a dilated bronchus next to an artery (long arrow).

Diagnosis is usually based on clinical presentation. Excessive salt excretion by sweat glands is characteristic.

Pulmonary manifestations, particularly recurrent pneumonia caused by viscous mucus and mucus plugging, cause the greatest morbidity and mortality. *Staphylococcus* and *Pseudomonas* are common organisms. Radiographs show hyperinflation, bronchitis with peribronchial infiltration, upper lobe-predominant bronchiectasis up to 2 cm in diameter (frequently containing fluid), interstitial disease, emphysema, mucous plugging and atelectasis, variable degrees of adenopathy, and enlarged pulmonary arteries due to hypertension (Fig. 9-17) .

Increased salivary secretions, nasal polyps, and sinusitis affect the upper respiratory tract. Pancreatic involvement produces pancreatic insufficiency, meconium ileus, pancreatitis, and diabetes mellitus. Liver involvement may produce billiary cirrhosis, leading to portal hypertension, varices, and hypersplenism. The gallbladder wall may thicken. Females have reduced fertility, and males have hypoplasia of the vas deferens, epididymis, and seminal vesicles.

Complications include pneumothorax due to rupture of emphysematous blebs, hemoptysis, lung abscesses, and empyemas. Death is usually the result of respiratory failure often associated with massive hemoptysis or cor pulmonale. Improved medical management including antibiotics and occasionally lung transplantation has improved survival, but life expectancy is reduced. A delayed presentation and a more mild course is seen in some patients who present as adults with cylindrical bronchiectasis as opposed to the younger patients who have cystic and varicose patterns.

4.5 SMALL-AIRWAYS DISEASE

- Chest radiographs are often normal in patients with small-airways disease, and CT results can even appear normal despite abnormal pulmonary function tests. Detection of subtle disease is best accomplished using expiratory HRCT which can demonstrate the structural and functional abnormalities to better advantage.

- **Asthma** is a hypersensitivity reaction, producing reversible bronchoconstriction causing dyspnea, coughing, and wheezing. *Intrinsic asthma* is caused by an autoimmune phenomenon related to infection, exercise, or drugs but not environmental antigens. *Extrinsic asthma* is an immediate hypersensitivity response with histamine release by mast cells. Allergens include pollens, animal fur, spores, dust, and chemicals. Bronchial wall edema and hypertrophy of bronchial smooth muscle and mucus glands leads to mucus plugging.

  Radiologic findings may include hyperinflation, bronchial wall thickening, and localized air trapping during acute exacerbations, although the radiograph is most often normal. Chronic changes can include bronchiectasis and scarring from recurring infections. Patients are predisposed to pneumonia and may have peripheral infiltrates due to airway obstruction or atelectasis from mucoid impaction. Complications include pneumomediastinum and pneumothorax.

- **Bronchiolitis** refers to inflammation, and sometimes fibrosis involving primarily the small airways, caused by damage to bronchiolar epithelium. *Proliferative bronchiolitis* is the result of an organizing intraluminal exudate, in contrast to *constrictive bronchiolitis* which involves the membranous and respiratory bronchial walls. **Bronchiolitis obliterans** is characterized by granulomatous inflammation within bronchioles and alveolar ducts, producing small-airways obstruction.

  Causes include pulmonary infections, smoke, toxic fume or dust exposure, drug toxicity, graft-versus-host and auto-immune disease, lung transplantation, and connective tissue disorders, but it is often idiopathic. Patients develop a non-productive cough, dyspnea, fever, or other nonspecific symptoms that do not respond to antibiotics. Radiologic findings include hyperinflation and bronchiolectasis. HRCT may show patchy air trapping on expiration, centrilobular branching structures and nodules (Fig. 4-12), mosaic perfusion with areas of hypoventilation, and decreased blood flow due to vessel constriction.

- **Swyer-James syndrome**, referring to a small, hyperlucent lung with diminished vascular supply, is believed to be a result of bronchiolitis obliterans occurring in early childhood as a complication of a viral infection (see Section 9.4).

- **Diffuse panbronchiolitis**, characterized by diffuse airway inflammation, affects primarily Asians. Patients present with bronchiectasis and bronchiolectasis and peripheral nodular opacities representing dilated opacified bronchioles.

- **Bronchiolitis obliterans with organizing pneumonia (BOOP)** also referred to as cryptogenic organizing pneumonia (COP), is the most common cause of proliferative bron-

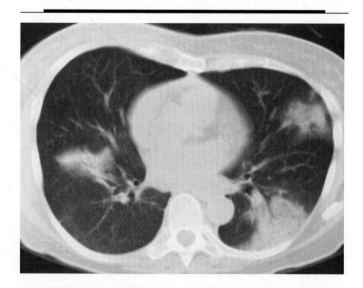

FIGURE 4-16   BOOP. CT showing focal areas of predominantly peripheral consolidation as a consequence of granulomatous bronchial inflammation. (With permission from Sagel SS, Slone RM. The lung. In: Lee JKT, Sagel SS, Stanley RJ, Heiken JP, eds. *Computed Body Tomography with MRI Correlation.* 3rd ed. New York: Lippincott-Raven, 1998.)

chiolitis. It is the result of polypoid granulation tissue obstructing bronchioles and alveolar ducts, with organizing pneumonia and inflammatory cells infiltrating the airspace and interstitium. It affects middle-aged men and women. Patients typically experience several weeks of upper respiratory symptoms and nonproductive cough.

Radiographs typically show bilateral patchy ground-glass infiltrates and areas of peripheral consolidation, presumably representing postobstructive pneumonitis, sometimes with pulmonary nodules, bronchial wall thickening, and dilation. The appearance often simulates bronchial pneumonia, but steroids rather than antibiotics are the treatment of choice (Fig. 4-16). Peripheral consolidation can also be seen with chronic eosinophilic pneumonia, sarcoidosis, and lymphoproliferative disorders.

4.6 PULMONARY EMPHYSEMA

- **Pulmonary emphysema** is a chronic condition characterized by progressive irreversible enlargement of airspaces distal to the terminal bronchiole with destruction of the alveolar walls and no obvious fibrosis. It results in loss of lung elastic recoil, causing airflow obstruction, air trapping, hyperinflation, hypoxemia, and hypercapnea (Fig. 4-17). Pulmonary function testing demonstrates an obstructive pattern, with elevated total lung capacity and residual volume, and reduced vital capacity (FEV_1) and diffusing capacity.

- **Chest radiographs** may demonstrate hyperinflation of the thorax and downward displacement and flattening of the diaphragm as a result of air trapping, but lung destruction is

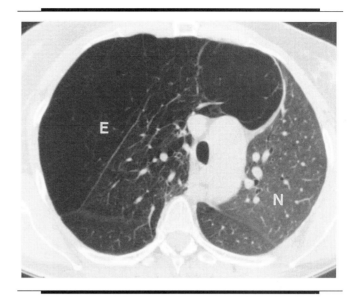

FIGURE 4-17 **Left lung transplant for emphysema.** HRCT illustrating the characteristic findings of advanced emphysema (E), including hyperinflation, reduced attenuation due to lung destruction, and attenuated vessels in contrast to the "normal" (N) transplanted lung. (With permission from Sagel SS, Slone RM. The lung. In: Lee JKT, Sagel SS, Stanley RJ, Heiken JP, eds. *Computed Body Tomography with MRI Correlation.* 3rd ed. New York: Lippincott-Raven, 1998.)

usually visible only in patients with moderate to advanced disease (Fig. 4-18). The clinical term **chronic obstructive pulmonary disease** should not be used to describe the morphologic abnormalities depicted on imaging studies.

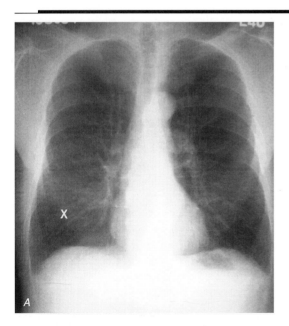

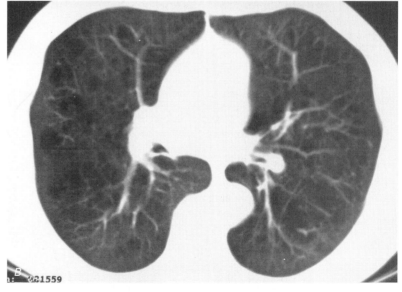

FIGURE 4-18 **Moderate emphysema.** (*A*) PA chest radiograph showing thoracic distention with downward displacement of the diphragm. The crossing of the tenth posterior and sixth anterior ribs (X), is normally about 1 cm above the dome of the right hemidiaphragm in medium-build patients. (*B*) CT showing moderate lung destruction as focal lucent defects without definable walls.

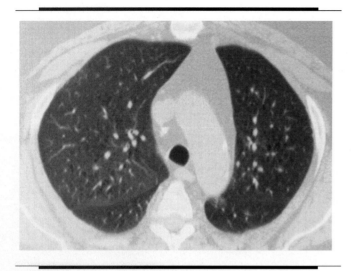

FIGURE 4-19   Mild emphysema. HRCT with 2-mm collimation showing tiny lucent defects characteristic of mild centrilobular pulmonary emphysema.

- **CT**, particularly HRCT, permits identification of destroyed lung tissue that correlates well with direct pathologic examination. CT characteristics of emphysema include areas of decreased attenuation without visible walls, pulmonary vessel distortion, and pruning. HRCT can reliably depict even mild emphysema that escapes detection by pulmonary function testing (Fig. 4-19). Images obtained in expiration accentuate areas of lung destruction and air trapping.

- Although pulmonary artery enlargement and mild pulmonary arterial hypertension are common in advanced emphysema,

pulmonary artery size is a poor indicator of pressure, and despite enlargement and advanced emphysema, significant pulmonary arterial hypertension is surprisingly uncommon.

- Pulmonary emphysema is often seen in combination with other pulmonary disease processes, and its presence can alter the appearance of diffuse and focal lung diseases. Pulmonary edema, for example, may take on a more focal, patchy appearance simulating pneumonia. This is because the edema primarily involves the areas of normal, better-perfused lung and spares the severely emphysematous, oligemic regions.

- Blebs and bullae are frequently observed in association with emphysema but can be seen as a localized process in otherwise normal lungs.

- **Compensatory emphysema** refers to decreased lung density and hyperinflation in normal lung adjacent to an area of volume loss due to atelectasis, pulmonary resection, or thoracic deformity. It is not true emphysema since there is no actual lung destruction.

- **Congenital lobar emphysema** is typically discovered within the first 6 months of life in association with respiratory distress. Initially fluid-filled, the overdistended, hyperlucent lobe produces a mass effect including pulmonary compression and mediastinal shift (Fig. 9-8). The left upper (40 percent) and middle (30 percent) lobes are the most common location. Treatment involves surgical resection (see Section 9.4).

- Four principal types of emphysema have been described pathologically: centrilobular, panlobular, paraseptal, and paracicatricial (Fig. 4-20). It is common for types to coexist.

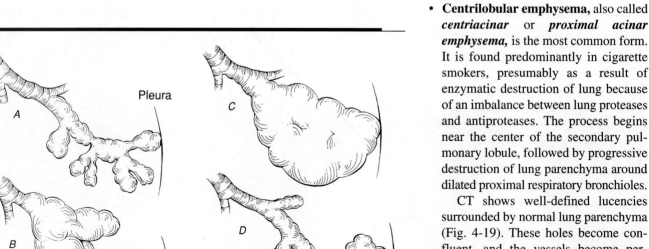

FIGURE 4-20   Pathologic types of emphysema. Pattern of involvement of the terminal and respiratory bronchioles. (*A*) Normal anatomy. (*B*) Centrilobular (central acinar) emphysema with destruction centered at the terminal bronchiole. (*C*) Panlobular emphysema affecting the entire lobule. (*D*) Paraseptal (distal acinar) emphysema affecting primarily the acinus.

- **Centrilobular emphysema,** also called *centriacinar* or *proximal acinar emphysema,* is the most common form. It is found predominantly in cigarette smokers, presumably as a result of enzymatic destruction of lung because of an imbalance between lung proteases and antiproteases. The process begins near the center of the secondary pulmonary lobule, followed by progressive destruction of lung parenchyma around dilated proximal respiratory bronchioles.

  CT shows well-defined lucencies surrounded by normal lung parenchyma (Fig. 4-19). These holes become confluent, and the vessels become peripherally attenuated as the destruction progresses. (Fig. 4-21). The apical and posterior segments of the upper lobes and superior segments of the lower lobes are most severely affected.

- **Panlobular emphysema**, also called *panacinar* or *diffuse emphysema,* affects the entire secondary pulmonary

It can accompany the centrilobular emphysema seen in smokers. It is seen in α_1-antitrypsin deficiency as a result of unchecked proteolytic digestion of lung parenchyma. There is usually a lower lobe predominance, presumably due to greater blood flow. An identical pattern of emphysema can be seen with intravenous injection of Ritalin or methadone.

α_1-**Antitrypsin deficiency** is a rare autosomal recessive disorder affecting young men and women. α_1-antitrypsin is a glycoprotein synthesized in the liver which is a proteolytic inhibitor of trypsin, bacterial proteases, and proteolytic enzymes. Homozygotic individuals may develop hepatic cirrhosis as a complication (see Section 9.6).

- **Paraseptal emphysema**, also called *distal acinar* or *localized emphysema*, involves the distal portion of the lobule; the pathogenesis is unknown. It can be seen in association with centrilobular or panlobular emphysema, or as an isolated phenomenon. Localized areas of destruction and airspace enlargement are seen within otherwise normal lung, primarily in the lung periphery, characteristically adjacent to the visceral pleura and interlobular septa (Fig. 4-24). The term **vanishing lung** describes patients with dyspnea and massive bullae (Fig. 4-25).

- **Paracicatricial emphysema**, also called *irregular* or *scar emphysema*, refers to airspace enlargement and lung destruction resulting from adjacent pulmonary fibrosis. There is no

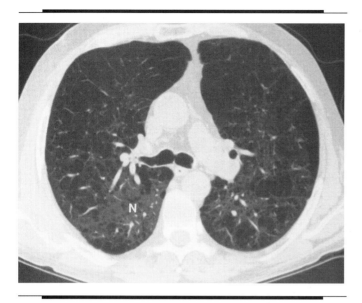

FIGURE 4-21 Advanced centrilobular emphysema. HRCT showing confluent parenchymal destruction in contrast to small areas of normal (N) and mildly emphysematous lung.

lobule, producing diffuse destruction (Fig. 4-22). CT shows widespread lung destruction and vascular distortion described as "simplification of lung architecture" (Fig. 4-23).

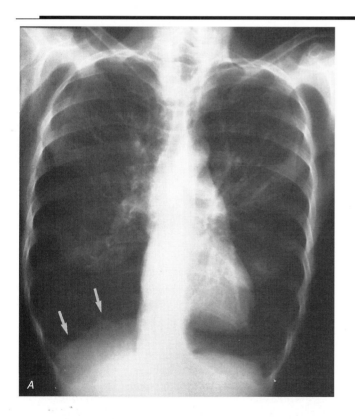

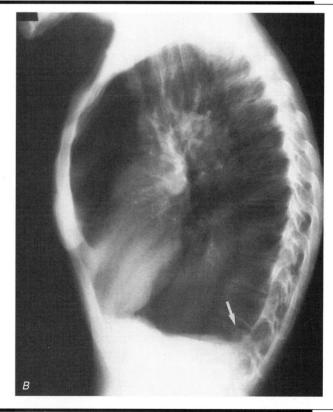

FIGURE 4-22 α_1-Antitrypsin deficiency emphysema. (*A*) PA and (*B*) lateral chest radiograph in a 59-year-old woman with advanced panlobular emphysema. Note dramatic thoracic distention with inversion of the diaphragm, revealing its costal insertions (arrows) on the PA image and pseudoblunting of the posterior costophrenic angle (arrow) on the lateral image.

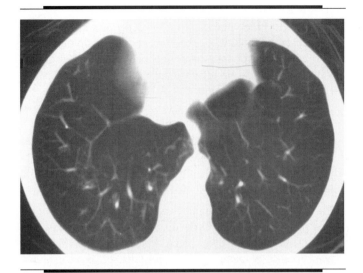

FIGURE 4-23   **Panlobular emphysema.** CT through the lung bases in a patient with α_1-antitrypsin deficiency, showing the characteristic pattern of lung simplification in panlobular emphysema. (With permission from Sagel SS, Slone RM. The lung. In: Lee JKT, Sagel SS, Stanley RJ, Heiken JP, eds. *Computed Body Tomography with MRI Correlation.* 3rd ed. New York: Lippincott-Raven, 1998.)

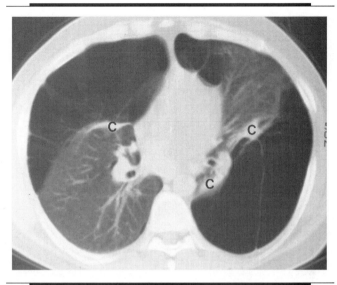

FIGURE 4-25   **Advanced bullous paraseptal emphysema.** CT showing large bulla compressing (C) underlying normal lung parenchyma.

consistent relationship to the acinus or secondary pulmonary lobule. Causes include inflammatory and infectious granulomatous disease, sarcoidosis, pneumoconiosis, and connective tissue disease. Associated traction bronchiectasis and honeycomb lung are often seen.

• **Medical management** options are palliative and include bronchodilators, steroids, supplemental oxygen, antibiotics, and smoking cessation. **Surgical management** options include lung volume reduction surgery and lung transplantation. (See Section 11.4, Figs. 11-28–35.)

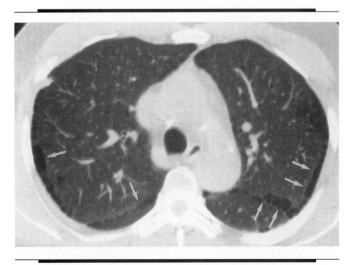

FIGURE 4-24   **Mild paraseptal emphysema.** CT showing subpleural lung destruction (arrows) along the periphery of the upper lungs and major fissures.

4.7   ENVIRONMENTAL LUNG DISEASE

• **Pneumoconiosis** refers to a group of lung diseases occurring as a result of exposure to inorganic environmental materials, typically occupational in nature. Foreign-body and inflammatory reactions often lead to interstitial nodules or fibrosis. Chest radiography may be used for surveillance, but CT, particularly HRCT, greatly increases the sensitivity and improves intraobserver agreement when assessing the lung parenchyma for occupational disease.

International labor organization (ILO) criteria for reporting these diseases are based on the shape, size, and distribution of parenchymal opacities and associated pleural abnormalities. The term ***B-reader*** refers to someone who has passed an ILO examination qualifying them to officially grade radiographs in conjunction with a standard comparison film set.

• **Silicosis** is caused by silicon dioxide dust inhalation. Exposed populations include sandblasters, stone grinders, and ceramic, foundry, and mine workers. The predominant abnormality is pulmonary nodules resulting from phagocytized dust and fibroblasts. The disease progresses slowly, over years. **Acute silicosis**, called silicoproteinosis, can develop after massive exposure, in which case pulmonary consolidation caused by abundant surfactant, similar to that observed in alveolar proteinosis, predominates. Fibrosis may develop (Fig. 1-18).

Simple silicosis refers to the presence of multiple discrete pulmonary nodules, typically only a few millimeters in diameter, with an upper lobe predominance and a slight posterior concentration. HRCT demonstrates a centrilobular and subpleural distribution; some nodules calcify. The nodules increase in size and number as the disease advances, eventu-

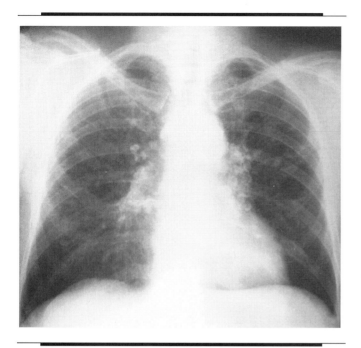

FIGURE 4-26 **Silicosis.** Chest radiograph showing predominantly upper lobe nodular opacities and eggshell calcification of hilar and mediastinal lymph nodes.

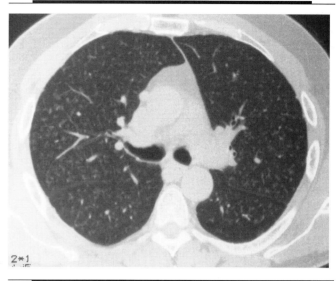

FIGURE 4-27 **Simple coal worker's pneumoconiosis.** HRCT showing multiple tiny nodular opacities with a predominantly upper lobe distribution in a 67-year-old man with a long history of occupational coal dust exposure.

ally becoming confluent, producing distortion and contraction of lung. Mediastinal adenopathy is common, classically with eggshell calcification (Fig. 4-26). There may be septal thickening as well.

Complicated silicosis, also called *progressive massive fibrosis*, refers to the formation of larger nodular opacities, termed *conglomerate masses*, by the coalescence of smaller silicotic nodules. They are usually symmetric and located in the upper lobes or superior segments, migrate toward the hila, and sometimes cavitate. The fibrosis produces upper lobe volume loss, paracicatricial emphysema, and progressive functional impairment. Otherwise, the pulmonary emphysema in these patients is a consequence of smoking rather than a primary manifestation of silicosis. Tuberculosis occurs with an increased incidence in patients with silicosis. The combination is called *silicotuberculosis*.

- **Coal worker's pneumoconiosis** is the result of incomplete clearing of inhaled dust containing inert coal and fibrinogenic silica dust. The radiographic appearance is nearly indistinguishable from that of silicosis, although pathologically the distinction can be made. Simple coal worker's pneumoconiosis refers to aggregates of "coal dust macules," measuring a few millimeters in diameter, found predominantly in the upper lobes (Fig. 4-27). As with complicated silicosis, fibrosis and progressive massive fibrosis may develop.

Anthrocosis is a pathologic term referring to the presence of coal dust or carbon from environmental pollution in the lung and lymph nodes, giving them a black color (black lung), but implies no clinical effect.

- **Asbestosis** refers to asbestos-induced pulmonary fibrosis in distinction from "asbestos-related pleural disease," which

refers only to pleural plaques that serve as a marker of asbestos exposure but do not impair pulmonary function (see Section 7.6, Fig. 7-15). The fibrosis may take 10 to 20 years to develop after initial exposure and is the main determinant of compensation in disability cases. Shortness of breath is the primary symptom. CT, particularly HRCT, is significantly more sensitive and also more specific than chest radiography for detecting asbestosis.

The earliest abnormality is typically in the posterior lung bases, presumably a consequence of fiber size and weight settling into the lower lungs. Septal thickening, parenchymal bands, subpleural curvilinear lines, nodules, and honeycombing develop. Traction bronchiectasis and pericicatrical emphysema can be seen in patients with advanced asbestosis (Fig. 4-28).

Areas of ground-glass attenuation due to mild fibrosis or edema may be seen. These changes may be more apparent on CT performed in the prone position, which also can demonstrate that they are fixed structural abnormalities and not simply subsegmental atelectasis and gravity-dependent blood flow secondary to less than full inspiration.

Asbestos-related pleural disease is almost always present in patients with parenchymal disease, although the absence of plaques does not exclude asbestosis. Fibrosis can occur as a result of a variety of lung diseases unrelated to asbestosis, and therefore even in association with pleural plaques it does not necessary indicate asbestosis.

Definitive diagnosis of asbestosis usually requires an open lung biopsy, but since there is no accepted treatment, diagnosis is usually based on a combination of clinical, physiologic, and radiologic information. Clinical information includes a reliable history of asbestos exposure at least 15 years earlier, restrictive pulmonary function, or reduced

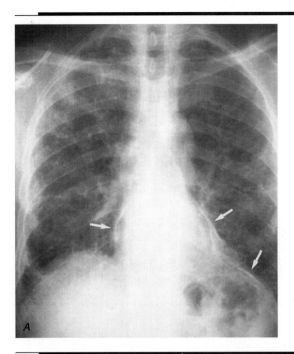
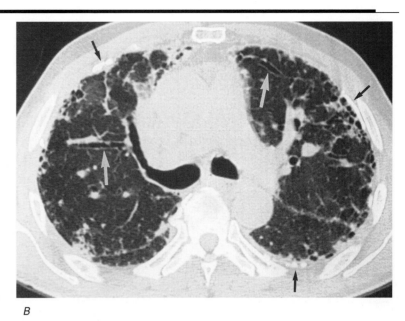

FIGURE 4-28   Advanced asbestosis. (*A*) Chest radiograph showing diffuse reticulonodular interstitial infiltrates and calcified pleural plaques on the hemidiaphragm and mediastinal pleura (arrows). (*B*) HRCT showing honeycombing in the lung periphery characteristic of fibrosis, calcified pleural plaques characteristic of prior asbestos exposure (black arrows), and traction bronchiolectasis (white arrows) in a patient with a long history of occupational asbestos exposure.

diffusing capacity. Phagocytized asbestos fibers termed *ferruginous bodies* are identified in sputum samples and biopsy specimens.

Other complications of asbestos exposure include development of mesothelioma (see Section 7.7) and bronchogenic carcinoma (see Fig.7-18).

- **Berylliosis** is a cell-mediated delayed-type hypersensitivity reaction to beryllium, which is used in the manufacture of fluorescent lamps, aircraft, and nuclear reactors. Alveolitis is seen in the acute form. Chronic exposure leads to a granulomatous response similar in appearance to that seen in pulmonary sarcoidosis, with small, diffuse parenchymal nodules that spare the apex and base, septal lines, bronchial wall thickening, areas of ground-glass attenuation, and hilar adenopathy which may calcify. Chronic berylliosis is a systemic disease involving multiple tissues and organs.

- Other causes of pneumoconiosis include **graphite dust** which can produce dense centrilobular nodules, septal thickening, and conglomerate masses. **Siderosis**, manifested as dense centrilobular nodules, is the result of iron oxide deposition and occurs in arc welders and iron miners. **Hard metals**, including tungsten, cobalt, and titanium, can produce pneumonitis and fibrosis. **Shaver disease** caused by aluminum dust is manifested as upper lobe reticulonodular fibrosis. **Stanosis** is caused by tin oxide, and **barytosis** by barium sulfate.

- **Extrinsic allergic alveolitis**, also called *hypersensitivity pneumonitis*, is an immunologically mediated response to

organic dust in the environment producing airway and parenchymal inflammation. The precipitating agent is primarily the associated fungal antigens (Table 4-1). This is in contrast to pneumoconioses caused by inorganic dust. Clinical testing demonstrates hypoxemia as well as reduced vital capacity and diffusing capacity during acute episodes.

Acute allergic alveolitis is an immune complex, hypersensitivity reaction to heavy antigen exposure producing airspace disease; radiography reveals areas of ground-glass attenuation and small, ill-defined centilobular opacities (Fig. 4-29). Symptoms may include headache, fever, chills, nonproductive cough, and shortness of breath several hours after exposure to the antigen, with resolution frequently occurring over several days. The lung volumes are typically normal, but airway inflammation may cause air trapping.

Subacute allergic alveolitis is the result of less intense but continuous exposure. Recurrent symptoms include fever, cough, myalgias, or arthralgias. Imaging studies demonstrate poorly defined centrilobular nodules and patchy ground-glass attenuation representing pneumonitis.

Chronic allergic alveolitis is a cell-mediated reaction to prolonged exposure, with development of a chronic cough and progressive shortness of breath months or years after initial exposure. Imaging demonstrates indistinct nodular centrilobular opacities, reduced lung volumes, and diffuse peripheral pulmonary fibrosis with relative sparing of the lung bases. Lymph node enlargement may occur, but pleural effusions are rare. Pericacatrical emphysema, honeycombing, and traction bronchiectasis occur with advanced fibrosis.

TABLE 4-1

Hypersensitivity pneumonitis	Extrinsic agent
Farmer's lung	Moist, moldy hay
Bird fancier's or pigeon breeder's lung	Particulate matter in excrement or feathers
Bagassosis	Moldy sugar cane
Mushroom worker's lung	Mushroom compost dust
Malt worker's lung	Mildewed barley
Maple bark disease	Moldy maple bark dust
Suberosis (cork worker's disease)	Mildewed cork dust
Sequoiosis	Redwood dust
Pandora pneumonitis	Air-conditioning and heating systems

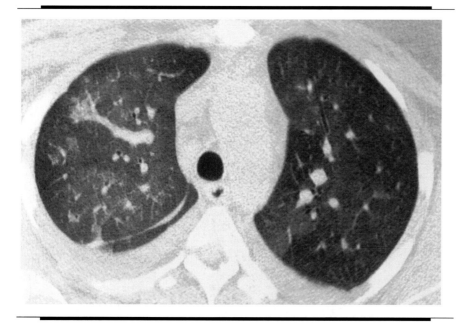

FIGURE 4-29   Hypersensitivity pneumonitis. HRCT showing patchy areas of ground-glass attenuation representing pneumonitis in a 32-year-old woman with extrinsic allergic alveolitis.

- **Noxious gas inhalation** can produce bronchial and pulmonary irritation and inflammation. It is usually a result of occupational accidents, and potential causative substances include chlorine, phosgene, ammonia, sulfur dioxide, toluene, and nitrous oxide *(silo filler disease)*. Acute symptoms include dyspnea, and recovery may take weeks. Imaging may reveal mild bronchitis and noncardiogenic edema. Bronchiolitis can develop as a complication.

4.8 FIBROSIS AND AUTOIMMUNE DISEASE

- **Pulmonary fibrosis** represents irreversible pulmonary scarring. Chronic inflammatory lung disease may resolve or organize and progress to fibrosis. Chemotherapy agents, radi-

ation therapy, infections, occupational lung disease, and collagen vascular diseases may produce pulmonary fibrosis (**Differentials 55–59**). Symptoms include progressive dyspnea and dry cough.

Pathologically it is often impossible to determine the specific cause of fibrosis, but the pattern and distribution can suggest a diagnosis. Idiopathic pulmonary fibrosis (IPF) is subpleural and lower lung zone predominant. Sarcoidosis is diffuse or upper lobe predominant and may have a peribronchovascular distribution. Asbestosis appears similar to IPF, but typically there are pleural plaques or thickening. Silicosis may have conglomerate fibrotic masses and nodules in the upper lung. Eosinophilic granuloma has upper zone predominant cystic spaces and relative sparing of the lung bases. Extrinsic allergic alveolitis causes diffuse involvement with randomly distributed areas of ground-glass attenuation and subpleural fibrosis.

- **Idiopathic pulmonary fibrosis**, or **fibrosing alveolitis**, is the cryptogenic form of the disease. Desquamative interstitial pneumonia (DIP) refers to the early inflammatory phase of the disease with intraalveolar inflammatory cells and usual interstitial pneumonia (UIP) to nonspecific interstitial pneumonitis and fibrosis. **Hamman-Rich syndrome** is the rapidly progressive form of IPF.

Early on, HRCT may demonstrate areas of ground-glass opacity representing active alveolitis which is primarily cellular. The severity and extent are good predictors of potential response to treatment. These areas eventually progress to irregular linear opacities, representing fibrosis, which is irreversible.

End-stage fibrosis produces disruption of the underlying lung architecture, with a honeycomb pattern of thick, irregular subpleural and basilar septal lines surrounding small cystic air spaces, and traction bronchiectasis. More severe cases may involve the entire lung and reduce lung volumes. Adenopathy may be present as a consequence of the inflammatory process. Pleural effusions are rare.

Connective Tissue Disease

- **Collagen vascular diseases** are chronic autoimmune inflammatory conditions. Scleroderma, rheumatoid arthritis, and lupus frequently produce chronic interstitial pneumonitis. CT

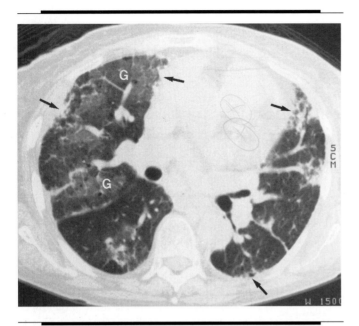

FIGURE 4-30   Lupus. HRCT showing areas of ground-glass attenuation (G) suggesting active alveolitis and areas of fibrosis with honeycombing (arrows). (With permission from Sagel SS, Slone RM. The lung. In: Lee JKT, Sagel SS, Stanley RJ, Heiken JP, eds. *Computed Body Tomography with MRI Correlation.* 3rd ed. New York: Lippincott-Raven, 1998.)

by joint involvement. Distal clavicular, glenohumeral, and superior rib erosions may be visible on chest radiographs. The fibrosis may progress slowly, rapidly, or remain stable, and is typically bilateral, peripheral, and lower lobe in distribution and indistinguishable from other causes.

Patients may have pulmonary nodules, termed **necrobiotic nodules**, which are peripheral and usually less than 1 cm in diameter but can exceed 5 cm and may cavitate. They are temporally related to subcutaneous nodules and may recede and recur. Arteritis, pulmonary hypertension, and bronchiolitis obliterans may also occur. Abnormalities may also be seen as a consequence of drug therapy. **Caplan syndrome** refers to fibrotic nodules occurring in coal miners with rheumatoid arthritis.

- **Sjögren syndrome** affects exocrine glands and is characterized by a dry mouth and eyes. It is often seen in association with other connective tissue disorders, particularly rheumatoid arthritis, scleroderma, polymyositis, or lupus and is termed **secondary Sjögren**. Patients have chronic bronchitis, recurrent pneumonia, and a higher incidence of chronic active hepatitis, cirrhosis, thyroiditis, bronchiectasis, and lymphoproliferative disorders such as pseudolymphoma. Patients may have pleural effusions and develop lipoid interstitial pneumonia or pulmonary fibrosis.

findings generally correlate well with the duration of symptoms and measures of pulmonary function. HRCT may detect pulmonary abnormalities despite normal chest radiographs and an absence of clinical symptoms, particularly in lupus patients.

- **Systemic lupus erythematosus** affects primarily young woman. African-Americans are affected more frequently than Caucasians. Small pericardial and chronic exudative pleural effusions are common and often lead to pleural fibrosis. Lower lobe-predominant septal thickening and areas of ground-glass attenuation are the most common pulmonary findings. Airspace nodules, bronchiectasis, and architectural distortion from fibrosis are less common. Patients may also develop cardiomyopathy, glomerulonephritis, polyarteritis, or pulmonary artery hypertension from vasculitis (Fig. 4-30).

- **Scleroderma** is seen most commonly in young women, and affects the gastrointestinal tract and skin. A dilated air-filled esophagus may be seen. Pulmonary involvement is usually limited to basilar interstitial fibrosis. Although sometimes attributed to aspiration, secondarily to esophageal dismotility, the fibrosis is likely a primary manifestation of the systemic disease (Fig. 4-31). A combination of **C**alcification in soft tissues, **R**aynaud disease, **e**sophageal dysmotility, **s**clerodactaly, and **t**elangectasias is referred to as **CREST** syndrome.

- **Rheumatoid arthritis** is more common in women, but the pulmonary manifestations are more common in men. Exudative pleural effusions, alveolitis, and basilar interstitial fibrosis are the most common findings and are usually preceded

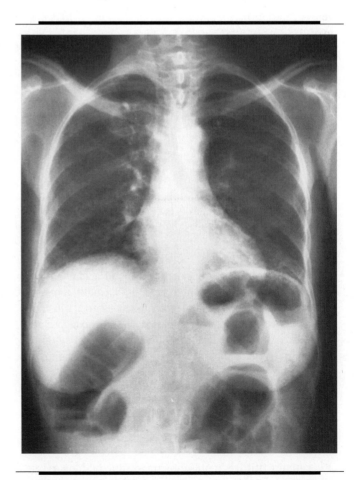

FIGURE 4-31   Scleroderma. Chest radiograph showing basilar fibrosis and atonic bowel.

- **Ankylosing spondylitis**, seen most frequently in young men, rarely involves the lungs, but when it does, bone abnormalities, including spinal fusion and syndesmophytes, are obvious. Apical and upper lobe interstitial and pleural fibrosis may be seen, as well as cavities and sometimes bronchiectasis. Patients have antibodies to HLA-B27. Heart block and aortic insufficiency are cardiovascular manifestations.

- **Dermatomyositis** is an uncommon connective tissue disorder that is a rare cause of interstitial pneumonitis and fibrosis.

- Other less common vasculites affecting the lung include polyarteritis nodosa, Churg-Strauss disease, allergic angiitis, and lymphoid granulomatosis.

4.9 IDIOPATHIC AND IATROGENIC LUNG DISEASE

- **Alveolar proteinosis** is the result of abnormal accumulation of surfactant in alveoli. The exact etiology is unknown but likely related to immunodeficiency, overproduction of surfactant by granular pneumocytes, or defective clearance by alveolar macrophages. This results in alveolar filling with periodic acid-Schiff (PAS)-positive phospholipid material. It is primarily an airspace disease but smooth septal thickening can also be seen.

  There is a wide age range, and men are affected more than women. Symptoms include dyspnea, cough, weight loss, weakness, and hemoptysis. Pulmonary function testing reveals a reduced diffusing capacity. Imaging studies demonstrate predominantly perihilar and lower lobe ground-glass attenuation and consolidation (Fig. 4-32). There is no adenopathy, cardiomegaly, or pleural effusions. There is slow progression with a variable course of clinical and radiologic improvement and exacerbation. Superimposed pneumonia is common. Organisms include *Nocardia*, mycobacteria, and cytomegalovirus (CMV). Treatment involves bronchopulmonary lavage.

- **Alveolar microlithiasis** is a rare disease of unknown etiology affecting middle-aged individuals. Patients are usually asymptomatic but may have dyspnea. Imaging features are disproportionately worse than clinical symptoms and include diffuse, fine, sandlike microcalcifications measuring less than 1 mm in diameter (**Differentials 21 and 66**). Some patients progress to interstitial fibrosis. The microliths may continue to enlarge, progress to pulmonary fibrosis, or become arrested. There is intense uptake on radionuclide bone scans.

- **Idiopathic pulmonary hemosiderosis** in children and young adults is characterized by recurrent episodes of hemoptysis due to pulmonary hemorrhage. Radiographic findings are similar to those for Goodpasture syndrome, but renal function is normal and antibasement antibodies are absent. Airpace disease is seen during acute episodes. Patients may develop iron deficiency anemia and hepatosplenomegaly. Hemosiderin deposition eventually leads to fibrosis.

- **Lymphangioleiomyomatosis** (LAM) is a rare disease of unknown etiology which affects primarily young women of

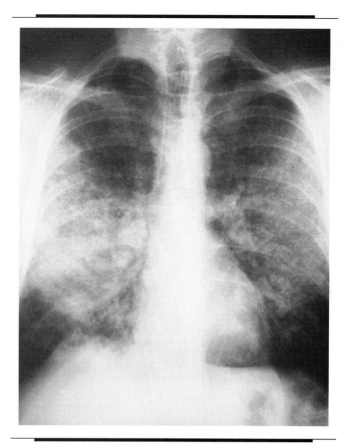

FIGURE 4-32 Alveolar proteinosis. Chest radiograph showing diffuse, predominantly airspace disease bilaterally with sparing of the apices and bases in a 42-year-old man. He was subsequently treated with bronchoalveolar lavage.

reproductive age. The disease is characterized by smooth muscle proliferation in the airway, leading to the development of pulmonary cysts and pneumothoraces, in lymphatics leading to chylothoraces and adenopathy, and to a lesser degree in arterioles and venules. It is exacerbated during pregnancy and is probably hormone-related. Shortness of breath, spontaneous pneumothorax, and chylous effusion are common (Fig. 4-33).

HRCT shows small, well-defined, thin-walled cysts, ranging from a few millimeters to several centimeters in diameter, uniformly distributed throughout otherwise normal lung. In addition to pulmonary cysts, septal thickening may result from lymphatic engorgement, smooth muscle proliferation, and fibrosis. The lung volumes are typically normal, or increased in advanced disease (Fig. 4-34).

Pulmonary artery pressure increases as the disease progresses, leading to cor pulmonale in some patients. Hemoptysis occurs in 40 percent. Medical therapy includes antiestrogen treatment with progesterone, or oophorectomy. LAM is uniformly fatal, typically within 10 years of diagnosis. Lung transplantation is an option for some patients.

- **Tuberous sclerosis** is an autosomal dominant neurocutaneous syndrome which rarely involves the lungs (1 percent), but when it does, it is indistinguishable radiologically and

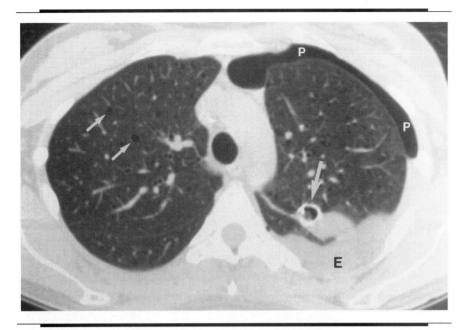

FIGURE 4-33   Mild lymphangioleiomyomatosis. HRCT showing multiple small, circular lucencies representing pulmonary cysts (small arrows) in a woman with a left pneumothorax (P) and chylous effusion (E). Note chest tube in the major fissure (large arrow).

can develop and metastasize to the lung. Skin nodules can mimic pulmonary nodules on chest radiographs. Skeletal findings include scoliosis, thin ribs, and notching from neurofibromas of the intercostal nerves. About one-fifth of patients develop pulmonary fibrosis, typically with a basal predominance. Upper lobe bullae are also common.

- **Löffler syndrome**, also called *acute eosinophilic pneumonia*, refers to acute transient pulmonary infiltrates and consolidation with peripheral blood and pulmonary eosinophilia that can be idiopathic or the result of an allergic reaction to a parasitic infection such as strongyloidiasis or schistosomiasis. Symptoms are absent or minimal. Underlying asthma is common. Imaging studies show focal nonsegmental, peripheral infiltrates which are migratory, changing over days and clearing within a month (**Differential 36**).

pathologically from LAM. Seizures, mental retardation, adenoma sebacium, CNS hamartomas, astrocytomas, and renal angiomyolipomas are sometimes associated.

- **Neurofibromatosis** is an autosomal dominant condition characterized by café-au-lait spots, subcutaneous neurofibromas, and cranial nerve schwannomas. Neurofibrosarcomas

- **Chronic eosinophilic pneumonia** is an idiopathic disease affecting middle-aged women more than men. Patients may experience coughing, wheezing, fever, malaise, or dyspnea, and almost all have peripheral blood eosinophilia. Imaging studies demonstrate peripheral bilateral nonsegmental alveolar infiltrates which change slowly, lasting a month or more (**Differential 37**). Treatment involves steroids.

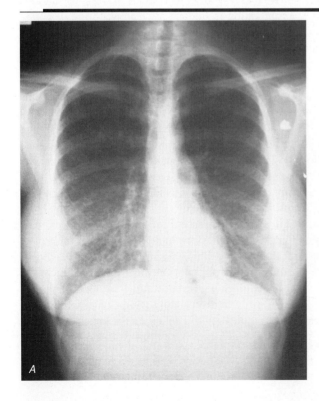

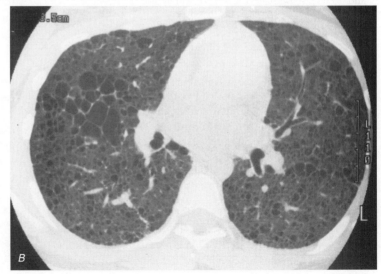

FIGURE 4-34   Advanced lymphangioleiomyomatosis. (*A*) Chest radiograph in a 19-year-old woman with shortness of breath, demonstrating increased lung volumes and a pattern of diffuse lung disease which appears to be interstitial. It is accentuated in the lung bases because of the overlying soft tissues of the chest wall. (*B*) HRCT showing innumerable pulmonary cysts of varying sizes with intervening normal lung parenchyma and no significant interstitial disease.

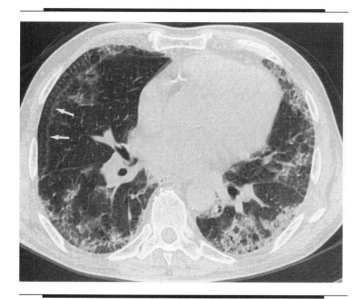

FIGURE 4-35 Amiodarone toxicity. HRCT demonstrating irregular interstitial thickening with associated architectural distortion characteristic of fibrosis. Note also subpleural bands (arrows). (With permission from Sagel SS, Slone RM. The lung. In: Lee JKT, Sagel SS, Stanley RJ, Heiken JP, eds. *Computed Body Tomography with MRI Correlation.* 3rd ed. New York: Lippincott-Raven, 1998.)

Other causes of pulmonary eosinophilia include tropical pulmonary eosinophilia (filaria), drugs, and *Aspergillus.*

• **Pulmonary amyloidosis** is a very rare disease characterized by extracellular accumulation of an unusual protein. It may be primary or secondary to an underlying chronic disease. Chest involvement can include tracheobronchial disease, pulmonary infiltrates, solitary, or multiple pulmonary nodules that may cavitate or calcify. Fibrosis and adenopathy can develop, but effusions are rare.

• **Drug-induced lung disease** is a potential complication of several chemotherapy and therapeutic agents. Toxic effects are often dose-related and cumulative. Pulmonary manifestations can include interstitial infiltrates, effusions, nodules, and fibrosis. A narcotic overdose often leads to edema. Methotrexate, aspirin, penicillin, bleomycin, and nitrofurantoin can cause eosinophilia and pulmonary infiltrates. Procainamide, isoniazide, and penicillin can result in pneumonitis and pleural effusions. In rare cases bleomycin causes pulmonary nodules indistinguishable from metastases. Busulfan, amiodarone, azothioprine, bleomycin, and cyclophosphamide can cause fibrosis, primarily within the posterior lung. HRCT is more sensitive than radiography in evaluating these complications and

may allow early detection of active inflammatory disease, permitting discontinuation of the drug before substantial fibrosis occurs.

• **Amiodarone hydrochloride**, used to treat refractory arrhythmias in patients at risk for sudden death, accumulates in the liver and lung and can cause severe progressive and potentially fatal pneumonitis. Ground-glass opacities on HRCT suggest reversible infiltrative lung disease, but findings may be nonspecific. Advanced disease is associated with irreversible fibrosis (Fig. 4-35). High-attenuation pleural and

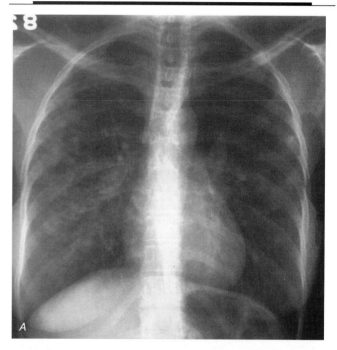

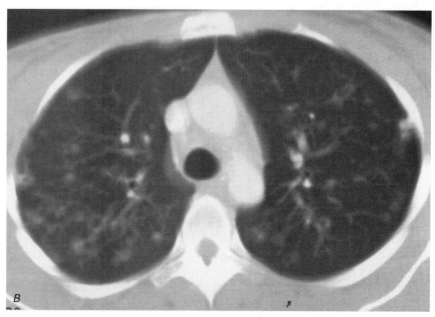

FIGURE 4-36 Histiocytosis X. (*A*) Chest radiograph in a 20-year-old woman showing nodular infiltrates bilaterally. (*B*) CT showing predominantly upper lobe nodules, some with cavitation.

parenchymal abnormalities may be seen, as well as increased attenuation of the liver due to iodine deposition.

- **Eosinophilic granuloma (EG)**, also called histiocytosis-X, is an idiopathic disease that may be systemic or affect primarily the lungs. Most patients are female cigarette smokers. Symptoms include dry cough, dyspnea, and pneumothorax. The most common findings are upper lobe-predominant interstitial nodules, pulmonary cysts, or a combination (Figs. 4-36 and 4-37). Fibrosis, interlobular septal thickening, and ground-glass opacity may also be seen. Irregularly shaped air collections representing pericicatricial emphysema may develop in advanced disease. There is no lymphadenopathy.

The nodules are usually less than 5 mm in diameter and often distributed in the center of secondary pulmonary lobules around small airways. It is likely that nodules progress to cavitary nodules, thick-walled cysts, and then to thin-walled cysts. When both nodules and cysts are observed, EG can be differentiated from other diseases such as granulomatous infections, silicosis, metastatic disease, and sarcoid. Geographic lytic bone lesions are most common in the skull but can sometimes be seen in the ribs or spine.

- **Sarcoidosis** is a systemic disease of unknown etiology characterized pathologically by widespread development of noncaseating epithelioid cell granulomas which may resolve or convert to fibrous tissue. The disease most commonly affects mediastinal lymph nodes and lung, but uveitis, cardiac, liver, spleen, skin, bone, and salivary involvement also occurs.

Laboratory studies may show anemia, leukopenia, elevated sedimentation rate, blood eosinophilia, hypercalcemia, hypercalcuria, and elevated levels of serum angiotensin converting enzyme (ACE). It may be an immunologically mediated response to as yet unidentified inhaled agents. Berylliosis is indistinguishable radiologically and pathologically from sarcoidosis.

One-half of cases are detected incidentally on routine chest radiographs. Patients with adenopathy alone are usually asymptomatic, but patients with pulmonary involvement may experience weight loss, fatigue, fever, cough, or shortness of breath. Hemoptysis is rare. The disease is generally more common in African-American, Puerto Rican, West Indian, and United Kingdom populations. Women are more susceptible than men. Diagnosis is usually confirmed by transbronchial biopsy which may demonstrate granulomas despite an absence of radiographically obvious peribronchial disease.

The chest radiograph is abnormal at some point in over 90 percent of patients (Fig. 4-38). Adenopathy is the most common manifestation and is seen by radiography in 80 percent of patients at some time during the course of the disease. Most have symmetric hilar, and classically right paratracheal, involvement. Subcarinal adenopathy is also common. Unilateral hilar adenopathy (<5 percent) and isolated paratracheal adenopathy are uncommon. Peripheral eggshell, lymph node calcification is occasionally seen (Fig. 4-39). Pleural effusions are exceedingly rare. Radiographic staging is outlined in Table 4-2.

Stage I disease resolves within a few years in most patients, and less than one-third of patients with stage I progress to develop lung disease. Adenopathy is usually present when there is pulmonary disease, and it typically decreases as lung disease progresses.

The **pulmonary manifestations** of sarcoidosis, which include interstitial infiltrates and nodules, are the result of deposition of noncaseating granulomas along the lymphatics lining the bronchovascular bundles and intralobular septa. Findings include 1- to 10-mm irregular interstitial and subpleural nodules throughout the lungs (Fig. 4-40) and confluent interstitial infiltrates which can be asymmetric. Cavitation is rare.

The midlung and upper lung zones are most commonly involved, and the lung periphery and bases are generally spared. HRCT demonstrates nodular, irregular thickening along bronchovascular bundles and interlobular septae similar to that characterizing lymphangitic carcinomatosis (Fig. 4-41).

Pulmonary involvement usually resolves but does progress to fibrosis in some patients (<20 percent), with resultant architectural distortion, traction bronchiectasis, pleural thickening, and pericicatricial emphysema (Fig. 4-42). The distribution is often patchy in contrast to the peripheral, lower lobe distribution of IPF.

Occasionally, pulmonary sarcoidosis may appear as diffuse ground-glass opacities or as consolidation termed cannonball, nummular, or **alveolar sarcoid**. The radiographic appearance is nonspecific and can be seen with pneumonia, bronchoalveolar cell carcinoma, BOOP, lymphoma, and Wegener granulomatosis (Fig. 4-43).

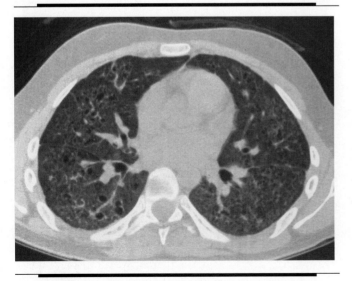

FIGURE 4-37   Histiocytosis-X. HRCT showing thin-walled cysts rather than nodules. (With permission from Sagel SS, Slone RM. The lung. In: Lee JKT, Sagel SS, Stanley RJ, Heiken JP, eds. *Computed Body Tomography with MRI Correlation.* 3rd ed. New York: Lippincott-Raven, 1998.)

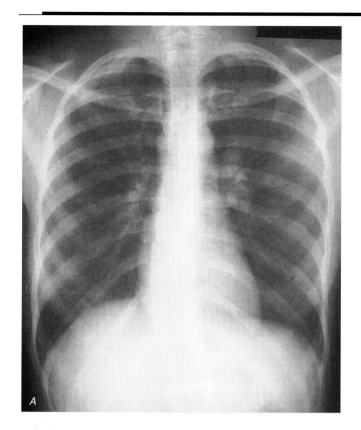

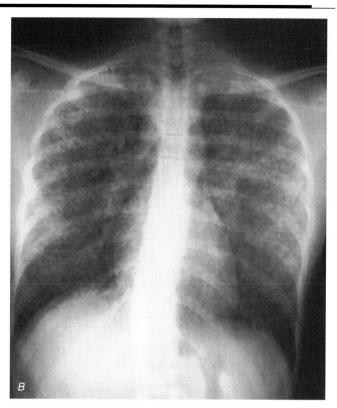

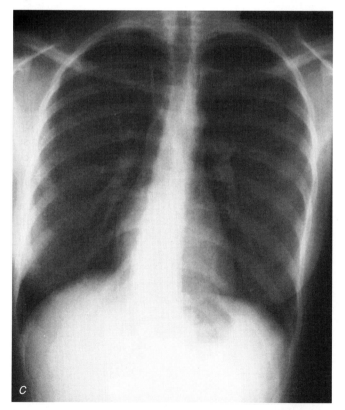

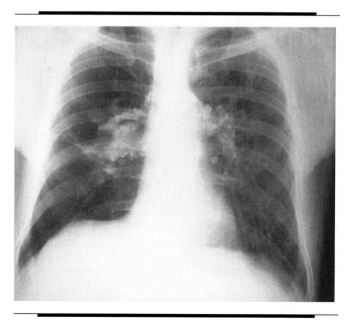

FIGURE 4-38   Stages of sarcoidosis. (*A*) Chest radiograph showing bilateral hilar and subtle right paratracheal lymphadenopathy.
(*B*) Subsequent radiograph showing right paratracheal and bilateral
hilar adenopathy and diffuse pulmonary sarcoidosis with small pulmonary nodules. (*C*) Essentially normal radiograph several years
after treatment.

FIGURE 4-39   Sarcoidosis. Chest radiograph showing peripheral
eggshell calcifications in hilar lymph nodes which can be seen in
sarcoidosis, silicosis, and treated lymphoma.

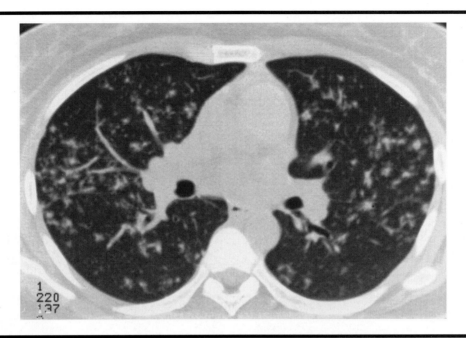

FIGURE 4-40   **Pulmonary sarcoidosis.** HRCT demonstrating ill-defined pulmonary nodules in a 39-year-old woman with sarcoidosis. (With permission from Sagel SS, Slone RM. The lung. In: Lee JKT, Sagel SS, Stanley RJ, Heiken JP, eds. *Computed Body Tomography with MRI Correlation.* 3rd ed. New York: Lippincott-Raven, 1998.)

Lofgren syndrome is a acute constellation of clinical symptoms in patients with sarcoid, including fever, erythema nodosum, arthralgias, and hilar adenopathy with focal pulmonary infiltrates.

Patients with pulmonary sarcoidosis are predisposed to superimposed bacterial and mycobacterial infections, and in patients with fibrosis, the cystic spaces may become infected with aspergillus, leading to hemoptysis. Death is directly

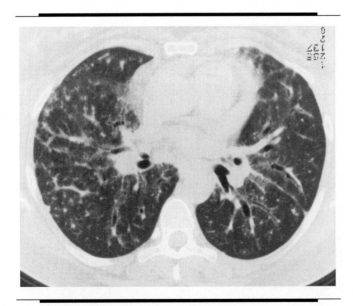

FIGURE 4-41   **Pulmonary sarcoidosis.** HRCT demonstrating a nodular infiltrate with a bronchovascular distribution in a 42-year-old woman. The bronchial margins and pleural interface are indistinct, and there are ill-defined nodular opacities in the lung parenchyma. The scan was obtained with the patient in a prone position. (With permission from Sagel SS, Slone RM. The lung. In: Lee JKT, Sagel SS, Stanley RJ, Heiken JP, eds. *Computed Body Tomography with MRI Correlation.* 3rd ed. New York: Lippincott-Raven, 1998.)

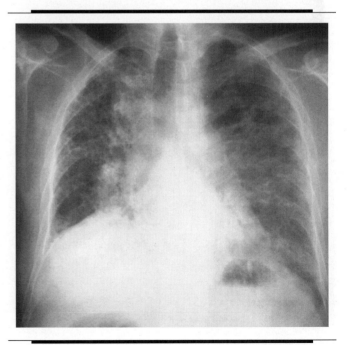

FIGURE 4-42   **Advanced pulmonary sarcoidosis.** PA chest radiograph showing mediastinal fullness, reduced lung volumes, and a reticulonodular pattern of pulmonary fibrosis. (With permission from Sagel SS, Slone RM. The lung. In: Lee JKT, Sagel SS, Stanley RJ, Heiken JP, eds. *Computed Body Tomography with MRI Correlation.* 3rd ed. New York: Lippincott-Raven, 1998.)

TABLE 4-2   RADIOLOGIC STAGING OF SARCOID

Stage	Findings	At presentation (%)	All radiologic abnormalities resolve (%)
0	Normal imaging	10	N/A
I	Adenopathy without pulmonary disease	50	65
II	Adenopathy and pulmonary disease	30	50
III	Pulmonary disease without adenopathy	10	20
IV	Pulmonary fibrosis	Rare	0

attributed to sarcoid in less than 5 percent of patients and may occur as a result of cor pulmonale, hemorrhage, mycetoma, or respiratory failure. Treatment involves steroids.

- **Sickle cell disease** produces a number of morphologic changes that can be depicted on imaging studies. Bone infarcts, sclerosis due to renal osteodystrophy, and central endplate compression fractures are common skeletal abnormalities. *Sickle cell lung*, also called "acute chest syndrome," is a syndrome of fever and pulmonary infiltrates in patients in whom no infectious organisms are recovered. HRCT may demonstrate predominantly intralobular septal thickening, parenchymal bands, pleural tags, traction bronchiectasis, and architectural distortion as a consequence of fibrosis, the severity and extent of which correlate with the number of prior episodes of pneumonia and acute chest syndrome.

4.10 METASTASIS AND DIFFUSE PULMONARY MALIGNANCY

- **Lymphangitic carcinomatosis** is the result of interstitial spread of carcinoma. In most cases, the tumor spreads hematogenously to the lungs, secondarily penetrating the interstitium and lymphatics, spreading along the intralobular septa, subpleural space, and connective tissue lining the bronchovesicular bundles, and producing a nodular interstitial pattern (Fig. 4-44). Pulmonary lymphangitic spread is most frequently observed secondary to adenocarcinoma of the

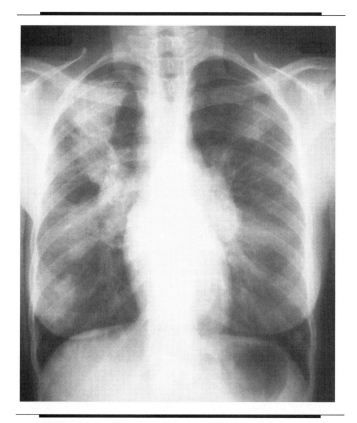

FIGURE 4-43   Alveolar sarcoidosis. Chest radiograph showing bilateral hilar and right paratracheal adenopathy and extensive pulmonary consolidation.

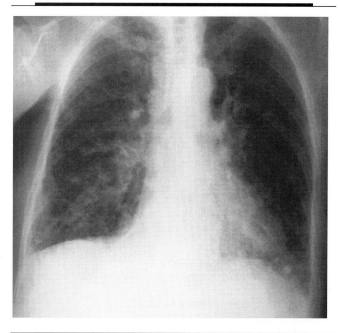

FIGURE 4-44   Lymphangitic spread of breast cancer. Chest radiograph showing diffuse nodular interstitial opacities throughout both lungs.

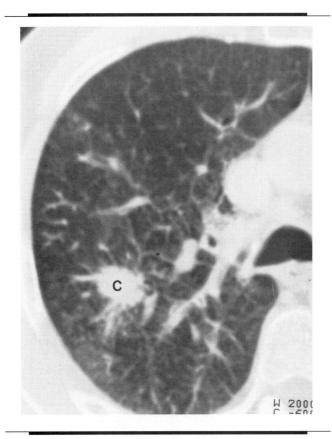

FIGURE 4-45   Local lymphangitic spread of lung cancer. CT showing a 2-cm spiculated bronchogenic carcinoma (C) with surrounding nodular interstitial thickening characteristic of local interstitial (lymphangitic) spread.

breast, lung, stomach, colon, prostate, and pancreas. Direct local lymphangitic spread can sometimes be seen around bronchogenic carcinomas (Fig. 4-45) .

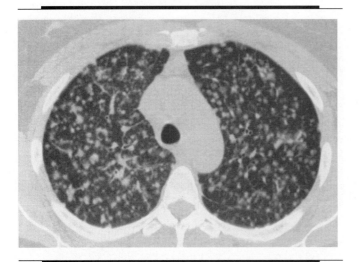

FIGURE 4-46   Bronchoalveolar cell carcinoma. HRCT showing innumerable small and ill-defined pulmonary nodules throughout both lungs representing disseminated bronchoalveolar cell carcinoma in a 48-year-old woman.

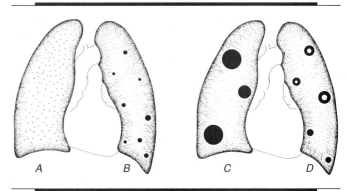

FIGURE 4-47   Patterns of pulmonary metastases. (*A*) Milliary metastases seen with melanoma and thyroid cancer. (*B*) Typical pattern with nodules of varying sizes and slight lower lobe predominance. (*C*) A few large pulmonary metastases can be seen with colon cancer and sarcomas. (*D*) Cavitary nodules seen most frequently with squamous cell carcinoma of the head and neck and cervix.

HRCT demonstrates irregular septal, subpleural, and bronchovascular thickening which becomes nodular as the disease progresses. The characteristic HRCT pattern of nodular septal thickening has been described as having a "beaded chain" appearance. Pathologic examination shows interstitial edema and fibrosis with lymphatic dilatation and tumor cells infiltrating connective tissue.

Both the central and peripheral lung may be involved, but it is more common in the lower lung zones and is often associated with adenopathy or pleural effusion. Although long-term survival following development of pulmonary lymphangitic carcinomatosis is unusual, modern radiation and chemotherapy treatment can dramatically impact disease progression, resulting in stable or only gradually progressive disease.

- **Bronchoalveolar cell carcinoma (BAC)** may appear as lobar consolidation, single or multiple pulmonary nodules (Fig. 4-46), or diffuse airspace disease. It is characterized by preservation of lung architecture with a well-differentiated adenocarcinoma arising from the bronchiolar and alveolar walls. Mucinous BAC may present as low-attenuation nodules and in some cases mimic alveolar proteinoses.

  An HRCT pattern of ground-glass opacity with superimposed smooth septal thickening and a patchy geographic distribution referred to as "crazy paving" has been reported as characteristic of alveolar proteinosis but may be seen with BAC as well.

- **Pulmonary metastases** are generally the result of hematogenous spread and are common in patients with sarcomas, melanoma, and renal cell, breast, and thyroid carcinoma. Because of the varying frequency of these primary malignancies, the most common primary cancers when pulmonary metastases are seen, in decreasing order of frequency, breast, renal, head and neck, and colon cancer. Most patients have multiple peripheral nodules of varying sizes (**Differential 19**), but other patterns can also be seen (Fig. 4-47). CT typically shows a peripheral distribution of smooth, round

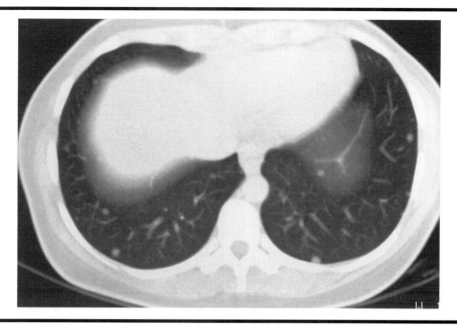

FIGURE 4-48 Metastatic thyroid cancer. CT showing multiple, small and well-defined pulmonary nodules that are primarily peripheral and lower lobe in distribution, characteristic of pulmonary metastases, in a 24-year-old woman with a history of thyroid cancer.

nodules and may demonstrate proximity to pulmonary arterial branches (Fig. 4-48).

Innumerable tiny metastases (milliary) are most common with thyroid carcinoma and melanoma (Fig. 4-49). Large metastases are most commonly due to sarcomas and to testicular, colon, and renal cell carcinoma (Fig. 4-50). Central necrosis and cavitation are most common with squamous cell cancers (Fig. 4.51) but can be seen with sarcomas, colon cancer, and melanoma (**Differential 27**).

Hemorrhagic pulmonary metastases typically have ill-defined margins and include choriocarcinoma, melanoma, thyroid and renal cell carcinoma. Endobronchial metastases can be seen with lymphoma and with lung, renal cell, breast, and colon cancers. Calcification is uncommon, occurring in less than 1 percent of pulmonary metastases, but can be observed in sarcomas and in breast, thyroid, testicular, ovarian, and particularly mucinous adenocarcinomas and also following radiation or chemotherapy.

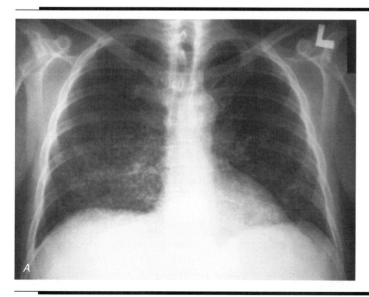
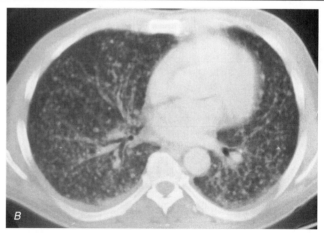

FIGURE 4-49 Metastatic melanoma. (*A*) Chest radiograph and (*B*) CT showing innumerable small pulmonary nodules characteristic of metastatic melanoma, metastatic thyroid cancer, and some infections.

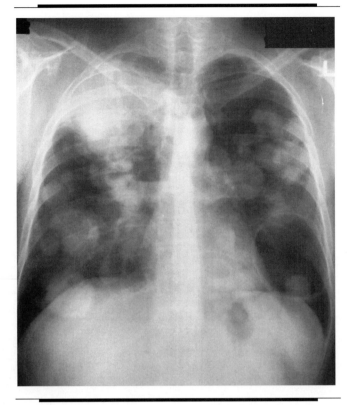

FIGURE 4-50   Metastatic testicular cell carcinoma. Chest radiograph showing dozens of pulmonary nodules of various sizes throughout both lungs, including one large cystic mass in the left lung base, in a 32-year-old man with brain and pulmonary metastases from choriocarcinoma of the testes.

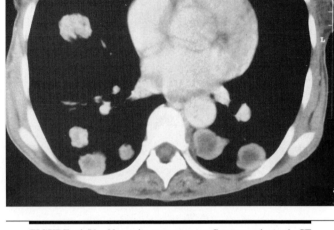

FIGURE 4-51   Necrotic metastases. Contrast-enhanced CT showing multiple pulmonary nodules with enhancing margins and low-density centers, characteristic of necrosis, in a 55-year-old woman with metastatic cervical cancer.

In most cases a solitary pulmonary nodule is more likely to represent a primary lung cancer, even in patients with a known extrathoracic primary cancer. The most likely causes of solitary metastases are sarcomas and colon, renal cell, testicular, and breast cancer.

Bibliography

Akira M. Uncommon pneumoconioses: CT and pathologic findings. *Radiology.* 1995;197:403–409.

Akira M, Yamamoto S, Yokoyama K, Kita N, Morinaga K, Higashihara T, Kozuk T. Asbestosis: High resolution CT pathologic correlation. *Radiology.* 1990;176:389–394.

Armstrong P, Wilson AG, Dee P, Hansell DM. *Imaging of Diseases of the Chest.* 2nd ed. St. Louis: Mosby-Yearbook; 1985.

Austin JHM, Müller NL, Friedman PJ, et al. Glossary of terms for CT of the lungs: Recommendations of the Nomenclature Committee of the Fleischner Society, *Radiology.* 1996;200:327–331.

Bouchardy LM, Kuhlman JE, Ball WC, Hruban RH, Askin FB, Siegelman SS. CT findings in bronchiolitis obliterans organizing pneumonia (BOOP) with X-ray, clinical, and histologic correlations. *J Comput Axial Tomogr.* 1993;17:352–357.

Corcoran HL, Renner WR, Milstein MJ. Review of high resolution CT of the lungs. *Radiographics.* 1992;12:917–939.

Foster WL Jr. Giminez, Roubidoux, MA, et al. The emphysemas: Radiolgic-pathologic correlations. *Radiographics.* 1993;13:311–318.

Fraser RG, Paré JAP, Paré PD, Fraser RD, Generoux GP. *Diagnosis of Diseases of the Chest.* Vols. 2 and 3. 3rd ed. Philadelphia: WB Saunders; 1989, 1990.

Garg K, Lynch DA, Newell JD, King JTE. Proliferative and constrictive bronchiolitis: Classification and radiologic features. *AJR Am J Roentgenol.* 1994;162:803–808.

Grenier P, Chevret S, Beiglman C, Braumer MW, Chastang C, Valeyre D. Chronic diffuse infiltrative disease: Determination of the diagnostic value of clinical data, chest radiography, and CT with Bayesian analysis. *Radiology.* 1994;191:383–390.

Grenier P, Cordeau M-P, Beigelman C. High resolution computed tomography of the airways. *J Thorac Imaging.* 1993;10:227–235.

Grenier P, Valeyre D, Cluzel P, Brauner MW, Lenoir S, Chastang C. Chronic diffuse interstitial lung disease: Diagnostic value of chest radiography and high-resolution CT. *Radiology.* 1991;179:123–132.

Gurney JW. The pathophysiology of airways disease. *J Thorac Imaging.* 1995;10:227–235.

Haaga JR, Lanzieri CF, Sartoris DJ, Zerhouni EA, eds. *Computed Tomography and Magnetic Resonance Imaging of the Whole Body.* 3rd ed. St Louis: Mosby-Year Book; 1994.

Hartman TE, Primack SL, Lee KS, Swensen SJ, Müller NL. CT of bronchial and bronchiolar diseases. *Radiographics.* 1994;14:991–1003.

Kang EY, Miller RR, Müller, NL. Bronchiectasis: Comparison of preoperative thin section CT and pathologic findings in resected specimens. *Radiology.* 1995;195:649–654.

Leung AN, Staples CA, Müller, NL. CHronic diffuse infiltrative disease: Comparison of diagnostic accuracy of high resolution and conventional C. *Am J Roentgenol.* 1991;157:693–696.

McGuinness G, Naidich DP, Leitman BS, McCauley DI. Bronchiectasis: CT evaluation. *Am J Roentgenol.* 1991;160:253–257.

McLoud T. Occupational lung disease. *Radiol Clin North Am.* 1991;29: 931–941.

Mogavero-Newmark G, Conces DJ, Kopecky KK. Spiral CT evaluation of the trachea and bronchi. *J Comput Axial Tomogr.* 1994;18:552–554.

Müller NL. Clinical value of high relolution CT in chronic diffuse lung disease. *Am J Roentgenol.* 1991;157:1163–1170.

Müller NL, Miller RR. Computed tomography of chronic diffuse infiltrative disease: Part I. *Am Rev Respir Dis.* 1990;142:1206–1215.

Müller NL, Miller RR. Computed tomography of chronic diffuse infiltrative disease: Part II. *Am Rev Respir Dis.* 1990;142:1440–1448.

Müller NL, Miller RR. Diseases of the bronchioles: CT and histopathologic findings. *Radiology.* 1995;106:3–12.

Naidich DP, Zerhouni EA, Siegelman SS, *CT and MRI of the Thorax.* 2nd ed. New York: Lippincott-Raven; 1992.

Putman CE, ed. *Diagnostic Imaging of the Lung.* New York: Marcel Dekker; 1990.

Rémy-Jardin M, Giraud F, Rémy J, Copin MC, Gosselin B, Duhamel. A. Importance of ground-glass attenuation in chronic diffuse infiltrative lung disease: Pathologic CT correlation. *Radiology.* 1993;289:693–698.

Sagel SS, Slone RM. The lung. In: Lee JKT, Sagel SS, Stanley RJ, Heiken JP, eds. In: *Computed Body Tomography with MRI Correlation.* 3rd ed. New York: Lippincott-Raven, 1998.

Stern EJ, Frank MS. CT of the lungs in patients with pulmonary emphysema: Diagnosis, quantification and correlation with pathologic and physiologic findings. *Am J Roentgenol.* 1994;162:791–798.

Stern EJ, Swensen SJ. *High-Resolution CT of the Chest: Comprehensive Atlas.* Philadelphia; Lippincott-Raven; 1996.

Swensen SJ, Aughenbaugh L, Douglas W, Myers JL. High resolution CT of the lungs: Findings in various pulmonary diseases. *Am J Roentgenol.* 1992;158:971–979.

Thurlbeck WM, Müller NL. Emphyema: Definition imaging, and quantification. *Am J Roentgenol.* 1994;163:1017–1025.

Webb WR, Müller NL, Naidich DP. *High-Resolution CT of the Lung.* 2nd ed. Philadelphia: Lippincott-Raven; 1996.

Chapter 5

MEDIASTINUM

Fernando R. Gutierrez

5.1 MEDIASTINAL COMPARTMENTS

- The mediastinum, bounded by the lungs laterally, the chest wall anteriorly, and the spine posteriorly, contains the heart and great vessels, central pulmonary vessels, tracheobronchial tree, thymus, esophagus, lymph nodes, and lymphatics. This diverse collection of respiratory, vascular, gastrointestinal, and lymphatic structures lays the framework for a vast array of pathology.

- **Chest radiographs** are the primary screening examination for mediastinal pathology. Enlargement or displacement of normal structures, abnormal contours, increased density, and discrete masses can be readily detected.

- Although the location and shape of an abnormalitiy can often suggest a specific diagnosis, further evaluation with **computed tomography (CT)** is usually necessary to fully characterize the nature of a lesion, whether vascular, cystic, or soft tissue. Intravenous (IV) contrast is generally indicated, although noncontrast images are useful when cystic lesions are suspected.

- In an effort to narrow the differential diagnostic possibilities, the mediastinum is often artificially divided into compartments. The **classic anatomic description** divides the mediastinum into four compartments. The superior mediastinum or thoracic inlet marks the cervicothoracic junction and is defined by an imaginary line between the sternal angle and the fourth intervertebral disk (**Differential 106***).

  The anterior mediastinum lies between the sternum and pericardium. The middle mediastinum contains the pericardium, heart, and roots of the great vessels. The posterior mediastinum lies posterior to the pericardium and anterior to the lower eight vertebral bodies.

- The divisions used in this book represent a modification of the classic nomenclature, typically used in radiology, that divides the mediastinum into three major compartments (Fig. 5-1).

  The **anterior mediastinum**, bounded anteriorly by the sternum and posteriorly by the brachiocephalic vessels, aorta, and anterior pericardium, contains the thymus, internal mammary arteries and veins, and fat (**Differential 107**).

  The **middle mediastinum** contains the heart, ascending and transverse portions of the aorta, superior and inferior vena cava, brachiocephalic vessels, trachea, main bronchi, lymph nodes, and central pulmonary arteries and veins (**Differential 108**).

  The **posterior mediastinum** extends from the posterior portion of the pericardium anteriorly to the paravertebral gutters posteriorly and is bounded laterally by the mediastinal pleura (medial parietal pleura). It contains the descending thoracic aorta, thoracic duct, esophagus, azygos and hemiazygos veins, autonomic and intercostal nerves, and fat (**Differential 109**).

5.2 PNEUMOMEDIASTINUM

- **Perforation** can establish a communication with an adjacent hollow structure, thus resulting in gas collections in potential distensible spaces of the mediastinum (Fig. 5-2).

  Communication can also be established with the peritoneum or retroperitoneum through the esophageal hiatus. The air initially accumulates anteriorly, emphasizing the value of the lateral radiograph in visualizing the retrosternal area.

---

*Please refer to Chapter 2, in which the differential diagnoses are discussed in numerical order.

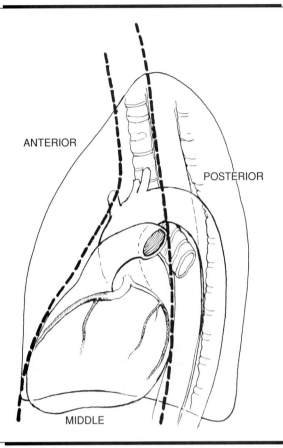

FIGURE 5-1   Mediastinal compartments. Lateral projection of the chest illustrating the most commonly used radiologic division of the mediastinum into anterior, middle, and posterior compartments.

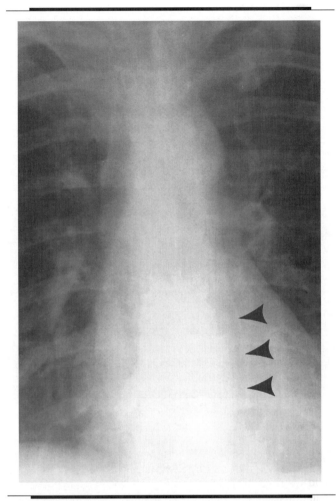

FIGURE 5-2   Pneumomediastinum. Chest radiograph demonstrating a small air collection along the left side of the mediastinum (arrowheads). Esophagoscopy had resulted in a small perforation.

The distinction of pneumomediastinum from pneumopericardium can be difficult to establish. One discriminator is that a pneumomediastinum can extend around the aortic knob into the potential spaces of the superior mediastinum. A pneumopericardium rarely extends to the level of the arch since the pericardial reflections end at the level of the ascending aorta.

While pneumomediastinum can result in pneumothorax, the opposite situation is uncommon. It may be difficult at times to distinguish a medial pneumothorax (air between visceral and parietal pleura) from a pneumomediastinum (air outside the parietal pleura). Lateral decubitus views can be helpful in making the differentiation.

Among the common causes of pneumomediastinum are barotrauma (volotrauma) and bronchial asthma. Barotrauma occurs in patients with mechanical ventilators when air dissects along the walls of the airway into the mediastinum or pleural space (**Differential 102**).

5.3 INFLAMMATORY DISEASE

- **Acute mediastinitis and mediastinal abscess** can result from a diversity of causes such as surgery, perforation of the esophagus during swallowing of sharp objects, endoscopy, or tracheal rupture during intubation. Additionally, the spread of infections from adjacent organs such as the lung can result in mediastinal infections that may ultimately result in abscess formation. Other causes of esophageal perforation include **Boerhaave syndrome** and tumor necrosis eroding the wall of the esophagus.

  Early during the infectious process, CT may demonstrate streaky, soft-tissue infiltration of the mediastinal fat. Later, if the disease progresses, drainable fluid collections and gas bubbles may be observed. If esophageal perforation is suspected, CT evaluation should be performed using water-soluble oral contrast material and IV contrast.

- **Fibrosing mediastinitis** is rare, occurring with infections of *Histoplasma capsulatum* which can result in exuberant fibrogenesis of the mediastinum causing compression or occlusion of mediastinal structures (Fig. 5-3). An immunologic response to the histoplasma organism has been postulated as the probable cause.

  Symptoms depend on the severity of the obstruction as well as the structures involved. Involvement of the trachea

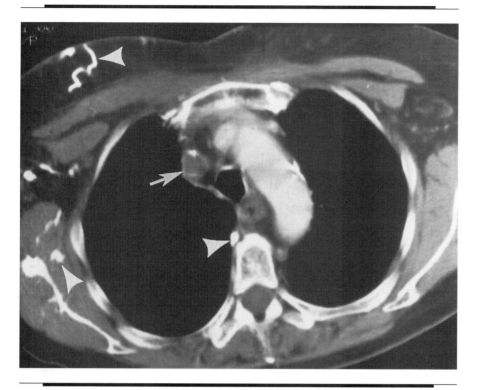

FIGURE 5-3   Fibrosing mediastinitis as a result of histoplasmosis. Chest CT demonstrating thrombosis of the SVC (arrow) and multiple collateral vessels in the mediastinum and chest wall (arrowheads).

The size of the lymph nodes varies depending on the method of measurement (short versus long axis). A maximum diameter of 1 cm along the short axis of the node has been advocated as the threshold for most mediastinal lymph nodes. This criterion is of limited value since large nodes may be benign and nodes smaller than 1 cm may contain malignant deposits. Whichever criteria is utilized to measure lymph node size, it must be remembered that normal-sized lymph nodes may or may not be pathologic since the internal architecture of the lymph node cannot be assessed even with state-of-the-art CT.

- Most mediastinal and hilar lymph node metastases arise from an intrathoracic neoplasm (bronchogenic carcinoma), usually on the ipsilateral side, or lymphoma. Extrathoracic tumors frequently associated with metastases to the hilar and mediastinal lymph nodes are breast, renal, testicular, head and neck cancer, and melanoma. Alternatively, inflammatory lesions such as sarcoidosis, tuberculosis, and fungal infections, as well as inhalational diseases such as silicosis, can cause adenopathy.

and major bronchi, superior vena cava and the pericardium can occur. Pulmonary infiltrates can be observed as a result of pulmonary infarction from arterial compression or pulmonary edema due to compression of the pulmonary veins.

Rarely, there may also be involvement of the retroperitoneum. Fibrosis of the mediastinum and retroperitoneum has also been reported as a complication of methysergide and other drug therapy. CT can demonstrate a conglomeration of calcified lymph nodes encroaching on the mediastinal structures.

5.4 MEDIASTINAL ADENOPATHY

- **Mediastinal adenopathy** is a common cause of mediastinal widening on chest radiographs. CT is more sensitive than plain radiography and may detect unsuspected adenopathy. With increasing size, mediastinal lymph nodes become less sharply defined, as they "blend" with the adjacent mediastinal fat. The anterior mediastinum is the most commonly affected compartment in patients with Hodgkin lymphoma.

- There is variation in the **normal size of lymph nodes** depending on their location within the mediastinum (Fig. 5-4). While subcarinal lymph nodes can have a normal diameter threshold of 12 mm, lymph nodes located in the cardiophrenic angle are usually 5 mm or less in diameter. Alternatively, a cluster of borderline enlarged lymph nodes should be suspected as being diseased.

- **Calcification** within mediastinal lymph nodes almost certainly excludes malignancy. The most common cause is healed granulomatous infections. Acquired immunodeficiency syndrome (AIDS) patients with *Pneumocystis carinii* infections can exhibit calcified mediastinal lymph nodes, apparently from a necrotizing granulomatous reaction. Inhalational disorders such as silicosis have been associated with lymph node calcification, either in an eggshell, central, or diffuse pattern. An eggshell pattern of calcification can also be seen with sarcoidosis and treated lymphoma. Rare causes of malignant calcified lymph nodes have been described in metastatic osteosarcoma, broncholalveolar cell carcinoma, and mucinous adenocarcinoma of the colon and ovaries (**Differential 99**).

- **Low-attenuation** mediastinal lymph nodes can be seen in cases of mycobacterial or fungal infections, as well as in aggressive malignancies with tumor necrosis within those nodes, such as from lung, testicular and ovarian primaries (**Differential 100**).

- **Enhancing lymph nodes** can be seen in angiofollicular lymph node hyperplasia (Castleman disease) and in highly vascular metastatic renal or thyroid carcinoma (**Differential 101**).

- **Sarcoidosis** is a systemic disease of unknown etiology that commonly presents incidentally on routine chest radiographs. Adenopathy is the most common manifestation,

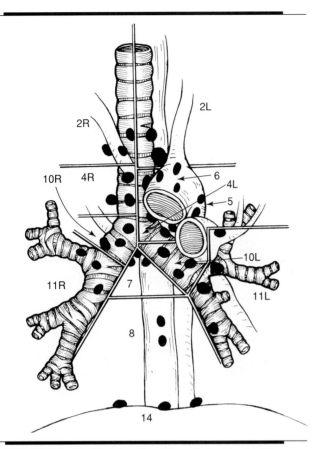

FIGURE 5-4   Modified American Thoracic Society classification of regional nodal stations. (2R) Right upper paratracheal nodes. Nodes to the right of the midline of the trachea, between the intersection of the caudal margin of the brachiocephalic artery with the trachea and the apex of the lung or above the level of the aortic arch. **(2L) Left upper paratracheal nodes.** Nodes to the left of the midline of the trachea, between the top of the aortic arch and the apex of the lung. **(4R) Right lower paratracheal nodes.** Nodes to the right of the midline of the trachea, between the cephalic border of the azygos vein and the intersection of the caudal margin of the brachiocephalic artery with the right side of the trachea or the top of the aortic arch. **(4L) Left lower paratracheal nodes.** Nodes to the left of the midline of the trachea, between the top of the aortic arch and the level of the carina, medial to the ligamentum arteriosum. **(5) Aortopulmonary nodes.** Subaortic and para-aortic nodes, lateral to the ligamentum ateriosum or the aorta or left pulmonary artery, proximal to the first branch of the left pulmonary artery. **(6) Anterior mediastinal nodes.** Nodes anterior to the ascending aorta or the innominate artery. **(7) Subcarinal nodes.** Nodes arising caudal to the carina of the trachea but not associated with the lower lobe bronchi or arteries within the lung. **(8) Paraesophageal nodes.** Nodes dorsal to the posterior wall of the trachea and to the right or left of the midline of the esophagus below the level of the subcarinal region (nodes around the descending aorta should also be included). **(9) Right or left pulmonary ligament nodes.** Nodes within the right or left inferior pulmonary ligament (not shown). **(10R) Right tracheobronchial nodes.** Nodes to the right of the midline of the trachea, from the level of the cephalic border of the azygos vein to the origin of the right upper lobe bronchus. **(10L) Left peribronchial nodes.** Nodes to the left of the midline of the trachea, between the carina and the left upper lobe bronchus, medial to the ligamentum arteriosum. **(11) Intrapulmonary nodes.** Nodes removed in the right or left lung specimen, plus those distal to the main stem bronchi or secondary carina (includes interlobar, lobar, and segmental nodes). **(14) Superior diaphragmatic nodes.** Nodes adjacent to the pericardium within 2 cm of the diaphragm.

seen by radiograph in 80 percent of patients at some time in the course of the disease. Most have symmetric hilar and classically right paratracheal involvement. Pulmonary involvement includes insterstitial infiltrates and nodules; it is variable, with adenopathy typically decreasing as lung disease progresses. (See Section 4.9 for a more complete discussion.)

- **Castleman disease** is a benign condition of uncertain etiology characterized by enlarged lymph node masses that can appear in various locations, predominantly in the mediastinum (Fig. 5-5). This entity has other synonyms such as giant lymph node hyperplasia, angiofollicular lymph node hyperplasia, lymphonodal hamartoma, and follicular lymphoreticuloma.

  There are two variants: the plasma cell (acute) form and the hyaline-vascular type which has a more chronic tendency. The lesion is usually discovered incidentally in asymptomatic patients or in individuals with nonspecific systemic symptoms such as low-grade fever or night sweats.

  Castleman disease usually affects young patients who present with mediastinal or hilar masses that exhibit diffuse contrast enhancement and are highly vascular on angiography. This imaging feature helps differentiate this condition from other mediastinal and hilar masses.

  Histologically, Castleman disease can be difficult to differentiate from thymoma or even malignant lymphoma. An association with Kaposi sarcoma has been described.

- **Hilar lymphadenopathy** can be very difficult to determine on plain radiography. Although CT is superior in assessing hilar anatomy, the use of intravenous contrast material frequently is necessary for proper identification of hilar structures. In general, lymph nodes greater than 5 mm in

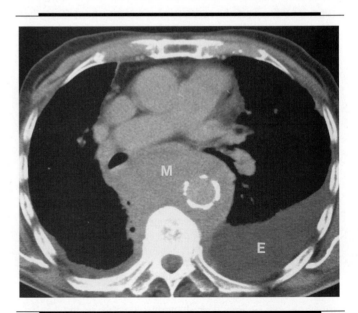

FIGURE 5-5   Castleman disease. Contrast-enhanced CT demonstrating a large posterior mediastinal mass (M) surrounding a calcified descending aorta and displacing vascular structures anteriorly. The mass enhances compared to pleural fluid (E).

size are considered abnormal in the hila. As is the case in the mediastinum, neoplastic and inflammatory nodes have similar appearances on CT.

Occasionally, hilar enlargement may be due to vascular causes. Bilateral pulmonary artery enlargement may be observed in pulmonary artery hypertension, left-to-right shunts, idiopathic dilatation of the pulmonary arteries, and congenital absence of the pulmonary valve. Unilateral pulmonary artery enlargement may be seen in pulmonary valve stenosis, pulmonary artery aneurysm, and surgical systemic-to-pulmonary-artery shunts (**Differentials 97 and 98**).

5.5 ANTERIOR MEDIASTINUM

- The most common anterior mediastinal masses are lymphomas, thoracic goiters, lesions of the thymus, and germ cell tumors (**Differential 107**).

- **Intrathoracic goiters** appear on chest radiographs as a superior mediastinal mass displacing the trachea. Radionuclide scintigraphy was the primary method of diagnosis in the past, but most cases are now diagnosed with CT which can distinguish it from other causes of a mediastinal mass and assess the relationship to vascular and other adjacent structures.

    Although in most cases the intrathoracic goiter is located in the anterior mediastinum anterior to the great vessels, in about 20 percent of cases it is located posterior to the trachea. On serial images, there is almost always continuity with the cervical thyroid. Intrathoracic goiters often have areas of low attenuation and calcification.

- **The thymus** is composed of two lobes which are frequently asymmetric. In younger patients, it has a triangular appearance and is isointense to muscle on CT. With increasing age, thymic tissue atrophies and is replaced by fat but can frequently exhibit streaky or nodular densities.

- **Thymic cysts** can be found anywhere along the development pathway of the thymus from the neck to the mediastinum. They can be congenital from the persistence of the thymopharyngeal duct or acquired from degeneration or inflammation. In general, they have a homogeneous fluid component on CT compared to cystic degeneration of malignant tumors which have a predominant soft-tissue attenuation. This differentiation may be difficult at times, requiring cytologic confirmation.

- **Cysts** can be seen in cases of Hodgkin lymphoma, probably as a result of thymic involution. They can persist or even enlarge following radiation or chemotherapy.

- **Rebound thymic hyperplasia** is a phenomenon that is more common in children and young adults, where a period of stress with thymic involution is followed by regrowth or overgrowth of the gland. Subsequently, there is a gradual return of the thymus to normal size. Despite an abnormal increase in size, the gland maintains its normal arrowhead configuration.

    This condition is a common finding in young patients after chemotherapy and may represent a diagnostic dilemma in patients with lymphoma or in patients being managed for Cushing syndrome. If the thymic shape is preserved and the enlargement correlates with the chemotherapy, follow-up imaging is usually all that is needed.

- **Thymomas** are neoplasms of thymic epithelial cells and lymphocytes usually located in the anterior mediastinum but rarely can be found in the posterior mediastinum or even in the neck. Cystic degeneration of the tumor can occur, with areas of necrosis or calcification. The size can vary, and at times they can fill the mediastinum.

    Rather than being a histologic classification, the term *invasive* or *noninvasive* refers to encapsulation of the tumor (noninvasive) or penetration of the capsule with subsequent invasion of the mediastinum. Approximately 30 percent of thymomas are invasive, and spread usually occurs by continuity. Distant metastases are extremely rare.

    Most thymomas are seen in patients in the fifth or sixth decade of life with no gender predilection. In patients with myasthenia gravis, the size tends to be smaller, apparently because of symptoms precipitating an early evaluation.

    Approximately 40 percent of patients with thymomas have myasthenia gravis (Fig. 5-6), whereas 15 percent of patients with myasthenia gravis have thymoma. The relationship between these two conditions is not clearly understood. Thymectomy, even in patients without thymoma, has been associated with symptomatic relief.

    Thymomas have also been associated with hypogammaglobulinemia, pure red cell aplasia, thyroid carcinoma, ulcerative colitis, and Crohn disease.

- **Thymic lymphoid hyperplasia** has also been associated with myasthenia gravis. In these cases, CT scans can vary from a normal to a symmetrically enlarged thymus.

- **Thymolipomas** are composed of fat and involuted thymic tissue and are usually seen at an earlier age than thymomas. They may grow to a significant size before diagnosis. CT demonstrates a mediastinal tumor composed mainly of fat and traversed by septations of soft tissue representing the residual thymic tissue. The high signal intensity characteristic of fat is seen on T1-weighted MR scans.

- **Thymic lymphoma** is common in patients with Hodgkin disease, particularly the nodular sclerosing variety (Fig. 5-7). The thymic enlargement can be diffuse or asymmetric, and cystic degeneration may occur. Calcification can develop after treatment.

    In contrast to thymoma, Hodgkin disease is usually accompanied by nodal enlargement in other parts of the mediastinum and elsewhere. Differentiation between thymic rebound hyperplasia and recurrent lymphoma can be a diagnostic challenge in younger patients after being treated for the disease.

- **Thymic carcinoma** is a rare malignant neoplasm that arises from the thymic epithelium. The basic pathologic distinction from invasive thymoma is the presence of malignant cytology and more local invasion.

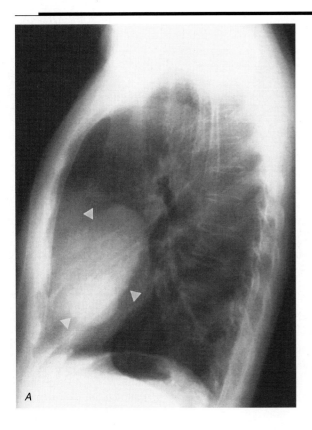

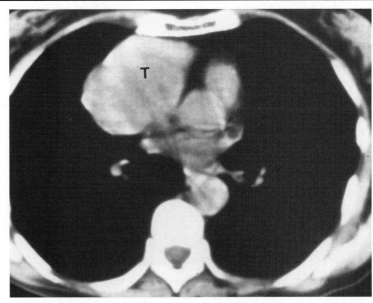

FIGURE 5-6   Thymoma. (*A*) Lateral chest radiograph showing a large anterior mediastinal mass (arrowheads) superimposed over the heart in a patient with myasthenia gravis. (*B*) CT demonstrating the thymoma (T).

Radiologically, it may be difficult to differentiate thymic carcinoma from other thymic neoplasms such as invasive thymoma. CT may show areas of necrosis, calcification, or cyst formation. They tend to be very anaplastic, infiltrating tumors which metastasize via lymphatic and hematogenous routes. There can be gross invasion of adjacent mediastinal structures, as well as distant metastases, and the prognosis is generally poor.

- **Germ cell tumors** arise from remnants of the primitive germ cell layers. They are usually found during the second to fourth decade of life and are located in the anterior mediastinum, in or adjacent to the thymus. They can be benign (mature teratoma), which is most common, or malignant and considered primary if no gonadal or retroperitoneal tumor involvement can be found.

  Mature teratomas are cystic and have well-defined walls. In approximately one-half of cases, fat can be detected within the tumor mass. In addition, areas of soft tissue, calcification, or even ossification can be found. They do not erode adjacent mediastinal structures.

  Seminomas and nonseminomatous tumors represent malignant germ cell tumors and may have radiographic characteristics similar to those of areas of soft tissue, necrosis, or even calcification. They can rapidly metastasize to lung, pleura, and bone and occur in both men and women. Primary gonadal tumors frequently metastasize to the mediastinum (Fig. 5-8).

5.6 TRACHEA

- The trachea is a tubular structure composed of 14 to 20 incomplete C-shaped hyaline cartilage rings completed by a posterior membrane. It extends from the cricoid cartilage to the carina, located at approximately the T5 level. In the cervical area it is located in the midline, deviating to the right within the thorax.

  The cartilage rings can become calcified as part of the aging process. This is frequently seen in elderly females,

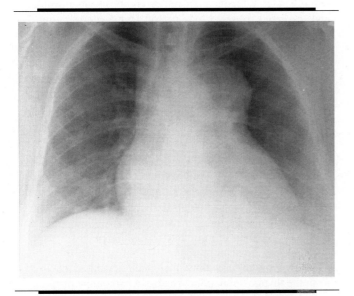

FIGURE 5-7   Hodgkin lymphoma. Chest radiograph demonstrating a large mediastinal mass in a 24-year-old woman.

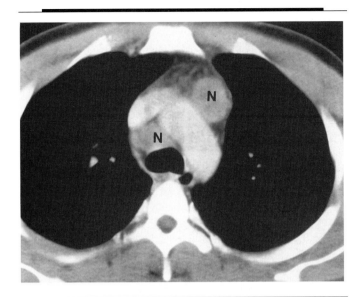

FIGURE 5-8 Metastatic testicular carcinoma. CT showing mediastinal adenopathy (N).

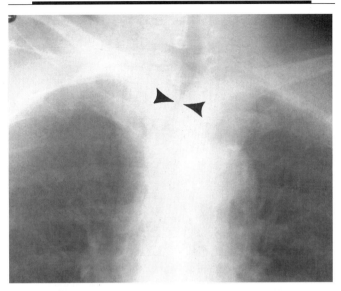

FIGURE 5-9 Tracheal narrowing. Focal tracheal narrowing (arrowheads) caused by scarring from a prior tracheostomy.

being present on CT in approximately 50 percent of patients in the seventh and eighth decades. The trachea can calcify prematurely in children and adults receiving coumadin therapy.

The carinal bifurcating angle is typically 60 to 75 degrees. The right mainstem bronchus has a steeper angle than the left. The mean transverse diameter of the trachea is approximately 15 mm for women and 18 mm for men.

- **Focal tracheal narrowing** occurs most commonly after iatrogenic injuries from prolonged endotracheal intubation or tracheostomy tube insertion. The incidence of this endotracheal intubation complication has decreased with the use of high-volume, low-pressure cuffs (Fig. 5-9). Stenotic lesions can occur at the stoma site (usually due to granulation) or near the tube tip.

- **Tracheomalacia** is a condition in which there is destruction of the tracheal cartilage resulting in increased tracheal compliance (Fig. 5-10). The usual causes are intrinsic and extrinsic compression of the trachea leading to wall degeneration and collapse when subject to negative or positive pressures during respiration. Fluoroscopy, ultrafast CT, or helical CT can be used to confirm the diagnosis.

- **Diffuse narrowing** of the trachea can occur with a variety of conditions that can narrow the trachea over a long segment (**Differential 30**).

  1. **Saber sheath trachea** is a condition in which the coronal diameter of the trachea is narrowed as compared to the sagittal diameter. The trachea has a normal diameter in the cervical region but assumes the saber sheath configuration below the thoracic inlet (Fig. 5-11). It is seen predominantly in men with emphysema.

  2. **Tracheopathia osteochondroplastica (TOP)** results in thickening of the tracheal cartilages with submucosal

osteocartilagenous nodules. Patients are usually middle-aged, presenting with cough and hemoptysis as common clinical complaints. The condition can extend into the

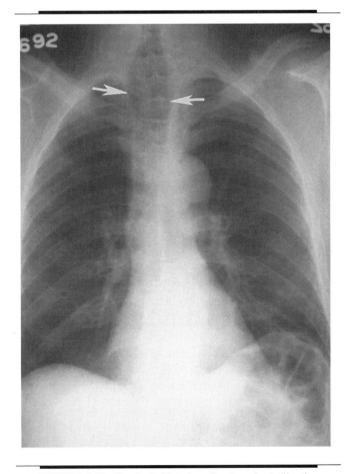

FIGURE 5-10 Tracheal dilatation. Focal tracheal dilatation (arrows) as a consequence of prolonged endotracheal intubation with an overdistended balloon.

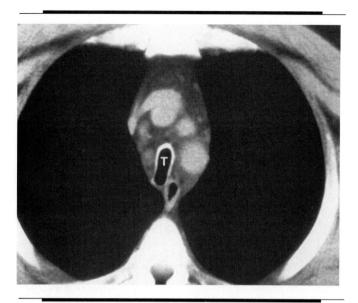

FIGURE 5-11 Saber-sheath trachea. CT demonstrating the narrowed transverse diameter of the trachea (T) at the level of the thoracic inlet with preservation of the anteroposterior diameter.

bronchi. Similar findings can also be found in amyloidosis (Fig. 5-12).

3. **Amyloidosis** of the tracheobronchial tree consists of deposition of a protein-polysaccharide complex in the submucosa that can lead to wheezing and stridor. Amyloid nodules can also be observed in the lung periphery. Areas of calcification can be present.

4. **Relapsing polychondritis**, which usually affects young and middle-aged adults, produces thickening and calcification of the tracheal cartilage, resulting in airway narrowing. There is usually diffuse thickening of the tracheobronchial wall, with lumen deformity and tracheal collapse.

    This condition is associated with inflammation and accelerated destruction of other cartilaginous structures such as the nose and ear lobes, resulting in clinical features of saddle nose and floppy ears. It can be associated with aortitis and arthritis. Airway involvement is the most common cause of death.

5. **Wegener granulomatosis** consists of acute necrotizing granulomas of the upper and lower respiratory tract, vasculitis, and glomerulonephritis. Males are more commonly affected than females, and the airway is most frequently affected. CT can demonstrate focal or diffuse tracheal narrowing with occasional cartilage distortion.

- **Acquired tracheomegaly** can be seen in a variety of conditions in which there is chronic inflammation of the trachea or retraction from adjacent fibrosis. Such conditions as cystic fibrosis and diffuse pulmonary fibrosis show progressive tracheal dilatation as the fibrotic changes ensue **(Differential 29)**.

- **Tracheobronchomegaly**, or Mounier-Kuhn syndrome, is a rare condition characterized by abnormal widening of the trachea and central bronchi associated with respiratory tract infections. It may be a congenital condition with an autosomal recessive pattern of transmission. It apparently represents a primary process in which there is progressive weakening of the walls of the airways. Patients may be asymptomatic or have relatively few symptoms, including chronic cough, hemoptysis, dyspnea, and repeated respiratory infections.

    The diagnosis is based on radiographic findings. It has been suggested that a coronal diameter of more than 26 mm in men and more than 23 mm in women on a posteroanterior chest radiograph is required for the diagnosis. These values represent the normal mean tracheal diameter plus three standard deviations. At times, the tracheal wall may have a corrugated appearance due to prolapse of the atrophic mucosa between the cartilage rings. Bronchiectasis may also be seen.

- **Tracheal tumors** are rare. While they can be seen at just about any age, when found in children they are mostly benign (hemangioma, papilloma), and in adults, mostly malignant (squamous cell and adenoid cystic carcinoma) (Fig. 5-13) **(Differential 32)**.

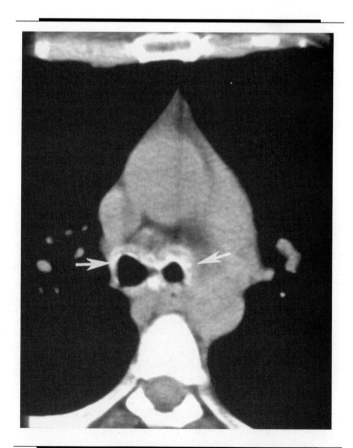

FIGURE 5-12 Tracheobronchopathia osteochondroplastica. CT just below the carina showing thickened, calcified bronchial walls (arrows).

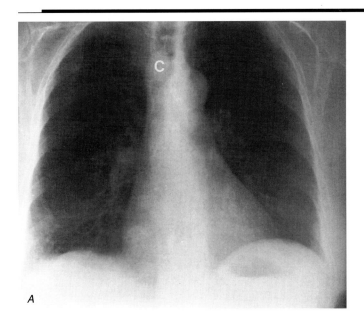

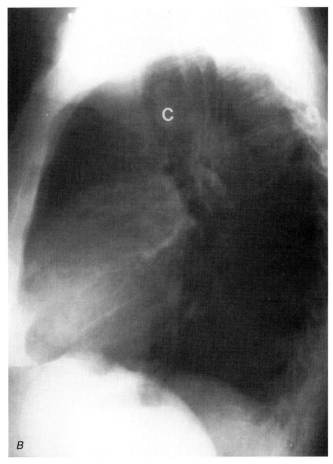

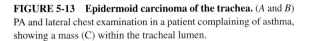

FIGURE 5-13   Epidermoid carcinoma of the trachea. (*A* and *B*) PA and lateral chest examination in a patient complaining of asthma, showing a mass (C) within the tracheal lumen.

The trachea may be involved by direct invasion from adjacent structures such as carcinoma of the esophagus or lung or rarely by metastases from distant primary cancers. Symptoms such as cough, asthma, and dyspnea, can have an insidious onset since it can take extensive luminal obstruction to develop symptomatology.

5.7 ESOPHAGUS

- The **esophagus** is a muscular tube which begins at the level of the cricopharyngeus muscle in the cervical region and extends along the posterior mediastinum down to the level of the gastroesophageal junction. At this level, it pierces the diaphragm to left of the midline and anterior to the aorta. The esophagus has no serosal covering. The proximal third of the esophagus is composed of striated muscle, while the distal third is composed of smooth muscle layers.

- **Esophageal duplication cysts** represent an embryologic defect consisting of doubling of the esophagus in some degree. They are usually located more posterior than bronchogenic cysts. The distal esophagus is the most common location. They have an epithelial lining that varies from squamous to columnar. Duplication cysts can be paraesophageal or intramural.

  On CT they appear as well-marginated spherical masses with near-water density and in close relationship to the esophagus. There is usually no visible communication with the esophageal lumen. The differential diagnosis includes neurogenic tumor, abscess, bronchogenic cyst, and leiomyoma.

- **Achalasia** is the result of a decrease in or absence of the ganglia in the myenteric plexus. **Chagas' disease**, caused by infection with *Trypanosoma cruzi*, can cause similar myenteric plexus abnormalities. The esophagus loses its normal peristaltic rhythm, resulting in various degrees of dilatation. There is difficulty in the normal passage of food through the lower esophagus into the stomach since there is failure of the sphincter to relax.

  Symptoms include dyspepsia, chest pain, regurgitation, and pulmonary symptoms related to aspiration pneumonia. Complications include the development of granulomatous lesions and a predisposition to esophageal carcinoma. Radiographically, a narrow distal esophagus is seen, accompanied by gross proximal dilatation (Fig. 1-10). Secondarily, inflammatory changes can develop in the mucosa as a result of chronic stagnation.

- **Esophageal varices** are usually located in the lower portion of the esophagus and gastric fundus. They are the result of portosystemic venous anastomosis secondary to **portal hypertension**. They appear as lobulated tubular densities in the retrocardiac region near the gastroesophageal junction (Fig. 5-14). A history of liver disease and intense enhancement after the administration of IV contrast, characteristic of vessels, help make the diagnosis on CT.

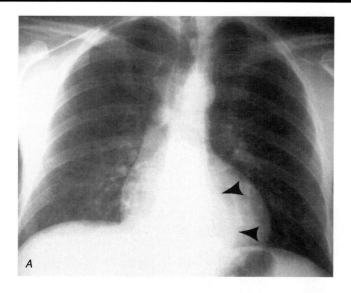

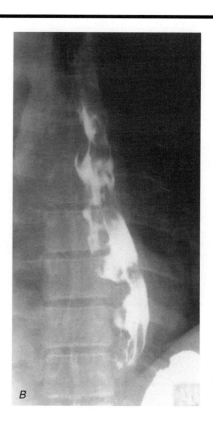

FIGURE 5-14   Esophageal varices. (*A*) Chest radiograph demonstrating a large paraspinal mass (arrowheads). (*B*) Corresponding esophagogram showing multiple varices indenting the esophageal lumen.

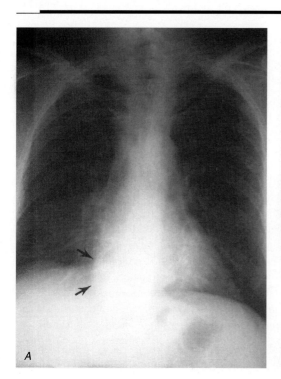

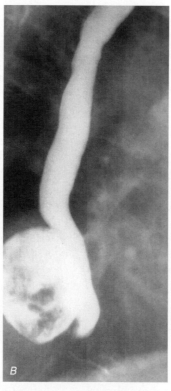

- **Esophageal diverticula** are believed to be acquired rather than congenital. They are usually found in adults, their incidence usually increasing with age. They are most common in the middle and distal third of the esophagus and are usually a consequence of abnormal esophageal peristalsis. Although most are asymptomatic, when they attain a large size, they can cause difficulties in esophageal emptying by compressing the adjacent normal esophagus.

  They are classified as **Zenker** or pulsion diverticuli when found in the upper third of the esophagus, as **traction diverticuli** in the midesophagus, and as **epiphrenic** or pulsion diverticuli in the distal esophagus. If large enough, they can be seen as a mediastinal mass on plain radiographs (Fig. 5-15).

- **Hiatal hernias** can be divided into sliding and paraesophageal types depending on whether the cardia remains normally located or not. They represent a common cause of a retrocardiac mass on plain films, usually with an air-fluid level. The vast majority of hiatal hernias are of the sliding type and their

FIGURE 5-15   Esophageal diverticulum. (*A*) Chest radiograph demonstrating a mass with an air-fluid level projecting just above the right hemidiaphragm (arrows). (*B*) Esophagogram showing a large distal esophageal diverticulum partially filled with food debris.

incidence increases with age. They are further discussed in Section 8.10.

- **Esophageal cancer** represents about 95 percent of all neoplasms of the esophagus and 1 percent of all cancers of the gastrointestinal tract. They infrequently present as mediastinal masses and frequently have lymphatic and mediastinal spread by the time of diagnosis. It is a disease of older people and affects males and blacks more commonly. Predisposing factors include alcohol consumption, smoking, achalasia, Barrett esophagus, and esophageal strictures, as well as exposure to tannins.

  The forms of spread are by direct extension to adjacent mediastinal organs. Lymphatic spread occurs to cervical, mediastinal, and upper abdominal nodes, and by blood-borne metastasis to the liver and lung. The chest radiograph is almost always normal, although proximal esophageal dilatation may be seen. An esophogram typically demonstrates a polypoid, ulcerated, or annular constrictive apple-core lesion with overhanging edges. Tumor necrosis can lead to fistula formation in adjacent structures. Fifty percent of esophageal cancers affect the middle third, 30 percent the distal third, and 20 percent the upper third.

  Adenocarcinoma has recently surpassed squamous cell as the most common cell type. Other malignant tumors are unusual. As a general rule, adenocarcinomas originate in columnar epithelium of Barrett esophagus or in the stomach with spread to the distal esophagus. The incidence of this type of cancer is on the increase.

  CT is a sensitive indicator for metastatic disease to the liver and adjacent mediastinal structures. Aortic invasion of esophageal carcinoma has been studied by determining the arc of periaortic fat obscuration. Prediction of mediastinal and upper abdominal lymph node involvement is not very accurate because of microscopic tumor involvement in normal-sized lymph nodes. The efficacy of CT staging is controversial, but the accuracy of CT staging of esophageal carcinoma is about 90 percent, with a lower detection rate for carcinomas near the gastroesophageal junction.

- **CT staging** of esophageal carcinoma:

  Stage I Intraluminal polypoid mass or localized wall thickening 3 to 5 mm. No adenopathy.

  Stage II Greater than 5 mm thickening of esophageal wall without adjacent or distant metastases.

  Stage III Wall thickening with direct extension into adjacent tissue with or without local or regional mediastinal adenopathy.

  Stage IV Any stage with distant metastatic disease.

5.8 CYSTIC LESIONS

- Cystic lesions of the mediastinum can be congenital, vascular, inflammatory, or neoplastic. They include bronchopulmonary foregut cysts (bronchogenic, esophageal duplication, and neuroenteric cysts), thymic cysts (Section 5.5), and pericardial cysts (**Differential 111**).

- **Bronchogenic cysts** are the most common type of congenital cyst of the mediastinum. They represent abnormal budding from the foregut or tracheobronchial tree and are usually in close proximity to the carina or right paratracheal region. Usually, communication with the foregut is lost, and they may have a stalk attaching them to the airway. They are typically smooth and spherical with a thin wall.

  They are lined by respiratory epithelium containing cartilage, smooth muscle, and mucous glands. They also contain fluid that can be serous, viscous, milky, or hemorrhagic, therefore having variable CT attenuation. Fluid-fluid levels may be identified due to layering of debris or milk or calcium. On MR, the T1 signal intensity is variable, and the T2 signal intensity is high (Fig. 5-16). They can demonstrate abnormal accumulation of ^{99m}Tc-MAA (macroaggregate albumen) on lung perfusion scanning.

  As a general rule, if the findings are typical and the patient is asymptomatic, conservative management is recommended. In cases of atypical radiographic presentation or if there are symptoms of compression, aspiration or surgery has been advocated.

- **Esophageal duplication cyst** is a rare type of duplication cyst that can appear at any age. Because of their similar location, they can be confused with bronchogenic cysts. They may have thicker walls and are located in the posterior mediastinum, attached to or near the esophagus, although this is not a specific finding (Fig. 5-17).

- **Neuroenteric cysts** are foregut cysts of the posterior mediastinum associated with vertebral column anomalies such as spina bifida and hemivertebra and can be attached by fibrous strands to the vertebrae. The appearance on CT is similar to that of other mediastinal cysts, although diagnosis can be suggested if vertebral anomalies are present. These anomalies may be located at a different level.

- **Pericardial cysts** are the result of an outpouching of the parietal pericardium that does not communicate with the pericardial sac. If they communicate with the pericardial sac, they are referred to as *pericardial diverticuli*. Most patients are asymptomatic, although chest pain, cough, and dyspnea have been described.

  These cysts are usually uniloculated spaces containing clear yellow fluid and located in the right anterior cardiophrenic angle, although they can be located in any part of the pericardium or extend to other areas of the mediastinum, making differentiation from a bronchogenic cyst difficult.

  Imaging typically reveals a rounded, smooth-walled structure adjacent to the right atrium with water attenuation values on CT (**Differential 110**). If the cyst contains clear fluid, MR will show low signal intensity on T1-weighted images and high signal on T2-weighted images. However, at times, the fluid may be proteinaceous, which can result in high signal intensity on T1 images.

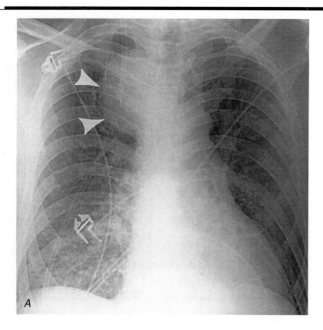
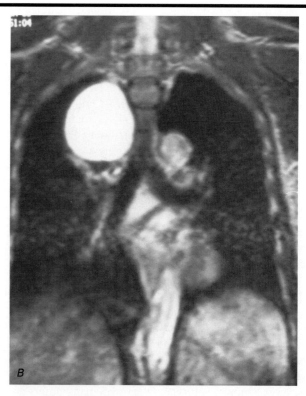

FIGURE 5-16   Bronchogenic cyst. (*A*) Chest radiograph showing a large right paratracheal mass with smooth margins (arrowheads) in an ICU patient. (*B*) Coronal T2-weighted MR demonstrating high signal intensity characteristic of fluid.

- A **mediastinal abcess** has clinical features, thick walls, and gas bubbles which can help differentiate it from other cystic masses. Other types of cysts may become secondarily infected.

- **Cystic intrathoracic goiters** show continuity with the cervical thyroid as a crucial differentiating feature.

- **Pancreatic pseudocysts** can dissect into the posterior mediastinum via the esophageal or aortic hiatus. Continuity with

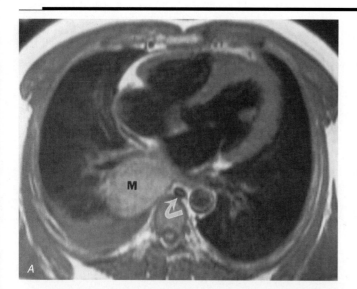
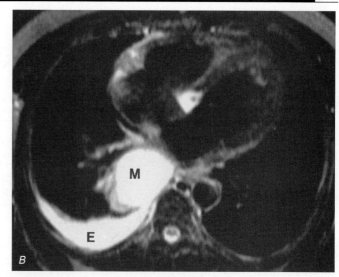

FIGURE 5-17   Esophageal duplication cyst. (*A*) T1-weighted and (*B*) T2-weighted MR demonstrating a cystic retrocardiac mass (M) adjacent to the esophagus (arrow). A pleural effusion (E) is also seen.

the pancreas and a history of pancreatitis should help identify this rare entity (Fig. 13-21).

- **Lymphangiomas (cystic hygromas)** are usually located in the neck, although in 10 percent of cases a mediastinal extension can be found. In less than 1 percent of patients, the lesion can be located exclusively in the mediastinum. They are benign tumors seen in young children. They are usually well-defined tumors consisting of proliferating lymphatics and can encompass other mediastinal structures. They are classified as capillary, cavernous, or cystic (hygromas), and mixed lesions are common.

Imaging characteristics include low signal intensity on T1-weighted MR images and high signal intensity on T2-weighted images because of the abundance of fluid-filled spaces. CT shows well-defined tumors with low attenuation values. Areas of hemorrhage or superimposed infection can exhibit higher attenuation values.

5.9 FATTY MASSES AND MESENCHYMAL TUMORS

- **Mesenchymal tumors** comprise several categories of tumors including those that arise from fat, lymphatics, blood vessels, muscle, and connective tissue.

- **Omental or abdominal fat** can herniate through the foramen of Morgagni, foramen of Bochdalek, or esophageal hiatus. Omental fat may contain streaky densities representing omental blood vessels. Continuity with the omentum establishes the proper diagnosis (Fig. 5-18).

- **Mediastinal lipomatosis** represents an abundant deposition of histologically normal fat that can result in smooth mediastinal widening without tracheal narrowing. It can be seen in obese patients and in patients undergoing steroid therapy or with Cushing disease. The fat deposition occurs primarily in the superior mediastinum but can be located in any mediastinal compartment and can extend into the atrioventricular grooves of the heart.

This condition represents diffuse or focal collections of unencapsulated fat. In general, the diagnosis can be established with plain radiographs because the deposition is smooth and symmetric without causing tracheal distortion. Frequently, it is associated with increased fat accumulation in the extrapleural areas and cardiophrenic angles. CT may be required to exclude a soft-tissue mediastinal mass.

- **Mediastinal lipomas** are rare. They typically have sharp margins and may be encapsulated or have thin soft-tissue septations. Additional areas of soft tissue or inhomogeneity should suggest other types of tumors such as a liposarcoma (Fig. 5-19), myelolipoma, or germ cell tumor. They usually do not compress adjacent mediastinal structures and should be differentiated from mediastinal lipomatosis in which the fat is not encapsulated.

- **Liposarcoma and lipoblastoma** typically have some soft-tissue stranding and infiltrating rather than smooth margins.

- **Teratomas and thymolipomas** can present as an inhomogeneous fatty mass in the anterior mediastinum and may contain calcium.

- **Hemangiomas** can arise from arterioles and venules, but most are of capillary origin. They are well-circumscribed developmental malformations composed of tangled interconnecting vascular spaces with endothelial cell proliferation and areas of thrombosis or fibrosis, leading to irregular contrast enhancement on CT. Punctate intravascular calcifications (phleboliths) may be seen.

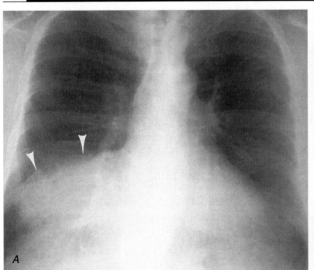
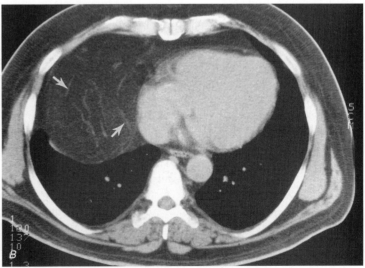

FIGURE 5-18 Morgagni hernia. (*A*) Chest radiograph demonstrating a large right cardiophrenic angle mass (arrowheads). (*B*) CT demonstrating a fatty mass with small blood vessels (arrows) indicative of omentum.

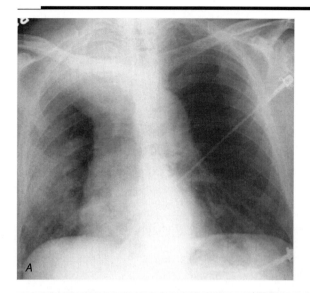
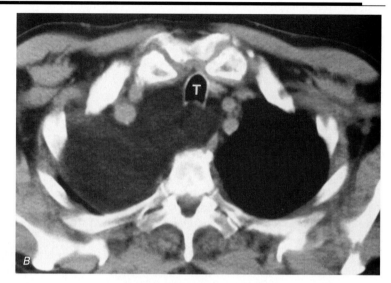

FIGURE 5-19   Mediastinal liposarcoma. (*A*) Portable chest radiograph in a 64-year-old male complaining of chest discomfort, demonstrates a large right paratracheal mass that fills most of the right lung apex. (*B*) Contrast-enhanced CT shows an infiltrating mass composed mostly of fat with soft tissue stranding throughout the tumor. T, trachea.

5.10   NEUROGENIC TUMORS

- Most posterior mediastinal masses are neurogenic tumors (**Differential 109**) and are divided into three major groups depending on whether they arise from the peripheral nerves (schwannoma, neurofibroma), sympathetic ganglia (ganglioneuroma, ganglioneuroblastoma, neuroblastoma), or paraganglia (chemodectoma, pheochromocytoma). Differentiating benign from malignant neurogenic tumors is not always possible with present imaging methods.

   The radiographic appearance is that of a well-defined posterior mediastinal mass which may be either smooth or lobulated. There is a wide variety in size. Calcification can be seen. There may be rib or vertebral scalloping from tumor compression.

- **Schwannoma**, also termed neurilemoma, is the most common type of peripheral nerve tumor. They tend to be encapsulated and are composed of Schwann cells. The nerve fibers do not course through the tumor. In general they are solitary, painless tumors, but can cause symptoms from pressure if large.

   Most patients are middle-aged, and these tumors affect males and females equally. They can occur in other areas of the body such as the head and neck. In the mediastinum, they can attain the largest sizes. These tumors do not recur after excision and do not tend to undergo malignant degeneration.

   The chest radiograph can reveal a well-demarcated paravertebral mass. Frequently, areas of low attenuation can be seen within the tumoral mass. Areas of increased vascularity can show increase gadolinium (Gd-DTPA) uptake on MR.

These tumors can enlarge intervertebral foramina if they involve the corresponding nerve root.

- **Neurofibroma** is a type of neurogenic tumor typically seen in younger patients. They can be single or multiple (neurofibromatosis) (Fig. 5-20). Solitary neurofibromas have a low incidence of malignant degeneration or recurrence after local excision; however, when multiple, the risk of malignant degeneration can be significant.

   The fundamental pathologic difference between these tumors and schwannomas is that neurofibromas contain Schwann cells that are tangled with the nerves, making it hard to dissect the tumor from the nerve. Collagen fibers or bundles are seen throughout the tumor.

   Approximately 30 percent of patients with neurofibromas have **neurofibromatosis**. Lateral meningoceles can also be seen in patients with neurofibromatosis. These represent an extrusion of the dura and arachnoid through an intervertebral foramen into the extrapleural thoracic gutter.

- **Malignant nerve sheath tumor** is a generic term that includes several types of tumors observed in patients with and without fibromatosis. The earlier the appearance of the neurofibromas, the higher the incidence of malignant transformation. They are very aggressive, with a high incidence of recurrence, particularly in patients with neurofibromatosis. As a general rule, patients with **von Recklinghausen disease** have a higher incidence of malignant nerve sheath tumors. This autosomal dominant disease is characterized by café-au-lait lesions of the skin, multiple peripheral nerve tumors, and dysplastic abnormalities of the skin, nervous system, endocrine organs, bones, and blood vessels.

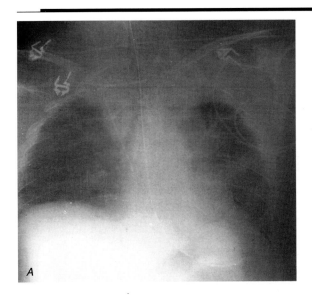
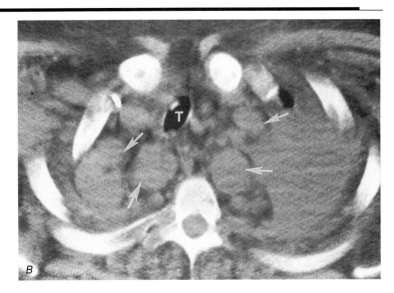

FIGURE 5-20   Neurofibromatosis. (*A*) Superior mediastinal widening seen on a portable chest radiograph in a 23-year-old patient with neurofibromatosis. (*B*) Large neurofibromas (arrows) are observed on a nonenhanced CT. T, trachea.

- **Tumors of sympathetic ganglia** include ganglioneuroma, ganglioneuroblastoma, and neuroblastoma. While nerve sheath tumors tend to have a lobulated appearance, ganglion cell tumors are elongated with tapered borders and oriented vertically along the direction of the sympathetic chain.

- **Neuroblastomas** are highly malignant undifferentiated tumors originating from sympathetic ganglia. They are seen almost exclusively in young children.

- **Ganglioneuroblastomas** also have malignant features, although they tend to have a better prognosis that neuroblastomas. Both tumors are observed in children, with less than 10 percent occurring in adults. Some have speckled calcifications.

- **Ganglioneuromas** are benign neoplasms found in teenagers and young adults.

- **Tumors of paraganglion cells** arise from aortic and pulmonary chemoreceptive glomera. When functional, signs and symptoms of overproduction of catecholamines such as flushing and systemic hypertension may be present. **Chemodectomas** or nonfunctioning paragangliomas are found near the aortic arch, in the region of the aortopulmonary window, or near the right pulmonary artery.

- **Pheochromocytomas** or functioning paragangliomas can be found in the posterior mediastinum or adjacent to the heart. The vast majority occur outside the chest. Because of their rich vascular supply, paraganglion cell tumors exhibit intense contrast enhancement on CT. An isointense signal is seen on T1-weighted MR images, and T2-weighted images show very high signal intensity.

- **Primitive neuroectodermal tumors (PNET)** are basically undifferentiated small, round cell sarcomas with clinical and radiographic characteristics similar to those of Ewing sarcoma. They can be found in bone or soft tissues of any part of the body including the thorax, and can frequently be quite large (Fig. 5-21).

  Symptoms include dyspnea, cough, fever, and weight loss. Associated pleural effusions, lung compression, or rib erosion may be present. The prognosis is poor, and metastases are frequent.

5.11 NON-NEUROGENIC POSTERIOR MEDIASTINAL MASSES

- A variety of conditions can present as posterior mediastinal masses, including vertebral abnormalities, lymphadenopathy, and mediastinal abscesses. Esophageal conditions such as hiatal hernia and esophageal varices can present as posterior mediastinal masses (**Differential 109**).

- **Vertebral abnormalities** such as **lateral intrathoracic meningocele** should be included in the differential diagnosis. This is a condition in which the spinal meninges protrude through the intervertebral foramina. They are frequently associated with neurofibromatosis.

  Plain films of the chest typically demonstrate a paravertebral mass associated with adjacent vertebral or rib scalloping or enlargement of the intervertebral foramina. CT or MR can confirm the diagnosis by identifying a fluid attenuation mass in communication with the spinal canal.

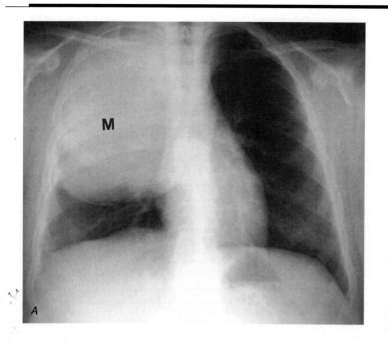
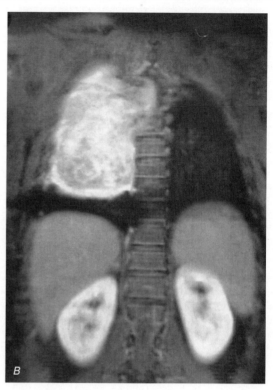

FIGURE 5-21   Primitive neuroectodermal tumor (PNET). (*A*) Chest radiograph showing a large posterior mediastinal mass in a child complaining of chest pain. (*B*) Coronal MR demonstrates tumor enhancement following gadolinium injection.

- **Infectious spondylitis**, or discitis, is characterized by a paraspinal mass associated with vertebral erosion and disk space narrowing. Tuberculosis and staphylococcus are the usual offending organisms.

- **Vertebral fractures**, particularly if they are associated with a paraspinal hematoma, should also be included in the differential diagnosis. These hematomas can dissect along the mediastinal plane and appear distant from the fracture site.

- **Mediastinal hemorrhage**, whether from spontaneous causes such as a bleeding aortic aneurysm or dissection or secondary to trauma, can cause chest pain. Clinical history and a high attenuation mass adjacent to the aorta are key elements in making the diagnosis. The MR appearance of a hematoma depends on the age of the thrombus.

- **Extramedullary hematopoiesis** is a rare cause of a posterior mediastinal mass resulting from expansion of the erythroid mass as a result of inadequate red cell formation. It has been described in the liver, spleen, spinal canal, and lymphatics. In the thorax it may be associated with subpleural masses, giving it a multilobulated appearance.

  Extramedullary hematopoiesis has been associated with a variety of diseases such as hemolytic anemias, carcinoma, and myelofibrosis. These masses are usually asymptomatic, although compression of adjacent structures may produce related symptoms.

Bibliography

Armstrong P, Wilson AG, Dee P, Hansell DM. *Imaging of Diseases of the Chest.* 2nd ed. St. Louis: Mosby-Year Book; 1995.

Brown LR, Aughenbaugh GL. Masses of the anterior mediastinum: CT and MR imaging. *Am J Roentgenol.* 1991;157;1171–1180.

Crylak D, Milne E, Imray TJ. Pneumomediastinum: A diagnostic problem. *Crit Rev Diagn Imaging.* 1984;23:75–117.

Ellis K, Austin JHM, Jaretzki A. Radiologic detection of thymoma in patients with myasthenia gravis. *Am J Roentgenol.* 1988;151:873–881.

Freeny PC, Stevenson GW. *Margulis and Burhenne's Alimentary Tract Radiology.* 5th ed. St. Louis: Mosby-Year Book; 1994.

Genereaux GP, Howie JL. Normal mediastinal lymph node size and number: CT and anatomic study. *AJR Am J Roentgenol.* 1984;142:1095–1100.

Goldwin RL, Heitzman ER, Proto AV. Computed tomography of the mediastinum: normal anatomy and indications for the use of CT. *Radiology.* 1977;124:235.

Heitzman ER, Goldwin RL, Proto AV. Radiologic analysis of the mediastinum utilizing computer tomography. *Radiol Clin North Am.* 1977;15:309.

Lee KT, Sagel SS, Stanley RJ, Heiken JP. *Computed Body Tomography with MRI Correlation.* 3rd ed. New York: Lippincott-Raven; 1998.

Reed JC. *Chest Radiology: Plain Film Patterns and Differential Diagnoses.* 4th ed. St. Louis: Mosby-Year Book; 1997.

Chapter 6

CARDIOVASCULAR DISEASE

Fernando R. Gutierrez

6.1 NORMAL THORACIC AORTA

• The aorta is an elastic artery that extends from the aortic valve to the iliac bifurcation at approximately L4. The aortic valve is composed of three cusps accompanied by sinuses (wall protrusions) just proximal to the tubular ascending aorta. The thoracic aorta is composed of the ascending, arch, and descending portions.

• The **ascending aorta** usually measures 2.6 to 2.8 cm in diameter, originates at the level of the third costal cartilage, and is surrounded by pericardium, making it a middle mediastinal structure.

• The **aortic arch** lies behind the manubrium and has a horizontal course as it arches to the left of the trachea to become the descending aorta at T4. It is not enveloped by pericardium and lies within the superior mediastinum. The diameter varies between 2.0 and 2.5 cm but can reach 3.5 cm after 60 years. There is little difference in diameter between sexes. The right brachiocephalic, left common carotid, and left sub-clavian arteries arise from the greater curvature of the aortic arch. Branching variants are common, including a common trunk for the brachiocephalic and left common carotid artery in 10 percent of the population and an aberrant right subclavian artery in 0.3 percent.

• The **descending thoracic aorta** lies in the left paravertebral region within the posterior mediastinum. Its diameter varies between 2.0 and 2.3 cm from a point near its origin to the diaphragmatic hiatus. Branches include pericardial, esophageal, bronchial, intercostal, and superior phrenic arteries.

• The histologic composition of the aorta allows for rapid expansion to absorb hydrostatic forces and quick recoil to maintain diastolic pressure. It consists of three layers: the ***tunica intima***, the innermost layer, composed of endothelium and connective tissue; the ***tunica media***, the middle layer mostly composed of elastic fibers, smooth muscle cells, and the vasa vasorum; and the ***tunica adventitia*** or outer wall, composed of connective tissue. The tunica media in the ascending aorta has more elastic fibers and a richer network of vasa vasorum than the rest of the aorta.

• The two major **functions** of the aorta include generation of the aortic pulse waveform and conducting systemic blood flow.

The **aortic pulse waveform** is generated as blood is ejected out of the left ventricle into the aorta during systole. The high elastic fiber content of the aorta allows propagation of the pulse pressure waveform. More peripheral arteries have less elastic fibers, making them behave more like semi-rigid tubes and allowing steeper changes in the arterial waveform.

The impulse phase of ventricular systole begins with the opening of the aortic valve when the aortic blood pressure is lower than the left ventricular pressure, allowing blood to rapidly accelerate into the ascending aorta. Initially, flow is turbulent as it passes across the aortic valve, with laminar flow established in the more distal ascending aorta. Vessel compliance and blood inertia allow passage of pressure waves and blood flow peripherally. Reversal or backward flow can be noted transiently in late systole.

- **Imaging of the aorta.** Plain radiographs may be helpful for screening, detecting aortic calcification and enlargement. Cross-sectional imaging, including computed tomography (CT), magnetic resonance (MR) imaging, and echocardiography, are the modalities of choice in the assessment of aortic abnormalities. Angiography is reserved for selected cases requiring additional anatomic or hemodynamic information.

6.2 CONGENITAL ANOMALIES OF THE AORTA

- **Hypoplastic ascending aorta**, commonly referred to as hypoplastic left heart syndrome, can result from aortic valve atresia, mitral valve atresia, or premature closure of the foramen ovale. The patent ductus serves as the source of systemic blood via the right heart.

  Hypoplasia of the left atrium, left ventricle, and ascending aorta is a hallmark feature. Once the ductus closes (usually within the first 2 weeks of life), severe heart failure ensues. The ascending aorta shows varying degrees of hypoplasia, its only role being to supply retrograde blood flow to the coronary arteries. This condition occurs predominantly in males.

  Radiographic features are moderate to severe cardiomegaly with vascular plethora and pulmonary edema (**Differential 118***). Angiography reveals lack of forward aortic flow and variable degree of aortic hypoplasia (Fig. 6-1).

  The untreated mortality rate approaches 95 percent in the first month of life. Treatment consists of prompt management of heart failure and maintenance of ductus patency. Surgical therapy has been attempted with a staged Norwood operation and, more recently, heart transplantation.

- **Supravalvular aortic stenosis** is congenital narrowing of the ascending aorta just above the coronary arteries. It is usually focal but may be diffuse and extend to the origin of the brachiocephalic arteries. **William syndrome** is a sporadic form accompanied by mental retardation and elfin fascies. Although associated with hypercalcemia of infancy, the majority of patients lack this feature.

- A **right aortic arch** is an aorta ascending to the right of the trachea. Several types are possible depending on embryologic development (Fig. 6-2).

  A **right aortic arch with mirror-image branching** is the most common form; branches are the left innominate, right common carotid, and right subclavian arteries (**Differential 135**). This type of aortic arch has a high association with congenital heart disease (98 percent) such as tetralogy of Fallot, truncus arteriosus, tricuspid atresia, and transposition of the great vessels. Because of its higher incidence, a cyanotic child with a mirror-image right arch usually has tetralogy of Fallot. The incidence of an associated vascular ring is low. A barium esophagram shows no posterior indentation.

---

*Please refer to Chapter 2, in which the differential diagnoses are discussed in numerical order.

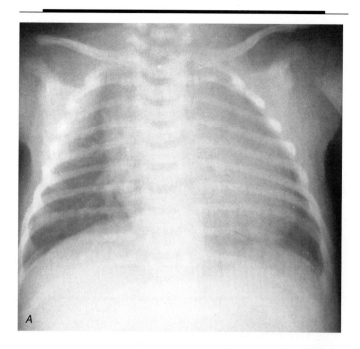

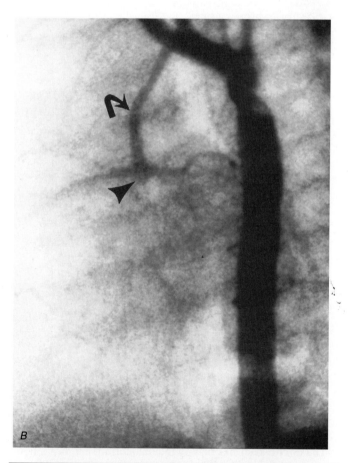

FIGURE 6-1   Hypoplastic left heart. (*A*) Chest radiograph in a 3-day-old infant brought to the hospital with tachypnea, demonstrating moderate cardiomegaly. (*B*) Aortogram in LAO projection with injection in the descending aorta, demonstrating a very hypoplastic ascending aorta (arrow) and no flow across the aortic valve (arrowhead).

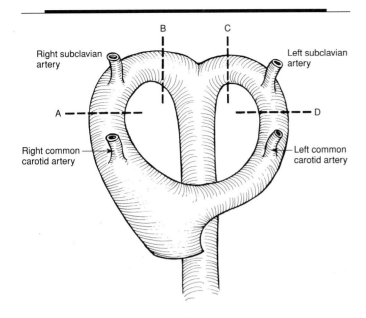

FIGURE 6-2 Edward hypothetical double aortic arch. Illustrating different development variants depending on the site of separation as noted by dotted lines. Lack of separation leads to a double aortic arch. (*A*) Left aortic arch with aberrant right subclavian artery. (*B*) Normal left aortic arch and right brachiocephalic trunk. (*C*) Right aortic arch with mirror-image branching. (*D*) Right aortic arch with an aberrant left subclavian artery.

A **right aortic arch with an aberrant left subclavian artery** is characterized by branching of the left common carotid, right common carotid, right subclavian artery, and left subclavian artery which passes posterior to the esophagus. The incidence of associated congenital heart defects is low. There is an indentation on the posterior wall of the esophagus (Fig. 6-3) which may be larger in patients with an aortic diverticulum (Fig. 6-4). Only when there is a left patent ductus is there a vascular ring, which is usually loose and asymptomatic.

- A **cervical aortic arch** is located at the base of the neck. It is related to formation of the aortic arch from the second or third brachial arch instead of the fourth. Patients usually present with a pulsatile mass in the supraclavicular fossa. Associated intracardiac abnormalities are rare. The diagnosis can be made from plain radiographs or cross-sectional imaging (Fig. 6-5).

- A **double aortic arch** is the result of lack of regression of a segment of the brachial aortic arches. There is persistence of the fourth brachial arches bilaterally, resulting in two arches passing on either side of the trachea before joining behind the esophagus to form a "vascular ring" encircling the trachea and esophagus (Fig. 6-6). The right arch tends to be higher and larger than the left which is frequently hypoplastic. A double aortic arch is generally an isolated anomaly, usually manifested by compression of the esophagus or trachea leading to stridor, dysphagia, or cough.

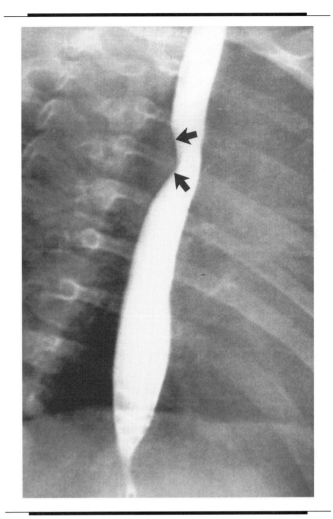

FIGURE 6-3 Right aortic arch and aberrant left subclavian. Esophagogram in a child in a steep RAO projection showing posterior esophageal indentation (arrows).

Plain films and a barium swallow demonstrate anterior tracheal indentation and posterior esophageal compression. MR can be used when additional anatomic information is required before surgical repair.

- An **aberrant right subclavian artery** can arise as the last branch of a left aortic arch before passing behind the esophagus to reach the right arm. An aortic diverticulum (**Kömmerell diverticulum**) may be present at the origin. It is usually an isolated anomaly, and patients are asymptomatic.

  Dysphagia lusoria describes swallowing difficulties resulting from esophageal compression, presumably from a rigid, atherosclerotic, aberrant subclavian vessel. A posterior esophageal indentation on an esophagram in a patient with a left aortic arch establishes the diagnosis.

- An **interrupted aortic arch** consists of congenital absence of a portion of the arch and no connection between the two sections, thus differentiating this entity from an *atretic* aortic arch where a fibrous band connects the segments. Infants show symptoms of congestive heart failure after ductus closure.

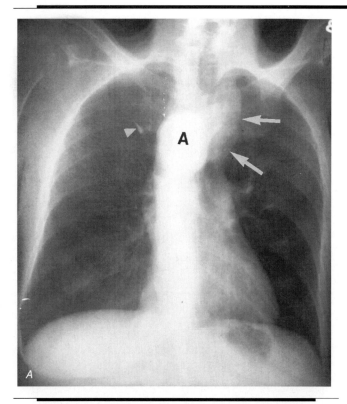

FIGURE 6-4   Right aortic arch. (*A*) Note large diverticulum at origin of left subclavian artery in an asymptomatic 73-year-old woman (arrows). Also note the accessory azygos fissure (arrowhead). (*B*) Lateral film demonstrating indentation of the posterior wall of the trachea (arrowheads) by aberrant left subclavian artery.

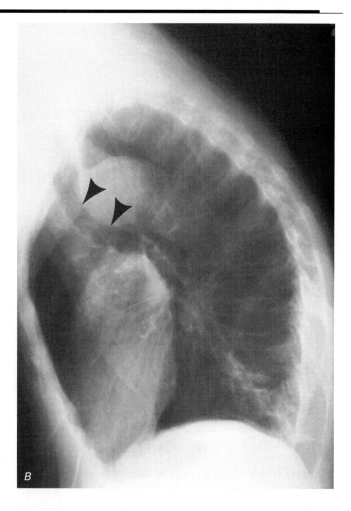

Classification depends on the segment absent. In **type A** the interruption occurs distal to the left subclavian artery and the distal aorta fills via the ductus arteriosus. In **type B**, the most common, the interruption occurs between the left common carotid artery and left subclavian artery, and in **type C** the interruption occurs between the brachiocephalic and left common carotid arteries.

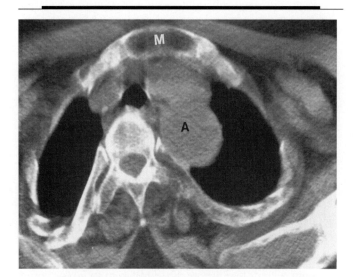

FIGURE 6-5   Cervical aortic arch. CT without intravenous contrast demonstrating a left aortic arch (A) projecting behind the manubrium of the sternum (M).

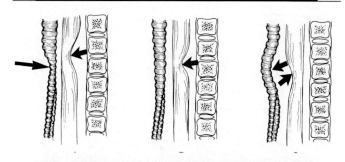

FIGURE 6-6   Tracheal and esophageal indentations seen in vascular anomalies. (*A*) Anterior tracheal and posterior esophageal indentation (arrow) due to a double aortic arch or right aortic arch with left ductus and aberrant left subclavian artery. (*B*) Posterior esophageal indentation (arrow) due to an aberrant subclavian artery. (*C*) Posterior tracheal and anterior esophageal indentations (arrows) seen with a pulmonary sling in which the left pulmonary artery arises from the right pulmonary artery.

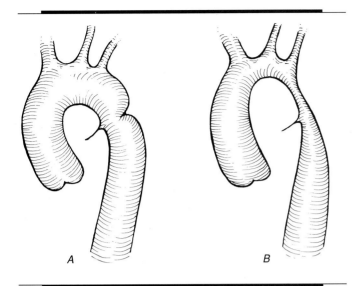

FIGURE 6-7 Aortic coarctation. (*A*) Adult and (*B*) infantile forms of aortic coarctation.

Chest radiographs usually demonstrate cardiomegaly and pulmonary venous hypertension. Echocardiography establishes the diagnosis and may identify associated intracardiac abnormalities such as ventricular septal defects (VSDs) and truncus arteriosus. Angiocardiography has been utilized for surgical planning. Treatment consists of prostaglandin E$_1$ infusion to keep the ductus open, followed by surgical repair. Results depend on the associated intracardiac abnormalities.

- **Coarctation of the aorta** is a congenital constriction usually occurring just beyond the origin of the left subclavian artery (juxtaductal position). Two major subtypes have been described depending on the relationship to the ductus arteriosus (Fig. 6-7).

  There is a high incidence of associated cardiac anomalies such as VSDs (35 percent), and patients can develop severe heart failure often requiring surgical correction. Coarctation of the aorta with an associated cardiac anomaly is one of the most common causes of congestive heart failure during the first week of life. With increasing age, there is progressive worsening, with an increasing pressure gradient across the coarcted segment.

- In the **adult type**, the stenotic region is located distal to the ductus. Depending on the severity, collateral vessels help supply blood to the more distal aorta. The proximal aortic arch has normal caliber. Sixty-five percent of patients have a bicuspid aortic valve. A higher incidence of coarctation occurs in males. Associated cerebral aneurysms and systemic hypertension predispose patients to hemorrhage.

  Radiographically, inferior rib notching (**Differential 94**), enlarged subclavian and internal mammary arteries (Fig. 6-8), and indentation of the distal aortic arch are seen. The lateral chest radiograph may demonstrate a calcified bicuspid aortic valve in adult patients.

- The **infantile type** exhibits long-segment narrowing proximal to the ductus arteriosus. As a result, the descending thoracic aorta receives blood from the right ventricle via the patent ductus arteriosus (PDA). When the PDA closes in the first few days of life, congestive heart failure develops.

  The usual radiographic manifestation is a newborn with cardiomegaly and congestive heart failure. It may take 5 or 6 years to develop radiographic rib notching. MR has proven useful in diagnosis and follow-up (Fig. 6-9).

- **Pseudocoarctation of the aorta** is a peculiar nonobstructive condition in which the aorta is "buckled" or "kinked" near the aortic isthmus. There is a high association with a bicuspid aortic valve, suggesting that this is a variant of coarctation. The chest radiograph may show significant deformity of the aortic isthmus, giving rise to the classic inverted "3" sign. There is no pressure gradient across the deformity and therefore no collateral circulation or rib notching.

6.3 ACQUIRED DISEASES OF THE AORTA

- With aging, the number of elastic and smooth muscle cells in the aorta decreases and there is an increase in the number of collagen cells and amount of mucoid ground substance. These histologic changes result in progressive enlargement of the aorta.

- **Arteriosclerosis** is a disease of the tunica intima, with the media secondarily affected. Atherosclerotic plaques progressively develop on the intimal surface and are more prevalent in the abdominal aorta. The ascending aorta is the least prone to age-related atherosclerosis. This may be explained by the presence of more elastic fibers and a richer vasa vasorum in

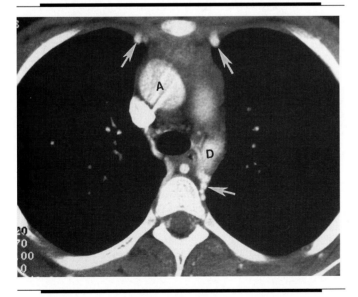

FIGURE 6-8 Coarctation of the aorta. Contrast-enhanced CT showing a normal-sized ascending aorta (A), small descending aorta (D), and large internal thoracic arteries and paraspinal collaterals (arrows).

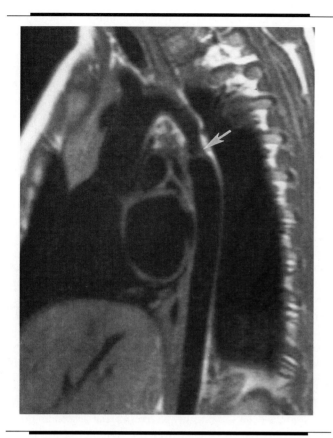

FIGURE 6-9   **High-grade infantile aortic coarctation.** Long-axis oblique T1-weighted MR image showing a focal area of aortic narrowing (arrow) and more proximal hypoplasia.

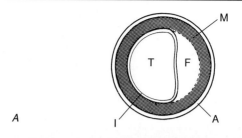

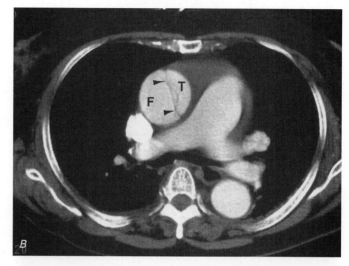

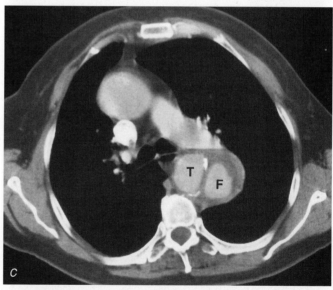

FIGURE 6-10   **Aortic dissection.** (*A*) Cross-sectional diagram showing displacement of the intima away from the media, creating a true (T) and a false (F) lumen. I, Intima; M, media, A, adventitia. (*B*) CT of Type A dissection with a true (T) and a false (F) lumen separated by the intima (arrowheads) in the ascending aorta. (*C*) Type B aortic dissection in another patient showing a true (T) and a false (F) lumen in the descending thoracic aorta.

this portion of the vessel. Type II hyperlipoproteinemia predisposes individuals to arteriosclerosis in the ascending aorta (**Differential 123**).

Other conditions associated with extensive ascending aortic disease are diabetes and syphilis. In luetic patients, however, the underlying media and adventitia are abnormal. The basic pathology is endoarteritis of the vasa vasorum, resulting in their destruction and replacement with granulation tissue.

- **Aortic dissection** develops as a result of a hematoma within the media separating the aortic wall into two layers (Fig. 6-10). There is usually an intimal tear allowing communication between the true and false lumens. Predisposing factors include hypertension, connective tissue disorders such as Marfan and Ehler-Danlos syndromes, a bicuspid aortic valve, coarctation (probably related to hypertension and a bicuspid valve), and pregnancy.

Most intimal entry sites are within the first few centimeters of the ascending aorta, gaining access to the media and propagating around the arch and frequently into the descending aorta with additional intimal tears (reentry points). The false lumen may remain patent long after surgical intervention for repair of the ascending aorta.

Aortic dissection is the most common aortic emergency, and 95 percent of patients survive the episode with proper treatment

resulting in a 10-year survival rate of 40 percent. Proximally, it can involve the aortic valve, rendering it insufficient. Mortality is usually from intrapericardial bleeding with cardiac tamponade. Aortic dissections are of two major anatomic types.

- In **type A dissection**, the ascending aorta is involved, often with an entry point in the aortic root. In rare cases, the ascending aorta is involved in a retrograde fashion. In general, this condition represents a surgical emergency. A homograft is placed to prevent retrograde dissection with hemorrhagic pericardial tamponade. (See Section 11.6.)

- **Type B dissection** characteristically involves only the descending aorta. The intimal tear is usually just distal to the origin of the left subclavian artery.

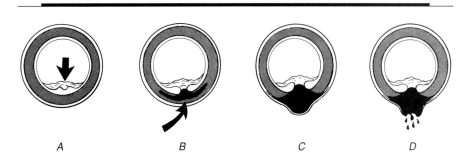

FIGURE 6-11   Progressive stages of a penetrating atherosclerotic ulcer. (*A*) Atherosclerotic plaque (arrow) on the surface of the aortic intima. (*B*) As the disease progresses deeper into the aortic wall, the tunica media will eventually be involved by the enlarging hematoma (curved arrow) (*C*) until there is disruption of the adventitia (*D*) with bleeding outside the aorta.

Plain films demonstrate widening of the superior mediastinum, (**Differential 105**), although it may be normal in about 15 percent of cases. Displacement of intimal calcifications can be a reliable sign, but must be interpreted with caution since the oblique course of the arch can simulate this finding. Comparison with prior chest radiographs to detect interval changes is crucial.

Cross-sectional imaging with two-dimensional echocardiography, CT, and MR is useful in noninvasive diagnoses. Precontrast CT images may demonstrate an acute hematoma within the aortic wall and displacement of the calcified intimal layer. CT with contrast demonstrates the intimal flap separating the true and false lumen, often with differential opacification. Angiography is used in cases requiring additional anatomic information for surgical planning; however, in cases of false lumen thrombosis, angiography may be falsely negative.

- **Penetrating atherosclerotic ulcers** have clinical findings similar to those of aortic dissection, yet the imaging features are different. It represents an atherosclerotic plaque that burrows into the media, causing bleeding and hematoma formation. Typically, an ulceration can be seen in the middle or distal thoracic aorta with an intramural hematoma (Fig. 6-11) outside the intimal layer. Angiographically, an ulceration of the aortic wall is seen. CT and MR are also helpful in the differentiation. (Fig. 6-12).

Penetrating plaques must be differentiated from type B aortic dissection, since aggressive surgical management may be indicated in the former; although most can be successfully treated medically with antihypertensive therapy. Close follow-up is recommended in patients treated conservatively.

- **Thoracic aortic aneurysms** can be congenital or acquired and usually occur at points of medial weakness. Hypertension often compounds the problem by further expanding the weakened wall. Aneurysms are described as saccular or fusiform depending on their morphologic characteristics.

- **Sinus of Valsalva aneurysms** can be congenital or acquired. In the congenital variant, separation of the media from the fibrous aortic valve annulus creates an aneurysm at the base of the aortic sinus. The right coronary sinus is most commonly involved, and the left is rarely involved. These aneurysms can become infected, producing aortic insuffi-

ciency and fistulization to the right heart with subsequent left-to-right shunting and high-output heart failure.

The acquired form of sinus of Valsalva aneurysm is seen in patients with Marfan syndrome, with dilatation of the aortic root and sinuses and loss of the sinotubular angle producing a "Florence flask" or "light bulb" aortic deformity.

- **Aneurysms of the ascending aorta** can be due to syphilis (luetic) or **Marfan syndrome**. Atherosclerotic aneurysms of

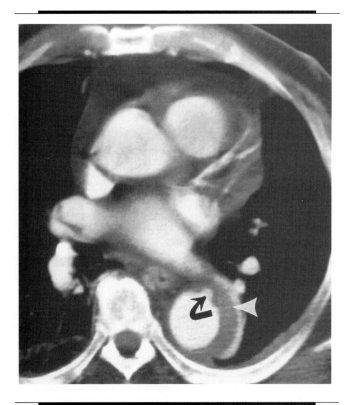

FIGURE 6-12   Penetrating atherosclerotic plaque. Contrast-enhanced CT depicting a penetrating atherosclerotic plaque burrowing into the aortic wall (arrow). A hematoma of the media is also present (arrowhead).

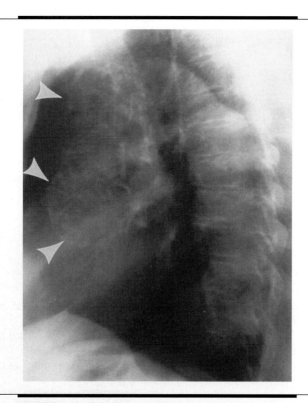

FIGURE 6-13 Syphilitic aortitis. Lateral radiograph demonstrating coarse, irregular calcification of the ascending aorta (arrowheads).

the ascending aorta are uncommon and are usually asymptomatic until they become large.

Luetic aortic aneurysms can occur at any level of the aorta but are most common in the ascending portion, presumably because of the rich vasa vasorum network (Fig. 6-13). Unlike cystic medial necrosis, they tend to spare the sinuses of Valsalva, although the coronary artery origins may be involved, causing angina pectoris.

Poststenotic jetting from **valvular aortic stenosis** can lead to ascending aortic aneurysm formation. **Takayasu disease** may in rare cases be manifested as an ascending aortic aneurysm (**Differential 134**).

- Most **aortic arch aneurysms** are atherosclerotic. Surgical repair of aortic arch aneurysms is technically difficult. Cross-sectional imaging demonstrates thickened aortic walls.

- **Descending aortic aneurysms** are usually arteriosclerotic and frequently associated with abdominal aortic aneurysms.

- A **traumatic** etiology should be suspected with aneurysms near the aortic isthmus. Only 3 percent of patients with traumatic pseudoaneurysms survive without prompt surgery. When chronic, these pseudoaneurysms can calcify and cause airway compression (Fig. 6-14). The aortic isthmus (just distal to the left subclavian artery near the ductus ligamentum) is the most common location of traumatic aortic injury, although the arch and ascending aorta may be involved in rare cases. (See Section 10.2 for more details.)

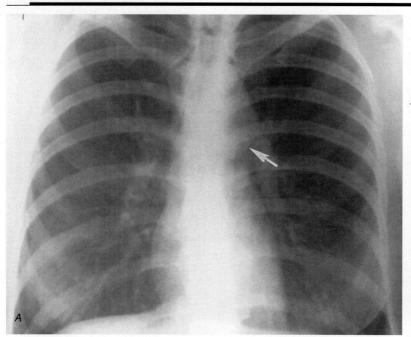

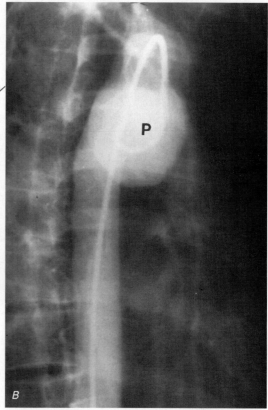

FIGURE 6-14 Chronic traumatic aortic pseudoaneurysm. (A) Frontal chest radiograph in a 34-year-old woman with a history of a motor vehicle accident 10 years earlier, demonstrating a calcified mediastinal mass silhouetting the proximal descending aorta (arrow). (B) Aortogram in the RAO projection confirms the presence of the pseudoaneurysm (P).

Emergency aortography should be performed in cases where a traumatic injury to the aorta is suspected. Alternatively, dynamic CT may play an important role in excluding aortic injury. Plain film findings of acute traumatic aortic injury can include a wide mediastinum, airway deviation, apical capping, irregularity of the aortic contour or adjacent mediastinum, and deviation of the nasogastric tube (Figs. 10-3 to 10-6).

- **Mycotic aneurysms** can occur at any level and usually are the result of spread from infection caused by valvular vegetations. They are frequently saccular and may expand rapidly.

6.4 CARDIAC IMAGING

- **Initial imaging evaluation** with plain chest radiographs excludes symptomatic thoracic entities such as a pneumothorax and provides important information regarding pulmonary vascularity, cardiac enlargement, pericardial calcification, and superior mediastinal appearance.

- **Two-dimensional echocardiography** is the tool of choice in assessing cardiac anatomy and hemodynamics. It is noninvasive, portable, and reliable. Doppler color flow can add additional information. Transthoracic two-dimensional echocardiography is usually adequate for most patients. When proper windowing becomes difficult because of emphysema or chest wall deformities, transesophageal echocardiography (TEE) may help further characterize problematic anatomic areas. One drawback is the invasiveness of the procedure, usually requiring patient sedation.

- **MR** can further characterize conditions not readily discerned with echocardiography. Besides traditional spin-echo sequences, gradient-recalled techniques combined with pharmacologic stress allow comparison of wall motion with myocardial perfusion. Cine velocity mapping has allowed fairly accurate calculation of blood flow in vessels and chambers. The role of cardiac MR is evolving.

- **CT** is also very effective in imaging the heart, pericardium, and pulmonary vessels. Faster scanners with improved resolution have created new applications.

- **Angiocardiography** remains the imaging technique of choice for surgical planning. Catheterization allows coronary angioplasty or valvuloplasty in the treatment of cardiac diseases.

6.5 CARDIAC ANATOMY AND MALPOSITIONS

- The heart is centered within the middle mediastinum and has three major surfaces. The diaphragmatic or inferior surface is composed mainly of the left ventricle, the anterior wall is composed mostly of the right ventricular free wall, and the left atrium comprises the posterior wall (Fig. 6-15A).

- **The pericardial sac** is a two-layered serofibrous membrane that envelops the heart and root of the great vessels, creating the pericardial cavity containing 30 to 50 ml of clear fluid. This allows the heart to move freely within the chest. The outer layer, composed of connective tissue (fibrous pericardium), anchors the heart to the diaphragm and adjacent mediastinal structures. This layer is lined with the serous (visceral) pericardium which reflects back on itself to cover the heart. It is separated from the epicardium by a thin layer of fat and secretes pericardial fluid.

- **The right atrium**, located between the superior vena cava (SVC) and the inferior vena cava (IVC) sits on the right hemidiaphragm and forms the majority of the right heart border on frontal chest radiographs. Just above it is the right atrial appendage, which at times can partially encircle the anterolateral wall of the ascending aorta. The atrial septum constitutes the posteromedial wall of the right atrium and separates the right and left atria. It has a thinner central portion called the fossa ovalis. Enlargement manifests itself primarily as an outward bulge of the right heart border on frontal chest radiographs (Fig. 6-15B).

- **The right ventricle** occupies a significant portion of the anterior surface of the heart and is composed of the inflow, apical, and outflow portions. Enlargement is most noticeable on the lateral chest radiograph by filling of the retrosternal clear space (Fig. 6-15C). The right ventricle has an irregular inner surface composed of *trabeculae carnae*. A distinguishing feature of the right ventricle is the septomarginal bundle or *moderator band* extending from the ventricular septum to the base of the anterior papillary muscle.

  Blood enters via the tricuspid valve and exits via the pulmonary valve. The *tricuspid valve* has three cusps that extend from the annulus into the right ventricle where they are anchored to corresponding papillary muscles by chordae tendineae. The *pulmonary valve* is composed of three semilunar cusps strengthened by fibrous tissue to prevent regurgitation. The pulmonary sinuses are areas of outpouching located between the wall of the pulmonary artery and the valve leaflets.

- **The left atrium** constitutes most of the dorsal surface of the heart and receives inflow from all four pulmonary veins. Enlargement is evident on the frontal chest radiograph by increased density over the right atrium and straightening of the left heart border caused by the enlarged atrial appendage. The enlarged left atrium projects posteriorly on the lateral image (Fig. 6-15D). There are no valves in the pulmonary veins. The left atrial appendage is a superior extension slightly narrower than the right atrial appendage and similarly is composed of a rough internal surface of *musculi pectini*.

- **The left ventricle** is a cylindrical chamber that constitutes most of the inferior and left lateral cardiac margins. The left ventricular myocardium is approximately three times the thickness of the right ventricle. When enlarged, the left heart border takes on a globular shape on the posteroanterior radiograph, and the base of the heart projects posteriorly on the lateral radiograph (Fig. 6-15E).

  Blood enters via the mitral valve which prevents regurgitation into the left atrium and exits via the aortic valve.

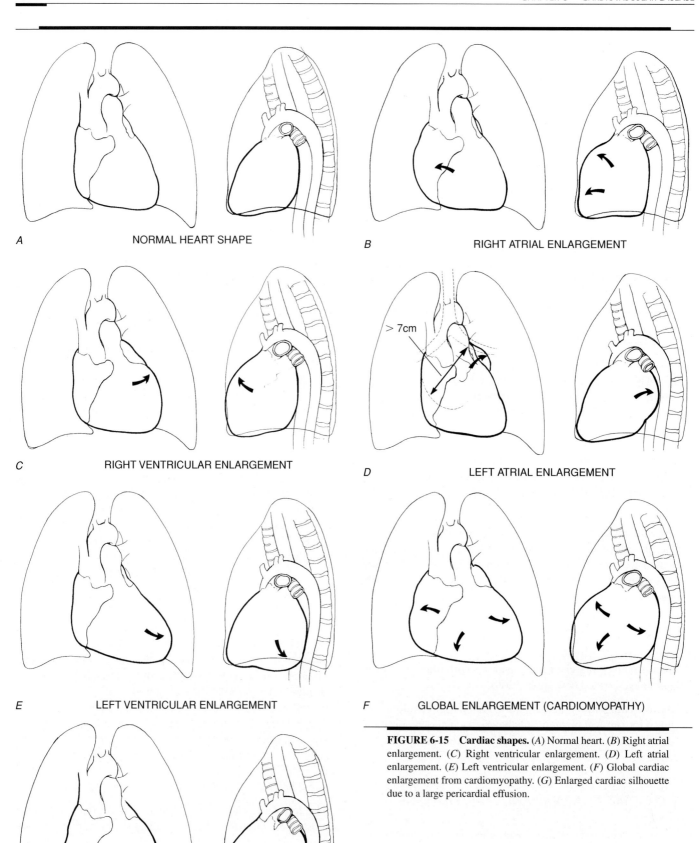

A   NORMAL HEART SHAPE

B   RIGHT ATRIAL ENLARGEMENT

C   RIGHT VENTRICULAR ENLARGEMENT

D   LEFT ATRIAL ENLARGEMENT

E   LEFT VENTRICULAR ENLARGEMENT

F   GLOBAL ENLARGEMENT (CARDIOMYOPATHY)

G   PERICARDIAL EFFUSION

FIGURE 6-15   **Cardiac shapes.** (*A*) Normal heart. (*B*) Right atrial enlargement. (*C*) Right ventricular enlargement. (*D*) Left atrial enlargement. (*E*) Left ventricular enlargement. (*F*) Global cardiac enlargement from cardiomyopathy. (*G*) Enlarged cardiac silhouette due to a large pericardial effusion.

The *mitral valve* is composed of a large anterior cusp and a smaller posterior cusp attached to their respective papillary muscles via *chordae tendineae*. The interventricular septum separates the left and right ventricles. The aortic valve has three cusps, the right, left, and posterior or noncoronary cusp.

- Cardiac blood supply is provided via the **coronary arteries** which are the first branches of the ascending aorta. The right coronary artery arises just above the right aortic cusp and after a short horizontal course under the right atrial appendage courses within the right atrioventricular groove. It provides branches for the sinoatrial node and the anterior (right) ventricular surface. It produces a posterior descending branch which supplies the inferior surface of the interventricular septum and ends as a posterolateral ventricular branch. The atrioventricular node branch also arises from the right coronary artery (Fig. 6-16).

  The left main coronary artery arises just superior to the left coronary sinus underneath the left atrial appendage. It divides into two main branches, the circumflex and the left anterior descending (LAD) arteries. The circumflex branch travels within the left atrioventricular groove and sends lateral and posterolateral branches to the left ventricular wall.

  The LAD branch courses within the superior interventricular groove above the ventricular septum which it supplies with septal perforator branches. The diagonal or anterolateral branches supply the anterolateral left ventricle.

- **Venous drainage** occurs via the great cardiac vein which parallels the LAD, the middle cardiac vein which parallels the posterior descending artery, and the little cardiac vein which parallels the right coronary artery. These three veins converge to form the *coronary sinus* which drains into the base of the right atrium.

- **Coronary dominance** describes the major coronary branch supplying the inferior cardiac surface. About 80 percent of patients have a right dominant system. About 10 percent of the population has a left dominant system. A small percentage of patients have a balanced system.

- **Cardiac malpositions.** The location of the heart is variable, and it can be left-sided (levocardia), midline (mesocardia), right-sided (dextrocardia), or external to the chest cavity (ectopia cordis). **Levocardia** is the usual situation in patients with situs solitus, and the right atrium sits above the liver. The left ventricular apex points anteriorly and to the left. In **mesocardia** the ventricular apex points toward the midline. This condition may be associated with congenital heart disease.

- In **dextrocardia** the bulk of the heart is located in the right hemithorax (**Differential 112**). It is important to be able to differentiate true *dextroversion*, in which the ventricular apex points to the right, from *dextroposition* of the heart, in which the heart is "pulled" into the right hemithorax by volume

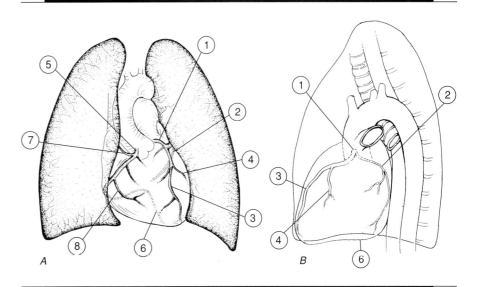

FIGURE 6-16   Normal coronary arteries. (*A*) frontal and (*B*) lateral projection showing the (1) left main, (2) left circumflex, (3) left anterior descending, (4) diagonal branches, (5) right main, (6) posterior descending, (7) branch to the sinoatrial node, and (8) right ventricular branch.

loss. Dextroversion is almost universally associated with congenital heart disease, whereas dextroposition is not.

- **Ectopia cordis** is a very rare condition in which the heart is partially or totally outside the thorax, usually in the abdomen (thoracoabdominal ectopia cordis). The sternum is usually cleaved, allowing the heart to be displaced through a diaphragmatic defect, sometimes under the abdominal skin through a midline abdominal defect. Complex congenital heart defects may also be present.

6.6 CARDIAC PHYSIOLOGY

- The **cardiac cycle** can be divided into six phases: isovolumetric contraction, systolic ejection, isovolumetric relaxation, rapid ventricular filling, diastasis, and atrial contraction. Blood flows from areas of high pressure to areas of low pressure.

- **Isovolumetric contraction** signals electrical activation of the ventricular myocardium, and as ventricular contraction begins, the ventricular pressure exceeds that in the atria, forcing mitral and tricuspid valve closure. During this phase, the ventricular volumes remain constant.

- **Systolic ejection** starts when intraventricular pressure exceeds aortic and pulmonary arterial pressures, forcing the aortic and pulmonary valves open. The ejection period has early, rapid and late, slower ejection phases. Ventricular volumes change significantly during the ejection phase. This period is primarily responsible for the first heart sound.

- **Isovolumetric relaxation** lasts from the time the aortic and pulmonary valves close until the semilumar valves open as the ventricular pressure drops below intra-atrial pressure. The second heart sound occurs as the aortic and pulmonary valves close.

- **Rapid ventricular filling** occurs when ventricular pressure falls below atrial pressure, allowing the atrioventricular valves to open and blood to enter the ventricles. During this early diastolic period, 85 percent of ventricular filling occurs. The third heart sound corresponds to this period, and coronary artery flow (a diastolic phenomenon) takes place.

- **Diastasis** is a period of slow ventricular filling in which a small amount of additional blood flows into the ventricular chambers. Flow through the mitral and tricuspid valves essentially ceases until the next phase.

- **Atrial systole** commences with electrical activation of the left atrium [the P wave of the electrocardiogram (ECG)] and atrial contraction. The contribution of ventricular filling from this part of the cycle is approximately 15 percent. Under high demand such as atrial fibrillation or exercise, this period may become augmented and therefore crucial. Enhanced atrial contraction is thought to be related to the fourth heart sound.

6.7   APPROACH TO CONGENITAL HEART DISEASE

- **Congenital heart disease** affects about 1 percent of the population. Evaluation includes a physical exam, plain radiographs, and noninvasive imaging (predominantly echo-cardiography) complemented by angiocardiography and potentially interventional treatment. Hypoplastic left heart syndrome and coarctation of the aorta (discussed in Section 6.2) are the most frequent causes of **congestive heart failure in newborns**; therefore, imaging should include adequate visualization of the left ventricle and aorta (**Differential 118**).

  Since the gamut of diseases is complex and extensive, an organized step-by-step approach should be followed so the differential diagnosis can be narrowed before the next imaging step is undertaken. This is probably the time when the radiologist's input to the cardiologist or referring physician has the greatest impact.

- The **imaging algorithm** usually starts with **two fundamental premises**: (1) information regarding the presence or absence of central cyanosis and (2) the state of the pulmonary vasculature as seen on the plain chest radiograph.

- **Cyanosis** is a bluish skin discoloration that occurs when significantly reduced hemoglobin (more than 5 g/100 ml) is being carried in the blood. It occurs when there is right-to-left shunting or because of mixing of the blood (from a univentricular heart) resulting in a significant amount of "deoxygenated" blood in the systemic circulation. This information is usually readily available after an initial physical exam and laboratory blood work have been performed.

- **Pulmonary vascularity.** Analysis should begin with an assessment of the pulmonary vessels from the main pulmonary artery and continuing to the distal vessels. Pulmonary vascu-

larity can be classified into four broad categories: normal, increased, decreased, and asymmetric.

- **Shunt vascularity (Differential 127)** occurs when significant blood flow is rerouted to the lungs. The lungs are a low-pressure system and have the potential capacity to accommodate extra blood flow with relative ease. It usually takes a 2-to-1 shunt before the augmented pulmonary plethora can be detected on radiographs. The three major causes of increased blood flow through the lungs include (1) a left-to-right shunt, (2) an admixture lesion, and (3) a high-flow state such as an arteriovenous fistula, anemia, or thyrotoxicosis.

- **Newborns** with septal defects do not usually have shunt vascularity during the first few days after birth because of high pulmonary arterial resistance. The pulmonary vascular resistance drops in the ensuing weeks as a result of thinning of the media and luminal enlargement. It may take 4 to 8 weeks after birth for the pulmonary resistance to drop to the point where significant left-to-right shunting is visible on a chest radiograph.

6.8   ACYANOSIS AND SHUNT VASCULARITY

- **Atrial septal defects (ASDs)** account for approximately 10 percent of congenital heart defects and are the most common congenital heart condition in adults. There is a 3:2 female predominance and an occasional familial tendency. ASDs have been described in the Holt-Oram syndrome, an autosomal dominant condition that also includes upper extremity anomalies. Typically, patients with ASDs remain relatively asymptomatic until adulthood. Pulmonary hypertension rarely develops during childhood. Elective repair is recommended.

  The radiographic findings of ASD are shunt vascularity and enlargement of the right ventricle with a normal-sized left atrium (Fig. 6-17). Smaller shunts may have a normal chest radiograph. Several different types of defects have been described based on location:

  Ostium secundum defects involve the central portion of the atrial septum or fossa ovalis and are the most common ASD.

  Sinus venosus defects are located in the superior portion of the atrial septum and are associated with partial anomalous venous return of the right upper lobe pulmonary vein.

  Ostium primum defects are located in the lower portion of the atrial septum and are associated with a cleft anterior mitral valve. They are frequently associated with trisomy 21, although less often than atrioventricular canals. There is no gender predilection. Angiographically, left ventricular injection demonstrates a "goose neck" deformity (Fig. 6-18). Patients with this type of defect usually have more severe and earlier symptoms than patients with a secundum ASD.

  Coronary sinus ASDs are a very rare anomaly and occur inferior and slightly anterior to the fossa ovalis. A coronary ASD is usually part of a developmental complex that includes absence of the coronary sinus and a persistent left

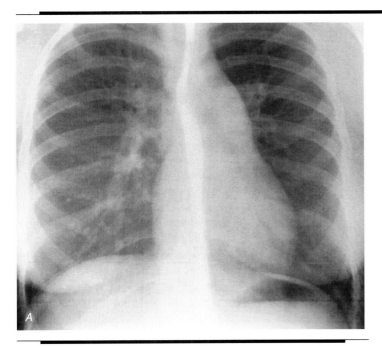
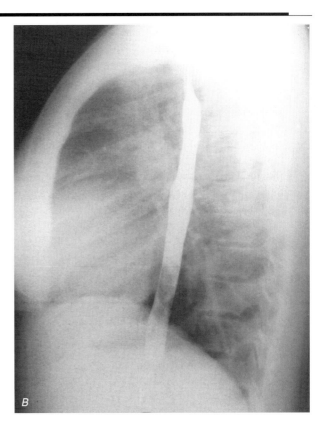

FIGURE 6-17 Atrial septal defect. (*A*) Frontal chest radiograph in a 28-year-old woman showing increased pulmonary (shunt) vascularity. Note the increased size of the lower lobe vessels. (*B*) Lateral view with barium showing a normal-sized left atrium and no esophageal indentation.

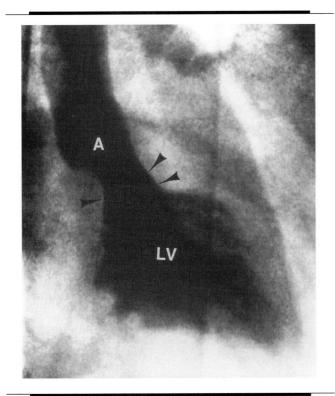

FIGURE 6-18 Primum ASD. Left ventriculogram in an RAO projection showing a "goose neck" deformity of the left ventricular outflow tract (arrowheads). LV, Left ventricle; A, ascending aorta.

SVC. Anatomically, this type of defect consists of "unroofing" of the coronary sinus.

- **Endocardial cushion defects** are related to faulty development of endocardial cushions and the atrioventricular septum. They represent a broad spectrum of anomalies varying from a simple primum ASD to a complete atrioventricular canal.

  Patients are frequently fatigued and dyspneic from shunting and associated mitral regurgitation, which complicates surgical repair. There is a frequent association with Down syndrome, particularly in patients with an anterioventricular canal. Infants are often critically ill with congestive heart failure. Pulmonary hypertension can develop at an early age. Cyanosis may be a clinical manifestation, and ECG features include prolonged PR intervals and left axis deviation.

- **Ventricular septal defects (VSDs)** are the most common congenital heart defects (about 20 percent of all cases) after bicuspid aortic valves. They are the most common lesion described with chromosomal syndromes, and the overall incidence is greater in females than in males. The size of the defect generally determines the magnitude of shunting. Defects are considered large when they are the size of the aortic orifice or larger. There are four types, classified by their septal location.

  Perimembranous, membranous, or **infracristal defects** are the most common (80 percent) and involve the perimembranous portion of the ventricular septum just below the aortic valve.

Muscular or **trabecular defects** are frequently multiple and are difficult to visualize from the right ventricle since they are hidden behind muscular trabeculae. When multiple, they have been described as "swiss cheese" defects.

Inlet muscular defects occur below the septal leaflet of the tricuspid valve and are considered part of the spectrum of atrioventricular canal defects.

Outlet, supracristal, or **conal** defects occur beneath the pulmonary valve and are relatively rare except in Far Eastern countries.

Radiographic features depend on defect size and patient age. Small defects may have a normal radiograph. Moderate left-to-right shunting (usually greater than 2 to 1) result in increased size of the pulmonary vessels and left atrial enlargement, differentiating VSDs from ASDs (**Differential 127**).

A progressive decrease in pulmonary vascularity may be related to the following: (1) Spontaneous closure of the defect (about 60 percent). Usually, the smaller the defect, the higher the incidence of spontaneous closure. Closure usually takes place in the first few years. (2) Development of increased pulmonary vascular resistance (Eisenmenger syndrome). Patients exhibit right ventricular hypertrophy and strain on the ECG. (3) Development of muscle bundles within the right ventricular chamber, causing an intraventricular pressure gradient and thus diminishing pulmonary perfusion.

MR can be used when echocardiography is limited, particularly in adults with emphysema, in children with chest deformities, and in poststernotomy patients. The exact size and location of the defect can be demonstrated and associated heart defects excluded.

Cardiac catheterization is primarily performed to document the location of the defect, measure the magnitude of the shunt, and estimate the pulmonary vascular resistance for surgical planning. In many cases, noninvasive imaging can provide this information.

Treatment varies depending on patient age and shunt magnitude. During infancy and in patients with heart failure, a trial of medical treatment is instituted. Larger defects, those that show no evidence of closure, or those with elevation of the pulmonary resistance, should be surgically corrected.

- **Patent ductus arteriosus (PDA).** The ductus arteriosus is a vascular channel connecting the left pulmonary artery and descending aorta just beyond the left subclavian artery, diverting the major proportion of the right ventricular output away from the high-resistance pulmonary circulation in the fetus.

Under normal circumstances, the ductus closes within the first few days of life by a combination of smooth muscle wall contractions and endothelial proliferation. Increasing Pa_{O_2} and the release of various vasoactive substances play important roles in complete closure and eventual formation of the ligamentum arteriosum. Conditions that lower the arterial Pa_{O_2} level or increase circulating prostaglandins delay normal closure.

Patent ductus arteriosus may be isolated or be part of other congenital defects such as coarctation or tetralogy of Fallot. The incidence of PDA is higher in people living at higher altitudes and in low-birth-weight premature infants. The clinical manifestations of PDA depend on the magnitude of the shunt, with smaller ones being clinically silent. Larger shunts are accompanied by tachypnea, tachycardia, and ventricular failure.

Radiographic findings depend on the size of the shunt and the age of presentation. Small infants with large shunts exhibit increased vascularity, high-output failure, and cardiomegaly with left atrial enlargement.

Infants may have a persistent bulge at the distal end of the ductus even after complete closure. This ductus "bump" may be evident for several weeks and should not be mistaken for a patent ductus. In rare cases this ductus diverticulum can be identified in adults during routine angiography.

Treatment varies with age of presentation. Pharmacologic closure with indomethacin, a vasoconstrictor, has had variable success. It is important to identify calcium in the wall of a PDA particularly in adults since this may complicate surgical closure. Alternatively, surgical closure by ligation carries a low morbidity and mortality. More recently, intravascular umbrella devices have been successfully employed (Fig. 12-13).

- **Partial anomalous pulmonary venous return (PAPVR)** represents a group of entities in which some of the pulmonary venous blood ends up in the right atrium or systemic veins. The condition may be isolated or associated with other congenital heart conditions. The clinical symptoms are variable, depending on the amount of venous return.

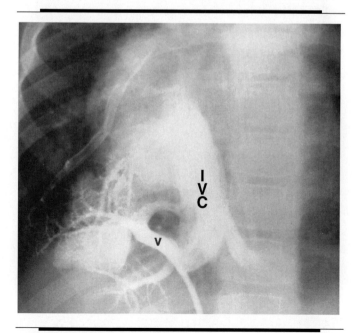

FIGURE 6-19 Partial anomalous pulmonary venous return (scimitar syndrome). Selective injection into the anomalous vein (V) just before drainage into the inferior vena cava (IVC).

Anomalous right upper lobe pulmonary venous return is associated with sinus venosus ASD. The anomalous vein drains into the upper part of the right atrium near the SVC confluence.

Anomalous right lower lobe venous drainage is usually part of the *hypogenetic lung syndrome spectrum* and represents a more primitive malformation than the other forms. Part or all of the right lung drains into the inferior vena cava and right atrium near the diaphragm. Radiographically, a characteristic curvilinear density may be seen in the right lower lobe (*scimitar syndrome*) (Fig. 6-19). This anomaly is accompanied by volume loss of the right hemithorax and ipsilateral mediastinal deviation. Respiratory infections are common.

Systemic drainage of the left upper lobe is usually an incidental finding in asymptomatic patients. The anomalous vein drains into the left innominate vein. This condition must be differentiated from a persistent left superior vena cava. **Left lower lobe partial anomalous venous return** is usually associated with pulmonary sequestration.

6.9 CYANOSIS WITH NORMAL OR DECREASED PULMONARY VASCULARITY

- **Cyanotic heart disease with normal or decreased pulmonary vascularity** consists of a group of diseases characterized by obstruction of blood flow through the right heart. The obstruction may occur from the tricuspid valve to the main pulmonary artery. An associated septation defect, usually an ASD or patent foramen ovale, provides relief by allowing communication between the pulmonary and systemic circulations, thus causing cyanosis. Patients exhibit normal or decreased vascularity on chest radiographs (**Differential 129**).

- **Tricuspid atresia** is the absence of a tricuspid valve without direct communication between the right atrium and right ventricle. The right ventricular cavity is usually hypoplastic, with the sinus portion incompletely formed; however, in cases with large VSDs, the right ventricular cavity may be well preserved. There is usually a VSD of variable size, and an ASD. This condition occurs in about 3 percent of patients with congenital heart disease.

  Associated anomalies are common, including a right aortic arch with mirror-image branching in about 5 percent of patients. Several major groups include tricuspid atresia with normally related great vessels (70 percent), transposition of great vessels (25 percent), and corrected transposition of great vessels (5 percent).

  Radiographically, most patients (70 percent) exhibit normal or decreased pulmonary vascularity. Cardiac size is usually normal or slightly increased, with a rounded ventricular contour. MR often shows fatty accumulation within the right atrioventricular groove around the atretic orifice. The hypoplastic right ventricle and VSD can also be seen. Cardiac catheterization is usually performed and may include balloon atrial septostomy to increase atrial mixing.

- **Ebstein anomaly** represents less than 1 percent of all cases of congenital heart disease. It has been reported in infants born to mothers treated with lithium during pregnancy. Anatomically, there is redundancy of the medial and posterior cusps of the tricuspid valve which are tethered to the right ventricular wall, forming a third or "atrialized" right heart chamber. The degree of redundancy can vary from mild to marked, with large amounts of tricuspid regurgitation. Associated anomalies are common, most frequently an ASD.

  Clinical symptoms are related to the degree of leaflet displacement and associated tricuspid regurgitation. Symptoms appearing at birth because of the normally elevated pulmonary resistance may soon subside only to recur later in life. With mild leaflet displacement, symptoms may be virtually absent, allowing survival well into adulthood. Larger displacement is accompanied by tricuspid regurgitation, right atrial enlargement, and right-to-left shunting across the atrial septum associated with cyanosis. Arrhythmias and heart block are common. Wolff-Parkinson-White (WPW) syndrome has been reported in 10 percent of cases.

  Plain films demonstrate variable cardiomegaly and right atrial enlargement, depending on the severity of tricuspid regurgitation (Fig. 6-20). Heart size varies from normal or slightly increased to massive enlargement, usually seen in newborns. The cardiac configuration has been described as "box-shaped." The pulmonary vascularity varies from normal to slightly decreased.

  Cardiac catheterization, MR, or echocardiography can demonstrate the three right heart chambers: right atrium, atrialized ventricle, and normally trabeculated right ventricular

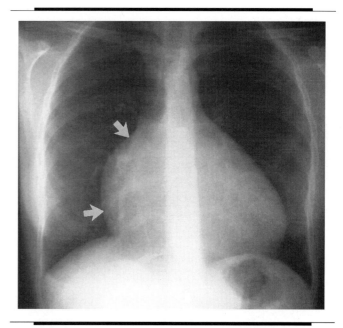

FIGURE 6-20 Ebstein anomaly of the tricuspid valve. Chest radiograph in a 32-year-old patient diagnosed with Ebstein anomaly. Note decreased pulmonary vascularity and right atrial enlargement (arrows).

chamber. Catheterization, which is rarely indicated, is associated with a high incidence of arrhythmias due to increased cardiac irritability.

Treatment usually consists of prophylactic antibiotic therapy and management of dysrhythmias. Surgical repair has met with limited success and is rarely indicated.

- **Tetralogy of Fallot** is the combination of right ventricular infundibular hypoplasia, overriding aorta, a VSD, and right ventricular hypertrophy. It is the most common cause of cyanotic heart disease in older patients (70 percent of cases). The most important component is hypoplasia of the right ventricular infundibulum which is deviated superiorly, anteriorly, and to the left, causing outflow stenosis. A VSD is located beneath the crista supraventricularis under the straddling aortic root. Spontaneous closure is excedingly rare. Right ventricular hypertrophy is secondary to elevated right ventricular pressures.

A right aortic arch with mirror-image branching occurs in approximately 25 percent of cases (**Differential 135**). The incidence is even higher among patients with more severe forms of stenosis or atresia. An ASD can be seen in association with tetralogy of Fallot (**pentalogy of Fallot**). Coronary arterial anomalies can be found in about 5 to 10 percent of cases, usually an aberrant left anterior descending branch arising from the right coronary artery. This anomaly has important surgical implications since the aberrant vessel crosses the right ventricular outflow tract, interfering with surgical ventriculotomy.

A persistent left SVC can be seen in up to 5 percent of cases. This anomaly also has important implications for surgical correction. Other congenital heart defects also have a high incidence of persistent left SVC. Pulmonary vascular

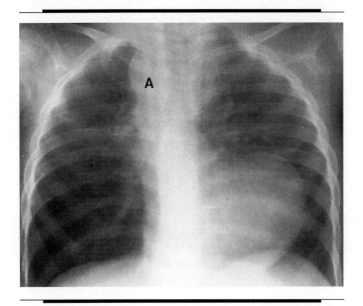

FIGURE 6-21   Tetralogy of Fallot. Frontal chest radiograph in a cyanotic infant illustrating a right aortic arch (A), decreased pulmonary vascularity with concave right ventricular outflow tract, and right ventricular hypertrophy with uplifting of the heart apex.

abnormalities such as peripheral pulmonary artery stenosis and enlarged bronchial arteries can also be frequently found.

Clinical features are variable and depend on the severity of the disease. "Pink" or acyanotic tetralogy occurs with mild infundibular stenosis and no net right-to-left shunt to cause cyanosis. Only when the pulmonary arterial resistance increases or the systemic arterial resistance decreases does the patient develop symptoms. Cyanosis associated with clubbing usually appears between 6 months and 1 year of age, probably as a result of the increasing physical activity of the child.

The **radiographic features** of tetralogy of Fallot are also variable, depending on the severity of the stenosis and the degree of right-to-left shunting. Plain films show normal or decreased vascularity with a small pulmonary outflow tract that may be flat or even concave in more severe cases. Also, the bronchial arteries may be well developed, causing disorganized perihilar vessels bilaterally. The heart size is usually normal or small. The ventricular apex tends to be elevated because of the ventricular hypertrophy and clockwise rotation and is described as "boot-shaped" (Fig. 6-21). The aorta may become enlarged from right-to-left shunting.

MR is comparable to echocardiography in demonstrating the intracardiac anatomy but is superior in demonstrating associated pulmonary arterial and aortic anomalies. In addition, MR can evaluate patients who have undergone palliative operations.

Angiocardiography is used to further determine anatomic detail prior to surgery planning. Aortography and at times selective coronary arteriography should be performed to determine the anatomy of the coronary arteries.

Surgical repair depends on the size and condition of the pulmonary arterial tree. Patients with multiple high-grade peripheral stenosis are not candidates for complete repair because of the inability to accept the cardiac output. A palliative systemicopulmonary anastomosis can be performed in cases where the pulmonary arterial cross-sectional area is inadequate. Definitive repair by a longitudinal right ventriculotomy, patch enlargement of the right ventricular outflow tract, and VSD patching can be performed at a later date after proper growth of the pulmonary arterial tree and after the patient's condition improves.

- **Tetralogy of Fallot with absence of the pulmonary valve** is a rare syndrome in which there is aneurysmal dilatation of the pulmonary arteries (**Differential 138**). It has been described in association with absence of PDA and the DiGeorge syndrome. Massive dilatation of the central pulmonary arteries may compress the airway, causing hyperinflation or atelectasis and respiratory distress. Pulmonary insufficiency can lead to right ventricular enlargement.

- **Pulmonary atresia with an intact ventricular septum** differs from tetralogy of Fallot because it lacks a VSD. There is fusion of the pulmonary valve leaflets and variable hypoplasia of the right ventricle. A right-to-left shunt occurs through an ASD or patent foramen ovale. The right atrium is usually

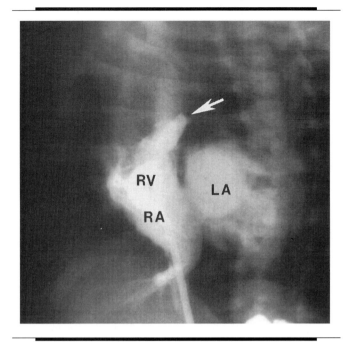

FIGURE 6-22   Pulmonary atresia with intact ventricular septum. Right atrial (RA) injection in the LAO projection demonstrating a right-to-left shunt into the left atrium (LA) across a patent foramen ovale. A hypoplastic right ventricular chamber (RV) is seen overlying the right atrium. The pulmonary valve is atretic (arrow).

enlarged and hypertrophied. Blood mixes within the left atrium before passing into the left ventricle and out the aorta. A PDA usually provides pulmonary flow. As the ductus closes in the infant, hypoxemia develops and death may occur if the condition is not treated promptly.

Radiographically, infants exhibit decreased pulmonary vascularity with variable cardiomegaly, mostly depending on the size of the right ventricle, and associated tricuspid insufficiency with concomitant right atrial enlargement. If the right ventricle is hypoplastic and tricuspid regurgitation is limited, the heart size may be normal. In cases of a well-developed right ventricular chamber and marked tricuspid regurgitation, cardiomegaly may be significant. This radiographic appearance may be very similar to that seen in Ebstein anomaly.

Angiography is helpful in surgical planning by determining the size, appearance, and function of the right ventricular chamber (Fig. 6-22). In severe cases, the right ventricle may be diminutive and have myocardial sinusoids that communicate between the ventricular chamber and coronary arteries.

Treatment consists of maintaining the ductus patent with prostaglandin E_1 to improve oxygenation and decrease acidosis, followed by surgery. A valvotomy can be performed in patients with larger right ventricles, whereas systemicopulmonary shunts are reserved for those with hypoplastic chambers. In the latter group, a second operation (a valvotomy or a Fontan procedure) can be performed at a later date depending on subsequent right ventricle growth.

6.10 CYANOSIS AND INCREASED PULMONARY VASCULARITY

- **D-transposition of the great arteries**, the most common cyanotic condition associated with increased pulmonary vascularity on the chest radiograph, represents 7 percent of all congenital heart malformations. Without proper treatment, the overall infant mortality can reach 90 percent by the end of the first year. In this entity, each great artery is misplaced, arising from the wrong ventricle. Anatomically, there is atrioventricular concordance, with the right atrium connected to the right ventricle and left atrium connected to the left ventricle, however, there is ventricle–great vessel discordance, with the right ventricle connected to the aorta and the left ventricle connected to the pulmonary artery. For survival, a septation defect is necessary. ASDs, VSDs, and PDA are common associated defects, causing increased pulmonary vascularity on the chest radiograph.

The systemic venous blood passes from the right atrium into the right ventricle and out the aorta (Fig. 6-23). A parallel circuit is present, with the pulmonary venous blood entering the left atrium and left ventricle. Once in the left ventricle, this oxygenated blood goes out the main pul-

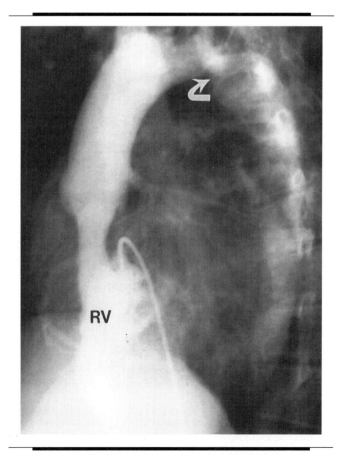

FIGURE 6-23   D-transposition of the great arteries. Right ventriculogram showing the aorta arising from the right ventricle (RV). A mild area of aortic coarctation is also present (arrow).

monary arteries to the lungs. A septation defect can connect these parallel circulations, allowing mixture and survival.

Frequent associated anomalies include VSD, subpulmonary stenosis, mitral valve abnormalities, and coarctation of the aorta. Radiographically, increased pulmonary markings, an "egg-shaped" heart, and a narrow superior mediastinum are distinguishing features. The narrow superior mediastinum is due to the anteroposterior relationship of the great arteries and thymic hypoplasia from cyanosis and stress. It usually takes several weeks before increased pulmonary vascularity is appreciated on the chest radiograph.

Early diagnosis and prompt therapy are imperative in neonates with this condition. Traditionally, cardiac catheterization with palliative atrial balloon septostomy was followed by an atrial baffle procedure (a Mustard or Senning operation) later in life. At present, once the definitive diagnosis is made with two-dimensional and Doppler echocardiography, infants can undergo an arterial switch operation. Prostaglandin infusion keeps the ductus open while surgical planning is undertaken.

In the **Mustard operation**, an atrial baffle is made with autologous pericardium, while in the **Senning procedure** the atrial walls and septum are used to form a baffle, avoiding any type of exogenous material. Residual intracardiac shunts, caval and pulmonary venous obstructions, and cardiac arrythmias are common complications. The **arterial switch procedure** has gained widespread popularity since it returns the great arteries and ventricles to their normal anatomic relationship. Among postoperative complications are stenosis of the aortic root and transplanted coronary arteries, aortic insufficiency, and postoperative dysrhythmias. Surgical results are better in younger infants, thus allowing their left ventricle to take over the pressure demands of the systemic circulation at an earlier age.

- **Double outlet right ventricle (DORV) without pulmonary stenosis** is a rare spectrum of anomalies in which both great arteries originate from the morphologic right ventricle. DORV varies from a simple VSD with relatively normally positioned great vessels to complete malposition of the great vessels (Taussig-Bing anomaly). If there is associated pulmonary stenosis, this entity clinically resembles tetralogy of Fallot. If there is no pulmonary stenosis and transposition of the great vessels, as they arise from the right ventricle, patients exhibit cyanosis clinically and shunt vascularity on the chest radiograph.

  The pathologic hallmark of DORV is separation of both semilunar and atrioventricular valves; thus, two infundibula are seen arising from the morphologic right ventricle. DORV is usually accompanied by a VSD, with different anatomic relationships to the aorta and pulmonary artery depending on the type.

- In true **Taussig-Bing anomaly**, the VSD is located underneath the pulmonary valve. Differentiation from transposition of the great vessels can be difficult, relying on the presence (or absence) of continuity between both semilunar and atrioventricular valves. Surgical repair of these complex conditions can be very difficult and require precise anatomic description preoperatively. Specifically, the exact location of the VSD and its relationship to the great vessels is crucial.

- **A single ventricle or univentricular heart** is characterized by a single ventricular chamber that receives blood from one or two atrioventricular valves (admixture lesion). A variety of complex anatomic malformations are included in this entity. In many cases, an accessory rudimentary chamber is also present. Most univentricular hearts are of the left ventricular morphology. The ventriculoarterial connections are variable, and multiple associated congenital anomalies may be present.

  Clinically, central cyanosis is a distinguishing feature, and infants experience poor growth, respiratory infections, and congestive heart failure.

  The chest radiograph usually demonstrates diffuse cardiomegaly and increased pulmonary vascularity (unless there is associated pulmonary or subpulmonary stenosis).

  Echocardiography and MR can be helpful in determining anatomic characteristics. A majority of patients exhibit a large left ventricle-type chamber with a rudimentary right ventricular chamber underneath the aortic valve. Pulmonary stenosis may be present, as well as either one (single-inlet) or two (double-inlet) atrioventricular valves connecting the atria to the single ventricle.

  Surgical treatment is variable and depends on associated lesions. Palliative operations are usually associated with limited success. Pulmonary artery banding may help alleviate this condition in patients without pulmonary stenosis, while systemic to pulmonary shunts can be attempted in patients with severe pulmonary stenosis. Somewhat better results have been obtained with the Fontan operation, although elevated pulmonary artery resistance is a surgical contraindication.

- **Persistent truncus arteriosus** is an uncommon condition accounting for approximately 2 percent of cardiac malformations. It consists of a single truncal vessel arising from the base of the heart and giving rise to the aorta and the pulmonary artery. There is also an associated VSD of the infundibular or supracristal type. The truncal valve is usually tricuspid but can also be quadricuspid or bicuspid, frequently resulting in truncal insufficiency.

  A mirror-image right aortic arch can be found in about one-third of cases. An interrupted aortic arch and an absent pulmonary artery have also been reported. Three types of truncus arteriosus have been described depending on the origin of the pulmonary arteries from the truncal vessel (Fig. 6-24).

  In **type I**, both pulmonary arteries arise from a common trunk (60 percent of all cases). In **type II** the left and right pulmonary artery arise separately and posteriorly from the trunk (30 percent). In **type III** the pulmonary vessels arise separately from the lateral walls of the trunk (10 percent).

  Clinical symptoms of heart failure are variable depending on the amount of pulmonary overcirculation and truncal insufficiency. Cyanosis may decrease as pulmonary vascular resistance decreases and pulmonary blood flow increases. Early corrective surgery (before high pulmonary resistance develops), particularly if there is no truncal insufficiency, offers a good chance for prolonged survival.

Radiographically, the combination of increased pulmonary vascularity and right aortic arch in a newborn with cyanosis is strongly suggestive of truncus. Evidence of pulmonary arterial hypertension with enlarged central vessels and distal pruning can be seen at an early age.

- **Total anomalous pulmonary venous return (TAPVR)** includes a variety of conditions in which the pulmonary veins drain into the systemic veins or right atrium instead of into the left atrium. An associated cardiac anomaly is present in about one-third of cases. The frequency is about 2 percent of congenital heart defects, with equal gender prevalence except in cases of TAPVR to the portal vein where there is male predominance. An interatrial communication is necessary to sustain life. TAPVR is frequently seen in patients with asplenia. Four major types have been described, depending on drainage:

  Type I is supracardiac, with the pulmonary veins draining into the SVC via the innominate vein. On plain films, patients exhibit increased pulmonary vascularity and a "snowman" or "figure 8" configuration of the superior mediastinum. This is the most common type, representing slightly more than one-third of all cases.

  Type II forms a connection at the cardiac level, either to the coronary sinus directly or to the right atrium. Multiple veins may connect to the right atrium.

  Type III or infradiaphragmatic drainage has an anomalous draining vein transversing the diaphragm through the esophageal hiatus before terminating in the portal vein, ductus venosus, hepatic vein, or inferior vena cava (IVC). The classic presentation is an infant with cyanosis and pulmonary venous obstruction.

  Type IV represents an anomalous connection at two or more of the above levels.

  As in other congenital heart conditions, two-dimensional and Doppler echocardiography have reduced the need for cardiac catheterization except in cases of complex associated heart defects, in cases of multiple sites of anomalous connections, or to precisely identify sites of venous obstructions.

- **Tricuspid atresia with a large VSD.** Although most cases of tricuspid atresia are characterized by either normal or decreased vascularity on the chest radiograph, shunt vascularity may be identified if there is a large VSD. This phenomenon occurs in approximately one-third of patients, who may exhibit cardiomegaly and radiographic signs of congestive heart failure.

  The VSD may spontaneously close in individuals with tricuspid atresia. Radiographically this phenomenon is mani-

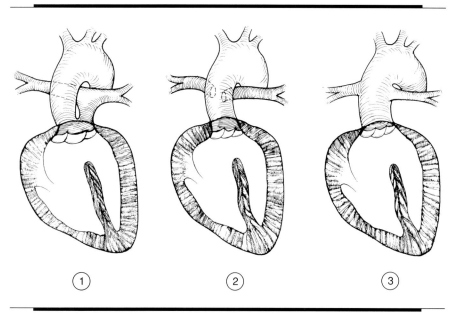

FIGURE 6-24   Types of truncus arteriosus. (1) Type I truncus in which the pulmonary trunk arises from the truncus. (2) Type II truncus in which the left and right pulmonary arteries arise close but separately from the posterior aspect of the truncus. (3) Type III truncus in which the pulmonary arteries arise from the lateral aspect of the truncus. Note the large septal defect between the right and left ventricles.

fested as a progressive decrease in the pulmonary vascularity on serial radiographs.

6.11 VALVULAR HEART DISEASE

- **Valvular heart disease** can be congenital or acquired. In some situations, as in aortic stenosis, a congenitally abnormal valve degenerates with "wear and tear," resulting in valvular heart disease. Acquired valvular heart disease is usually due to chronic degenerative changes or an inflammatory process, particularly infections caused by group A *β-hemolytic streptococcus*, an organism that carries antigens that cross-react with antigens in cardiac tissues.

- **Rheumatic heart disease** has become rare as the incidence of rheumatic fever has dropped significantly in western countries. It most commonly affects the mitral valve (85 percent of all cases), aortic valve (45 percent), tricuspid valve (15 percent), and rarely the pulmonary valve. When present, aortic and tricuspid valvular heart lesions are found in combination with mitral valve disease. After recovery from the acute episode, there is usually a latent asymptomatic period ranging from 3 to 30 years.

- **Aortic stenosis (AS)** is usually the result of a bicuspid aortic valve or rheumatic heart disease. In the case of bicuspid aortic valves, progressive degenerative changes occur along "stress lines," eventually leading to calcification and stenosis. Other causes are rheumatic fever, collagen vascular disease, and rheumatoid arthritis. Clinically, patients with AS have a prolonged, silent course for many years. Once symptoms develop, there is a rapidly progressive downhill slope, emphasizing the need for early diagnosis.

Calcification in the aortic valve area on radiographs should prompt echocardiography (**Differential 123**). The lateral chest radiograph is the best single view for seeing the calcifications (Fig. 6-25). In the case of a bicuspid aortic valve, about 50 percent of patients demonstrate calcification on the lateral chest radiograph by 50 years of age. Poststenotic dilatation of the aortic root due to the "jetting " effect from the stenotic valve may be seen. Left ventricular enlargement may be present with associated aortic regurgitation.

The normal valve area in adults is approximately 2 cm^2/m^2. A valve area of 0.6 cm^2/m^2 is considered severe, and 0.4 cm^2/m^2 is considered critical. Syncope, decreased ejection fraction, and congestive heart failure are poor prognostic factors.

Heyde syndrome (aortic stenosis and gastrointestinal bleeding) is thought to be due to angiodysplasia of the colon. Approximately one-quarter of patients with proven vascular ectasia of the colon on colonoscopy have AS.

Treatment of significant stenoses consists of valve replacement. Valvotomy and valvuloplasty procedures can produce aortic insufficiency and are limited to poor surgical candidates.

- **Mitral stenosis (MS)** is most commonly the result of rheumatic heart disease. Cases of congenital mitral stenosis (parachute mitral valve) are exceedingly rare. Frequently, patients with mitral stenosis also have some degree of concomitant mitral insufficiency.

Pathologically, patients with MS have scarring of the mitral valve leaflets with retraction of the subvalvular apparatus and chordae tendineae. Calcification is frequently present pathologically although a rare finding on plain films.

Clinically, dyspnea from pulmonary venous hypertension and fatigue from reduced cardiac output can develop. In severe MS, dyspnea at rest and pulmonary edema may be present. Hemoptysis, atrial fibrillation, and systemic embolization are frequent complications.

Plain radiographs demonstrate the characteristic "mitral heart" with progressive cardiomegaly and right ventricular and left atrial enlargement (**Differential 119**). Enlargement of the left atrial appendage causes straightening of the left heart border and focal bulging below the main pulmonary artery. The pulmonary arteries progressively enlarge, and there is pulmonary vascular redistribution from venous hypertension (Fig. 6-26). On rare occasions, left atrial calcifications can be seen, as a result of calcified mural thrombi. Pulmonary calcification due to hemosiderosis is rare.

Treatment consists primarily of rheumatic fever prophylaxis. The incidence of rheumatic fever has decreased significantly in the United States in the past 25 years as a result of improved hygiene and better prophylaxis. Diuretics, digitalis, and anticoagulants are used once heart failure and atrial fibrillation develop. Balloon commissurotomy and surgical valve replacement are employed in patients with significant gradients.

- **Calcification of the mitral valve annulus** alone is common but seldom clinically important. Secondary pulmonary venous and arterial hypertension can develop as severity of disease increases.

- **Mitral valve prolapse** is a common valvular abnormality found in approximately one-third of the population. It is transmitted as a familial autosomal dominant trait. This condition is frequently seen in Marfan and Ehlers-Danlos syndromes and in cardiac disorders such as secundum ASD and Ebstein anomaly. Although most patients with mitral valve prolapse are in fact asymptomatic, atypical chest pain and palpitations are frequent complaints. A midsystolic click and a systolic murmur are common at auscultation.

Complications of mitral valve prolapse include superimposed endocarditis, rupture of the chordae tendineae, mitral valve insufficiency, ventricular arrythmias, and cerebral emboli.

- **Pulmonary valvular stenosis (PVS)** is a congenital condition in which there is commissural fusion. It represents approximately 6 percent of congenital heart defects. Rheumatic pulmonary valvulopathy is extremely rare. Occasionally a dysplastic pulmonary valve is seen with thickening and rigidity but no commissural fusion. A bicuspid pulmonary valve is frequently observed in patients with tetralogy of Fallot.

Malformations of the pulmonary valve can be associated with the following systemic disorders: Noonan syndrome (male Turner), neurofibromatosis, leopard and Laurence-Moon-Biedl syndrome, maternal rubella, and trisomies 13, 15, and 18. An acquired form can be found in patients with carcinoid syndrome.

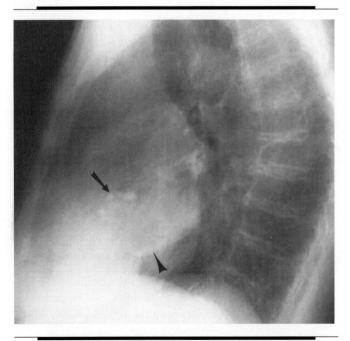

FIGURE 6-25   Calcific aortic stenosis. Lateral chest radiograph demonstrating calcification of the aortic valve (arrow) and mitral valve annulus (arrowhead).

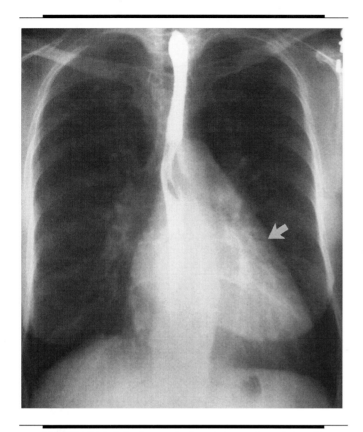

FIGURE 6-26   Mitral stenosis. Frontal chest radiograph in a 42-year-old female with mitral stenosis. Note straightening of the left heart border and enlarged left atrial appendage (arrow).

On plain films, the heart remains of normal size despite significant pressure gradients, except in patients with heart failure. Pulmonary vascularity is frequently asymmetric, with prominence of the main and left pulmonary arteries as a result of poststenotic jetting. Calcification of the pulmonary valve is rare. Gradient-recalled MR images can show the "negative" jetting of blood.

- **Supravalvular pulmonary stenosis** affects one or more branches of the pulmonary artery above the valve. It can be observed in patients with a VSD, William syndrome, tetralogy of Fallot, and rubella embryopathy. Radiographically, distortion or "sausagization" of the pulmonary arteries may be observed.

6.12 CORONARY HEART DISEASE

- Although the most common cause of coronary disease is acquired, several congenital entities are worth mentioning: abnormal origin of the left coronary artery from the pulmonary artery and single coronary artery origin with the left branch passing between the aorta and the main pulmonary artery, among others.

   White-Bland-Garland syndrome consists of a congenital anatomic variant in which the left coronary artery originates from the pulmonary artery (Fig. 6-27). During intrauterine

life, and shortly after birth, there is usually enough oxygen perfusion of the myocardium because of high pulmonary artery resistance. As the pulmonary arterial resistance drops after birth, myocardial perfusion drops and ischemia ensues. Frequently, infants develop congestive heart failure, and Q waves can be seen on the electrocardiogram.

- **Atherosclerosis** is a multifactorial process in which heredity, diet, smoking, emotional stress, physical inactivity, diabetes, and hyperlipidemia play an important role. Atherosclerosis of the coronary arteries is the most common cause of ischemic heart disease.

   The major complications of ischemic heart disease are cardiac failure, arrythmias, myocardial infarction leading to ventricular aneurysm, interventricular septal rupture, papillary muscle dysfunction or rupture, and systemic embolization.

- **Left ventricular aneurysms** can be divided into *true aneurysms*, which are by far the most common, and *false aneurysms*, which are contained ruptures. Both can occur

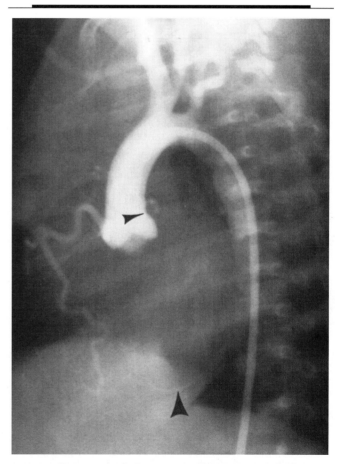

FIGURE 6-27   White-Bland-Garland syndrome. Aortogram obtained in the LAO projection in an infant admitted with congestive heart failure and an abnormal electrocardiogram. This early image clearly demonstrates the ascending aorta and right coronary artery, but the left coronary artery (small arrowhead) is not visualized. Note the collateral circulation from the right coronary artery (large arrowhead) supplying the left ventricular base.

as a complication of myocardial infarction and may calcify. True aneurysms usually involve the anterolateral wall and false aneurysms the posterobasal wall. Large true aneurysms may require elective resection, whereas false aneurysm repair is a surgical emergency.

- **Coronary artery aneurysms** are usually atherosclerotic and associated with abdominal aortic aneurysms. They predispose patients to myocardial ischemia. Other causes of coronary artery aneurysms are congenital, periarteritis nodosa, and Kawasaki disease.

- **Coronary artery calcification** is associated with a 50 to 75 percent incidence of hemodynamically significant disease although not necessarily at the site of the calcification (**Differential 123**). The mortality rate for coronary artery disease in patients with calcification is no different than in those without calcification. The calcium is usually in the intimal layer, except in rare cases of Möckenberg sclerosis where it is in the media.

 There are discrepancies between coronary angiography and postmortem studies, usually involving underestimation of the severity of the disease. It has been postulated that underestimation results from the diffuse nature of atherosclerosis where "normal" areas of comparison are also diseased.

 Arterial stenoses with less than 50 percent diameter narrowing (equivalent to a 75 percent cross-sectional narrowing) are generally not considered hemodynamicaly significant, although the number of stenoses and their lengths can affect distal perfusion. A 75 percent diameter narrowing in a vessel represents about a 90 percent cross-sectional narrowing. Mortality is directly related to the number of major coronary vessels involved.

 Although extremely rare, other disease entities can cause coronary artery stenosis besides atherosclerosis, including dissection, syphilis, trauma, periarteritis nodosa, and Kawasaki disease.

- The principal indication for **coronary arteriography** is angina pectoris or clinical suspicion of coronary disease. The procedure is generally performed to establish the severity and extent of the condition. Frequently, diagnostic catheterization is followed by angioplasty or another invasive procedure.

 Cardiac catheterization is usually performed utilizing the Judkins femoral approach technique and ventriculography, followed by hand-injected selective artery injections in multiple planes. Imaging is performed with 35-mm cineangiography, with high-resolution digital imaging used for immediate viewing during the procedure. Although biplane facilities are desirable, such as for imaging congenital heart defects, single-plane systems utilizing C-arm technology are adequate for most catheterization laboratories.

 Left ventriculography is usually performed by injecting 40 to 45 ml of contrast at a rate of 12 to 15 ml/s through a pigtail-type catheter. Standard views are left anterior oblique (LAO) and right anterior oblique (RAO) with a 6-in image intensifier.

 Although cardiac catheterization is a very safe procedure, potential complications such as arrythmias, arterial occlusion, embolization, and myocardial infarction can occur. The mortality rate is below 0.2 percent and is usually related to the patient's condition and the complexity and length of the procedure.

- **Percutaneous transluminal coronary angioplasty (PTCA)** has become a common, safe procedure for the treatment of coronary artery disease. The overall success rate varies between 80 and 90 percent. Restenosis remains a major problem occurring in approximately 30 to 40 percent of patients after 6 months. With multivessel PTCA, there is approximately a 50 percent chance of restenosis in at least one lesion. Presently, most coronary artery interventional procedures involve the placement of intracoronary stents for vessel patency. Other procedures such as atherectomy and laser angioplasty are now performed less frequently compared to a few years ago.

6.13 PERICARDIUM

- **Pericardial (celomic) cysts** are usually unilocular and smooth, are without a pedicle, and contain transudative fluid. They are usually less than 3 cm in diameter and are located in the right cardiophrenic angle; they are usually clinically silent but can be associated with pain, dyspnea, and cough, perhaps related to compression of adjacent structures. Diagnosis is usually made by detecting a cardiophenic angle mass on plain radiographs, CT images, or echocardiography (**Differential 110**).

- **Pericardial diverticula** are similar in appearance to pericardial cysts except they communicate with the pericardial cavity. Their size can vary with body position, presumably as a result of filling and emptying with fluid.

- **Congenital absence of the pericardium** is a rare condition in which all or part (usually the left) of the pericardium is absent. The symptoms are usually nonspecific, such as pain or dyspnea, and can be exacerbated in the left lateral decubitus position. Torsion of all or part of the heart due to the unrestricted mobility of the heart has been associated with this condition. Radiographically, exaggerated leftward displacement of the heart with the presence of lung between the heart and left diaphragm should suggest the diagnosis. CT can demonstrate an abnormal separation between the ascending aorta and main pulmonary artery with lung tissue between these two structures and no vascular attachment to the anterior chest wall (Fig. 6-28).

- **Acquired pericardial conditions** encompass a range of conditions. **Pericardial fat necrosis** is a nondescript condition that can cause sharp, pleuritic chest pain. CT can demonstrate an area of soft tissue infiltration of the pericardial fat. Treatment generally involves anti-inflammatory therapy.

- **Pericardial effusion** refers to excess fluid in the pericardial cavity as a result of inflammation, fluid retention, infection, or hemorrhage (**Differential 116**). Most pericardial effusions arise from the visceral pericardium. Radiographically, peri-

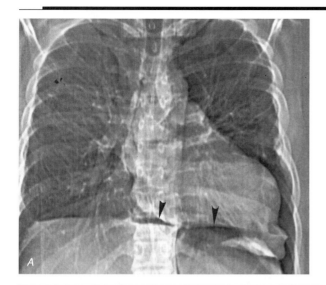
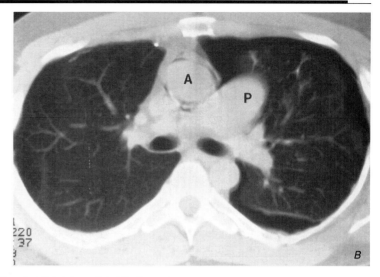

FIGURE 6-28 **Congenital absence of the left side of the pericardium** in a 32-year-old admitted to the emergency room with shortness of breath and a pneumothorax. (*A*) CT topogram shows a left pneumothorax, air dissecting inferior to the heart (arrowheads), and cardiac displacement to the left. (*B*) CT at the level of the great vessels showing air dissecting around the aortic root (A). P, Pulmonary trunk.

cardial effusions, depending on their size, can demonstrate an enlarged, globular ("water bottle") cardiac silhouette (Fig. 6-15*G*). Lateral radiographs may demonstrate a "fat pad sign" with separation of the pericardial fat layers by the effusion. Echocardiography is the usual mode of diagnosis. CT or MR can be helpful in cases where large amounts of pericardial fat make echocardiography difficult (Fig. 6-29).

Because of the fibrinolytic and anticoagulant properties of the pericardial serosa, as well as the constant beating motion of the heart, blood within the pericardial cavity usually remains liquid and mixes with the rest of the fluid. However, particularly after trauma, pericardial adhesions and loculations may form. In the absence of inflammation or trauma, malignancy is the usual cause of hemopericardium.

- **Cardiac tamponade** refers to a pathophysiologic continuum in which there is significant compression of the heart by accumulating pericardial contents, reducing cardiac filling. In its more severe form, this condition can become a life-threatening emergency. If rapidly accumulating (e.g., in aortic dissection with pericardial rupture), as little as 150 ml can be lethal in minutes. Symptoms are variable and nonspecific such as chest discomfort, cough, dyspnea, and weakness.

Physical signs include tachycardia, distant heart sounds, hypotension, and jugular venous distention. Pulsus paradoxus, an important physical finding associated with tamponade, is described as an exaggeration of the normal (<10 mmHg) systolic fall in arterial pressure during inspiration that returns in expiration. With pulsus paradoxus, inspiration improves right heart dynamics at the expense of left heart dynamics, reversing on expiration. Treatment consists of prompt evacuation.

Chest radiographs can demonstrate diffuse enlargement of the cardiac silhouette with clear lungs (**Differential 114**).

Comparison with prior radiographs may show interval enlargement of heart size. Echo-Doppler cardiography, particularly with TEE, can eliminate the need for invasive hemodynamic measurement. Although the ventricular systolic function appears good, collapse of the right ventricular free wall during early diastole is a fairly specific indicator of tamponade physiology. The right atrial chamber may also exhibit diastolic collapse. An inspiratory shift of the ventricular septum into the left ventricle may also be seen. Catheterization

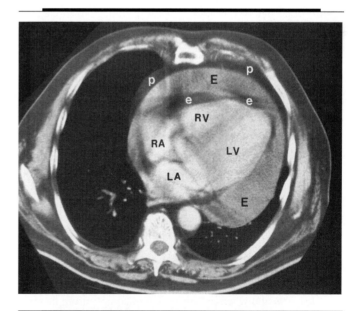

FIGURE 6-29 **Pericardial effusion.** CT showing a large pericardial effusion (E) separating the epicardial (e) and pericardial fat (p). LV, left ventricle; RV, right ventricle; RA, right atrium; LA, left atrium.

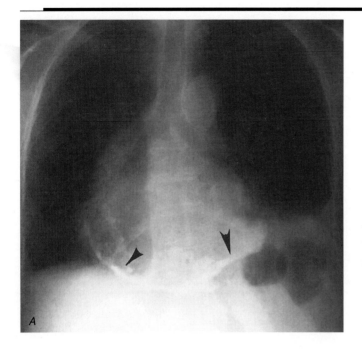
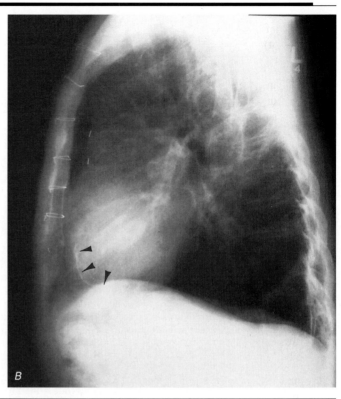

FIGURE 6-30   Calcifications. (*A*) Chest radiograph showing a large amount of pericardial calcification (arrowheads) in a patient with constrictive pericarditis. (*B*) Lateral chest radiograph showing a thin rim of myocardial calcification in a characteristic apical location in this patient with a calcified apical aneurysm following myocardial infarction. Note hemoclips and sternal wires as evidence of prior coronary bypass surgery.

usually demonstrates equilibration of central circulatory diastolic pressures.

- **Constrictive pericarditis** is a form of cardiac compression with important similarities to and differences from cardiac tamponade. Constrictive pericarditis is usually secondary to a scarred, nondistensible pericardium. Physiologically, constrictive pericarditis restricts diastolic filling of the ventricles. Management consists of surgical removal of the abnormal pericardium. Subtotal pericardiectomy may be effective in high-risk patients.

Causes include infection (viral, tuberculosis), trauma (surgery, penetrating wounds, blunt trauma, pericardial defibrillating pads), radiation (therapeutic, accidental), neoplasia (primary or secondary), vasculitis or connective tissue disease, drugs (Methysergide, Procainamide), myocardial infarction (Dressler syndrome), asbestosis, and idiopathic causes.

Although constrictive pericarditis resembles tamponade hemodynamically, there are certain differences. Kaussmaul sign (inspiratory jugular venous distention) is characteristic of constriction only. Pulsus paradoxus is rare in constrictive pericarditis and when present is due to complicating factors. Symptoms are a reflection of systemic venous congestion, fluid retention, and decreased ventricular stroke volume. At times it may resemble congestive heart failure (dyspnea, orthopnea, pedal edema, ascites).

Imaging of the pericardium can demonstrate thickening or calcification. Approximately, one-third to one-half of cases demonstrate calcification on a chest radiograph, best seen on the lateral radiograph (Fig. 6-30). The calcification is characteristically denser over the right heart and left atrioventricular groove and diaphragmatic surface of the ventricles (**Differential 123**). Although the presence of alveolar pulmonary edema is rare, left atrial enlargement and pulmonary vascular redistribution may be observed. CT and MR may show pericardial thickening (>4 mm) as well as vena cava thickening (particularly the IVC) and enlarged atria with small tubelike ventricles. CT and MR can aid in surgical planning by revealing the distribution of the pericardial thickening and any associated myocardial fibrosis.

Echocardiography can demonstrate pericardial thickening comparable to MR or CT. Echocardiography with Doppler recordings is ideally suited to determining associated hemodynamic changes. No single echo or Doppler sign, however, is pathognomonic of constriction. It is important to differentiate constriction from restrictive myocardial dynamics.

Cardiac catheterization can demonstrate diastolic pressure equilibration and an early halt to ventricular filling in a "square root" diastolic configuration.

6.14 CARDIAC TUMORS

- Tumors of the heart can be divided into primary (benign or malignant) and secondary (metastatic) (**Differential 115**).

- **Primary tumors** of the heart are rare, the majority are benign, and they can occur at any age. The most common primary benign tumor of the heart is **myxoma**, which usually appears as a polypoid, pedunculated left atrial mass attached to the atrial septum. Less commonly, myxomas can be located in the right atrium or right ventricle and rarely in the left ventricle. Although they are considered benign, they have been known to recur after resection. They are rare in children.

    Sarcomas are the second most common primary cardiac neoplasm. The most common is angiosarcoma of the right atrium (Fig. 6-31). These tumors are usually aggressive and can involve the pericardium early.

    Rhabdomyoma is the third most common primary heart tumor. This tumor is benign and is the most common intracardiac neoplasm in childhood. Often multiple, rhabdomyoma usually arises in the ventricles near the septum or crista supraventricularis. If large enough, it can produce obstruction to intracavitary blood flow. About one-half of these tumors have been described in patients with tuberous sclerosis.

- **Lipomatous hypertrophy** of the atrial septum can be considered an intracavitary benign neoplasm of the heart. Other rare benign primary tumors of the heart are **hamartoma, fibroma,** and **fibromyxoma**.

- **Metastases** are the most common cardiac malignancies and are twice as common as primary tumors. Common metastatic tumors to the heart are lung, breast, melanoma, and lymphoma. Metastases to the endocardium (**carcinoid**), myocardium, and pericardium have all been described. Although most metastatic tumors to the heart are asymptomatic and found at autopsy, if large enough, they can cause obstruction or arrythmias.

- Intracavitary tumors of the heart are very rare (bronchogenic, ovarian). Most of them first involve the pericardium by direct invasion (lung, breast, melanoma, esophagus, lymphoma). In children and adolescents, osteogenic sarcoma and chondrosarcoma may metastasize to the heart.

    Plain films can demonstrate cardiac enlargement that may cause distortion of the heart silhouette in large pericardial masses. Associated pericardial effusions may in part explain the cardiomegaly.

- Echocardiography is the imaging modality of choice for intracavitary tumors, whereas CT and MR are better methods of assessing intramural and pericardial masses as well as any extracardiac extension of the disease. In addition, MR may be indicated in cases of intracavitary tumors, other than classic pedunculated left atrial myxoma, to determine the extent of involvement.

Bibliography

Abrams HL. *Coronary Arteriography: A Practical Approach.* Boston: Little Brown; 1983.

Adams, FH, Emmanoulides GC, Riemenschneider TA. *Heart Disease in Infants, Children and Adolescents.* Baltimore: Williams & Wilkins; 1989.

Chen JTT. *Essentials of Cardiac Roentgenology.* Boston: Little Brown; 1987.

Cosh JA, Lever JV. *Rheumatic Disease and the Heart.* Berlin: Springer-Verlag; 1988.

Curtiss EI, Reddy PS, Uretsky BF, Cecchetti AA. Pulsus paradoxus: Definition and relation to severity of cardiac tamponade. *Am. Heart J.* 1988;115:391–398.

Elliot LP. *Cardiac Imaging in Infants, Children and Adults.* Philadelphia: JR Lippincott; 1991.

Gedgaudas E, Moller JH, Castaneda-Zunica WR, Amplatz K. *Cardiovascular Radiology.* Philadelphia: WB Saunders; 1985.

Knaus R. *The Practice of Echoradiography.* New York; John Wiley;1985.

Kubicka RS. How to interpret coronary arteriograms. *Radiographics.* 1986;6:661–701.

Rienmüller R, Gürgan M, Erdmann E, Kemkes BM, Kreutzer E, Weinhold G. CT and MR evaluation of pericardial constriction. *J. Thorac. Imaging.* 1993;8:108–121.

Spindola-Franco H, Fish BG. *Radiology of the Heart: Cardiac Imaging in Infants, Children, and Adults.* New York: Springer-Verlag; 1985.

Spodick DH. *The Pericardium: A Comprehensive Textbook.* New York: Marcel Dekker; 1997.

Swischuck LE. *Plain Film Interpretation in Congenital Heart Disease.* 2nd ed. Baltimore: Williams & Wilkins; 1979.

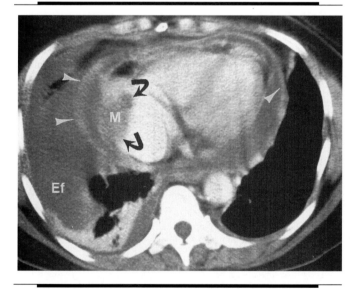

FIGURE 6-31   Angiosarcoma of the right atrium. CT demonstrating a sessile mass attached to the lateral wall of the right atrium (M, arrows). Note thickening and enhancement of the pericardium (arrowheads). There is a large right pleural effusion (Ef) which was proven to be malignant.

Chapter 7

THE PLEURA

Richard M. Slone

7.1   PLEURAL ANATOMY

- The **visceral pleura** covering the lung includes mesothelial cells lining the surface, underlying connective tissue, and a vascular layer. Blood is supplied by both pulmonary and bronchial arteries.

- The **parietal pleura** lines the thoracic cavity, mediastinum, and diaphragm. There is an overlying layer of connective tissue and extrapleural fat of variable thickness along the chest wall surface just beneath the endothoracic fascia. Only the parietal pleura is innervated with sensory nerves. Blood is supplied by systemic vessels.

- The **pleural space** normally contains a small amount of pleural fluid (about 10 ml), primarily produced and resorbed by the parietal pleura, providing lubrication.

- The pleural layers, in combination with the innermost intercostal muscle, are typically indistinguishable and appear as a thin line called the "**intercostal stripe**" on computed tomography (CT) images. The intercostal fat between ribs separates the intercostal stripe from the internal and external intercostal muscles.

- The **inferior pulmonary ligament** represents a union of the parietal pleura covering the mediastinum and visceral pleura at the hilum. It courses inferoposteriorly from the inferior pulmonary vein adjacent to the inferior vena cava (IVC) and azygos vein on the right and the descending aorta and esophagus on the left. It divides the medial pleural space into anterior and posterior compartments, demonstrated when pleural effusions are present.

The ligament widens inferiorly and may continue to the diaphragm, merging with the parietal pleura. A complete inferior pulmonary ligament tethers a collapsed lower lobe to the mediastinum. Paraesophageal varices and lymphadenopathy within the ligament can simulate parenchymal pathology.

Pleural Fissures

- **Pleural fissures** are clefts in the lung formed by the interface of visceral pleura covering the lobes (Fig. 7-1). They act as barriers to the spread of infection, thereby creating a sharply marginated border to a pneumonia or neoplasm, sometimes simulating atelectasis.

The **major fissure** separates the lower lobes from the rest of the lung. The upper portion is typically concave toward the anterior chest, and the inferior portion is concave toward the posterior chest. Fat may enter the inferior margin of the fissure.

The **minor fissure**, present only on the right, extends from the anterior chest wall to the major fissure posteriorly, is typically convex upward, and separates the middle and right upper lobes.

The major fissures are partially incomplete in over one-half of patients, and the minor fissure even more frequently. It therefore may not extend all the way to the hilum. This anatomic variability allows air, infection, and neoplastic disease to spread easily between lobes.

- The **anterior junction line** is seen as an oblique line projecting over the lower trachea and great vessels on PA chest radiographs (Fig. 7-2). It represents contact between the pleural surfaces of the right and left lungs anterior to the mediastinum. This line is formed by two layers of visceral and parietal pleura and may have fat within it.

- The **posterior junction line** is seen as an oblique line coursing a short distance in the superior mediastinum and terminating at the aorta, often projecting over the trachea on posteroanterior (PA) chest radiographs. It represents contact between the pleural surfaces of the right and left lungs and contains two layers of visceral and parietal pleura.

- The **azygoesophageal line** seen projecting over the spine on PA chest radiographs represents the interface between the right lung posterior to the mediastinum and the lateral surface of the esophagus and descending aorta.

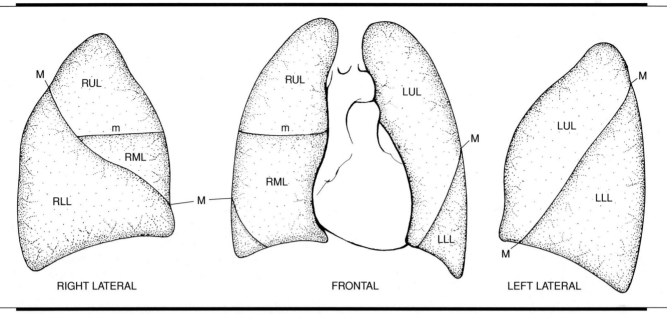

M   RUL   RUL   LUL   M

m   m   LUL

RML   M

RML   LUL

RLL   M   LLL   LLL

M

RIGHT LATERAL   FRONTAL   LEFT LATERAL

FIGURE 7-1   Normal pleural fissures. Anterior and lateral views of the lung surface showing the location of the major (M) and minor (m) fissures separating the upper, middle, and lower lobes. RUL, Right upper lobe; RML, right middle lobe; RLL, right lower lobe; LUL, left upper lobe; LLL, left lower lobe.

• **Accessory fissures** represent invaginations of the visceral pleura between pulmonary segments, forming accessory lobes (Fig. 7-3). The pulmonary segments and bronchial and arterial anatomy remain normal. The *inferior accessory fissure* separates the medial basal segment from the rest of the lower lobe.

The *superior accessory fissure* arises below the superior segmental bronchus, usually at or just below the level of the minor fissure, and separates the apical segment of the lower lobe from the basal segments. The *left minor fissure* separates the lingula from the anterior segment of the left upper lobe and may be cephalad or caudal to the minor fissure.

• The **azygos fissure**, present in 1 percent of individuals, results from the right posterior cardinal vein failing to migrate over the apex of the right lung, thereby entrapping a portion of the right upper lobe. The pleural septum, comprised of four pleural layers, is convex toward the chest wall and runs obliquely from the apex to the azygos vein (Fig. 7-4).

The intrapulmonary course of the azygos vein is higher than that of the normal azygos and may mimic a pulmonary nodule. The "azygos lobe" varies in size and shares its normal bronchovascular supply with the right upper lobe. A *left azygos lobe* formed by the left superior intercostal vein is exceedingly rare.

7.2 IMAGING THE PLEURA

• **Chest radiography** is the primary technique for detecting most pleural abnormalities, such as effusions and

Posterior junction line

Paratracheal stripe

Azygoesophageal recess

Right paraspinal line

Left subclavian

Aortic line

Anterior junction line

Left paraspinal line

FIGURE 7-2   Mediastinal lines. Location of the various pleural interfaces and reflections as seen on a PA chest radiograph.

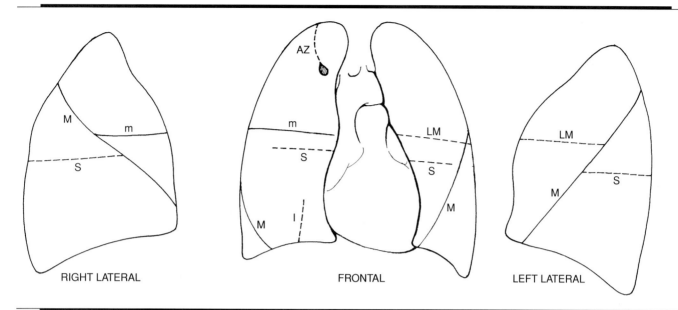

RIGHT LATERAL

FRONTAL

LEFT LATERAL

FIGURE 7-3 Accessory fissures. Anterior and lateral views showing the location of the inferior accessory fissure (I), superior accessory fissure (S), left minor fissure (LM), and azygos fissure (AZ) relative to the major (M) and minor (m) fissures.

pneumothoraces. The appearance of extrapleural, pleural, and peripheral parenchymal lesions overlap.

A **pleural location** is suggested by a lenticular or crescentic shape, tapering or obtuse angle at the chest wall interface, and well-defined margin with the adjacent lung.

An **extrapleural location** is confirmed by the presence of an associated extrapleural soft tissue mass, bone destruction, or displaced extrapleural fat (**Differential 86***).

Lesions forming an acute angle with the chest wall are typically **parenchymal** in origin. Exceptions include pedunculated pleural lesions or loculated pleural fluid collections that bulge into the lung or parenchymal lesions that infiltrate the pleura and create an obtuse angle with the chest wall.

- **Computed tomography (CT)** can be helpful in confirming the presence and extent of a pleural lesion, characterizing the abnormality, and distinguishing between pleural and pulmonary parenchymal processes.

  CT is also useful in assessing the relative amounts of consolidation and pleural fluid and determining whether

there is associated interstitial lung disease. When a large effusion is present, performing a CT following drainage of the fluid optimizes assessment of the underlying lung.

The fat content of lipomas, calcifications, and extrapleural fat thickening in asbestos-related pleural disease, and the

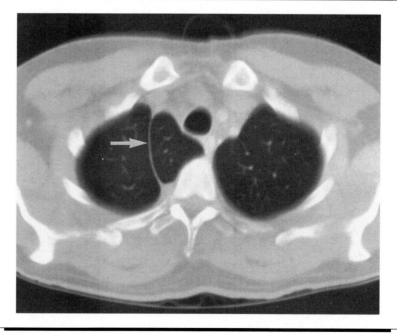

FIGURE 7-4 Azygos fissure. CT through the lung apex showing the azygos fissure (arrow) created by entrapment of the azygos vein. The fissure is composed of two layers of visceral and two layers of parietal pleura.

*Please refer to Chapter 2, in which the differential diagnoses are discussed in numerical order.

water density of loculated effusions, can help distinguish benign from malignant lesions.

Intravenous (IV) contrast is generally not necessary, but it can help differentiate consolidation and atelectasis, which demonstrate marked enhancement, from pleural tumors and metastases, which are enhanced compared to pleural fluid. Contrast also defines areas of necrosis and demonstrates peripheral enhancement in an abscess or empyema.

- **Magnetic resonance imaging (MR)** plays a secondary role to CT in evaluating the pleura. The multiplanar imaging capability is useful in evaluating the extension of peripheral parenchymal or pleural-based tumors such as bronchogenic carcinoma and mesothelioma into the chest wall, lung apex, or diaphragm.

  MR may be useful in distinguishing benign from malignant pleural lesions. Signal hypointensity relative to skeletal muscle on T2-weighted images suggests a benign pleural process. Hyperintensity on T2-weighted images or gadolinium-enhanced T1-weighted images suggests an inflammatory or malignant process.

- **Ultrasound** can be extremely helpful in corroborating the presence of pleural fluid and in guiding aspiration, although it cannot evaluate parenchymal disease.

7.3 PNEUMOTHORAX

- **Pneumothorax**, referring to air in the pleural space, is typically the result of a defect in the visceral pleura. **Chest radiography** is the principal technique for detecting and evaluating pneumothoraces. Diagnosis is based on visualization of the thin, white visceral pleural line (Fig. 7-5).

  Artifacts including tubing, sheets, and skin folds can sometimes simulate a pneumothorax but lack the absence of peripheral vascular markings and radiolucency.

  Detection is greatly limited in the semierect or supine position since the air collects anteriorly; therefore patients should be radiographed erect if at all possible. A decubitus film accomplishes the same goal and is very sensitive for small pneumothoraces.

  The conspicuity of a pneumothorax is increased on *expiratory films* in which normal lung decreases in volume and increases in density relative to the fixed pleural air collection.

- **CT** can be helpful in complex cases such as differentiating a large bulla from a pneumothorax, assessing the adequacy of chest tube positioning, or when extensive subcutaneous air obscures radiographic findings (Fig. 7-6).

- **Causes** include penetrating trauma, iatrogenic puncture from a central line (Fig. 7-7) or thoracentesis, rupture of a pulmonary cyst bullae or bleb, or dissection from a pneumomediastinum or pneumoperitoneum (**Differential 70**). Symptoms include pleuritic chest pain and shortness of breath.

- A small pneumothorax may be asymptomatic and resolve spontaneously over one or several days, but larger pneumo-

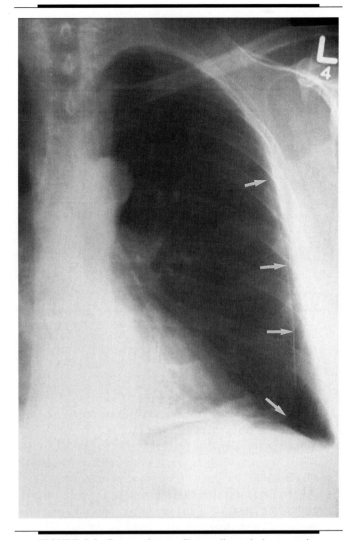

FIGURE 7-5   Pneumothorax. Chest radiograph demonstrating the thin visceral pleural line (arrows) and peripheral lucency with lack of vascular markings.

thoraces often produce hypoxemia, necessitating chest tube placement for treatment. Reexpansion may be delayed if there is underlying lung disease, if there is pleural thickening, or if the pneumothorax is chronic. Rapid reexpansion of a chronically collapsed lung can cause *reexpansion pulmonary edema*.

- A primary **spontaneous pneumothorax** can occur in otherwise healthy individuals in the absence of a known traumatic event. This occurs more frequently in tall, thin males in their third to fourth decade. Apical bullae and emphysematous lesions may warrant resection to prevent recurrences.

- A **tension pneumothorax** occurs when air is able to enter but not exit the pleural space. Clinically there is progressive dyspnea and hypoxemia, and radiographically there is ipsilateral hyperinflation of the hemithorax, downward displacement of the diaphragm, and contralateral shift of the mediastinum. This can occur despite incomplete collapse of the lung in patients with fibrosis or emphysema.

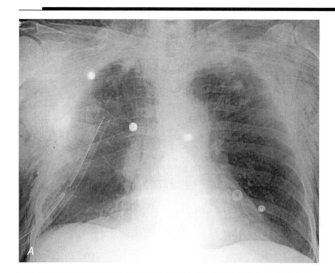
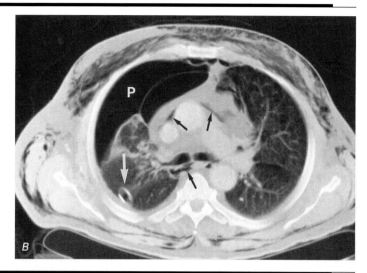

FIGURE 7-6 **Subcutaneous emphysema, pneumomediastinum, and pneumothorax.** (*A*) Portable chest radiograph showing a right chest tube and extensive subcutaneous emphysema. Air adjacent to the pectoralis muscles produces lines radiating from the attachment on the humerus. (*B*) CT reveals extensive subcutaneous emphysema, a pneumomediastinum (black arrows), a large right pneumothorax (P), and a chest tube located within the major fissure (white arrow). With permission from Slone RM, Gierada DS.: Pleura, chest wall and diaphragm. In: Lee JKT, Sagel SS, Stanley RJ, Heikan JP (eds). *Computed Body Tomography with MRI Correlation.* Philadelphia: Lippincott-Raven; 1998.

- A **bronchopleural fistula** refers to a communication between the airways and pleural space and can occur as an immediate or delayed complication of pulmonary surgery, cancer, trauma, or infection. When present following pneumonectomy, air is seen in the postpneumonectomy space and fluid can be aspirated into the remaining lung.

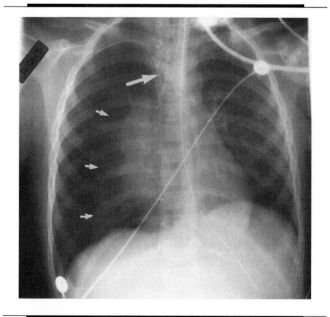

FIGURE 7-7 **Large pneumothorax.** Portable chest radiograph showing near-complete collapse of the right lung (small arrows) following placement of a right subclavian central venous catheter (large arrow).

7.4 PLEURAL FLUID

- **Pleural effusions** are the most common pleural pathology and develop when the rate of fluid production is increased, such as in heart failure, or when resorption is impaired, such as in lymphatic obstruction by tumor. The most common causes are congestive heart failure, pneumonia, tumor, and pulmonary embolism (**Differentials 72 and 73**). Clinical symptoms may include dyspnea and occasionally chest pain, depending on the etiology.

  The cause may be systemic (hypoalbuminemia), thoracic (parapneumonic), or abdominal (pancreatitis) in etiology. Patients with massive ascites may develop pleural effusions as a result of transdiaphragmatic flow of ascites through lymphatic channels or diaphragm defects.

  Effusions can easily obscure significant underlying lung disease such as pneumonia or tumor (Fig. 7-8). A unilateral pleural effusion in an older patient without symptoms of infection or evidence of heart disease is usually malignant, due either to primary lung cancer or pleural metastases.

  Effusions are classified clinically as transudates or exudates, according to their biochemical composition. This distinction is important in clinical differential diagnosis.

- **Transudates** are the result of increased capillary hydrostatic pressure or decreased colloid osmotic pressure and result from systemic rather than pleural pathology, such as congestive heart failure or a hypoproteinemic state such as cirrhosis (**Differential 75**).

  Transudates typically have a homogeneous, near-water attenuation on CT and are bilateral. They are typically clear fluid with a total protein content <3 g/dl, specific gravity

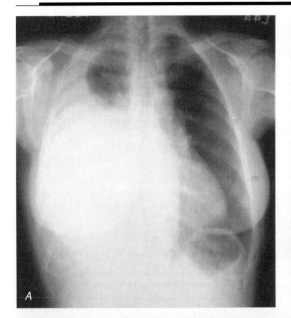

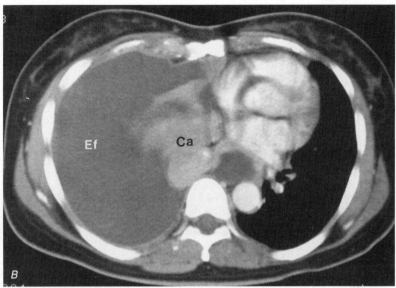

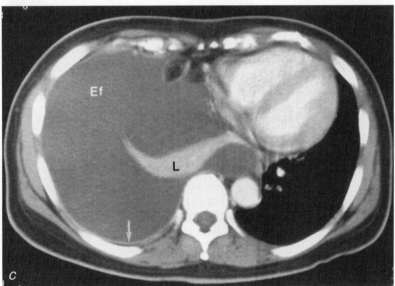

FIGURE 7-8 Malignant pleural effusion. (*A*) Chest radiograph showing a large right pleural effusion with contralateral shift of the mediastinum. (*B* and *C*) CT demonstrating a central obstructing lung cancer (Ca), a large pleural effusion (Ef) with enhancing atelectatic lung (L) tethered to the mediastinum by the inferior pulmonary ligament. Note the thickened enhancing pleura (arrow) characteristic of an exudate.

<1.016, lactodehydrogenase (LDH) concentration <200 units/L, pleural fluid/serum protein ratio <0.5, and LDH ratio <0.6.

- **Exudates** are the result of a local pathologic process involving the pleura, most commonly infection or tumor (**Differential 76**). The pathophysiology involves disruption of the pleura or lymphatic obstruction. Thickening of the parietal pleura usually indicates that an effusion is exudative.

  Exudates are typically opaque with a total protein content >3 g/dl, specific gravity >1.016, LDH concentration >1000 units/L, pleural fluid/serum protein ratio >0.5, and LDH ratio >0.6. They may have a high white blood cell count (>15,000 cells/ml) or a low glucose level (<40 mg/dl). They may be bloody or chylous.

- **Bilateral** pleural effusions are usually transudates, although in some situations, such as congestive heart failure, they may

be primarily right-sided. The smaller amount of fluid often seen on the left probably is a result of cardiac motion, which stimulates lymphatic resorption.

- **Unilateral** effusions are often exudates. Left-sided pleural effusions can be observed following rupture of the esophagus, a dissecting aneurysm, and traumatic injury of the aorta. Pancreatitis typically leads to left-sided effusions but may cause isolated right-sided effusions.

- Pleural thickening or enhancement on CT usually indicates an exudate. Pleural thickening, however, may not always be observed with a malignancy or parapneumonic effusion. Pleural thickening and effusion resulting from a malignancy may be either malignant (as a result of neoplastic spread to the pleura itself) or benign.

- Imaging often suggests an explaination for an effusion, particularly when the cause is pulmonary disease; however, *thoracentesis* is the mainstay for diagnosing the composition of pleural effusions and determining whether the pleural space is infected or contains blood or malignant cells.

- **Hemothorax** is suggested by pleural fluid with an inhomogeneous appearance on CT, including fluid levels or higher attenuation (Fig. 7-9). The increased attenuation is due to a high protein content, which can be seen with other complex fluid collections. A hemothorax can lead to significant pleural fibrosis (fibrothorax) and calcification. Causes include trauma, malignancy, pulmonary embolism, and pleural endometriosis (**Differential 77**).

- **Chylothorax** refers to an effusion containing lymphatic fluid, which has a high triglyceride content, and can result in CT attenuation less than that of water. Chylous effusions are uncommon and may result from damage to the thoracic duct, slow leakage from pleural lymphatics, or communication of the pleural space with chylous ascites.

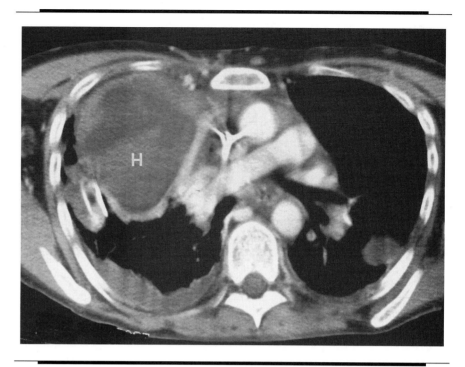

FIGURE 7-9   Hemothorax. Contrast-enhanced CT showing a loculated fluid collection (H) with areas of soft tissue and fluid density.

About one-half of chylothoraces are related to tumors, mostly lymphoma. Surgery is the most common traumatic cause of chylothorax (**Differential 78**). Transection of the lower thoracic duct may produce an isolated right effusion, and transection of the upper duct, an isolated left effusion.

Location of Fluid

- In the **erect position**, fluid initially collects in the posterior costophrenic sulcus and is visible on the lateral projection when 50 ml is present. As the volume exceeds 200 ml, blunting of the lateral costophrenic angle can be appreciated on the PA examination and the diaphragm becomes obscured. A lateral decubitus examination is the most sensitive, being able to detect less than 10 ml of fluid. CT is also sensitive for detecting small pleural effusions and frequently demonstrates fluid not appreciated on radiographs (Fig. 7-10).

- Blunting of the lateral costophrenic angles with preservation of the posterior angle almost always indicates scarring rather than a small effusion, likely as a sequela of prior infection or organized effusion.

  The interface between the lung and the effusion is usually concave, termed a **meniscus**, with higher extension laterally. A sharp, horizontal interface indicating an air-fluid level is diagnostic of a hydropneumothorax.

- In the **supine position**, mobile pleural fluid initially collects in the posteromedial hemithorax, which is the most dependent portion of the pleural space. As the volume approaches 500 ml, a diffuse opacity develops on the affected side. Vessels are seen through the fluid, but not air bronchograms

unless there is associated atelectasis or infection. The degree of opacity decreases progressively in the cephalad direction on semierect examinations and obliterates the diaphragm with increasing size.

As an effusion increases in size, it conforms to the pleural space and may extend laterally, displacing the lung away from the thoracic wall. The lateral aspect of the major fissure may become filled with fluid, noted as a superiorly marginated opacity pointing toward the hilum. A large effusion may be seen circumferentially.

- Pleural effusions usually cause some **atelectasis** of the underlying lung. Large pleural effusions result in lower lobe collapse with upward displacement of the collapsed lobe, as opposed to the posteromedial location of typical lower lobe collapse caused by other etiologies.

  A very large effusion may opacify the entire hemithorax and can create a mass effect, collapsing the lung and resulting in a contralatereal shift of the mediastinum. This is in contrast to an opaque hemithorax with an ipsilateral mediastinal shift due to collapse alone.

- A **lateral decubitus examination** can be used to confirm the mobility of fluid and distinguish pleural fluid collections from pleural masses or parenchymal lesions. Movement of the fluid may reveal underlying pulmonary pathology.

- Pleural fluid may collect in a subpleural location. A **subpulmonic** effusion can be overlooked, mimicking elevation of the hemidiaphragm. Air in the stomach may make the presence of an effusion obvious on the left, and the peak of the diaphragm is more lateral with a subpulmonic effusion. Decubitus positioning confirms an effusion if it is mobile.

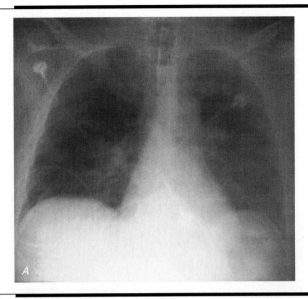
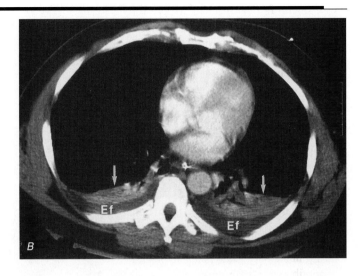

FIGURE 7-10   Small pleural effusions with atelectasis. (*A*) Portable chest radiograph without obvious pleural or parenchymal disease. (*B*) CT obtained the same day revealing small bilateral pleural effusions (Ef) with associated atelectasis (arrows).

• **Adhesions** may lead to loculation of fluid, which does not change appearance with changes in patient position. Fluid loculated within a fissure may produce a *pseudotumor*, which can simulate an intrapulmonary mass in one projection, although a characteristic lenticular shape is usually seen

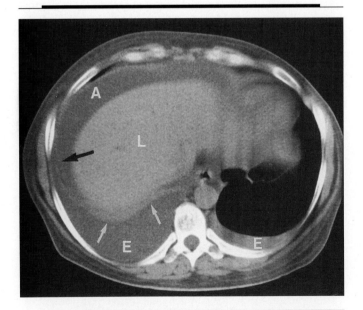

FIGURE 7-11   Pleural effusion and ascites. CT through the dome of the liver (L) and lung base showing bilateral pleural effusions (E); there is a thin strip of atelectatic lung in the right base (white arrows) separated from the ascites (A) around the liver by the diaphragm (black arrow). Note how the effusion extends behind the crus of the right hemidiaphragm and is primarily posteromedial in location. The ascites forms a sharp interface with the liver, spares the bare area, and is primarily anterolateral in location.

in the other. The sharp pleural margins and water density on CT should be a clue to its correct etiology.

• Several signs have been described to distinguish pleural fluid from ascites on CT (Fig. 7-11).

Displaced crus sign: Pleural fluid lies posterior to the diaphragmatic crus, displaces the diaphragm away from the spine, and decreases in the caudal direction. Ascites is anterolateral to the crus, displace the diaphragm toward the spine, and increase in volume in the caudal direction.

Diaphragm sign: The diaphragm can be visualized when both ascites and pleural fluid are present. Ascites is inside the diaphragm, and effusions outside. An exception occurs with large effusions which may invert the hemidiaphragm. A partially collapsed lower lobe within a pleural effusion can simulate the diaphragm.

Bare area sign: The right coronary ligament restricts peritoneal fluid from moving posteromedially to the liver on the right and the splenorenal ligament adjacent to the spleen on the left. Fluid adjacent to these areas is pleural, although massive ascites may extend medially beneath the hemidiaphragms above these areas on either side.

Interface sign: There is often a sharp margin between ascites and the liver or spleen and a hazy interface between pleural fluid and the diaphragm.

7.5 PLEURAL INFECTIONS

• An **empyema** is an infected exudative pleural effusion containing pus (WBC count >5000/mm^3) that most commonly occurs as the result of an infected parapneumonic effusion, particularly following pyogenic bacterial pneumonia but also with tuberculosis or fungal infections.

Infection can also occur as a complication of trauma, esophageal perforation, septic pulmonary infarction, or spread from osteomyelitis or an abscess. Iatrogenic pleural infection may follow thoracic surgery, thoracentesis, or percutaneous biopsy.

- The incidence of **parapneumonic pleural effusions** is dependent on the infecting organism, ranging from about 10 percent for pneumonias caused by pneumococcus to over 50 percent of those caused by *Staphylococcus pyogenes*.

  Most parapneumonic effusions are composed of thin, sterile fluid from visceral pleura inflammation and increased capillary permeability and resolve with antibiotics. However, some become infected and progress to an empyema, in which large numbers of white cells accumulate in the pleural space with fibrin deposition. Pleural thickening impairs fluid resorption and promotes loculation.

  Fluid may also accumulate in subpleural bullae as a result of adjacent pneumonitis, analogously to a parapneumonic pleural effusion. Diagnosis may require comparison with prior examinations to confirm preexisting bullous disease.

- **Empyemas** generally have smooth walls and a lenticular shape with obtuse margins that conform to the pleural space. They usually form a sharp border with the adjacent lung, which is frequently compressed, resulting in displacement and bowing of peripheral pulmonary vessels and bronchi around its circumference (Figs. 7-12 and 1-17).

  CT can depict the pleural fluid and thickening of the adjacent pleural surfaces which become organized with fibrosis

and vascular ingrowth. The extrapleural fat may be edematous, resulting in elevation of the parietal pleura away from the chest wall.

- A **lung abscess**, representing a localized area of lung necrosis, usually has thick, irregular walls, especially internally, and a spherical or oblong shape which forms an acute angle with the chest wall when peripheral. Lung destruction results in abrupt termination of bronchi and vessels at the margin of the abscess, and the parenchyma surrounding the abscess is often infected (Fig. 3-18).

  Identification of a central lung abscess is typically not difficult, although differentiation from a cavitary neoplasm may be problematic. Distinguishing an empyema from a peripheral lung abscess may be difficult with radiographs. CT can reliably distinguish between an abscess and empyema.

  Differentiation is crucial because proper therapy for an empyema requires thoracostomy tube drainage, whereas a lung abscess is appropriately managed with antibiotics and postural or bronchoscopic drainage.

- An air-fluid level can be seen in a lung abscess due to communication with the bronchial tree or in an empyema resulting from a bronchopleural fistula. Consolidated lung, pleural fluid, and septated collections may be associated with either an abscess or an empyema, and in some cases an empyema and a lung abscess coexist, typically with both being the result of a necrotizing pneumonia.

  IV contrast helps demonstrate the so-called *split-pleura* sign, the marked thickening and enhancement of visceral and parietal pleural layers seen in over two-thirds of empyemas.

- **Chest tube drainage** is the treatment of choice for management of empyemas. CT may be needed to clarify the exact site and extent of the empyema and its relationship to the tube. An improperly drained empyema is much more commonly a consequence of tube malposition than of the tube being clogged with fibrin or debris.

  A persistent air leak may be caused by inadvertent lung puncture by the tip of the tube. Potential complications may be signaled by noting the tube tip abutting the mediastinum and its contained vessels. The pleural surfaces have a remarkable capacity to heal, and an uncomplicated pleural peal often resolves following catheter drainage.

- Improper treatment of an empyema usually results in progressive organization of the fibrous pleural lining surrounding the loculated pleural fluid. This thickened inelastic membrane traps the lung and contracts the hemithorax. The pleura may eventually calcify, particularly if the empyema was a tuberculous infection. Effective therapy then requires surgical pleural decortication.

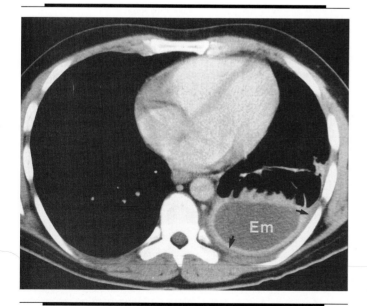

FIGURE 7-12 Empyema. CT showing an oval pleural-based fluid collection (Em) with an enhancing wall, extrapleural edema (arrows), and displacement and compression of the lung. With permission from Slone RM, Gierada DS. In: Lee JKT, Sagel SS, Stanley RJ, Heikan JP (eds). *Computed Body Tomography with MRI Correlation.* Philadelphia: Lippincott-Raven; 1998.

7.6 PLEURAL PLAQUES

- **Apical lung fibrosis** and adjacent pleural thickening are commonly observed as a senescent change, possibly related to relative ischemia, or as result of prior granulomatous infections such as tuberculosis or histoplasmosis. Asymmetry raises suspicion of a superior sulcus tumor but can be seen as a sequela of infection. Comparison with prior films or evaluation with CT is mandated. Pain or bone erosion is an ominous finding. MR may be helpful in better assessing the adjacent vessels and brachial plexus when a mass is identified.

• **Pleural thickening** may be focal or diffuse and is usually the result of a preceding inflammatory or infectious process (**Differential 79**). Normal anatomic structures such as the phrenic bundles or intercostal veins should not be mistaken for small pleural plaques. Peripheral pulmonary disease and occasionally a process involving the spine can extend into the paraspinal soft tissues and present as pleural disease.

  Localized pleural thickening is often the result of fibrous material deposited as a consequence of a prior organized effusion, hemothorax, or empyema.

  Benign causes of **diffuse pleural thickening** include prior surgery, radiation therapy, asbestos exposure (Fig. 7-13), drug reactions, and collagen vascular disease. Circumferential fibrous visceral pleural thickening, referred to as a *fibrothorax*, may restrict ventilatory excursion and reduce lung volumes. Calcification is common.

• **Malignant neoplasms**, including metastases, mesothelioma, and lymphoma, also can be manifested as thickened pleura. When nodularity, a thickness over 1 cm, or mediastinal pleural involvement is seen, a malignant etiology should be suspected.

• **Pleural calcification** is often associated with pleural thickening and is most commonly the result of asbestos exposure but may be due to prior infection or hemorrhage, particularly if unilateral (**Differential 80**). A prior tuberculous empyema

may cause dense, unilateral pleural thickening with calcification and is often accompanied by substantial parenchymal disease and volume loss.

  Large calcified plaques can simulate parenchymal disease and present a confusing appearance on standard radiographs. Oblique radiographs, fluoroscopy, or CT can be used to profile and confirm the plaques and exclude the presence of pulmonary disease. Pleural calcifications alone probably have no detectable effect on lung volumes or pulmonary function.

  Hypercalcemia from pancreatitis and secondary hyperparathyroidism in patients with chronic renal failure can occasionally cause pleural calcifications which may involve the diaphragm. Diffuse calcification can be seen as a consequence of prior pleurodesis, in which the apparent "calcification" represents talc. Bilaterally symmetric disease, particularly with calcified plaques on the diaphragm, is almost pathognomonic of asbestos-related pleural disease.

• **Extrapleural fat**, located outside the parietal pleura yet within the endothoracic fascia, is present to a varying degree in most adults. It is typically smooth, symmetric, thickest over the lung apex and midhemithorax, oriented along the long axis of the posterior fourth through eighth ribs, and associated with generalized fat deposition in the mediastinum and subcutaneous tissues (Fig. 7-14).

  Abundant extrapleural fat in obese individuals can simulate pleural thickening on chest radiographs, but the density and location is well demonstrated and characteristic on CT. Chronic pleural processes often produce localized expansion of the adjacent extrapleural fat layer. Increased density within the fat suggests an active pleural process.

• **Asbestos dust exposure** is associated with pleural inflammation leading to effusions, focal plaque formation, diffuse pleural thickening, pulmonary fibrosis, and malignant neoplasms of the lung, pleura, and stomach.

  Asbestos-related pleural plaques are the most frequent manifestation of asbestos exposure. They are often observed in pipe fitters and shipyard workers. The latent period between exposure and radiologic demonstration of the plaques is approximately 20 years. They are composed of hyalinized collagen in the submesothelial layer of the parietal pleura and are actually extrapleural.

  The plaques have sharp margins and range in thickness up to 15 mm (Fig. 7-15). They are typically bilateral and most common in the paravertebral and posterolateral midportion of the chest between the fourth and eighth ribs. They may occur overlying the mediastinum, diaphragm, and pericardium.

• **Plaque calcification** is common and may be punctate, linear, or cakelike, especially along the diaphragmatic surface where it is almost pathognomonic of prior asbestos exposure. Calcified and noncalcified plaques frequently coexist.

  Benign asbestos-related pleural plaques can occasionally be large and irregular and resemble mesothelioma. Benign pleural plaques may enlarge on serial examinations, confounding the distinction from malignancy. However, visceral and mediastinal pleura involvement is rare and should raise the suspicion of mesothelioma.

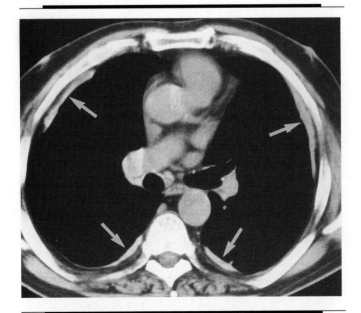

FIGURE 7-13 Pleural plaques. CT showing bilateral soft tissue density pleura-based plaques (arrows) with associated thickening of the extrapleural fat characteristic of a chronic process.

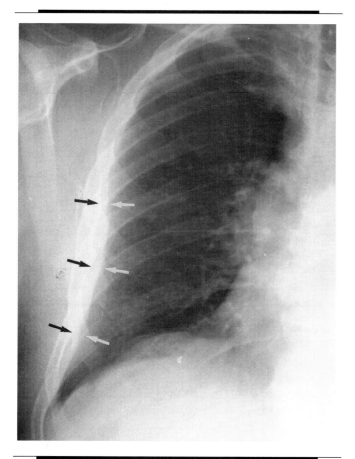

FIGURE 7-14 **Extrapleural fat simulating a pleural plaque.**
PA chest radiograph showing a strip of soft tissue separating the
lung edge (white arrows) from the chest wall (black arrows) charac-
teristic of a pleural plaque. CT demonstrated bilateral symmetric
thickening of extrapleural fat. With permission from Slone RM,
Gierada DS. In: Lee JKT, Sagel SS, Stanley RJ, Heikan JP (eds).
Computed Body Tomography with MRI Correlation. Philadelphia:
Lippincott-Raven; 1998.

- A chronic **pleural effusion** may be the first abnormality to
  develop in a patient with substantial asbestos exposure after
  a latency of 8 to 10 years. These effusions are typically exudates and may be hemorrhagic. Such effusions may also be
  the first sign of a mesothelioma or lung cancer.

- **Asbestosis** refers to pulmonary fibrosis caused by asbestos
  exposure and should not be used to describe asbestos-related
  pleural abnormalities. Although there is a correlation between the severity of pleural disease and the presence of
  asbestosis, most patients with plaques do not have interstitial
  pulmonary disease.

- Bakelite- and mica-related pneumoconioses can produce
  interstitial lung and pleural disease similar to that associated
  with asbestos exposure. Talcosis results in large, unusually
  shaped pleural plaques, and the entire lung may become
  encased with calcification.

- Patients exposed to asbestos have an increased incidence of
  bronchogenic carcinoma. The most common cell type is

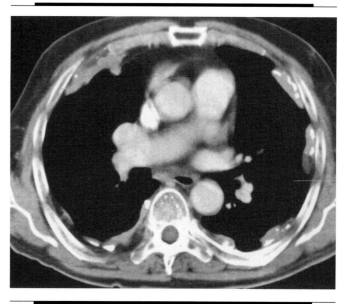

FIGURE 7-15 **Asbestos-related pleural disease.** CT image in a
patient with a history of asbestos exposure, showing bilateral calcified pleural plaques. With permission from Slone RM, Gierada DS.
In: Lee JKT, Sagel SS, Stanley RJ, Heikan JP (eds). *Computed Body
Tomography with MRI Correlation.* Philadelphia: Lippincott-Raven;
1998.

adenocarcinoma. The risk is dose-related, and there is a
latency period of 20 years. Smoking greatly increases the risk
when combined with asbestos exposure. This synergistic
effect leads to more than a 50-fold increased risk of developing bronchogenic carcinoma.

- **Rounded atelectasis** refers to a focal spiral infolding of lung
  seen exclusively adjacent to pleural thickening. It usually
  occurs in the posterior lower lobe and is most commonly
  associated with asbestos-related pleural disease. Patients usually are asymptomatic, and the finding is often incidental.

  This infolding is typically 4 to 7 cm in diameter, may be
  more lucent centrally or contain air bronchograms, and has
  irregular margins with bronchi and vessels curving into the
  mass at the edge closest to the hilum, producing a "comet
  tail" appearance. The adjacent lung may demonstrate compensatory hyperinflation, and there may be other signs
  indicative of volume loss.

  There is usually little change with time, although resolution may occur following a pneumothorax or pleural effusion.
  It may simulate bronchogenic carcinoma, requiring percutaneous biopsy to corroborate the diagnosis in equivocal cases.

7.7 PLEURAL TUMORS

- The most common benign tumors involving the pleura are lipomas and fibrous tumors. Metastatic disease is the most common malignant neoplasm. Primary pleural tumors, such as
  mesothelioma, are rare. Bronchogenic carcinoma, thymoma,

and lymphoma also may directly invade the pleura (**Differentials 81 and 82**).

- Features suggesting malignancy include pleural thickening over 1 cm, disseminated pleural nodules, extension into the fissures or mediastinal pleural involvement, and associated effusion or volume loss of the ipsilateral hemithorax. Definitive diagnosis usually requires biopsy.

Benign Tumors

- **Lipomas** are usually asymptomatic incidental findings. Some may extend from the chest wall into the pleural space, protruding into the pleural surface and simulating a peripheral pulmonary lesion. CT allows a definitive diagnosis based on homogeneous fat attenuation (Fig. 1-15). A capsule or small bands of fibrous soft tissue are sometimes identified.

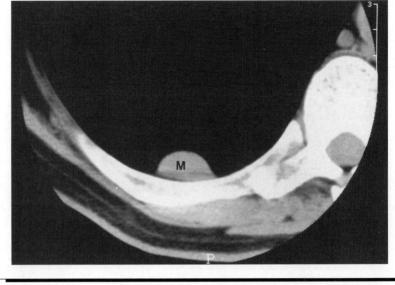

FIGURE 7-16   Benign fibrous tumor. CT showing a pleura-based soft tissue mass (M) incidentally discovered on a chest radiograph. CT-guided biopsy confirmed the diagnosis.

- **Fibrous tumors of the pleura** (previously called benign mesothelioma) are rare, but they are the most common benign pleural tumor (Fig. 7-16). These tumors are indolent and slow-growing, occur equally in men and women, and are found in all ages. There is no relationship to asbestos exposure. Most are asymptomatic and discovered incidentally, but patients with large tumors may present with a cough, chest pain, or dyspnea. Clinical findings may include hypertrophic pulmonary osteoarthropathy, clubbing, or hypoglycemia.

  The vast majority of these tumors are benign, but some are histologically malignant and can invade the chest wall or mediastinum. They do not metastasize outside the thorax. Treatment is surgical, although local recurrence is common and can occur as late as 15 years after resection.

  Features suggesting the diagnosis include a solitary, sharply defined, soft tissue pleura-based mass without evidence of chest wall invasion. They are usually sessile or lobulated, but some are attached to the pleural surface by a pedicle or stalk, allowing mobility which is pathognomonic. An associated effusion is rare.

  Most of these tumors arise from the visceral pleura and may occur within a fissure, simulating a pulmonary nodule. Calcification occurs in approximately 10 percent. They may grow to be very large, displacing bronchi, producing atelectasis, and almost filling a hemithorax.

  There is homogeneous contrast enhancement on CT. Large tumors may have low-attenuation areas as a result of cystic necrosis or hemorrhage. They have a low signal intensity on T1-weighted images and high signal intensity on T2-weighted MR images.

- **Thoracic splenosis** is the result of ectopic splenic tissue being displaced into the thorax following a traumatic dia-

phragm injury. The splenic fragments become supplied by the pleural vessels and appear as pleural masses. The CT appearance is nonspecific. Splenic tissue can be diagnosed with sulfur colloid or heat-labeled red blood cell scintigraphy.

Pleural Metastases

- **Pleural metastases** account for the majority of malignant pleural neoplasms. They typically involve both the visceral and parietal pleura and almost always cause an associated effusion, which is the first manifestation in most cases (Fig. 7-17). A unilateral effusion in a patient over age 50 without underlying cardiopulmonary disease is malignant in most cases.

  Pleural metastases occur as a result of hematogenous spread from tumor emboli lodged in distal branches of the pulmonary arteries. Adenocarcinoma is the most likely cell type to metastasize to the pleura. Most pleural metastases are the result of lung or breast carcinoma and lymphoma. Invasive thymomas and lung and breast cancer may invade the pleura by direct spread.

  Pleural metastases usually appear as small, lenticular masses having obtuse margins with the chest wall. They enhance with contrast, improving differentiation from fluid on CT. They may progress to encase the entire hemithorax and extend into the fissures, making differentiation from mesothelioma difficult.

Malignant Tumors

- **Mesothelioma** is a rare, rapidly growing, highly malignant tumor of the pleura. It has an extremely poor prognosis. The mean survival following diagnosis is less than 1 year, and less than 10 percent of patients survive more than 3 years.

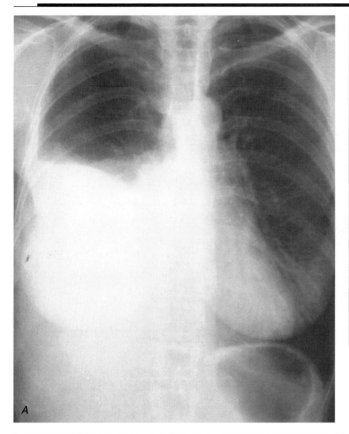

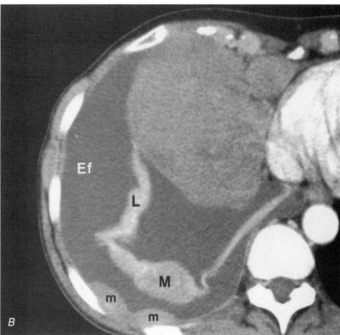

FIGURE 7-17   **Malignant pleural effusion.** (*A*) Chest radiograph showing a large right pleural effusion. (*B*) CT showing a large pleural effusion (Ef) with pleural metastases (M) involving the visceral pleura of the collapsed right lower lobe (L) and parietal pleura lining the thoracic space (m). With permission from Slone RM, Gierada DS. In: Lee JKT, Sagel SS, Stanley RJ, Heikan JP (eds). *Computed Body Tomography with MRI Correlation.* Philadelphia: Lippincott-Raven; 1998.

This tumor is more common in men than women, with a peak in the fifth and sixth decades of life. Clinical symptoms, including chest pain, dyspnea, cough, weakness, and weight loss, are late findings. Hypertrophic pulmonary osteoarthropathy is unusual.

The vast majority of patients have had occupational exposure to asbestos, but the risk is poorly related to the duration or degree of asbestos exposure. There is a 20- to 40-year latent period after initial exposure. Crocidolite is the most carcinogenic and fibrogenic type of asbestos. Chrysotile, amosite, anthophyllite, and tremolite are more benign.

Lung cancer is actually much more common than mesothelioma in patients exposed to asbestos. Mesothelioma is not smoking-related.

Almost all patients develop an ipsilateral pleural effusion as the initial radiolographic manifestation. The effusion is usually exudative and often hemorrhagic.

The tumor may appear as a focal mass or diffuse nodular pleural thickening between the lung and chest wall. Both the visceral and parietal pleura are involved, and extension into the fissures and along the mediastinal pleural surface is common (Fig. 7-18). Calcification is extremely rare.

As the tumor progresses, it may invade the lung, pericardium, mediastinum, ipsilateral chest wall, and occasion-ally the contralateral chest. It may penetrate the diaphragm and involve the peritoneal cavity or retroperitoneum. It is often advanced at diagnosis with circumferential involvement of the lung, ipsilateral volume loss, and fixation of the mediastinum.

Asbestos-related pleural disease is seen in the contralateral hemithorax in about one-half of patients. Asbestosis (pulmonary fibrosis) is uncommon. The pleural plaques themselves do not undergo malignant degeneration but are simply an indicator of prior asbestos exposure.

Surgical resection, either by a pleurectomy or extrapleural pneumonectomy, radiation therapy, and chemotherapy have all been advocated for the treatment of mesothelioma but with a high perioperative morbidity and little impact on survival. Operative morbidity is high.

The rare patient with a potentially resectable tumor typically has normal extrapleural fat and muscle with preservation of intercostal spaces and normal signal characteristics in the chest wall on MR. Rib displacement, extrapleural soft tissue infiltration, infiltration of the mediastinal soft tissues, or an extensive interface with the mediastinum is generally associated with unresectability.

- **Liposarcomas** are exceedingly rare and are typically more heterogeneous than a lipoma, with substantive areas of soft tissue density and infiltration of adjacent tissues (see Fig. 5-20). Inflammatory changes following infarction of a lipoma can produce a similar appearance.

- **Lymphoma**, including Hodgkin and non-Hodgkin disease, may involve the pleura but is rarely the initial manifestation of disease. It is more common with recurrence or by direct extension from the mediastinum or chest wall. A paraspinal location is common. Diffuse pleural involvement may occur.

  Lymphomatous involvement of the lymphatic channels and lymphoid aggregates found beneath the visceral pleura may appear as subpleural nodules or plaques. Mediastinal adenopathy may cause lymphatic obstruction leading to a pleural effusion, which occurs in up to one-third of patients with Hodgkin disease at presentation. **Leukemia** also may cause pleural thickening.

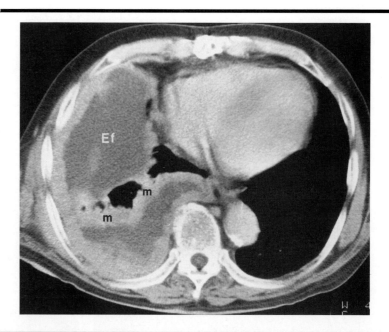

FIGURE 7-18   Mesothelioma. CT showing a circumferential pleural-based tumor extending along the visceral pleura within the major fissure (m). There is an associated malignant pleural effusion (Ef).

Bibliography

Armstrong P, Wilson AG. Dee P, Hansell DM. *Imaging of Diseases of the Chest.* 2nd ed. St Louis: Mosby-Year Book; 1995.

Dynes MC, White EM, Fry WA, Ghahremani GG. Imaging manifestaations of pleural tumors. *Radiographics.* 1992;12:1191.

Fraser RG, Paré JAP, Paré PD, Generoux GP. *Diagnosis of Diseases of the Chest.* Vol. 4, 3rd ed. Philadelphia: WB Saunders; 1991.

Freundlich IM, Bragg DG. *A Radiologic Approach to Diseases of the Chest.* 2nd ed. Baltimore: Williams & WIlkins; 1997.

Friedman AC, Fiel SB, Fisher MS, Rasecki PD, Lev-Toaff AS, Caroline DT. Asbestos-related pleural disease and asbestosis: A comparison of CT and chest radiography. 1998;150:268–275.

Goodwin JD, Tarver RD. Accessory fissure of the lung. *Am. J. Roentgenol.* 1985;144:39–47.

Halvorsen RA, Fedyshib PJ, Korobkin M, Foster WLJ, Thompson WM. Ascites or pleural effusion? CT differentiation: Four useful criteria. *Radiographics.* 1986;6:135–149.

Hanna JW, Reed JC, Choplin RH. Pleural infections: A clinical radiologic review. *J. Thorac. Imaging.* 1991;5(3):68.

Henschke CI, Davis SD, Romano PM, Yankeleviz DF. Pathogenesis, radiologic evaluation and therapy of plural effusions. *Radiol. Clin. North Am.* 1989;27:1241–1245.

Jones RN, McCloud T, Rockoff SD. The radiographic pleural abnormalities in asbestos exposure: Relationship to physiologic abnormalities. *J. Thorac. Imaging.* 1988;3(4):57.

Kawashima A, Libshitz HI. Malignant pleural mesothelioma CT manifestations in 50 cases. *Am. J. Roentgenol.* 1990;155:965.

Lesur O, Delorme N, Fromaget JM, Bernadac P, Polu JM. Computed tomagraphy in the etiologic assessment of idiopathic spontaneous pneumothorax. *Chest.* 1990;98(2);341–347.

Leung AN, Müller NL, Miller R. CT in differential diagnosis of diffuse pleural disease. *Am. J. Roentgenol.* 1990;154:487–492.

Light RW. *Pleural Diseases.* 3rd ed. Baltimore, Williams & Wilkins, 1995.

Matthay RA, Coppage L. Shaw C, Filderman AE. Malignancies metastatic to the pleura. *Invest. Radiol.* 1990;25:601.

McCloud TC, Flower CDR. Imaging of the pleura: Sonography, CT, and MR Imaging. *Am. J. Roentgenol.* 1991;156:1145–1153.

Müller NL. Imaging of the pleura. *Radiology.* 1993;186:297–309.

Patz EFJ, Shaffer K, Piwnica-Worms DR, Jochelson M, Sarin M, Sugarbaker DJ, Pugatch RD. Malignant pleural mesothelioma: Value of CT and MR imaging in predicting resectability. *Am. J. Roentgenol.* 1992;159:961.

Reed JC. *Chest Radiology.* 4th ed. St.Louis: Mosby-Yearbook, 1997.

Sofranik RN, Gross VH, Spizarny DL. Radiology of the pleural fissures. *Clin. Imaging,* 1992;16:221.

Wechsler RJ, Steiner RM, Conant EF. Occupationally induced neoplasms of the lung and pleura. *Radiol. Clin. North Am.* 1992;30:1245.

Chapter 8

CHEST WALL AND DIAPHRAGM

Richard M. Slone

8.1 CHEST WALL

- The chest wall includes the thoracic cage, muscle, fat, vessels, nerves, and lymphatics. Disease may arise within or spread to involve any of these tissues. Physical examination and radiography are limited in detecting and characterizing lesions involving the chest wall, especially in obese patients.

- **Computed tomography (CT) and magnetic resonance imaging (MR)** can distinguish between fat, soft tissue, and bone densities, display the individual components of the chest wall in cross section, and play complementary roles in assessing chest wall pathology. CT has higher spatial resolution and depicts cortical bone destruction better. MR allows direct multiplanar imaging, better soft tissue characterization, and better assessment of vascular flow.

- **Intravenous (IV) contrast** can be helpful in defining the relationship of tumors to vessels but can also lead to artifacts in the axilla, chest wall, and lower part of the neck on the side of injection. Transient enhancement of normal thoracic wall veins on the side of contrast injection, particularly in the periscapular and supraclavicular regions, may be seen on CT images because of retrograde flow.

    Enlarged **collateral vessels** in the chest wall suggest superior vena cava (SVC) obstruction or occlusion of another major vein in the thorax or abdomen. They appear on CT as round or tubular structures which enhance after IV contrast administration (see Fig. 5-3).

- Infections as well as benign and malignant tumors may involve the soft tissue and bone of the chest wall. Metastases are more common than primary malignancies, and almost any primary tumor can metastasize to the soft tissue or bones of the thoracic skeleton (Fig. 8-1).

    Chest wall lesions account for 2 percent of all primary tumors. Primary soft tissue tumors of the chest wall are more common than primary bone tumors, and most are malignant. Common benign lesions include osteochondromas, fibrous dysplasia, lipomas and desmoid tumors and common malignancies are chondrosarcoma, malignant fibrous histiocytoma (MFH), Ewing sarcoma, and rhabdosarcoma.

    Bronchogenic and breast carcinoma, thymoma, lymphoma, and mesothelioma may involve the chest wall by direct extension. In all cases of peripheral lung pathology, the chest wall should be carefully examined for evidence of involvement (**Differential 88***). Bone destruction is a definitive observation, however, soft tissue infiltration, stranding in fat, and pleural thickening are less reliable indications. Pain is indicative of parietal pleural involvement.

    Advances in chest wall reconstruction have facilitated potentially curative extensive resections of malignant neoplasms involving the chest wall, including both primary lesions and invasion by lung cancer.

8.2 THORACIC SKELETON

- The **thoracic skeleton** includes components of the axial skeleton (vertebral bodies, ribs, and sternum) and appendicular skeleton (clavicles and scapula). The **costovertebral articulations** include articulation of the head of each rib with the inferior articular facet of the vertebral body above and the superior articular facets of the vertebral body below. The

---

*Please refer to Chapter 2, in which the differential diagnoses are discussed in numerical order.

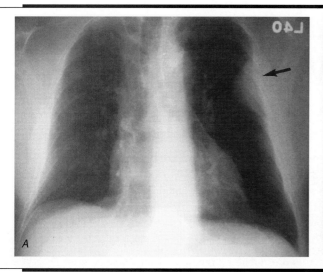 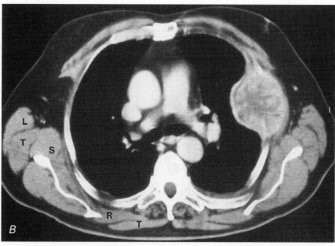

FIGURE 8-1   Metastatic renal cell cancer. (*A*) Chest radiograph showing a pleural-based mass with rib destruction (arrow). (*B*) CT with intravenous contrast demonstrating a large vascular chest wall mass displacing lung medially and soft tissues laterally. L, Latissimus dorsi; T, teres major; S, subscapularis; R, rhomboid; T, trapezius muscles. (With permission from Slone RM, Gierada DS. Pleura, chest wall, and diaphragm. In Lee JKT, Sagel SS, Stanley RJ, Heiken JP, eds. *Computed Body Tomography with MRI Correlation.* 3rd ed. Philadelphia: Lippincott-Raven; 1998.)

tubercle arising just beyond the neck of the rib articulates with the articular facet on the transverse process of the vertebral body. The posterior rib is called the ***angle of the rib***, and the remainder the ***shaft*** or ***body***.

• The **sternum** consists of the manubrium, body, and xiphoid. The first costal cartilage articulates with the side of the manubrium just below the sternoclavicular joint. The second costal cartilage articulates with the manubrium and sternal

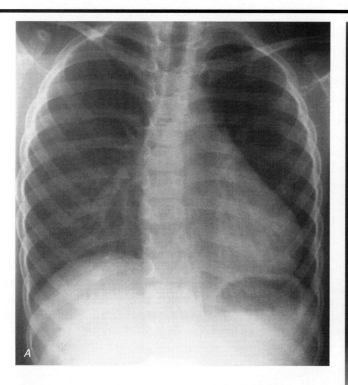 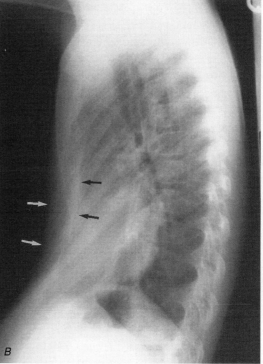

FIGURE 8-2   Pectus excavatum. (*A*) Chest radiograph showing leftward displacement of the heart. (*B*) Lateral radiograph demonstrating inward displacement of the lower sternum (black arrows) and costal cartilages with posterior displacement of the heart. White arrows denote anterior chest wall surface.

body at the sternal angle, the third through sixth costal cartilages with the body of the sternum, and the seventh at the junction with the xiphoid.

- **Degenerative changes** are common with advancing age and may develop prematurely as a consequence of overuse or trauma. Osteophyte formation and sclerosis are common along the vertebral endplates and glenohumeral, sternoclavicular, acromioclavicular, facet, and costovertebral joints. Spurs can mimic a pulmonary nodule. A vacuum phenomenon is occasionally observed in intervertebral and sternoclavicular joints.

- **Normal variants** include *cervical ribs* arising from the transverse processes of C7, which are directed caudal in contrast to the transverse processes of the thoracic vertebrae. They may be large or small, unilateral or bilateral. Other common anomalies include *hypoplastic, bifid,* or *fused ribs*. An *intrathoracic rib* is a particularly rare anomaly.

  Unfused spinous processes termed *spina bifida occulta* are a common normal variant, particularly in the upper thoracic spine. *Episternal ossicles* are posterior and cephalad to the cranial border of the manubrium. They range up to 15 mm in diameter, may be single or paired, and symmetric or asymmetric. A midline *sternal foramen* can be seen on CT as a small, corticated hole in the body of the sternum.

- **Chest wall deformities** include **pectus carinatum**, characterized by anterior protrusion of the sternum due to overgrowth of coastal cartilages. The sternum is often wider and longer than normal. **Pectus excavatum** is characterized as an inward depression of the sternum and lower costal cartilages with a normal manubrium and first and second ribs. This may cause compression and displacement of the heart and mediastinal structures (Fig. 8-2). The heart may appear enlarged and the right hilum indistinct. The lateral radiograph confirms the depressed sternum.

- **Scoliosis** of the thoracic spine is common and when advanced can lead to distortion of the chest wall and mediastinum, making interpretation of the underlying lung difficult (Fig. 8-3). Although usually idiopathic, a search should be made for underlying vertebral body anomalies such as hemivertebrae.

- **Thoracic outlet syndrome** refers to neurological or vascular symptoms caused by compression of the subclavian vessels or brachial plexus at the thoracic outlet. The cervicoaxillary canal can be narrowed as a result of trauma or congenital abnormalities of the clavicle or first rib.

- **Sternocostoclavicular hyperostosis**, sometimes accompanied by chronic pain and anterior chest swelling, is characterized by hyperostosis and soft tissue ossification between the clavicle, sternum, and upper ribs. Bone overgrowth may lead to a thick, wide sternum, sometimes simulating Paget disease or chronic osteomyelitis.

- **Costochondritis** (Tietze syndrome), which includes chest pain, tenderness, swelling of the costal cartilage, and some-

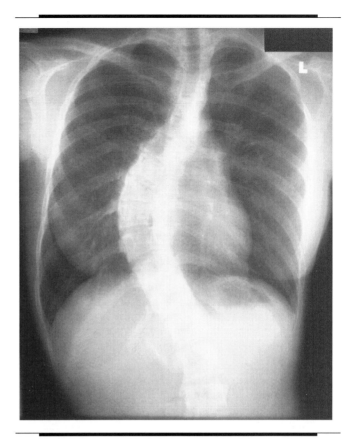

FIGURE 8-3 Scoliosis. Chest radiograph in a 26-year-old woman showing severe scoliosis with resultant alteration of the mediastinal contour. The scoliosis is idiopathic since there are no underlying causative vertebral anomalies.

times mild focal cartilaginous enlargement, can clinically mimic a chest wall mass.

- **Inferior rib notching** is most commonly associated with aortic coarctation or atherosclerotic obstruction and neurofibromas (**Differential 94**). **Superior rib notching** can be seen with rheumatoid arthritis, hyperparathyroidism, or neurofibromatosis (**Differential 95**).

- **Compression fractures** of the thoracic vertebrae in elderly adults occur as a consequence of osteopenia, typically osteoporosis, and are a common cause of back pain (**Differential 90**). Multiple fractures can cause a kyphotic deformity leading to atelectasis and pneumonia. The chronicity should be established by comparison with prior examinations. Bone destruction suggests a pathologic fracture, usually a metastasis.

- **Shoulder dislocations**, separations, and fractures are an occasional explanation for a patient with chest pain, although in almost all cases the diagnosis has already been made. An unrecognized anterior dislocation is occasionally detected on films obtained in the intensive care unit (ICU).

- **Rib fractures** are a common consequence of trauma. Isolated fractures can be the result of an underlying metastasis and should be suspected when acute fracture margins are indistinct. Multiple traumatic fractures usually involve contiguous ribs. Nondisplaced fractures may be very difficult to visualize on standard chest radiographs. Rib detail films obtained with a low kVp to accentuate subject contrast and multiple projections or spot films can help reveal a fracture if one is present. Associated complications may include pneumothorax, a pulmonary contusion, or an extrapleural hematoma. Atelectasis and pneumonia can develop as a consequence of splinting.

- **Callous formation** around healing fractures may simulate a pulmonary nodule and is a common problem in patients following cardiac and lung transplantation, when there is a high clinical suspicion of postoperative pulmonary pathology. CT can be used to confirm the etiology if required.

- The **clavicles** are a frequent site of fracture and often heal with deformity. Posterior dislocation of the clavicular head can damage the great vessels. Anterior dislocation is more common and easier to diagnose clinically. **Distal clavicular bone resorption** can be seen as a consequence of trauma, rheumatoid arthritis, and hyperparathyroidism (**Differential 96**). **Hypoplastic clavicles** can be observed with cleidocranial dysostosis.

- **Mediastinitis** is uncommon but carries a high mortality if untreated. CT is required as it is difficult to diagnose by radiograph. Treatment involves antibiotics, debridement, and drainage. Retrosternal air should be gone by 1 week, and mediastinal fluid by the end of 3 weeks following an uncomplicated sternotomy.

- **Osteomyelitis**, or septic arthritis of the sternum or sternoclavicular joint, is a rare complication of median sternotomy. Dehiscence or nonunion is more common but is difficult to diagnose on radiographs. Fractured sternal wires may be an indirect sign. Separation or bone destruction is usually evident on CT.

- **Discitis** as a result of hematogenous spread of infection to the intervertebral disk results in loss of disk height and eventual endplate destruction (Fig. 8-4). The vertebrae become sclerotic and may fuse after the infection heals. **Tuberculosis** (Pott disease) can involve the spine and classically destroys the vertebrae and intervertebral disk.

- **Radiation therapy** may result in localized osteoporosis, sclerosis, or even aseptic necrosis of the bones contained in the radiation port. Modern three-dimensional treatment planning has greatly reduced the incidence of this complication.

- **Diffuse skeletal sclerosis** can be caused by widespread metastases, particularly breast and prostate cancer but also metabolic bone disease such as myelofibrosis, sickle cell disease, renal osteodystrophy, or osteopetrosis (**Differential 93**; Fig. 8-5).

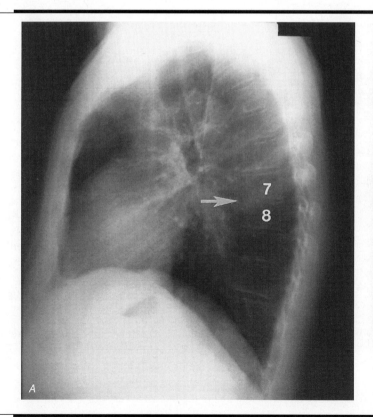
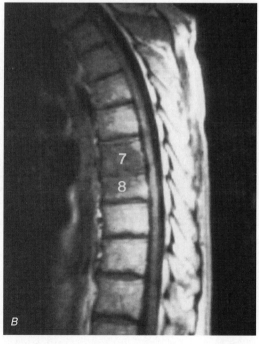

FIGURE 8-4 Discitis. (A) Lateral chest radiograph in a patient with back pain and fever showing obliteration of the anterior intervertebral disk space at T7-8. (B) T1-weighted MR confirming intervertebral disk destruction and edema in the adjacent vertebral bodies.

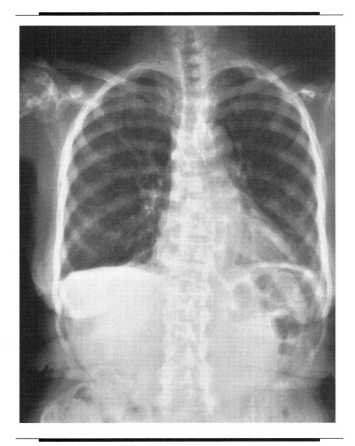

FIGURE 8-5 Sickle cell disease. Chest radiograph showing diffuse mottled sclerosis throughout the axial and appendicular skeleton due to multiple bone infarcts. There are also central endplate compression fractures and absence of the spleen.

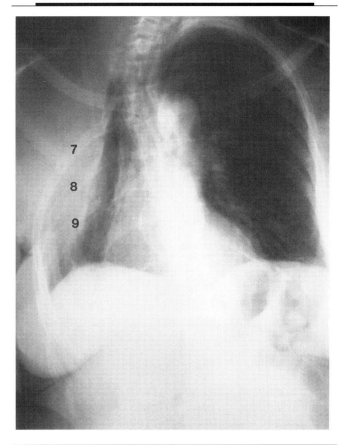

FIGURE 8-6 Thoracoplasty. Chest radiograph showing resection of the first through sixth right ribs and associated chest wall collapse as prior treatment for tuberculosis in a 50-year-old woman.

- Following **thoracotomy**, the ribs may be slightly splayed, or a rib is partially resected, typically the fifth rib. The rib may begin to regenerate from the remaining periosteum, producing a wavy appearance.

- **Thoracoplasty** refers to surgical resection or collapse of the upper chest wall, originally devised as a means to compress underlying lung tissue and treat patients with tuberculosis (Fig. 8-6). The appearance can be bizarre and can mimic massive trauma. Associated pleural thickening and calcification are common. Thoracoplasty is currently a treatment of last resort for some patients with a chronic empyema and insufficient lung to obliterate the pleural space.

8.3 BONE TUMORS

- Plain film **radiography** and radionuclide **bone scintigraphy** are used for detection of fractures and bone tumors. Although plain radiographs are sufficient for assessing multiple or nonaggressive lesions, **CT** or **MR** is more useful for solitary, aggressive appearing bone lesions and for evaluating bone involvement by adjacent tumors. MR is more sensitive in detecting bone marrow involvement, and CT is better at identifying bone destruction. Primary benign and malignant

tumors of the ribs have an equal incidence, but tumors of the sternum are more often malignant than benign.

- **Benign bone tumors** seen in the thorax include enostosis (bone islands), simple bone cysts, giant cell tumors, aneurysmal bone cysts, fibrous dysplasia, hemangiomas, osteochondromas (exostoses), and eosinophilic granuloma.

- **Bone islands** appear as focal sclerotic areas and commonly occur in the cancellous bone of the ribs, shoulder girdle, and spine (**Differential 91**). They can mimic pulmonary nodules.

- **Osteochondromas** (exostoses) are the most common benign bone tumors of the ribs. They appear as lobulated exophytic projections of cortical bone and have a cartilaginous cap. Rapid growth or pain suggests malignant degeneration to chondrosarcoma (Fig. 8-7).

- **Fibrous dysplasia** is the second most common benign rib tumor. Typically discovered in adulthood, approximately one-half of cases of monostotic fibrous dysplasia occur in the ribs. It typically appears as a central, expansile, fusiform, lytic lesion with thinning of the cortex. The fibrous matrix produces a "ground-glass" appearance centrally. Contiguous ribs may be involved (Fig. 8-8).

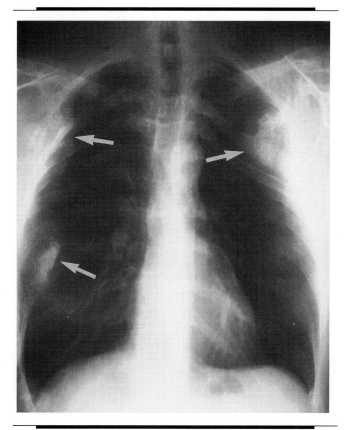

FIGURE 8-7 Multiple exostosis. Chest radiograph showing multiple exophytic bone lesions arising from the ribs and scapula in a young man with hereditary multiple exostosis.

- **Enchondromas** are benign bone lesions which are typically well-defined, expansile, and lobulated and contain diffuse or stippled calcification.

- **Aneurysmal bone cysts** appear as expansile lytic lesions sharply demarcated by a thin shell of periosteum. Most are seen in patients younger than 20 years old.

- **Hemangiomas**, benign lesions, have internal trabeculations and an intact cortical margin.

- **Hematopoietic disorders**, including thalassemia, hereditary spherocytosis, and myelosclerosis, can produce hypertrophy of the medullary cavity of the ribs, resulting in bone expansion. **Extramedullary hematopoiesis** can result in a paraspinal mass.

- **Eosinophilic granuloma** is a benign destructive bone lesion of unknown etiology that frequently involves the ribs and sternum, although the skull is the most common site. It typically appears as a lytic defect with well-defined margins and cortical scalloping. Pulmonary involvement, manifest as upper lobe nodules and cysts, is uncommon.

- **Bone metastases** from lung, breast, prostate, thyroid, or renal carcinomas and multiple myeloma are the most common cause of destructive bone lesions in the adult chest. Skeletal metastases generally appear as areas of lytic destruction. Thyroid cancer, renal cell carcinoma, and myeloma

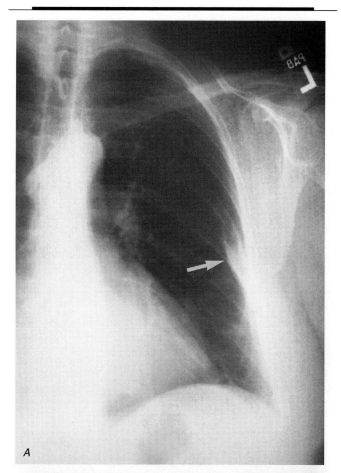

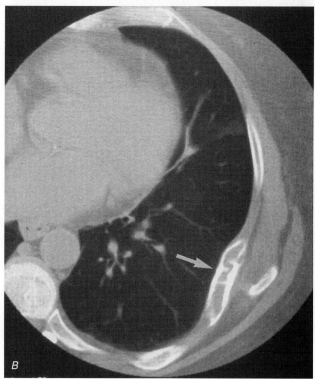

FIGURE 8-8 Fibrous dysplasia. (*A*) Chest radiograph and (*B*) CT showing an expansile lytic lesion involving the left posterolateral sixth rib (arrow). There is no cortical disruption or extraosseous soft tissue component. A biopsy confirmed the diagnosis.

often have an accompanying extraosseous soft tissue component (Fig. 8-9). Pathologic fractures are common (**Differential 92**). **Sclerotic metastases** can be observed with prostate and breast cancer and lymphoma (Fig. 8-10).

- **Primary malignant tumors**, such as a chondrosarcoma, osteosarcoma, plasmacytoma, lymphoma, or Ewing sarcoma, are much less common. Lymphoma, bronchogenic carcinoma, and breast carcinoma may invade bone directly.

- **Chondrosarcomas** often appear as large, lobulated masses with poorly defined margins and associated cortical bone destruction. They have a mottled pattern of internal calcification and an associated soft tissue mass and frequently involve an anterior rib near the costal cartilage junction.

- **Ewing sarcomas** exhibit variable lytic and blastic bone destruction and a soft tissue mass (Fig. 8-11). They are most common in children and young adults.

- **Diffuse sclerosis** may be due to widespread bone metastases, typically prostate cancer in men or breast cancer in women (Fig. 8-12). **Paget disease** can involve the thoracic spine, clavicles, or humerus. It is characterized by sclerosis, thickened trabeculae, and expansion of the involved bone.

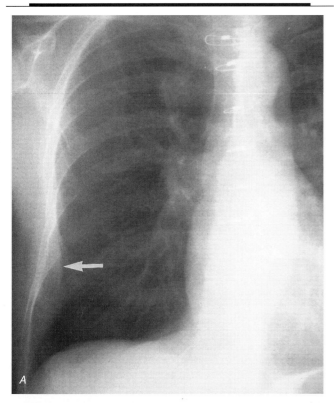

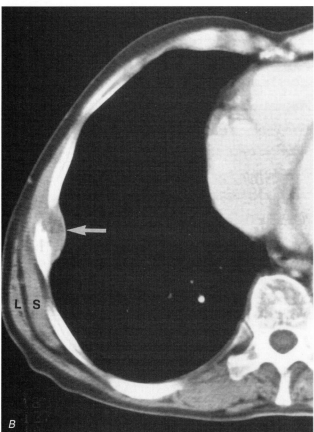

FIGURE 8-9   Rib metastasis. (*A*) Chest radiograph showing a pleural-based opacity (arrow). (*B*) CT demonstrating subtle rib destruction and an extraosteal, extrapleural soft tissue mass (arrow). Diagnosis: metastatic lung cancer. L, Latissimus dorsi; S, serratus anterior muscles.

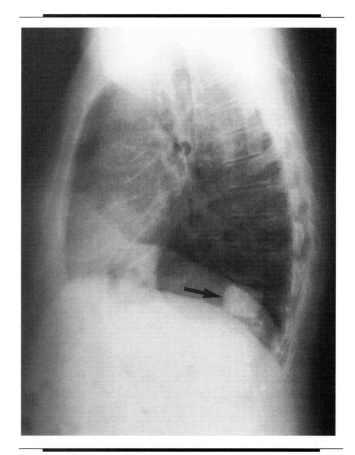

FIGURE 8-10   Metastatic prostate cancer. Lateral chest radiograph showing a sclerotic T12 vertebral body (arrow) in an 87-year-old man with prostate cancer.

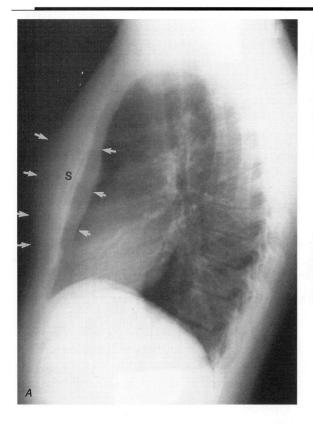

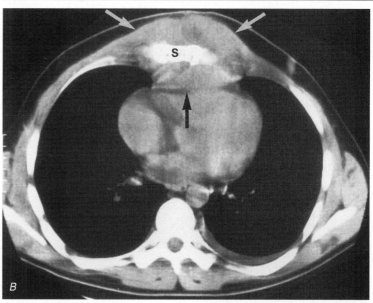

FIGURE 8-11   Ewing sarcoma. (*A*) Lateral chest radiograph and (*B*) CT showing a large soft tissue mass (arrows) arising from the sternum (S) in a 13-year-old boy.

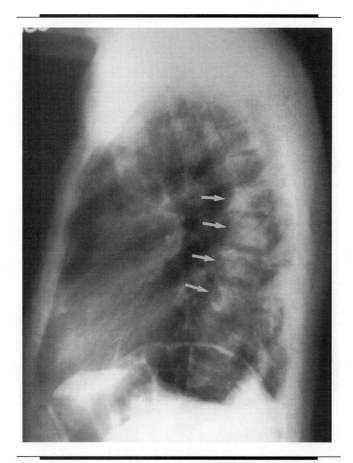

FIGURE 8-12   Bone metastases. Lateral chest radiograph showing diffuse irregular sclerosis of the thoracic vertebral bodies (arrows) representing metastatic prostate cancer.

8.4 SOFT TISSUE AND INFECTIONS

- The musculature of the chest wall provides respiratory and upper extremity movement. The external, internal, and innermost intercostal muscles insert between the ribs and the subcostal muscles from the angle of the rib to the internal surface of the next lower rib. The intercostal nerve, artery, and vein run in the costal groove between the internal and innermost muscle. The transverse thoracic muscle is sometimes seen behind the sternum on lateral chest radiographs. It connects the second through fifth costal cartilages with the lower sternum and lies deep to the internal thoracic vessels.

- The anterior axillary fold consists of the pectoralis major and minor muscles, and the posterior axillary fold consists of the subscapularis, latissimus dorsi, and teres major muscles. The serratus anterior lines the lateral chest wall. The long thoracic nerve and thoracodorsal and lateral thoracic vessels run lateral to this muscle.

- The superficial **back muscles** include the trapezius, latissimus dorsi, levator scapula, and rhomboids. The intermediate muscles include the inferior and superior serratus, and the deep erector spinae muscles include the ileocostalis, longissimus, multifidus, and spinalis.

- **Asymmetry** of the soft tissues can produce a differential density falsely attributed to pulmonary or pleural disease. Soft tissue abnormalities can produce either increased density (breast implants, soft tissue infection) or decreased density (mastectomy or Poland syndrome) (Fig. 8-13).

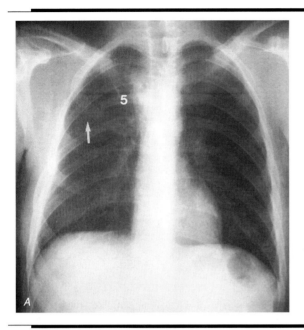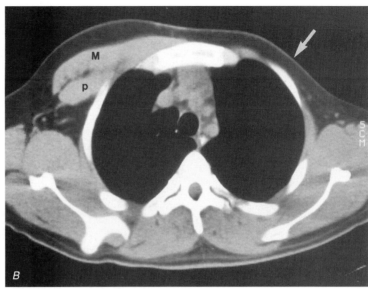

FIGURE 8-13   Poland syndrome. (*A*) Chest radiograph in a 19-year-old man demonstrating a relatively lucent left hemithorax. Note evidence of a prior right 5th rib thoracotomy (arrow) performed to resect a paratracheal mass shown to be histoplasmosis. (*B*) CT showing absence of the left pectoralis muscles (arrow). M, Pectoralis major; p, pectoralis minor muscles. (With permission from Slone RM, Gierada DS. Pleura, chest wall, and diaphragm. In Lee JKT, Sagel SS, Stanley RJ, Heiken JP, eds. *Computed Body Tomography with MRI Correlation.* 3rd ed. Philadelphia: Lippincott-Raven; 1998.)

- **Subcutaneous emphysema** is a common finding following thoracic surgery or chest tube placement. It appears as linear lucencies tracking between tissue planes (Fig. 7-6).

- Soft tissue **calcification** can be seen as a result of myositis ossificans, dermatomyositis, calcified lymph nodes, injection granulomas, and degenerating fibroadenomas in the breast.

- **Cellulitis, fasciitis, and abscesses** of the chest wall may occur as a result of surgery, trauma, or direct extension from osteomyelitis or pulmonary, pleural, or mediastinal infections (**Differential 88**). The risk is increased with age, diabetes, surgery, and trauma and in immunocompromised patients.

    Fungi such as *Blastomyces*, **bacteria** including *Staphylococcus* and *Klebsiella*, higher-order bacteria (*Nocardia, Actinomyces*), and **mycobacteria** are common organisms. Skin fistulae, air-fluid levels, or an associated empyema are clues to the presence of a chest wall infection. An adjacent pulmonary process or rib destruction is often seen.

    With *actinomycosis*, swelling, draining sinus tracts and fistulas, periosteal reaction, and bone destruction are common (Fig. 8-14). Individuals with poor dental hygiene and immune suppression are predisposed to this condition. Surgical debridement is typically required.

    Infected pleural fluid may extend directly through the thoracic wall and appear as a subcutaneous mass. Such an *empyema necessitatis* is most commonly secondary to tuberculosis but also may occur as a consequence of actinomycosis or blastomyocosis or following thoracentesis of a pyogenic empyema.

The extent and severity of chest wall infections are difficult to assess by physical examination or radiography alone. **CT** and **MR** are both useful in assessing their presence and extent. They often appear as an ill-defined infiltrating mass sometimes indistinguishable from a neoplastic process. Fluid collections should be readily apparent.

CT cannot only demonstrate contiguity of the subcutaneous abscess with a pleural space collection but also can show areas of lung destruction beneath the pleural disease that are obscured on conventional radiographs. Hypervascularity of an abscess wall can be seen on images obtained following IV contrast administration.

8.5 SOFT TISSUE TUMORS

- Both **CT and MR** can identify the presence and extent of soft tissue infiltration and assess bone involvement by chest wall tumors. Neither size nor sharpness of the border is a reliable diagnostic criterion of malignancy. Rapid growth, invasion of adjacent structures, and ancillary findings such as pulmonary metastases suggest malignancy (**Differential 89**).

    Masses with inhomogeneous density or signal intensity and irregular, infiltrative margins are suspicious for a malignancy, but chest wall infection, hematoma, and a desmoid tumor may have similar findings. Benign tumors are more likely to appear homogeneous, have smooth margins, and have a capsule or pedicle, but malignant neoplasms may have some of these features. Biopsy is usually required for diagnosis.

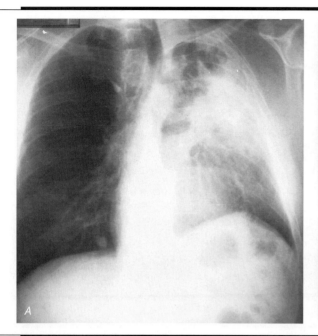
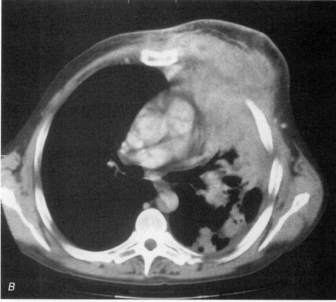

FIGURE 8-14   Pulmonary actinomycosis with chest wall involvement. (*A*) Chest radiograph in a 37-year-old man complaining of left chest swelling for 3 weeks. (*B*) CT confirms masslike pulmonary consolidation with contiguous chest wall involvement. (Figure courtesy of J. Root, M.D. with permission from Slone RM, Gierada DS.: Pleura, chest wall, and diaphragm. In Lee JKT, Sagel SS, Stanley RJ, Heiken JP, eds. *Computed Body Tomography with MRI Correlation.* 3rd ed. Philadelphia: Lippincott-Raven; 1998.)

- **Primary soft tissue tumors** are typically of mesenchymal origin, arising from fat, fibrous, vascular, neural, muscular, or dermal tissues and include basal and squamous cell carcinoma, hemangiomas, lipomas, fibromas, desmoid tumors, lymphomas, MFH, and sarcomas. **Metastatic cancer**, especially melanoma, can involve the soft tissues of the chest wall.

- A **lipoma** is the most common soft tissue tumor involving the chest wall (Fig. 8-15). It may be subcutaneous, intramuscular, or extrapleural, in which case it can displace pleura and mimic a pleural or pulmonary mass (Fig. 1-15). A transmural lipoma can widen an intercostal space and produce pressure erosion on adjacent ribs.

  These tumors usually have sharp margins, little architecture except for a thin capsule or septations, and occasionally small calcifications. They are easily diagnosed on CT or MR by their characteristic fat content. They have no malignant potential but may be resected for cosmetic reasons.

- **Neurogenic tumors**, including schwannomas, neurofibromas, neuroblastomas, and sarcomas (Fig. 8-16), can arise from the intercostal nerves. Plexiform neurofibromas in patients with neurofibromatosis may infiltrate the chest wall.

These tumors often have a low attenuation on CT because of abundant lipid content, a myxoid matrix, hypocellularity, and regions of cystic degeneration. Malignant degeneration may occur in patients with neurofibromatosis.

- **Hemangiomas** are benign vascular tumors found in the skin, soft tissues, and bones of the chest wall. They contain tortuous

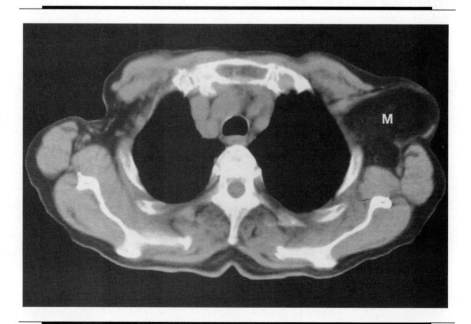

FIGURE 8-15   Lipoma. CT in an 85-year-old woman showing a fat attenuation mass in the left axilla (M). The mass displaces adjacent structures and has no significant stromal components or septations. The appearance is characteristic of a benign lipoma.

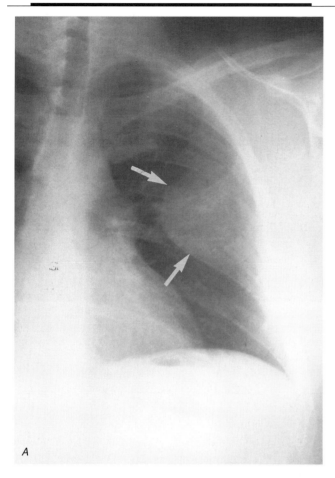

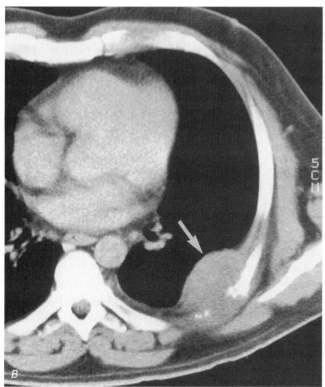

FIGURE 8-16 Chest wall sarcoma. (*A*) Chest radiograph and (*B*) CT showing a soft tissue mass with rib destruction arising from an intercostal nerve (arrows).

vessels, which are enhanced following contrast administration, possibly containing phleboliths. MR can clearly demonstrate their extent when flow-sensitive sequences are used.

- **Localized lymphangioma** is a cystic mass of sequestered ectatic lymphatic tissue that may be confused with a hemangioma. They are usually observed in the neck but may extend into the mediastinum, chest wall, or axilla. MR can define the extent of infiltration of adjacent tissues. Internal septations are frequent. Recurrence following incomplete excision is common.

- **Arteriovenous malformations** are seen as tubular structures exhibiting signal voids from flowing blood on T1-weighted spin-echo images, and high signal intensity from flowing blood on gradient-echo images.

- Other benign lesions commonly encountered include fibromas and sebaceous cysts, which are typically subcutaneous. Pedunculated moles and neurofibromas can simulate pulmonary nodules on chest radiographs.

- **Desmoid tumors** are a benign form of fibromatosis or a low-grade fibrosarcoma. Almost half occur in the chest wall or shoulder. They lack a capsule, infiltrate extensively into surrounding tissue, and recur when inadequately excised. An association is seen with Gardner syndrome and pregnancy.

- **Malignant fibrous histiocytoma (MFH)** is one of the more common primary soft tissue tumors seen in older adults. It typically appears as a lobulated soft tissue mass.

- **Lymphoma** may involve the chest wall by extension from adjacent lymph nodes, breast or rib involvement in non-Hodgkin disease, or the thymus in Hodgkin lymphoma. Invasion can impact therapy by altering the radiation ports chosen. MR is more sensitive than CT for detecting chest wall involvement by lymphoma.

- **Liposarcomas** are typically nonhomogeneous, contain soft tissue components in addition to fat, and are generally large and infiltrating. They are usually distinguished confidently from a benign lipoma, although a well-differentiated liposarcoma might appear similar.

- Other sarcomas affecting the soft tissues of the thorax include ***rhabdomyosarcoma, leiomyosarcoma***, and ***neurofibrosarcoma***.

8.6 AXILLA, SUPRACLAVICULAR FOSSA, AND BRACHIAL PLEXUS

- The **supraclavicular fossa** or "subclavian triangle" represents the thoracic outlet or root of the neck. It contains the scalene muscles, subclavian vessels, and supraclavicular lymph nodes. Supraclavicular nodes are seldom seen and should never be more than 1 cm in diameter. They can be enlarged as a result of infection or tumor.

- **The axilla** contains the axillary artery and vein, branches of the brachial plexus, and lymph nodes. Axillary lymph nodes drain the arm, breast, and thoraco-abdominal wall. Nodes lateral to the pectoralis minor are designated level 1, those under the muscle as level 2, and those medial to it as level 3. Enlarged nodes due to lymphoma are often large, bulky, and homogeneous (Fig. 8-17). Central necrosis can be observed with melanoma, squamous cell cancer, and tuberculosis.

- The anterior scalene muscle separates the subclavian vein (anterior) from the subclavian artery. Lateral to the teres major muscle the axillary artery and vein become the basilic vein and brachial artery, and medial to the first rib they become the subclavian vessels.

- Primary tumors are rare in the axilla and supraclavicular fossa. They include lipoma, liposarcoma, MFH, rhabdomyosarcoma, and cystic hygroma which appear as smooth, sharply outlined water-density masses. More commonly, involvement is the result of local extension of lung, breast, or head and neck cancers.

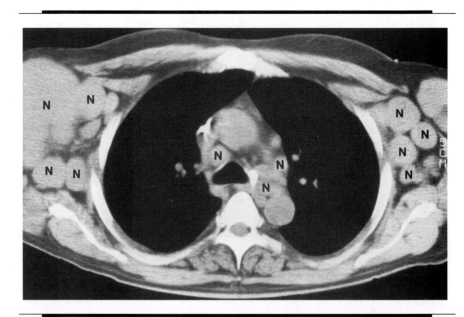

FIGURE 8-17   Adenopathy. CT in a 49-year-old man with chronic lymphocytic leukemia and lymphoma, demonstrating mediastinal and massive axillary adenopathy (N).

- The **brachial plexus** is formed by the nerve roots from C5 through T1. It passes between the anterior and middle scalene muscles. Laterally, it is enclosed by the axillary artery and vein in the axillary sheath.

    CT may detect enlarged axillary and supraclavicular lymph nodes not palpable on physical examination. It is important that the field of view include the axillary soft tissues and supraclavicular fossa in such patients. Helical CT, with sagittal and coronal reconstructions, can be used to image the brachial plexus and surrounding structures, including the subclavian artery and scalene muscles.

    MR is the modality of choice for evaluating the brachial plexus in patients with pain, neurologic deficit, or muscular atrophy and for assessing the extent of neoplasms such as superior sulcus tumors (Fig. 1-20). The plexus is well demonstrated on direct sagittal and coronal images. Axial images best depict the nerve roots near the spine.

    Schwannomas, neurofibromas, and neurofibrosarcomas may arise from the brachial plexus. Secondary neoplastic involvement can occur as a result of metastatic breast cancer or by direct extension of superior sulcus lung carcinoma, lymphoma, myeloma, or chest wall sarcoma.

    Trauma involving the proximal nerves may result in nerve root avulsion and formation of a pseudomeningocele. Injury to the more distal regions can cause hematoma, neural edema, or neural disruption with distortion and formation of a posttraumatic neuroma.

    Radiation fibrosis may involve the brachial plexus or axillary vessels and usually occurs within 2 years of treatment. It is often difficult to differentiate from tumor

recurrence, and a biopsy may be needed to corroborate or help exclude recurrence.

8.7 BREAST

- **Breast cancer** is the second leading cause of cancer death in women, occurring in approximately 10 percent. Survival is increased by early detection. The incidence in men is 1 percent of that of women. Chest radiography has no role in evaluating breast disease other than in identifying pulmonary metastases. Bone metastases may occasionally be detected.

- **Screen-film mammography** is the technique of choice for evaluating the breast and detecting breast carcinoma. Ultrasound can be used to determine if a mass is cystic or solid. Stereotactic needle biopsy or needle localization for surgical resection may be necessary to determine the diagnosis of suspicious lesions.

- **CT** is very helpful in staging breast cancer, particularly if chest wall invasion or internal mammary adenopathy, liver, or adrenal metastasis is suspected. Internal thoracic adenopathy can occur without axillary lymph node involvement. An incidental breast mass may be discovered on a CT examination performed for other reasons, but the appearance is usually nonspecific and mammography or biopsy is usually required for further evaluation.

- **Mastitis**, inflammatory breast cancer, and postradiation effects can have the same CT appearance. Inflammatory breast cancer causes edema, skin thickening, lymphadenopathy, and often ipsilateral arm swelling (Fig. 8-18). Diagnosis is made by punch biopsy of the skin showing invasion of dermal lymphatics.

- **Radiation therapy** may produce skin thickening up to 1 cm, inflammatory changes, and increased attenuation in the residual breast tissue and subcutaneous fat. These changes typically occur in the first few months following therapy and may resolve on follow-up. They should be confined to the radiation port.

  Radiation ports used to treat the breast are tangential to the chest wall to minimize radiation to the lung, but it is common to observe pulmonary fibrosis in the peripheral lung adjacent to the chest wall. The fibrosis persists and may have a nodular appearance, simulating metastasis or lymphangitic spread.

- **Deformities and scarring** from surgery or radiation complicate the evaluation of postoperative examinations. There is an asymmetric absence of breast and fatty tissue and, depending on the type of surgery (lumpectomy, radical or modified mastectomy), adjacent muscles and lymph nodes. In addition to increased lucency of the hemithorax, the orientation of the ipsilateral axillary fold is often more horizontal.

  Hematomas and seromas are common, and residual portions of muscle may remain at the sternal or costal attachment and should not be mistaken for recurrent tumor. The overlying skin following surgery should be less than 5 mm thick.

- **Breast reconstruction** has become an important component of breast cancer treatment, and superimposed surgical changes compound the postmastectomy appearance. The transverse rectus abdominis musculocutaneous (TRAM) flap technique is a common reconstruction technique involving transfer of fat, skin, and rectus abdominis muscle onto the chest wall.

- **Local recurrence** occurs in up to 30 percent of patients within 5 years, depending on the initial mode of treatment. Tumor may recur in the subcutaneous tissues, axilla, pectoral muscles, or internal mammary nodes and subsequently invade the chest wall, mediastinum, or sternum. CT and MR are valuable in documenting and assessing the extent of recurrent breast carcinoma.

- **Breast implants** are common. A unilateral implant may mimic a focal pulmonary process on radiographs, although the lateral view can confirm the chest wall location of the increased opacity. MR in conjunction with mammography is the procedure of choice for diagnosing breast implant rupture.

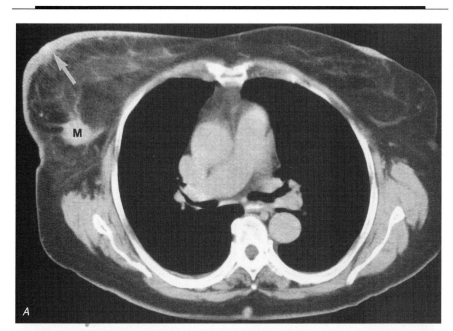

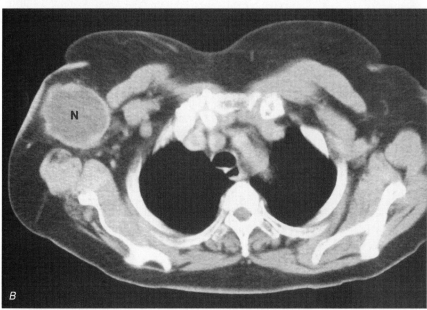

FIGURE 8-18 Inflammatory breast cancer. (*A*) CT in a 69-year-old woman showing a mass (M) and significant skin thickening around the nipple (arrow). (*B*) Higher image shows a large necrotic axillary lymph node (N). (With permission from Slone RM, Gierada DS. Pleura, chest wall, and diaphragm. In Lee JKT, Sagel SS, Stanley RJ, Heiken JP, eds. *Computed Body Tomography with MRI Correlation.* 3rd ed. Philadelphia: Lippincott-Raven; 1998.)

8.8 DIAPHRAGM

- **The diaphragm** is a thin, domed, musculotendinous structure separating the thorax from the abdomen and is the primary muscle of respiration. The right hemidiaphragm is typically 1 to 2 cm higher than the left hemidiaphragm.

The **muscular diaphragm** is composed of three groups: (1) the sternal portion of the diaphragm arising from the xyphoid process, (2) the costal slips from the ribs, and (3) the crura from the upper three lumbar vertebrae. All three converge on the **central tendon**. There are three major openings for the inferior vena cava (IVC), esophagus, aorta, and accompanying azygos, hemiazygos, and thoracic ducts.

The **lateral arcuate ligaments** are thickened bands of fascia overlying the quadratus lumborum muscles and are adjacent to the posterior pararenal space extending from the transverse process of L1 to the middle of the twelfth rib. A portion of the lumbar diaphragm is attached and can be mistaken for nodules or tumor implants.

- **Fluoroscopy** is useful in studying the movement of the diaphragm, particularly when paralysis is suspected. A *sniff test* refers to fluoroscopic observation of the diaphragm while the patient rapidly inhales through their nose. This maneuver accentuates abnormal movement of the diaphragm since it is almost an entirely diaphragm-dependent action. As intrathoracic pressure is reduced, a paralyzed hemidiaphragm is pulled up in contrast to the normal hemidiaphram which actively moves down. Paradoxical movement is diagnostic.

- Because of its thinness and its shape, the diaphragm is difficult to depict in its entirety on cross-sectional imaging studies; however, CT and MR examinations may be useful in assessing congenital or acquired defects in the structural integrity of the diaphragm. Peridiaphragmatic lesions also can be localized and characterized.

On **CT**, the crura, sternocostal attachments, and portions adjacent to abdominal fat are demonstrated. Segments in contact with the liver, spleen, or other upper abdominal viscera may be difficult to differentiate. Spiral CT with multiplanar reconstructions improves depiction of the normal and abnormal diaphragm.

The direct multiplanar imaging capability of **MR** is advantageous in assessing the diaphragm and peridiaphragmatic processes. Hernias and eventrations may be more readily recognized in coronal or sagittal planes. The feasibility of imaging normal diaphragmatic motion with fast gradient-echo MR has been demonstrated and may be useful for investigating functional diaphragmatic abnormalities.

- Disease in the chest, in the abdomen, or intrinsic to the diaphragm may alter its normal shape and position. **Bilateral elevation** is usually due to a poor inspiratory effort, obesity, or brain injury (**Differential 85**).

- **Unilateral elevation** of the hemidiaphragm can be seen as a consequence of abdominal organ enlargement (gastric distention, hepatomegaly, splenomegaly) or a unilateral decrease in lung size (lobar collapse, surgical resection), or hemidiaphragm paralysis. It can also be mimicked by the presence of a subpulmonic effusion (**Differential 84**).

- **Focal eventration** is a localized bulge in the diaphragm due to intrinsic thinning and weakness. It is most common in the anterior portion of the right hemidiaphragm. The exact etiology is unknown, but possibilities include congenital muscle deficiency or acquired focal diaphragmatic dysfunction secondary to ischemia, infarction, or neuromuscular disease.

- **Downward displacement** or flattening of the diaphragm can be seen in obstructive lung disease such as asthma, emphysema, and cystic fibrosis (**Differential 83**).

- **Free air** below the diaphragm is abnormal and can be observed as a result of bowel or stomach perforation, recent surgery, percutaneous feeding tube placement, paracentesis, or peritoneal dialysis (Fig. 13-1).

- **Anterior diaphragmatic lymph nodes** along the central portion of the diaphragm drain the diaphragm, anterior mediastinum, and anterosuperior liver. They reside posterior to the xiphoid and behind the seventh ribs and costal cartilages in the cardiophrenic angles. Up to two lymph nodes, less than 5 mm in diameter, normally may be visible on CT. Lymphadenopathy is often associated with lymphoma or lung, breast, or colon cancer. Lymphadenopathy at other locations or liver metastases are usually present.

- **Cardiophrenic angle masses** include pericardial fat and pericardial cysts differentiated by their characteristic CT attenuation values (Fig. 1-16). Morgagni hernias, anterior diaphragmatic adenopathy, portosystemic varices in patients with portal hypertension, and pleural and peripheral pulmonary processes (**Differential 110**).

- The **retrocrural space** contains the aorta, azygos vein, thoracic duct, nerves, and lymph nodes which drain the posterior mediastinum, diaphragm, and lumbar region. **Lymphadenopathy** is suggested when discrete soft tissue masses larger than 6 mm are present on CT and is often accompanied by upper abdominal para-aortic lymphadenopathy. Lymphoma is the most common malignant process.

Vascular masses, such as esophageal varices or aortic aneurysm, can also appear as retrocrural masses and are easily confirmed with CT. Extension of disease from the spine, such as malignancy, infection, or fracture with hematoma, can produce a retrocrural abnormality.

Azygos vein enlargement can occur with anomalous interruption, thrombosis, or obstruction of the IVC and should not be mistaken for retrocrural lymphadenopathy (**Differential 140**).

- Primary **tumors of the diaphragm** are rare. The appearance is generally nonspecific. Most are benign lipomas, neurofibromas, or mesothelial or teratoid cysts. Malignant fibrous or muscular sarcomas are extremely rare. Nodular infoldings of the lateral hemidiaphragms can mimic peritoneal tumor implants, and the attachment to the xiphoid or crura can mimic adenopathy or masses on CT.

- Small fat attenuation masses can be noted on CT within the diaphragmatic muscle, which are consistent with lipomas too small for clinical or radiographic detection. They may represent age-associated lipomas or small diaphragm defects.

8.9 HERNIAS

- Diaphragmatic hernias are common, occur in a variety of forms, and may be congenital or acquired.

- **Congenital** diaphragmatic hernias occur as a result of failure of closure of the pleuroperitoneal fold during the first trimester and have an incidence of roughly 1 in 2000 live births. They are much more common on the left side. Associated congenital anomalies are common. Communication between the abdomen and thorax may allow abdominal contents to enter the chest.

- **Bochdalek hernias** are the most common congenital diaphragmatic hernias. Located in the posterolateral diaphragm, they are the result of incomplete closure of the embryonic pleuroperitoneal membrane. The left-sided preponderance is thought to be due to earlier closure of the right pleuroperitoneal membrane and protection of right-sided defects by the liver.

  These hernias usually appear as a soft tissue mass bulging upward from the posterior aspect of a hemidiaphragm on the chest radiograph. The defect can usually be demonstrated on CT, and the contents defined without difficulty. Small defects may contain only retroperitoneal fat, and larger defects can contain the stomach, intestines, spleen, kidney, or liver.

  Similar-appearing and far more common **acquired focal diaphragmatic defects** or discontinuities, with or without herniated fat or viscera, can be seen in up to 5 percent of adults. Increasing incidence with age, weight gain, and emphysema suggests that the majority of posterior diaphragm defects are acquired and not true Bochdalek hernias.

- **Morgagni hernias**, which are anteromedial in location, are much less common than Bochdaleck hernias. They represent herniation through the sternocostal trigone due to failed fusion of the sternal and costal fibrotendinous elements of the diaphragm. Associated with obesity, they usually contain omental fat, are covered by both peritoneum and parietal pleura, and appear as an asymptomatic right cardiophrenic angle mass. The transverse colon is more frequently involved than the stomach, small bowel, or liver.

- **Hiatal hernias** representing herniation of the stomach through the esophageal hiatus, is a frequent finding in adults. The typical manifestation is that of an oval retrocardiac mass with an air-fluid level. This acquired abnormality is secondary to laxity and stretching of the phrenoesophageal ligament and widening of the esophageal hiatus. Obesity and increased intra-abdominal pressure are contributing factors.

  The majority (90 percent) can be reduced or are reversible and are called *sliding hiatal hernias*. Some are *paraesophageal*, in which case the stomach herniates up next to the distal esophagus.

Patients may be asymptomatic or have symptoms of gastroesophageal reflux. A very large hernia or "intrathoracic stomach" warrants elective surgical repair as it can become incarcerated or undergo volvulus. When marked ascites occurs in a patient with a hiatal hernia, fluid may extend into the lower posterior mediastinum, mimicking a mediastinal abscess, necrotic tumor, or foregut cyst.

- **Traumatic disruption of the diaphragm** can result from penetrating or blunt trauma and often goes undetected initially. It can enlarge over time and has a high risk of eventual incarceration and strangulation. Herniation most often occurs on the left side and involves the stomach but can involve the bowel, omentum, spleen, or liver. Radiographs may show an irregular diaphragm contour and bowel or abdominal organs above the diaphragm. CT may show discontinuity of the diaphragm, organs, or peritoneal fat above the diaphragm and focal constriction of the stomach or bowel at the site of herniation. (See Section 11.3 for more details.)

Bibliography

Brink JA, Heiken JP, Semenkovich J, Teefey SA, McClennan BL, Sagel SS. Abnormalities of the diaphragm and adjacent structures: Findings on multiplanar spiral CT scans. *Am. J. Roentgenol.* 1994;163:307–310.

Demos TC, Solomon C, Posniak HV, Flisak MJ. Computed tomography in traumatic defects of the diaphragm. *Clin. Imaging.* 1989;13:62.

Fortier M, Mayo JR, Swensen SJ, Munk PL, Vellet DA, Müller NL. MR imaging of chest wall lesions. *Radiographics.* 1994;14:597–606.

Fraser RG, Paré JAP, Paré PD, Fraser RS, Genereux GP. *Diagnosis of Diseases of the Chest.* Vol. 4, 3rd ed. Philadelphia: WB Saunders, 1991.

Gale ME. Bochdalek hernia: Prevalence and CT characteristics. *Radiology.* 1985;156:449–452.

Gierada DS, Curtin JJ, Erickson SJ, Probst RW, Strandt JA, Goodman LR. Fast gradient echo magnetic resonance imaging of the normal diaphragm. *J. Thorac. Imaging.* 1997;12:70–74.

Israel IS, Mayberry JC, Primack S. Diaphragmatic rupture: Use of helical CT scanning with multiplanar reformations. *Am. J. Roentgenol.* 1996; 167:1201–1203.

Jafri SZH, Roberts JL, Bree RL, Tabor HD. Computed tomography of chest wall masses. *Radiographics.* 1989;9:51.

Kuhlman JE, Bouchardy L, Fishman EK, Zerhount EA. CT and MR imaging evaluation of chest wall disorders. *Radiographics.* 1994;14:571–595.

Mirvis SE, Keramati B, Buckman R, Rodriguez A. MR imaging of traumatic diaphragmatic rupture. *J. Comput. Assist. Tomogr.* 1988;12:147–149.

Padovani B, Mouroux J, Seksik L, et al. Chest wall invasion by bronchogenic carcinoma: Evaluation with MR imaging. *Radiology.* 1993;187:33–38.

Panicek DM, Benson CB, Gottlieb RH, Heitzman ER. Diaphragm: Anatomic, pathologic and radiologic considerations. *Radiographics.* 1988;8:385.

Parienty RA, Marichez M, Pradel J, Parienty I, Demange P. Pararenal pseudotumors of the diaphragm: Computed tomographic features. *Gastrointest. Radiol.* 1987;12:131–133.

Posniak HV, Olson MC, Dudiak CM, Wisniewski R, O'Malley C. MR imaging of the brachial plexus. *Am. J. Roentgenol.* 1993;161:373–379.

Rapoport S, Blair DN, McCarthy SM, Desser TS, Hammers LW, Sostman HD. Brachial plexus: Correlation of MR imaging with CT and pathologic findings. *Radiology.* 1988;167:161–165.

Sharif HS, Clark DC, Aabed MY, Aideyan OA, Haddad MC, Mattson TA. MR imaging of thoracic and abdominal wall infections: Comparison with other imaging procedures. *Am. J. Roentgenol.* 1990;154:989–995.

Sherrier RH, Sostman HD. Magnetic resonance imaging of the brachial plexus. *J. Thorac. Imaging.* 1993;8:27–33.

Slone RM, Gierada DS. Pleura, chest wall, and diaphragm. In: Lee KT, Sagel SS, Stanley RJ, Heiken JP (eds.). *Computed Body Tomography with MR Correlation.* 3rd ed. Philadelphia: Lippincott-Raven; 1998.

Tarver RD, Conces DJJ, Cory DA, Vix VA. Imaging the diaphragm and its disorders. *J. Thorac. Imaging.* 1989;4(1):1–18.

Wechsler RJ. *Cross-sectional Analysis of the Chest and Abdominal Wall.* St. Louis: CV Mosby; 1989.

Worthy SA, Kang EY, Hartman TE, Kwong JS, Mayo JR, Müller NL. Diaphragmatic rupture: CT findings in 11 patients. *Radiology.* 1995;194: 885–888.

Chapter 9

CONGENITAL PULMONARY DISEASE AND PEDIATRICS

Matthew J. Fleishman

9.1   PEDIATRIC CHEST IMAGING

- Pathology in the pediatric thorax is distinct from adult chest disease. Although infection and inflammatory disease comprise the majority of abnormalities, the clinical appearance and radiographic manifestations often differ in children, as maturation of the tracheobronchial tree and lung parenchyma are ongoing through the age of 8.

- The normally prominent thymus and developing thoracic skeleton require recognition of an evolving standard of normalcy. Congenital and developmental abnormalities are more frequently encountered, whereas primary neoplasms, metastatic disease, and acquired conditions such as coronary artery disease and emphysema are unusual. The inability of small children to cooperate with examinations creates technical challenges in both plain film and cross-sectional imaging.

- Given the small thoracic diameter in the neonate and young child, there is no significant magnification difference between anteroposterior (AP) and posteroanterior (PA) radiographs. Accordingly, supine AP radiographs are generally obtained in children up to 4 years old. Immobilization is usually required. Well-collimated AP and lateral chest radiographs result in a gonadal dose of about 1 mrem.

- **Fluoroscopy** is often useful in the evaluation of possible foreign body airway obstruction, particularly in very young children where paired inspiratory and expiratory radiographs may be difficult to obtain. Changes in lung volume, excursion of the hemidiaphragms, and movement of the mediastinum may be observed.

- **Computed tomography (CT)** of the thorax is performed as in adults, and 5-mm collimation is typically used in small children. Low osmolar (nonionic) intravenous (IV) contrast is preferred, if needed, as it is better tolerated with a lower incidence of nausea and vomiting, less sensation at the injection site, and a lower risk of tissue necrosis in the event of extravasation. A rough guide to contrast volume is 2 ml/kg or 1 ml/lb of body weight. CT of the entire thorax results in a skin dose of about 2 rem.

- **Magnetic resonance imaging (MR)** examinations are useful in the evaluation of congenital heart disease, bronchopulmonary foregut malformations, and occasionally for tumor staging, such as for neuroblastoma. CT and MR examinations in children 6 months to 4 years old generally require closely monitored sedation.

- **Radionuclide scintigraphy** can be used to evaluate cardiac shunts, congenital anomalies of the pulmonary arteries, and pulmonary embolism.

9.2   AIRWAY DISORDERS

- **Airway disorders** are common in children and include asthma, aspiration injuries, congenital lesions, and acquired conditions.

- **Asthma** may be defined as a disorder of airway hypersensitivity producing reversible bronchoconstriction, precipitated by an abnormal response to a wide range of stimuli. The immediate hypersensitivity response is IgE-mediated, resulting in the release of histamines, leukotrienes, and prostaglandins. The agents responsible for smooth muscle contraction and inflammatory response are within airways. Asthma is the cause of more missed school days and health provider visits than any other childhood disease. Affected children are typically symptomatic by the age of 5.

Chest radiographs in acute asthma are often normal, and obtaining radiographs in uncomplicated asthma is of questionable value. Positive findings primarily relate to air trapping: hyperinflation, flattening of the diaphragm, and widening of the retrosternal clear space. Perihilar infiltrates and peribronchial thickening may be seen. Bacterial pneumonias and mycoplasma infection occur with greater frequency and may precipitate acute exacerbation. Atelectasis may result from mucous plugging. Pneumomediastinum and pneumothorax may be observed in young children.

- **Choanal atresia** is the most common congenital anomaly of the upper airway. The lesion is an obstruction of the posterior nasal airways; it is most commonly bilateral and usually osseous in nature, although it is composed of membranous soft tissue in 10 percent of cases. As infants are obligate nose breathers, inadequate communication between the nose and pharynx results in severe respiratory distress. Symptoms include poor sucking and swallowing, cyanosis, and apnea during feeding. The diagnosis is suggested by the inability to pass a catheter through the nose into the pharynx. CT can confirm and characterize the obstruction. Associations include craniofacial anomalies, esophageal atresia, congenital heart disease, and ocular defects. Treatment is surgical.

- **Croup** or **acute laryngotracheobronchitis** is an acute viral syndrome of the subglottic airway, producing inspiratory stridor, low-grade fever, and a characteristic "barking" cough. The primary causative agents are parainfluenza virus, respiratory syncytial virus, adenovirus, and influenza types A and B. Peak incidence is in children 6 months to 3 years old. AP and lateral airway radiographs reveal hypopharyngeal distention, a normal epiglottis and aryepiglottic folds, and symmetric "steeple" or "funnel-shaped" narrowing of the subglottic region beginning 1 to 2 cm below the piriform sinuses. The disorder is self-limited, and treatment is supportive.

- **Acute epiglottitis** is a true respiratory emergency, most commonly caused by infection with *Haemophilus influenzae* type B. *Streptococcus* and *Staphylococcus* species are additional causative agents. The peak incidence is in children 3 to 6 years old, but the disease also affects adults and immunocompromised patients. Symptoms include fever, dysphagia, and respiratory distress with a protruding tongue and drooling. Children often assume a "bolt upright" stance with the head thrust forward.

   Lateral soft tissue airway radiographs are specific, revealing thickening of the epiglottis and aryepiglottic folds, obliteration of the vallecula, and distention of the hypopharynx. Although acute epiglottitis predominantly involves the supraglottic portions of the airway, the frontal view may demonstrate subglottic edema indistinguishable from the typical appearance of croup. Angioneurotic edema and retropharyngeal hematoma can have a similar appearance. Radiographs should be obtained in the upright position, and the child should be accompanied by personnel skilled in emergent airway management, as intubation is sometimes required. Treatment is supportive, with airway management and antibiotics.

- **Laryngomalacia** is a common self-limited disorder of inspiratory stridor occurring in the first year of life, resulting from hypermobility and collapse of the upper airway. The condition abates as the attachments of the arytenoid tissues strengthen with age. The diagnosis is established by direct observation of the laryngeal soft tissues during respiration. On lateral airway fluoroscopy and radiography, the supraglottic larynx collapses on inspiration, with anterior bending of the aryepiglottic folds and posterior bending of the epiglottis.

- **Tracheomalacia** is a softening of the upper airway, resulting in buckling and collapse of the trachea and producing stridor which may occur on both inspiration and expiration. Wheezing, cough, and dyspnea are common. Intrinsic weakness of the tracheal cartilage may be idiopathic or related to prematurity, chondromalacia, polychondritis, or congenital absence or hypoplasia of one or more cartilaginous rings. Extrinsic causes of tracheomalacia include vascular rings, mediastinal tumors, tracheoesophageal fistulae, and foreign bodies. Fluoroscopically, tracheal collapse is observed on expiration. Symptoms improve with growth and maturation of the trachea, but reconstructive surgery, stenting, and tracheotomy may be required.

- In **bronchial atresia**, a normal bronchus ends blindly within the lung parenchyma. Lung distal to the atretic bronchus is initially fluid-filled but is eventually aerated via the pores of Kohn, resulting in a focal area of emphysema. The lesion may be discovered incidentally when a small area of isolated emphysema is detected on CT. The airway proximal to the stenosis fills with secretions, creating a **mucocele** often seen as a smooth branching opacity on chest radiographs (Fig. 9-1). The left upper lobe is the most common location. Surgical resection is necessary in the case of recurrent infections.

- **Primary tracheal stenosis** is a generally lethal congenital disorder in which there are one or more complete, rather than the normally incomplete, horseshoe-shaped rings of tracheal cartilage. Affected infants are cyanotic at birth, and intubation beyond the vocal cords is not possible. Esophageal atresia and a distal tracheoesophageal fistula may be associated. The trachea is markedly narrowed on both the frontal and lateral radiographs, and the diagnosis is confirmed by bronchoscopy.

- Congenital **bronchial stenosis** is uncommon. Acquired bronchial stenosis occurs most often in the right main bronchus from granulation tissue formed in response to frequent suctioning in the intubated infant. Postobstructive infection and emphysema may result and are often the presenting features on chest radiographs. Repeated bronchial dilatation or surgical reconstruction may be required to preserve lung function.

- **Tracheobronchomegaly** or **Mounier-Kuhn syndrome** is abnormal enlargement of the trachea and major bronchi. It is probably congenital in origin and related to atrophy or dysplasia of the supporting structures of the major airways. It can be associated with Ehlers-Danlos. Manifestations typically occur in adulthood, with progressive exertional

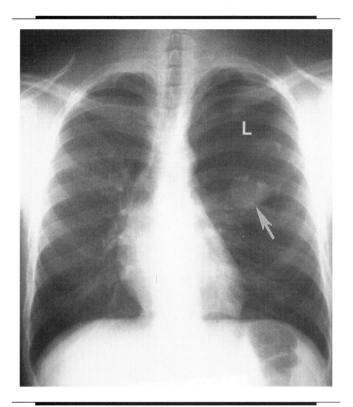

FIGURE 9-1 Bronchial atresia and regional hyperinflation. Chest radiograph in an asymptomatic 17-year-old showing a lucent left upper lung (L) with diminished vascular markings and a central opacity representing a bronchocele (arrow) in the blind-ending apicoposterior bronchus. Hyperinflation is due to collateral ventilation and air trapping.

dyspnea, difficulty in expectoration of copious secretions, and recurrent pneumonias, resulting in secondary bronchiectasis. The redundant membranous portions of the airways may produce obstruction on inspiration.

- **Congenital bronchiectasis** or **Williams-Campbell syndrome** is a rare disorder of bronchial wall cartilage, probably autosomal recessive, which produces bronchiectasis in the midlung and lower lung. Unlike immotile cilia syndrome, there is no association with sinus disease, otitis, or abnormal situs.

- **Angioneurotic edema** is an autosomal dominant deficiency of C1-esterase inhibitor resulting in increased vascular permeability and edema involving the airway, gastrointestinal (GI) tract, and extremities. Airway compromise is most common in children, producing stridor which may be life-threatening.

- In **tracheal bronchus**, a small segment of lung is aerated via a bronchus arising directly from the trachea. The pulmonary arterial and venous supplies are normal. Stenosis of the tracheal bronchus may result in recurrent pneumonia with bronchiectasis. If the condition is symptomatic, surgical resection of the tracheal bronchus and the involved pulmonary segment is performed. **Tracheal diverticulum** is a

blind-ending tracheal airway serving no lung parenchyma. Accessory cardiac bronchus is a rare congenital variant. Hemoptysis is a common clinical complication.

9.3 PEDIATRIC AIRWAY MASSES

- **Foreign bodies** may lodge in the esophagus or airways, producing cough and wheezing. Children younger than 3 years old are typically involved, and a high index of suspicion is required for unwitnessed aspiration events. Hyperinflation of the obstructed lung or segment may be observed, caused by a "check valve" mechanism in which air may pass by the obstruction on inspiration but is trapped by collapse of the airway around the foreign body during expiration.

  The relative hyperinflation is often more obvious on expiratory or decubitus radiographs or on fluoroscopic observation. The heart and mediastinum shift *away* from the affected side on expiration. In unrecognized cases, recurrent postobstructive pneumonia and bronchiectasis may develop. Postobstructive atelectasis or collapse is more common in older children and adults.

  Coins are commonly ingested or aspirated foreign bodies. The distinction between an esophageal and a tracheal location can usually be inferred from their orientation on frontal radiographs. Coins within the trachea are usually seen "on-edge," aligning with the flexible soft tissue portion of the posterior trachea, whereas coins in the esophagus are seen *en face* on the frontal film (Fig. 9-2).

- **Neoplasms** of the pediatric airways are rare, with benign lesions much more common than malignancy.

- **Juvenile neuroangiofibroma** is a benign vascular mass of the nasopharynx which may be locally invasive, occurring almost exclusively in adolescent boys. The appearance is that of recurrent epistaxis. The lesion arises within and widens the pterygopalatine fossa and may extend into the nasal cavity via the sphenopalatine foramen, into the orbit via the inferior orbital fissure, or into the middle cranial fossa via the pterygomaxillary fissure. The mass usually deforms the posterior maxillary wall.

  The lesion is supplied by branches of the ascending pharyngeal and internal maxillary arteries, demonstrating intense enhancement on CT and MR. A characteristic "salt-and-pepper" appearance is noted on MR, with punctate low-signal areas representing flow void within vessels. Tumor extent is best evaluated with postcontrast fat saturation MR. Preoperative embolization is often performed. Biopsy is strictly contraindicated.

- **Laryngocele** is an air- or fluid-filled cavity arising from the saccule of the laryngeal ventricle and extending into the lateral soft tissues. It may be confined by the thyrohyoid membrane (internal laryngocele) or protrude through it (external laryngocele). Best seen with CT and MR, the lesion appears as a cystic anterior neck mass arising at the level of the laryngeal ventricle. External laryngoceles protrude just below the angle of the mandible. Symptoms include stridor.

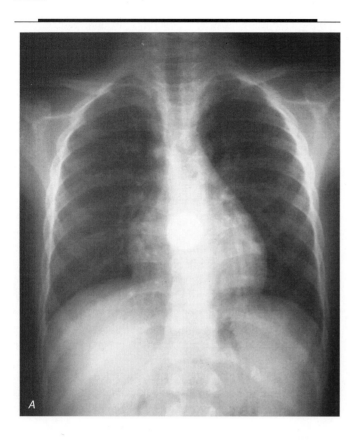

Uncommonly, the lesion may become infected and is then called a **pyolaryngocele**.

- **Laryngotracheal papillomatosis** is due to infection with human papillomavirus, probably acquired during passage through the birth canal. The lesions begin at and are most common around the larynx but may spread into the tracheobronchial tree, "dropping" from the more superior lesions. Cavitation is common. The papillomas may enlarge to significantly narrow or obliterate the airways. In small airways, they may produce obstruction. Treatment involves steroids and laser excision, but recurrence is common.

- **Neurofibromas** and **fibromas** are benign mesenchymal tumors usually occurring in the supraglottic region around the arytenoids and aryepiglottic folds. Typically submucosal in location, they appear as smooth masses on airway radiographs and demonstrate enhancement on CT and MR.

- Subglottic **hemangioma** is a benign hamartomatous neoplasm occurring in children 1 to 2 years old. Cutaneous hemangiomas are present in one-half of cases. Symptoms

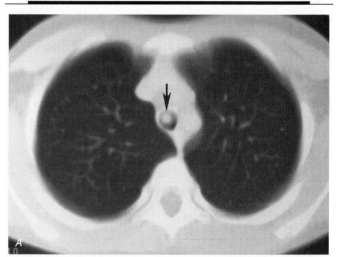

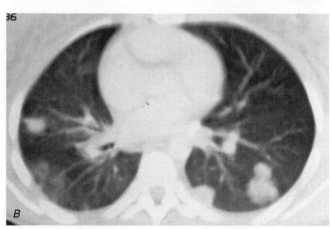

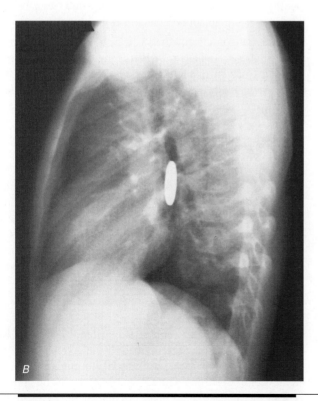

FIGURE 9-2   Coin in esophagus. (*A*) AP and (*B*) lateral chest radiograph showing the coin within the mediastinum. Coins in the trachea tend to orient edge-on in the frontal projection because of the soft posterior wall of the trachea.

FIGURE 9-3   Mucoepidermoid carcinoma of trachea. (*A*) CT showing the soft tissue mass (arrow) within the tracheal lumen. (*B*) Lower image revealing multiple parenchymal masses representing "drop metastases."

include hoarseness, cough, dysphagia, and wheezing. An asymmetric, eccentric, smooth, enhancing mass is seen on CT and MR, producing subglottic narrowing. These neoplasms typically regress by 18 months of age, but when symptomatic may be treated with steroids or laser excision. Surgical excision is rarely required.

- Tracheal **lymphangioma** or **cystic hygroma** is a benign lymphatic malformation which may occur around the larynx. Symptoms are similar to those of a subglottic hemangioma. Spontaneous regression is uncommon, and laser excision is often employed.

- **Hematomas** of the airway may produce significant obstruction and occur with anticoagulation and hemophilia.

- **Malignant neoplasms** of the pediatric airway are exceedingly uncommon. Bronchial carcinoids, salivary-type mucoepidermoid carcinoma (Fig. 9-3), and adenoid cystic carcinoma are rarely observed. Leiomyosarcoma, fibrosarcoma, and rhabdomyosarcoma of the airways have been described.

- **Calcification** of the tracheobronchial tree can be seen in children and adults on long-term anticoagulation therapy.

9.4 DEVELOPMENTAL THORACIC ANOMALIES

- In **pulmonary agenesis**, there is complete absence of the lung. The pulmonary artery and lung bud are absent. Newborns may be asymptomatic or suffer respiratory distress with cyanosis. The size of the chest remains normal, with the heart and mediastinum shifted toward the agenetic side (Fig. 9-4). Half of patients have congenital heart disease such as tetralogy of Fallot. There is often associated airway obstruction and poor handling of secretions.

- In **pulmonary aplasia**, the pulmonary artery and lung parenchyma are absent, but a blind-ending bronchial stump persists which may be a source of recurrent infection of the contralateral lung.

- **Pulmonary hypoplasia** may be associated with partial anomalous pulmonary venous return, termed the **pulmonary venolobar** or **scimitar syndrome**. There is hypoplasia of part or all of the right lung, with a small right pulmonary artery and partial pulmonary venous drainage below the diaphragm to the inferior vena cava (IVC) or to the hepatic or portal veins (Fig. 9-5). Associated cardiac anomalies include atrial septal defects (ASDs), tetralogy of Fallot, and truncus arteriosus.

  Radiographic findings include a small right chest and hilum, a rightward mediastinal shift with pleural angle blunting, and a scimitar vein in the right lower chest (seen on frontal radiographs in only one-third of cases). Pulmonary agenesis, aplasia, and unilateral hypoplasia most commonly involve the right lung.

- **Bilateral pulmonary hypoplasia** is incompatible with life. The cause may be idiopathic or secondary to conditions of oligohydramnios, such as bilateral renal agenesis (Potter

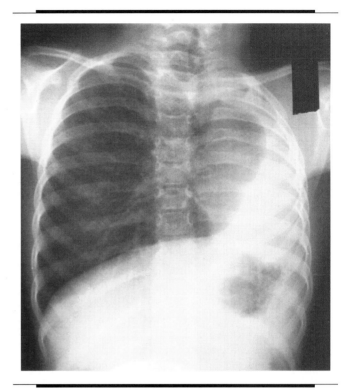

FIGURE 9-4 Pulmonary agenesis, left lung. Absent left lung with ipsilateral shift of the mediastinum and compensatory hyperinflation of the right lung.

syndrome) and amniotic fluid leak. Fetal exposure to normal volumes of amniotic fluid is required for lung development in utero. Severe chest wall abnormalities, including bone

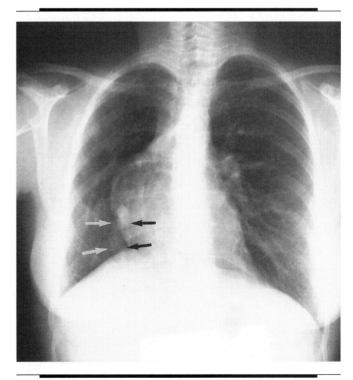

FIGURE 9-5 Scimitar syndrome. Chest radiograph showing a small right lung, ipsilateral mediastinal shift, and abherant pulmonary vein (arrows).

dysplasias and neuromuscular disorders, also may result in bilateral pulmonary hypoplasia.

Unilateral pulmonary hypoplasia is most commonly caused by a **congenital diaphragmatic hernia**, usually affecting the left hemidiaphragm and primarily the left lung. Herniation of abdominal contents into the hemithorax occurs because of failed closure of the pleuroperitoneal canal, preventing development of the ipsilateral lung. Shift of the mediastinum can also result in hypoplasia of the contralateral lung (Fig. 9.6). Elevated pulmonary vascular resistance and persistent fetal circulation following delivery are additional consequences. Infants are seen to have severe respiratory distress in the early days of life. The abdomen is often scaphoid. Bowel loops may be seen within the chest, and a nasogastric tube may appear within an intrathoracic stomach.

Associated anomalies include malrotation, neural tube defects, cardiac and genitourinary (GU) malformations, and intrauterine growth retardation. Treatment includes high-frequency ventilation with 100 percent oxygen, surfactant therapy, and sometimes extracorporeal membrane oxygenation (ECMO) aimed at stabilizing respiratory function and advancing lung maturity *prior to* surgical correction of the diaphragmatic defect. Despite therapeutic advances, about one-half of patients die. If recognized by prenatal ultrasound, in utero surgical repair of the diaphragmatic hernia can be attempted.

Acquired pulmonary hypoplasia may occur as a result of postviral bronchiolitis obliterans (**Swyer-James** or **MacLeod**

syndrome) or from necrotizing bronchiolitis following inhalational injuries, radiation therapy, or massive thromboembolism and infarction. The radiographic appearance is of a hyperlucent, small to normal-sized lung and hemithorax, with a small hilum and attenuated pulmonary vascularity. Cylindrical bronchiectasis and early termination of the bronchial tree are observed. On ventilation-perfusion scanning, extensive,

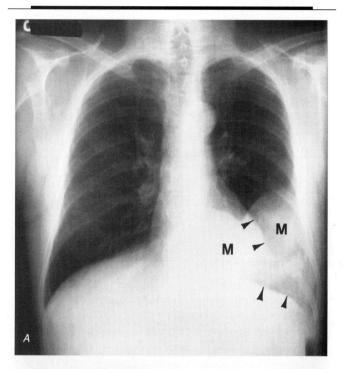

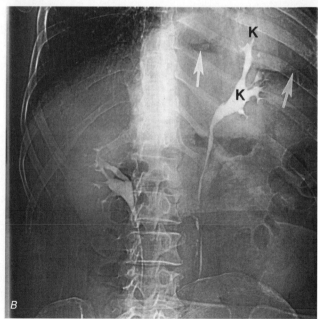

FIGURE 9-7   Bochdalek hernia. (*A*) Chest radiograph showing a smooth, lobulated mass (M). Preservation of the diaphragm and cardiac interface with the lung (arrowheads) confirms a posterior location. (*B*) Abdominal film from an intravenous urogram showing herniation of the left kidney (K) above the hemidiaphragm (arrows) into the left hemithorax.

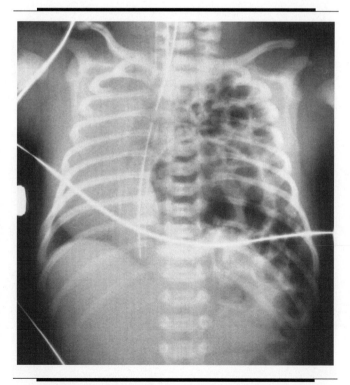

FIGURE 9-6   Congenital diaphragmatic hernia. The left hemithorax is filled with cystic lucencies representing herniated bowel. Also note contralateral mediastinal shift evidenced by a displaced nasogastric tube and diminished size of the right lung.

patchy, matched defects are seen, with air trapping on delayed ventilation images. Usually affecting an entire lung, the process may be limited to a lobe or segment, simulating the appearance of congenital lobar emphysema.

- **Bochdalek hernia** is the most common form of diaphragmatic hernia, representing a communication between the abdomen and thorax via the pleuroperitoneal canal. The defect is located posterolaterally and is most often left-sided (85 percent of cases). Herniated contents include bowel, spleen, kidney, and omental fat (Fig. 9-7). The radiographic findings relate to the volume and composition of the abdominal contents displaced into the thorax and range from a fatty posterior thoracic mass to an opacified hemithorax containing bowel.

- **Morgagni hernia** is considerably less common than Bochdalek hernia (<5 percent of diaphragm hernias). It usually occurs on the right side through an anterior defect in the sternocostal trigone or foramen of Larrey. The heart is thought to "protect" the occurrence of left-sided defects and hernias. The hernia generally contains a small portion of liver or omentum and occasionally bowel, typically colon.

  The radiographic appearance is that of a retrosternal mass which may be solid or of mixed solid and cystic composition when bowel is present. Contrast GI studies can confirm the presence of bowel in the hernia. Fat and liver herniation are readily identified on CT (Fig. 5-18).

- **Congenital lobar emphysema** is the isolated and progressive hyperinflation of one or more pulmonary lobes. The left upper lobe is most often affected (40 percent of cases), followed by the middle (30 percent), right upper (20 percent), and lower lobes (10 percent). Two lobes are involved in 5 percent of cases. The etiology is uncertain but is probably related to dysplasia, hypoplasia, or immaturity of bronchial cartilage in the involved lobes, endobronchial obstruction by webs, or extrinsic bronchial compression. Symptoms of tachypnea, wheezing, and infection occur in infancy, typically appearing by the age of 6 months. Boys are affected three times more often than girls.

  Immediate postnatal radiographs demonstrate a focal opacity in the involved lobe representing retained fluid. Follow-up radiographs show clearing of fluid and developing hyperlucency, progressing to lobar hyperinflation with compression of adjacent lung and contralateral mediastinal shift (Fig. 9-8). Associated cardiac lesions include ventricular septal defect (VSD) and patent ductus arteriosus (PDA). Occasionally, the entity goes unrecognized in childhood and lobar emphysema is first detected incidentally on radiographs obtained for other reasons. Surgical resection is usually undertaken to alleviate respiratory distress caused by compression of remaining normal lung tissue.

- **Pulmonary sequestration** is an abnormal congenital mass of lung lacking a normal communication with the tracheobronchial tree and pulmonary arterial system. The etiology is likely related to a lung bud that became isolated from the bronchopulmonary foregut. The arterial supply is via

a systemic vessel, usually arising from the thoracic or abdominal aorta.

The diagnosis is suggested by radiographs showing recurrent or persistent consolidation, sometimes including cystic lesions. CT and ultrasound may demonstrate the anomalous systemic artery; angiography is rarely necessary. Recurrent infections are common and provide indication for surgical resection. Asymptomatic lesions may be observed. Intralobar and extralobar forms are recognized and are best distinguished on the basis of their differential venous drainage.

Extralobar sequestration is usually located in the posterior basal segments, most often on the left (90 percent of cases) and more common in boys. Venous return is via systemic vessels, usually the inferior vena cava or azygos vein. The extralobar form has a separate visceral pleural covering distinct from the surrounding normal lung (Fig. 9-9).

Intralobar sequestration also occurs in the lower lobes, more commonly on the left (60 percent of cases) than on the right. Venous return is usually via the pulmonary veins or occasionally directly into the left atrium. The intralobar form resides within normal lung parenchyma and has no separate pleural covering. Collateral air drift via the pores of Kohn may lead to infection.

- **Congenital cystic adenomatoid malformation (CCAM)** represents a spectrum of cystic and solid lesions arising from the anomalous development and abnormal proliferation of terminal respiratory structures lacking mature alveoli. The cystic mass interferes with normal alveolar development in the remaining lung. CCAM usually involves one lobe and may enlarge after birth. Most often, symptoms appear in the first month of life (70 percent of cases), with respiratory distress secondary to the large space-occupying mass and

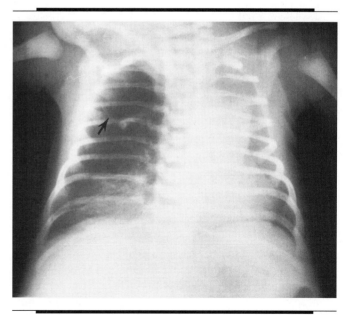

FIGURE 9-8 Congenital lobar emphysema. Chest radiograph demonstrating hyperlucency and hyperinflation of the right upper lobe. Note incidental azygos fissure (arrow).

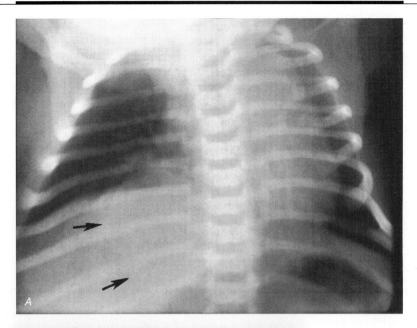

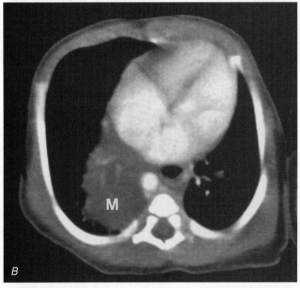

FIGURE 9-9 Pulmonary sequestration. (*A*) Chest radiograph showing a subtle opacity in the medial right lung base (arrows). (*B*) Contrast-enhanced CT demonstrating a soft-tissue mass (M) in the posterobasal right lower lobe.

hypoplasia of the remaining uninvolved lung. The remaining majority of cases appear by the first year of life with unresolving or recurrent consolidation and infection.

The radiographic appearance is that of an unresolving parenchymal mass with a variable cystic component (Fig. 9-10). The detection of cysts is dependent on the degree to which spaces within the lesion are air-filled by communication with the tracheobronchial tree. Three types are recognized based on their cystic content. Type I is most common and is composed of one or more large (>2 cm) air-filled cysts. Type II consists of small cysts (<2 cm) mixed with a solid mass. Type III appears as a solid mass without cysts.

The prognosis for type I CCAM is favorable. Surgical lobectomy is usually curative. Infants with the larger type II and III lesions often die of pulmonary hypoplasia and respiratory insufficiency. Differential diagnostic considerations include diaphragmatic hernia and staphylococcal pneumonia.

- **Bronchogenic cysts** are common bronchopulmonary foregut malformations, probably secondary to ectopic bronchial bud development. Typically large, round to oval and fluid-filled, they are asymptomatic unless infection occurs. These cystic lesions may communicate with the tracheobronchial tree, particularly when complicated by infection, in which case an air-fluid level is seen.

These cysts are lined with columnar respiratory epithelium and contain mucoid material of variable density. Bronchogenic cysts occur most commonly in the mediastinum and around the hilum (about 85 percent of cases) and, less commonly, within the pulmonary parenchyma (15 percent). Pulmonary parenchymal lesions typically involve the lower lobes, the right more than the left, and occur more commonly in boys.

CT demonstrates a nonenhancing mass. When the diagnosis is suspected, several *precontrast* images should be obtained through the lesion for purposes of comparative attenuation measurement, as the intrinsic attenuation of the cyst may be considerably higher than that of water owing to its mucinous content. With MR, the lesion is characteristically bright on T2-weighted sequences (Fig. 5-16).

- **Esophageal duplication cysts** are another common form of bronchopulmonary foregut malformation. They are typically round or tubular in configuration, are right-sided, and are located distally within the esophageal wall. By definition, they are surrounded by two muscular layers and contain squamous epithelium. Esophageal duplication cysts rarely communicate with the true esophageal lumen and are usually fluid-filled (Figs. 9-11 and 5-17). Symptoms relate to the size and location of the cyst and may include respiratory distress, dysphagia, GI bleeding, and infection. Radiographs may reveal a mass in the middle mediastinum. CT or MR can confirm the intramural location and cystic nature of the lesion.

- **Neurenteric cysts** develop as a result of failed separation of the pulmonary and notochordal elements during the third week of gestational development. There is a characteristic stalk-like connection between the cyst and the meninges or spinal cord which may or may not provide patent communication. Less commonly, there is persistent communication between the lesion and portions of the GI tract.

The typical lesion is a paravertebral posterior mediastinal mass, more often right-sided, with associated spinal and ver-

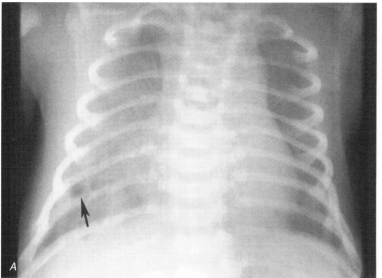
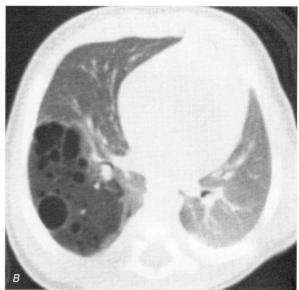
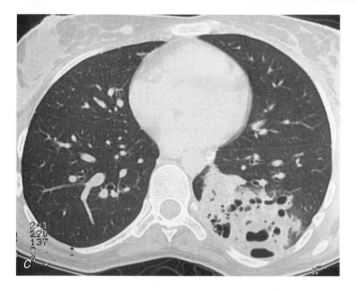

tubes which are easily malpositioned in newborns and small infants (Fig. 9-13).

- **Hyaline membrane disease (HMD)** is the most common form of respiratory distress in the premature newborn. It occurs almost exclusively in premature infants and in infants of diabetic mothers, with the greatest incidence in infants delivered by cesarean section. Girls are affected twice as often as boys. The disorder is chiefly related to a relative lack of surfactant, an agent secreted by type II pneumocytes, cells that are underrepresented in the premature lung. The relative lack of surfactant results in stiff lungs in which damaged cells, mucus, and debris fill the alveolar spaces.

FIGURE 9-10 CCAM. (A) Chest radiograph revealing a faint cystic lesion in the right lung base (arrow). (B) CT demonstrates a complex low-attenuation right lower lobe mass with large cysts characteristic of a type I CCAM. (C) CT from an adult with a CCAM in the left lower lobe.

tebral anomalies including scoliosis, hemivertebrae, and spina bifida. Neurologic symptoms are common. MR is best suited to defining the relationship of the cyst to the neural axis.

9.5 THE NEONATAL CHEST

- **Chest radiographs** are often obtained to help assess the cardiopulmonary status of newborns with respiratory distress. Hyaline membrane disease, transient tachypnea of the newborn, and pneumothorax are common causes (Fig. 9-12). Examinations are also valuable for assessing the location of catheters, endotracheal tubes, and nasogastric

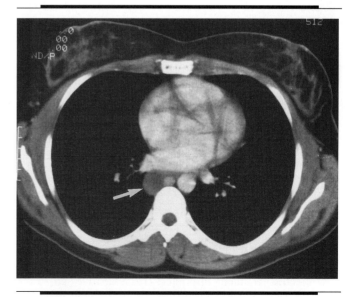

FIGURE 9-11 Esophageal duplication cyst. CT showing a water-density mass (arrow) posterior to the left atrium and adjacent to the esophagus.

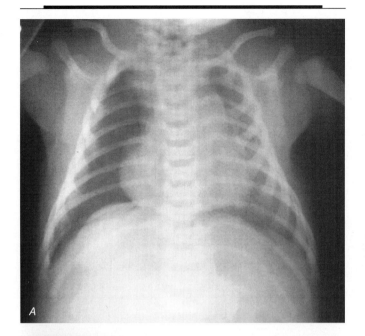

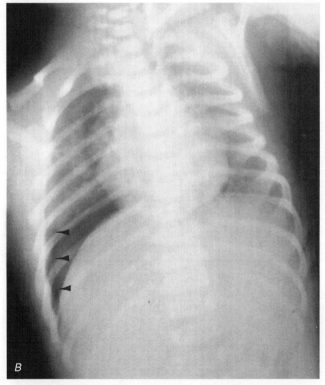

FIGURE 9-12   Newborn with pneumothorax. (*A*) AP supine chest radiograph showing lucent right hemithorax and sharp costophrenic angle. (*B*) Left lateral decubitus radiograph demonstrating the visceral pleural margin (arrowheads).

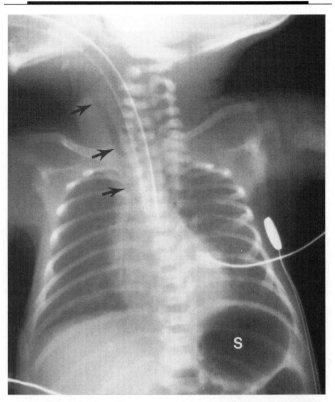

FIGURE 9-13   Endotracheal tube malposition. Chest radiograph showing an endotracheal tube entering the esophagus. The infant's head is turned to the right, revealing the trachea (arrows) anterior to the intubated esophagus. Note also gaseous distention of the stomach (S).

Respiratory distress occurs within the first few hours of life. The lungs are hypoinflated with diffuse and bilaterally symmetric granular infiltrates and extensive air bronchograms (Fig. 9-14*A*). Effusions are uncommon. Treatment includes supplemental oxygen and surfactant replacement. In most infants, there is gradual improvement and clearing

of infiltrates in the first few days of life, with resolution in 7 to 10 days.

Complications of HMD include pulmonary interstitial emphysema, pneumothorax, and bronchopulmonary dysplasia. Infants with severe respiratory distress, hypoxemia, and acidosis require ventilatory support with positive end expiratory pressure (PEEP) or continuous positive airway pressure (CPAP) to keep the collapsed terminal air spaces open. Positive-pressure ventilation leads to a variety of complications related to distention and rupture of the abnormal alveoli in immature lungs.

Gas may leak into the interstitium of the lung, manifesting as innumerable tiny cystic lucencies referred to as **pulmonary interstitial emphysema** (Fig. 9-14*B*). From this location, gas may dissect out toward the lung periphery, rupturing through the visceral pleura to cause **pneumothorax** and, if large enough, may produce tension. Because the lungs are stiff, often only partial collapse is observed. If gas dissects toward the hilum of the lung, **pneumomediastinum** and **pneumopericardium** may result.

As a consequence of persistently elevated pulmonary vascular resistance, the ductus arteriosus, which normally closes in the early hours or days of life, may remain patent. This results in persistent fetal circulation and congestive heart

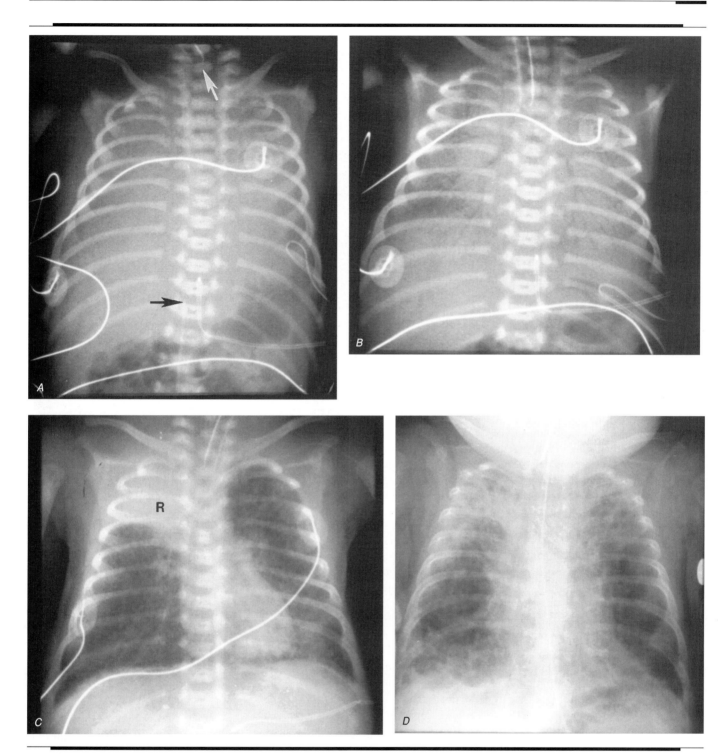

FIGURE 9-14   HMD and complications. (*A*) Postnatal chest radiograph demonstrating diffuse ground-glass infiltrates. An umbilical vein catheter (black arrow) and a endotracheal tube tip (white arrow) are seen. (*B*) After a short period of mechanical ventilation, air bronchograms are evident. Subtle cystic lucencies are seen bilaterally, indicative of pulmonary interstitial emphysema. (*C*) Diffuse cystic lucencies of pulmonary interstitial emphysema are now more extensive, and atelectasis has developed in right upper lobe (R). (*D*) After more than 4 weeks of therapy, the child remains intubated, the lungs are hyperinflated, and large, "bubbly" areas characteristic of bronchopulmonary dysplasia have developed bilaterally.

failure. Mucous plugging of airways by secretions and debris also leads to transient episodes of segmental and subsegmental **atelectasis** (Fig. 9-14*C*).

• **Bronchopulmonary dysplasia** is a chronic lung disease resulting from prolonged neonatal exposure to high oxygen concentrations and barotrauma from positive-pressure mechanical ventilation. It occurs in <20 percent of neonates affected by HMD. The entity can be defined radiographically as chronic hyperinflation, fibrosis, and "bubbly" cystic changes predominating in the upper lobes that persist after 1 month of age (Fig. 9-14*D*). Pathologically, there is destruction of the alveolar epithelium, with edema, hemorrhage, exudative necrosis, and fibrosis. The radiographic appearance of the chest generally returns to normal by 5 years of age. Pulmonary function tests remain abnormal, and there is an increased incidence of infection and reactive airways disease into young adulthood.

- **Wilson-Mikity syndrome** is an uncommon disorder seen in premature infants and is radiographically similar to bronchopulmonary dysplasia but unrelated to HMD. Chest radiographs are normal at birth. Respiratory distress, hyperinflation with "bubbly" lucent areas and reticular infiltrates develops at the age of 2 weeks. Probably secondary to pulmonary immaturity, it is felt to represent alveolar injury by room air or perhaps a sequela of viral infection.

- **Transient tachypnea of the newborn**, or "wet lung," is the most common form of respiratory distress occurring in full-term infants, often those delivered precipitously or by cesarean section. Amniotic fluid is retained within the lungs, either because it is inadequately expelled by chest compression or suctioning during delivery or because of impaired resorption. Mild respiratory distress begins in the early hours of life. Chest radiographs demonstrate hyperinflation, mild cardiomegaly and edema, pleural thickening, and small effusions. Symptoms resolve and radiographs become normal in 1 to 2 days.

- **Meconium aspiration** occurs in term and post-term infants in whom meconium stains the amniotic fluid, often in response to prenatal stress. Aspiration of the meconium-stained amniotic fluid results in chemical pneumonitis and bronchial obstruction with air trapping by the thick meconium and resulting reactive inflammatory exudate.

  Radiographically, there is hyperinflation with multifocal areas of atelectasis and coarse, nodular infiltrates. Effusions are uncommon. Pneumothorax and pneumomediastinum may result from air blockage and alveolar rupture. As in HMD, elevated pulmonary vascular resistance may cause persistent fetal circulation with a PDA. Therapy is supportive to allow resolution of the chemical pneumonitis. Symptoms and radiographic resolution typically occur within 2 days.

- **Neonatal pneumonia** is the result of a pulmonary infection acquired in utero following premature rupture of the membranes or via transplacental innoculation, by aspiration during passage through the birth canal, or soon after birth. The most common pathogen is **group B β-hemolytic streptococcus**, usually acquired during vaginal delivery, an infection with a 50 percent mortality. *Staphylococcus, Klebsiella, Pseudomonas, Chlamydia* (Fig. 9-15) and *Pneumococcus* are additional causative agents.

  The radiographic pattern is the most protean of those for the neonatal processes, as many cases appear identical to

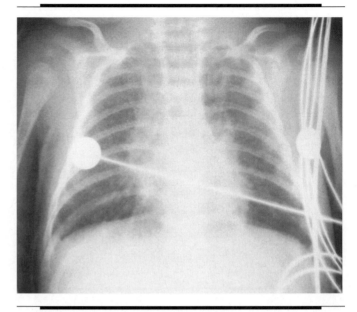

FIGURE 9-15 *Chlamydia* **pneumonia.** Chest radiograph demonstrating coarse, symmetric, bilateral interstitial infiltrates.

HMD, while others simulate the appearance of transient tachypnea of the newborn or meconium aspiration. Patchy bilateral infiltrates, atelectasis, and hyperaeration are typical. Pleural effusions may become complicated by empyema, particularly with *Staphylococcccus* and *Klebsiella* infections.

9.6 DIFFUSE PARENCHYMAL LUNG DISEASE

- **Primary pulmonary lymphangiectasia** is an uncommon and generally fatal disorder caused by failed regression of subpleural and interlobular pulmonary lymphatics during gestation, resulting in abnormally dilated and hypertrophic lymphatic channels. The pulmonary form may occur as an isolated abnormality or in association with hemihypertrophy, intestinal lymphangiectasia, or generalized angiomatosis.

  Pulmonary lymphangiectasia may also occur with anomalous pulmonary venous return and hypoplastic left heart, presumably related to increased lymphatic flow in the face of venous obstruction. Infants suffer respiratory distress from birth. Radiographs have the appearance of interstitial edema with venous congestion, hyperinflation, reticulonodular infiltrates, and focal areas of atelectasis. The diagnosis can be confirmed by lung biopsy.

- **Pulmonary histiocytosis**, also called **Langerhans cell histiocytosis** or **eosinophilic granuloma**, is an idiopathic systemic disease with variable expression, ranging from solitary bone lesions or skin disease to a multisystem process leading to organ failure and death. The pathologic hallmark is Birbeck granules in the cytoplasm of histiocytes. Pulmonary manifestations are present in one-half of patients.

  In young children with the severe systemic form, **Letterer-Siwe syndrome**, pulmonary involvement and symptoms are mild in comparison to the lytic osseous destruction, hepatosplenomegaly, and lymphadenopathy. In older children, typical symptoms of pulmonary involvement include nonproductive cough, dyspnea, and chest pain.

The most severe pulmonary disease is seen in adolescent boys, manifesting as a predominantly upper lobe nodular interstitial infiltrate which may progress to fibrosis. Hyperinflation and spontaneous pneumothorax are also observed. Symptoms and radiographic manifestations are more pronounced in smokers. Diabetes insipidus occurs in association with pulmonary involvement in about one-fourth of patients. In adolescents, the course of the disease is usually indolent and may remain stable, regress, or progress to end-stage fibrosis.

- **Pulmonary hemosiderosis** is the result of alveolar hemorrhage with the deposition of iron and hemosiderin in alveolar macrophages. It is commonly idiopathic, probably autoimmune, but may occur secondary to cardiac disease, such as mitral stenosis or vasculitis, or in association with milk allergy. When associated with glomerulonephritis, the condition is known as **Goodpasture syndrome**.

Radiographs reveal transient patchy bilateral alveolar infiltrates. With repeated episodes of hemorrhage, a reticular interstitial infiltrate may develop, progressing to fibrosis. Infants and young children develop anemia, fever, dyspnea, hepatosplenomegaly, weakness, and hemoptysis. Clubbing and pulmonary hypertension may develop. The prognosis is poorest in the idiopathic form, with children succumbing to respiratory insufficiency within several years.

- **Sarcoidosis**, a systemic granulomatous disease of unknown etiology, is rare in children younger than 15 years of age. More than 80 percent of pediatric cases occur in the southeastern and south central United States, suggesting a geographic antigenic origin. The majority of patients are young adolescents. Half are asymptomatic, the disease being initially recognized on routine radiographs. Symptoms may include generalized malaise, weight loss, cough, and dyspnea.

The radiographic pattern in children is similar to that in adults, with bilateral hilar and paratracheal lymphadenopathy present in nearly all cases. Reticulonodular interstitial infiltrates and the alveolar form of parenchymal disease also occur. The radiographic grading system is identical to that used in adults (see Section 4.9; Figs. 4-38–4-43).

- **Collagen vascular diseases** are uncommon in children but include juvenile rheumatoid arthritis, polyarteritis nodosa, systemic lupus erythematosis, dermatomyositis, and scleroderma. Pulmonary involvement typically results in restrictive lung disease and, occasionally, pulmonary hypertension. The radiographic appearance is similar to that in adults, including basilar interstitial infiltrates which may progress to fibrosis, pleural effusions, and pulmonary nodules in some disorders (see Section 4.8).

- There are numerous thoracic symptoms of **sickle cell disease**. The impaired immune function, propensity for pulmonary and osseous infarctions, and cardiac changes associated with sickle cell disease have a variety of thoracic radiographic manifestations. The presence of fetal hemoglobin F delays the appearance of clinical and radiographic abnormalities in children with homozygous hemoglobin S disease until 2 to 3 years of age.

Acute chest syndrome refers to the pulmonary infiltrates, effusions, fever, and chest pain that occur during acute sickle cell crises. These symptoms are due to hemorrhagic infarction, difficult to distinguish clinically or radiographically from pneumonia. Functional asplenia renders children with sickle cell disease more susceptible to *pneumococcal* pneumonia. Children with hemoglobin SS or SC disease are also more susceptible to *Mycoplasma pneumoniae* infection.

Cardiomegaly and **congestive heart failure** occur as a result of chronic anemia and high-output states. Pericarditis may also occur as a component of the acute chest syndrome. **Bone infarcts** may be recognized as sclerotic lesions in the proximal humerus, sternum, and ribs. In the thoracic spine, end-plate infarctions lead to central depressions resulting in characteristic H-shaped vertebral bodies. In children younger than 10 years, the splenic shadow may be enlarged on the frontal chest radiograph. In older children, the spleen becomes small, sometimes calcifying.

- α_1-**Antitrypsin** is a plasma glycoprotein with a broad range of protease inhibitor activities. The production of α_1-antitrypsin is governed by two autosomal codominant alleles, allowing for wide variation in the degree of enzyme deficiency. Marked α_1-antitrypsin deficiency results in panacinar pulmonary emphysema in adults (see Section 4.6).

Pulmonary disease and symptoms are rarely manifest in children, but homozygous enzyme deficiency is associated with juvenile hepatic cirrhosis. Early recognition is essential to improve the outcome. Therapeutic strategies include smoking cessation, immunization against influenza, *Pneumococcus*, and *Haemophilus* infections, and experimental replacement therapy with α_1-protease inhibitors.

- **Drowning** causes nearly 10,000 deaths annually in the United States, and more than one-half of the victims are children. Most incidents occur in private backyard swimming pools, and boys are involved three times as often as girls. **Near-drowning** is defined as immersion resulting in severe respiratory distress that is not fatal within 24 hours of the event. The pathophysiology of large-volume fresh- and saltwater aspiration differs in experimental models, however, there is no significant clinical difference given the small volumes of aspirated fluid observed in practice.

Patients suffer hypoxemia, hypercapnia, and acidosis, often complicated by hypothermia. Radiographs demonstrate alveolar edema with variable atelectasis caused by airway obstruction from aspirated particulate matter and bronchospasm from chemical pneumonitis (Fig. 4-8). Therapy consists of oxygen administration and positive-pressure mechanical ventilation.

- **Immotile cilia syndrome** is an autosomal recessive disease characterized by ultrastructural and functional abnormalities of cilia. Ciliary dysfunction results in impaired transport of

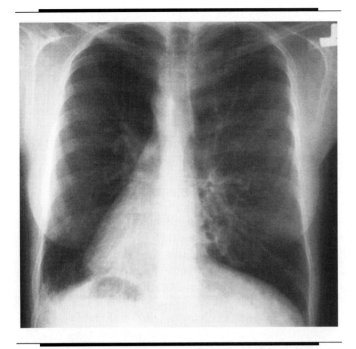

FIGURE 9-16   Kartagener syndrome. Chest radiograph showing situs inversus with a right-sided cardiac apex, a right aortic arch, and a right-sided gastric air bubble. Note bronchiectasis in the left lower lobe.

mucus, leading to recurrent infection and chronic inflammation affecting the sinuses and lungs and male infertility. Sinus opacification is a frequent finding, and the frontal sinuses are often hypoplastic. Nasal polyps, obstruction, and chronic otitis are frequent. Chronic mucus impaction and infection result in bronchiectasis. Other findings include atelectasis, recurrent infiltrates, and variable situs abnormalities. When associated with situs inversus, the disorder is known as **Kartagener syndrome** (Fig. 9-16).

- **Oxygen toxicity** occurs with prolonged exposure to elevated inspiratory concentrations of oxygen. Concentrations above 80 percent precipitate toxicity after 36 to 48 hours, with lower concentrations causing damage at a slower rate. Concentrations below 50 percent appear safe for extended periods. Bronchopulmonary dysplasia (see Section 9.5) represents the fibrosis resulting from prolonged mechanical ventilation and oxygen toxicity in neonates with HMD. In previously well children, prolonged hyperoxia produces tracheobronchitis, atelectasis, edema, and alveolar hemorrhage. Early exudative and subsequent proliferative phases may result in irreversible lung changes identical to those in acute respiratory distress syndrome (ARDS) (see Section 4.3).

9.7 INFLAMMATORY LUNG DISEASE

- **Cystic fibrosis (CF)** (see Section 4.4) is an autosomal recessive metabolic disorder characterized by abnormal exocrine gland function affecting the respiratory, GI, and reproductive tracts. The gene responsible for CF has been localized to the long arm of chromosome 7, and the pathophysiology relates to abnormal chloride transport in exocrine epithelial cells. Neonates may develop meconium ileus and intestinal obstruction. The diagnosis is established by the sweat test, in which a chloride concentration above 60 mEq/L is diagnostic of cystic fibrosis.

Severe respiratory disease eventually develops in all patients, but there is wide variability in age of onset, extent, severity, rate of progression, and complications of pulmonary disease. Upper respiratory involvement includes sinusitis, nasal polyps, and recurrent otitis. In the lower respiratory tract, recurrent bronchitis and pneumonias lead to purulent cough, hemoptysis, dyspnea, and hypoxemia due to mucus impaction, bronchiectasis, atelectasis, and pulmonary hypertension. *Pseudomonas* species are the most significant pathogens, and antibiotic resistance is problematic. There is a propensity for pneumothorax and invasive infections, including allergic bronchopulmonary aspergillosis and mycosis.

Chest radiographs demonstrate hyperinflation with upper lobe interstitial infiltrates and patchy areas of confluent infiltrate with atelectasis (Fig. 9-17). Mucus impaction in dilated airways may be recognized as tubular branching opacities. Air-fluid levels may be seen within bronchiectatic airways. Pulmonary arterial and right heart enlargement may be seen, along with hilar adenopathy from chronic infection. CT shows the severity of bronchiectasis, peribronchial thickening, mucus impaction, hilar adenopathy, and pulmonary arterial enlargement to better advantage.

Aggressive antimicrobial treatment, chest physical therapy, and general nutritional and supportive care have improved median survival and quality of life, but most patients with CF succumb to respiratory failure or other pulmonary complications. Lung transplantation, which must be performed bilaterally to prevent spread of infection from the native to the transplanted organ, is a promising option for some patients but remains limited in availability.

- **Chronic granulomatous disease** of childhood includes a variety of heritable disorders of white blood cell microbicidal function. The most common defect is an X-linked disorder, more common and severe in boys, but other metabolic defects demonstrate non-sex-linked heritability. Neutrophils, eosinophils, monocytes, and macrophages phagocytize offending organisms, but the oxidative mechanism for destroying these pathogens is impaired. The organisms are then able to proliferate, forming abscesses and granulomas.

The disease is characterized by recurrent bacterial and fungal infections, lymphadenopathy, hepatosplenomegaly, and infectious dermatitis. Acute, chronic, and recurrent respiratory tract infections are prominent features and a frequent cause of mortality. Radiographs demonstrate patchy, multifocal, and recurrent infiltrates, pleural effusions, pleural thickening or empyema formation, hilar lymphadenopathy, and cavitation within parenchymal abscesses. Fibrosis and honeycombing may develop. Gallium scans may be helpful in localizing infection and in distinguishing active lung disease from chronic scarring.

The most common pathogens include *Staphylococcus aureus, Klebsiella, Escherichia coli, Serratia, Aspergillus,*

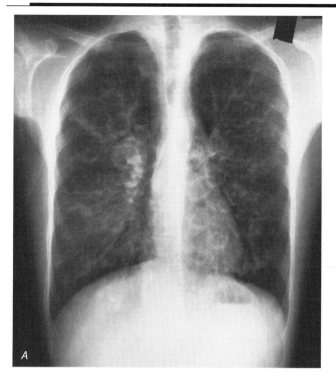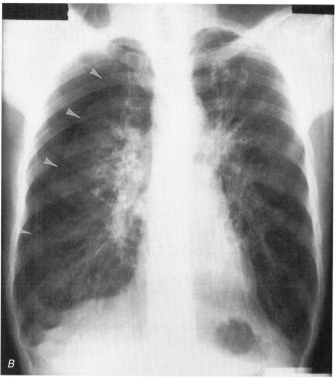

FIGURE 9-17   Cystic fibrosis. (*A*) Chest radiograph in a 20-year-old showing cystic bronchiectasis throughout both lungs. (*B*) Chest radiograph in an adult with cystic fibrosis featuring a right pneumothorax (arrowheads). Note hyperinflation, coarse interstitial markings, and predominately upper lobe bronchiectasis.

Nocardia and *Candida* species, and *Pneumocystis carinii.* The diagnosis is established by the nitroblue tetrazolium (NTB) test, a histochemical assay of neutrophil function. Management is by aggressive antimicrobial therapy, but the long-term prognosis is guarded.

- **Obliterative bronchiolitis (OB)** is the process of airway scarring following injury to the distal bronchial tree. Most commonly a sequela of viral infection, OB may also result from inhalational injuries, radiation therapy, thromboembolic disease, recurrent gastric aspiration, or connective tissue disorders, or as a component of lung destruction in bronchopulmonary dysplasia. Cough, wheezing, chest pain, and dyspnea are out of proportion to radiographic abnormalities, which are often normal. A unilateral hyperlucent lung with a small hilum and attenuated vascularity may be seen (Swyer-James syndrome). CT may reveal bronchiectasis.

- **Bacterial pneumonias** are a common cause for hospital admission in children. The clinical manifestation of viral and bacterial infections are frequently difficult to distinguish and are more nonspecific in infants. Empiric antimicrobial therapy is often instituted for the typical symptoms of high fever, tachypnea, cough, chest pain, lethargy, and decreased activity. Bacterial pneumonias may accompany or follow viral respiratory tract infections, probably as a result of impaired mucosal ciliary action. The most common pathogens are *Streptococcus pneumoniae, H. influenzae,* and *Staphylococcus aureus* (Fig. 9-18).

It is difficult to distinguish bacterial pathogens clinically or radiographically. *Haemophilus* tends to occur in 6- to 12-month-old infants, whereas *Pneumococcus* predominates in older children and adolescents. Radiographs demonstrate segmental or lobar consolidation, often with air bronchograms. Pleural effusions are common and, when present, argue against a purely viral infection. *Haemophilus* and *Staphylococcus* pneumonias are the most often complicated by empyema. Lung abscesses and postinfectious pneumatoceles are most commonly encountered with *Staphylococcus.*

- ***Chlamydia trachomatis*** is an avian pathogen that infects humans as an intracellular parasite. It is acquired during passage through the birth canal. Neonates develop respiratory distress, occasionally complicated by pulmonary hemorrhage. One-third of patients have chlamydial conjunctivitis. Radiographs demonstrate hyperinflation with diffuse bilateral perihilar interstitial infiltrates (Fig. 9-15).

- ***Mycoplasma pneumoniae*** is the most common pathogen to produce **atypical pneumonia**, so named because of the lack of response to usual antibiotic regimens. Its peak incidence is in children 5 to 15 years old, and it may also occur as a local outbreak among schoolmates and families. Symptoms range from a mild upper respiratory illness to a severe pneumonia with a nonproductive cough and high fever. Extrapulmonary symptoms, such as skin rash, malaise, headache, gastroenteritis, and myalgia frequently accompany the infection.

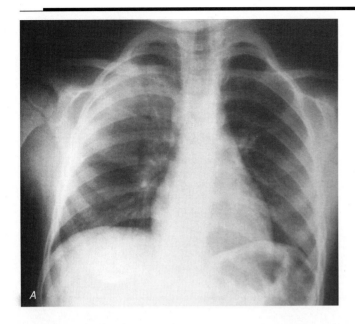
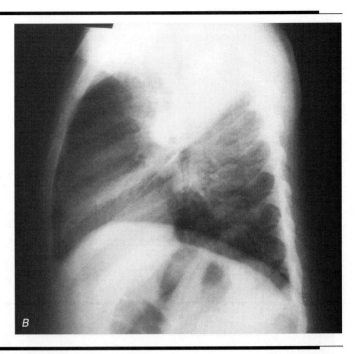

FIGURE 9-18   **Lobar pneumonia.** (*A*) PA and (*B*) lateral chest radiographs in a 5-year-old boy showing opacification and air bronchograms in the posterior segment of the right upper lobe characteristic of consolidation due to bacterial pneumonia. *Pneumococcus* was identified.

Radiographs demonstrate early reticular interstitial infiltrates which may progress to patchy or focal consolidation over a period of weeks. Small pleural effusions develop in 20 percent of cases. The relationship between severity of symptoms and radiographic abnormalities is frequently incongruous.

- **Pertussis**, or **whooping cough**, is caused by *Bordetella pertussis*, an organism that has been largely eradicated through childhood immunization. Children less than 5 years old are usually affected, and this condition is more common in girls. Radiographs show peribronchial infiltrates and patchy atelectasis favoring the middle and right lower lobes, often with hilar adenopathy. The pattern of infiltrates may produce the appearance of a "shaggy heart." The infection is often accompanied by a virulent bronchitis, which was formerly an important cause of bronchiectasis.

- **Round pneumonia** is characterized by a masslike spherical infiltrate frequently having unsharp edges and air bronchograms and almost always occurring in the posterior lower lobes (Fig. 9-19). The appearance probably represents a phase of consolidation in which organisms spread rapidly and centripedally via the pores of Kohn and canals of Lambert. *Pneumococcus* and other *Streptococcus* species are the most common pathogens producing this appearance.

- **Pneumatoceles** are transient, thin-walled parenchymal lung cysts, probably the result of severe overdistention and contained rupture of small airways or alveoli. In children, they are most commonly the sequelae of *Staphylococcus* infection. *Klebsiella* and *Pneumococcus* are less frequent

causative agents. Pneumatoceles also occur following lung trauma and as a complication of hydrocarbon aspiration.

- **Lung abscess** is the consequence of a necrotizing pneumonia in which inflammation and lung destruction result in the formation of a thick-walled cavity filled with purulent mate-

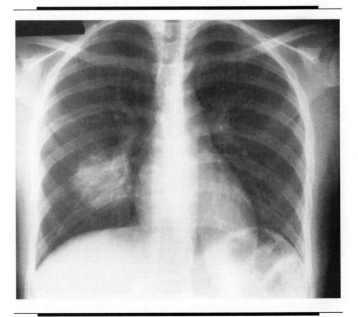

FIGURE 9-19   **Round pneumonia.** Chest radiograph showing a round masslike area of consolidation containing air bronchograms in the right lower lobe.

rial. Pneumonias caused by *Staphylococcus, Klebsiella,* and *Pseudomonas* are those most commonly complicated by the development of lung abscess. Lung abscess may also result from hematogenous seeding, as in septic emboli from bacterial endocarditis, or from aspiration, which may occur with neurologic disorders and structural abnormalities of the trachea and esophagus.

Radiographs and CT images reveal a thick-walled, fluid-filled parenchymal cavity. The cavity may contain air if there is communication with the tracheobronchial tree. In contrast to empyema, equal diameter of the cavity on the frontal and lateral projections aid in its localization to the lung parenchyma (see Fig. 3-18). On CT, there is an acute angle between the lesion and the pleura.

- **Aspiration pneumonia** occurs in children with neurologic and neuromuscular disorders such as seizure, coma, and swallowing dysfunction, as well as with structural and functional abnormalities of the esophagus such as tracheo-esophageal fistula and gastroesophageal reflux. Aspiration may also result from near-drowning or as a complication of general anesthesia. Chemical pneumonitis and airway obstruction from particulate matter may be followed by bacterial superinfection. Chronic aspiration leads to basilar interstitial infiltrates and bronchiectasis.

- **Actinomycosis** occurs in immunocompromised patients and in devitalized tissues of normal hosts and is caused by *Actinomyces israeli*, a gram-positive anaerobe. Patients with poor oral hygiene are predisposed to this condition, as the pathogen is a component of oral flora. Pulmonary infection usually results from aspiration. Sulfur granules are present within the infected material.

Chest radiographs demonstrate focal consolidation which frequently extends across fissures or into the chest wall. Cavitation is common. Pleural thickening, empyema, and rib and spine destruction may occur adjacent to the pulmonary consolidation (Fig. 9-20).

- **Viral infection** is the most common cause of lower respiratory tract infection in children. Although responsible for a large number of physician visits, most cases are mild and self-limited and are treated on an outpatient basis. In infants and immunocompromised children, viral infections can cause severe and life-threatening disease. Respiratory viruses are highly contagious, have short incubation periods, and spread in an epidemic fashion. The typical pathogens tend to produce pneumonia in infants, whereas older children suffer less serious respiratory tract infections.

Infection with **respiratory syncytial virus**, which is the most common viral agent, peaks in midwinter, along with **influenza** outbreaks. **Parainfluenza** infection peaks in the fall. **Adenovirus** infection is most common in winter and spring. Typical symptoms include high fever, coryza, cough, and tachypnea. Radiographs typically demonstrate mild hyperinflation with patchy perihilar and peribronchial infiltrates. Subsegmental atelectasis occurs frequently and favors the middle and right upper lobes. Effusions are distinctly uncommon and, if present, suggest bacterial infection. The radiograhic findings usually resolve within 2 days.

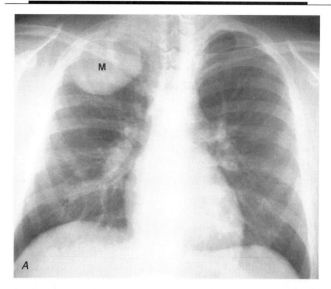
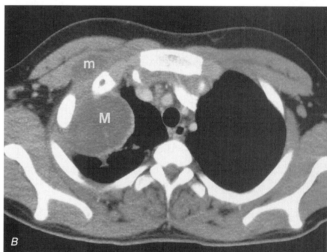

FIGURE 9-20 Actinomycosis of lung and chest wall. (*A*) Chest radiograph showing a large soft-tissue mass (M) in the right lung apex. Acute pleural margins suggest a primary parenchymal process. (*B*) CT shows a low-attenuation thick-walled mass (M) in the right upper lobe, directly abutting the anterolateral pleura and invading the anterior chest wall with spread (m) beneath the right pectoralis muscles.

- **Human immunodeficiency virus (HIV)** is an RNA retrovirus predisposing patients to opportunistic infections of all types. Almost 90 percent of affected children acquire the disease from their mothers during the perinatal period, although only one-third of babies born to HIV-positive mothers become infected with the virus. Others acquire the infection through contaminated blood products. The pulmonary manifestations of HIV disease in children relate to the increased propensity for pyogenic bacterial infections, opportunistic infection with *P. carinii* and cytomegalovirus, and the development of lymphocytic interstitial pneumonitis.

- ***Pneumocystis carinii*** **pneumonia (PCP)** is the most common opportunistic pulmonary infection in both children and adults with HIV disease. The infection begins as an alveolar inflammatory process, progressing to involve the interstitium. Symptoms of high fever, nonproductive cough, severe dyspnea, and hypoxemia rapidly progress to respiratory failure. The course of the disease is most severe in infants.

Radiographs typically demonstrate diffuse alveolar and interstitial infiltrates with hyperinflation and patchy areas of consolidation. Spontaneous pneumothorax may occur. Pneumatoceles may develop after successful therapy. In some patients, radiographs are normal or minimally abnormal despite severe clinical respiratory symptoms. The diagnosis may be supported by positive lung gallium scans. The pathogen is usually identifiable by bronchoalveolar lavage.

- **Cytomegalovirus (CMV)** is a DNA virus of the herpes family and is another common cause of opportunistic pulmonary infection in children with HIV disease. In infants, acquired and congenital infection are distinguished by documentation of disease onset after the age of 1 month. CMV can be acquired from healthy carriers who shed the virus in all types of body fluids. Pulmonary infection results in fever, nonproductive cough, dyspnea, and hypoxemia and is often fatal. Radiographs demonstrate diffuse nodular interstitial infiltrates frequently predominating at the lung bases.

- **Lymphocytic interstitial pneumonitis (LIP)** is a common complication of pediatric HIV infection, second only to PCP, and is uncommon in adults. Demonstration of LIP is a criterion for establishing the diagnosis of aquired immunodeficiency syndrome (AIDS). The exact etiology of LIP is uncertain, but it may be a direct response to pulmonary infection by HIV itself or secondary to an as yet unidentified pathogen. Pathologically, there is lymphocytic proliferation within the interstitium and adjacent to bronchioles. Symptoms include cough with respiratory distress and dyspnea less dramatic than that seen with PCP. Radiographs demonstrate bilateral reticulonodular interstitial infiltrates predominating at the lung bases (Fig. 9-21). The disease process may progress to fibrosis.

- **Bronchiolitis** is a common highly contagious form of viral respiratory tract infection almost always caused by **respiratory syncytial virus**. Its peak incidence is in 2- to 6-month-old infants but it is seen in children up to 2 years old. Defined as respiratory infection with hyperinflation and wheezing, it is often accompanied by cough and rhinorrhea. Fever is variable. Radiographs reveal marked hyperinflation and perihilar infiltrates.

- **Varicella-zoster virus** may cause severe pneumonia in immunocompromised patients but also occurs in some normal children following chickenpox. When pneumonia develops, it represents the sequela of extensively disseminated viral infection and has a mortality rate approaching 10 percent.

  The radiographic pattern is distinct from that of other viral pneumonias, revealing innumerable tiny pulmonary nodules which may evolve into confluent round areas of consolidation. Hilar adenopathy and small effusions may accompany the acute infection. In some patients, the pulmonary nodules may calcify into tiny 2- to 3-mm lesions.

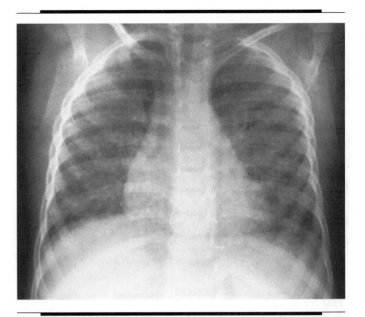

FIGURE 9-21   Pulmonary lymphocytic interstitial pneumonitis. Chest radiograph in a 3-year-old HIV-positive boy with CMV infection, demonstrating hundreds of tiny lung nodules representing biopsy-proven lymphocytic interstitial pneumonitis.

- **Histoplasmosis** is caused by the fungus *Histoplasma capsulatum*. This fungus is a dimorphic organism existing in a mycelial form in the soil and transforming into a yeast within the alveoli. The organism is present worldwide but is endemic in the central United States, with high rates of infection. Infection results from inhalation of spores from a contaminated source. In the lungs, the organism is ingested by macrophages, where they proliferate and are often carried to local lymph nodes. More than half of infections are asymptomatic. When present, symptoms are that of a mild respiratory infection or flulike illness.

  A disseminated, severe pneumonia can occur in infants and immunocompromised children or in normal children with massive exposures. Radiographic findings in acute infection range from normal to mild basilar infiltrates, often with hilar adenopathy. Milliary infiltrates may be seen in severe exposures. Calcification of healed parenchymal and hilar lesions represents the permanent manifestation of prior infection.

  Complications include **fibrosing mediastinitis**, in which an exuberant host reaction results in a fibrotic reaction that constricts the central airways and pulmonary vessels, a process that is rare in children. **Broncholithiasis** may result from erosion of calcified granulomas into the airways, producing wheezing, atelectasis, and postobstructive pneumonia (Fig. 3-27). **Pericarditis** may develop from direct pericardial infection or spread from adjacent mediastinal disease and may result in constrictive pericardial disease.

- **Mucormycosis** occurs almost exclusively in immunocompromised children, typically those with leukemia, lymphoma, or diabetes. The infection is characterized by fungal invasion

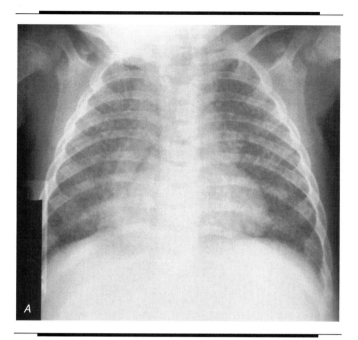

FIGURE 9-22   Miliary tuberculosis. Chest radiograph revealing innumerable tiny pulmonary nodules in a 1-year-old child with miliary tuberculosis.

of vessels, resulting in pulmonary infarction. Radiographs demonstrate a single large or multiple consolidative masses which tend to grow insidiously up to but not across pleural boundaries, frequently cavitating.

- **Mycobacterial infection** in children is chiefly caused by *Mycobacterium tuberculosis*. The infection is usually acquired by inhalation of bacilli within aerosolized droplets from actively infected individuals. In **primary infection**, the inhaled organism is phagocytized within alveoli and carried to regional lymph nodes. **Reactivation** may be precipitated by other illnesses, surgery, malnutrition, hormonal changes of puberty, or steroid therapy. The typical adult symptoms of fever, night sweats, and cough are often absent or minimal in children, who usually manifest only a mild cough. A high index of suspicion is needed to establish the diagnosis, which is usually confirmed by a positive tuberculin skin test and an abnormal chest radiograph.

  The radiographic appearance of tuberculous infection includes hilar and paratracheal lymphadenopathy, parenchymal consolidation and collapse, cavitation, pleural effusion, and thickening. **Miliary disease**, the result of hematogenous dissemination, is more common in infants and younger children (Fig. 9-22). As in adults, multiple drug therapy is necessary and drug-resistant organisms are becoming increasingly problematic.

9.8 PARENCHYMAL LUNG NEOPLASMS

- **Primary lung neoplasms** are exceptionally rare. **Pleuropulmonary blastoma** is a highly malignant primary mesenchymal neoplasm which appears as a large, lobulated mass associated with symptoms of cough, dyspnea, or chest pain. Brain metastases are common, and the prognosis is poor. Primary pulmonary parenchymal **lymphoma** is uncommon in all age groups. Primary **rhabdomyosarcoma, leiomyosarcoma, fibrosarcoma**, and **bronchogenic carcinomas** identical to those occurring in adults have all been reported.

- **Metastatic disease** far exceeds primary lung neoplasm in frequency, probably comprising more than 95 percent of all lung malignancies. **Wilm tumor, osteosarcoma, Ewing sarcoma, soft tissue sarcomas, rhabdomyosarcoma**, and malignant gonadal and extragonadal **germ cell tumors** are the most common neoplasms that produce lung metastases. **Lymphoma, leukemia, neuroblastoma, medulloblastoma**, and **ependymoma** are additional primary tumors with some propensity for pulmonary metastases. Children are rarely symptomatic from these lesions, except when the pulmonary tumor burden is large. One exception is the tendency of pneumothorax to occur with pulmonary metastases from osteosarcoma.

  As expected, the typical radiographic pattern is that of multiple pulmonary nodules. Cavitation may be seen with some entities. Pleural disease may also be encountered, particularly in lymphoma and leukemia. Pulmonary lesions from osteosarcoma, germ cell tumors, and Wilm tumor may be resected in an attempt to achieve a surgical cure.

Bibliography

Armstrong P, Wilson AG, Dee P, Hansell DM. *Imaging of Diseases of the Chest,* 2nd ed. St. Louis: Mosby–Year Book; 1995.

Fishman AP, Elias JA, Fishman JA, Grippi MA, Kaiser LR, Senior RM. In AP Fishman (ed): *Pulmonary Diseases and Disorders,* 3rd ed. McGraw-Hill, 1998.

Fraser RG, Paré JAP, Paré PD, Fraser RS, Genereux GP. *Diagnosis of Diseases of the Chest,* 3rd ed. vol. 2. Philadelphia: WB Saunders Co., 1989.

Grainger RG, Allison DJ. *Diagnostic Radiology—A Textbook of Medical Imaging,* 3rd ed. New York: Churchill Livingstone, 1997.

Silverman FN, Kuhn JP. *Essentials of Caffey's Pediatric X-ray Diagnosis.* Chicago: Year Book Medical Publishers Inc., 1990.

Sutton D. *Textbook of Radiology and Imaging,* 6th ed. New York: Churchill Livingstone, 1998.

Chapter 10

CHEST TRAUMA

Andrew J. Fisher

10.1 DEMOGRAPHICS, RADIOGRAPHIC TECHNIQUE, AND EVALUATION

- **Trauma** including homicide is the leading cause of death in patients under 40 years of age and the fourth leading cause of death overall, trailing cardiovascular disease, cancer, and stroke. Trauma leads to more lost life years than cancer and coronary artery disease combined and is estimated to cost the United States over $240 billion in medical, morbidity, and mortality costs annually. Although penetrating trauma from gunshot wounds and stabbings may be more dramatic, almost 80 percent of trauma is due to a blunt mechanism, including falls, motor vehicle collisions (MVCs), and industrial injuries.

- **Thoracic trauma** is a contributing factor in approximately one-half of blunt trauma cases, and the cause of death in roughly one-third. Three-fourths of patients with severe thoracic injuries have multiple associated injuries. As for all trauma patients, a systematic and rapid evaluation is warranted. Initial attention should be directed toward exclusion of life-threatening injuries and evaluation of interventions such as endotracheal tube (ETT) and thoracostomy tube placement. This examination is followed by a systematic search for less critical injuries and complications.

- **Radiographic evaluation** should begin immediately after the trauma service has assessed the victim and addressed airway, breathing, and circulatory concerns. The backboard should be removed as long as the patient is not in extremis or severely unstable. Depending on the site and mechanism of injury, the radiographic evaluation varies. Typically, limited views of the cervical spine, chest, and pelvis are obtained before assessing the appendicular skeleton.

A **supine chest radiograph** can be obtained if the patient has a known or suspected axial skeleton fracture or is extremely unstable; otherwise, an erect anteroposterior (AP) radiograph should be obtained (Fig. 10-1). Supine chest radiographs cause the mediastinum to appear broadened, posing difficulties in excluding aortic and other mediastinal injuries. Supine positioning also limits diaphragmatic excursion and consequently pulmonary aeration.

Consequently, if the patient is conscious and alert, the chest radiograph should be obtained upright during inspiration, with the patient leaning slightly forward.

In addition to positioning, quality radiographs should have limited overlying material and the site of penetrating injury localized with radiopaque markers. Results should be clearly and rapidly conveyed to the emergency department physicians. Once initial plain radiographs have been obtained, additional studies such as computed tomography (CT) or angiography can be performed as warranted.

- **CT in the trauma setting** serves several roles. Neurologically, it is valuable in assessing patients for closed head injuries or in further evaluating spinal fractures. It can confirm plain radiographic findings of pulmonary injuries and pneumothoraces and has a role in evaluating the abnormal mediastinum for hematoma and potential aortic injury. In the abdomen and pelvis, CT demonstrates parenchymal organ injuries and the potential need for consequent intervention. Penetrating trauma to the abdomen that breaches the peritoneum mandates surgical evaluation, bypassing cross-sectional imaging.

Approach to Trauma Radiographs

- As in the clinical evaluation, radiographic examination should be initially directed at excluding life-threatening injuries and evaluating interventions. This examination is followed by a more systematic search for other injuries requiring intervention and finally nontraumatic disease.

- **Life-threatening thoracic injuries** may include acute aortic injury and other vascular trauma; cardiac contusion, rupture,

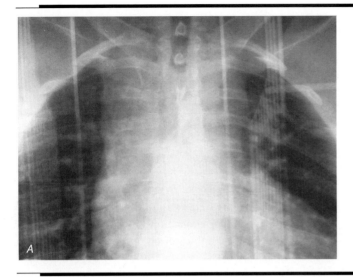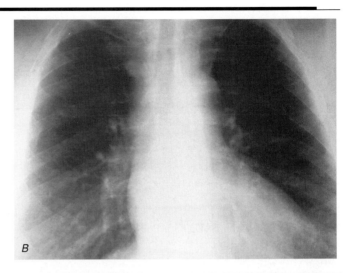

FIGURE 10-1   Supine and erect chest radiographs. (*A*) AP supine chest radiograph following a MVC in a morbidly obese 36-year-old male showing a markedly widened superior mediastinum and inability to discern the aorta. (*B*) The mediastinum appears normal on an AP erect chest radiograph obtained minutes later.

or tamponade; tension pneumothorax; flail chest; tracheobronchial injury; and spinal fractures and dislocations. Other less emergent but serious injuries include pulmonary contusions and lacerations, spinal and brachial plexus injuries, other fractures and dislocations, pleural fluid collections, and diaphragmatic disruption.

- **Evaluation of interventions** performed in the field might include ETT, tracheostomy tube, or nasogastric (NG) tube placement. Intubation of the esophagus is a relatively common finding with gastric distention and diminished pulmonary aeration. Excessive fluid resuscitation may result in pulmonary edema. Chest tube position and adequacy of pneumothorax decompression should be assessed on follow-up radiographs.

- Indirect chest involvement in trauma includes noncardiogenic pulmonary edema particularly from closed head injuries; air, pellet, or fat embolism (Fig. 10-2); and aspiration on loss of consciousness. Integration of other findings is essential.

- **Special patient situations** do occur. In **intoxicated patients**, the clinical examination may be less helpful at localizing injury, and radiographic evaluation plays an essential role. Aspiration pneumonia must be considered. In **pregnant patients**, the desire to limit radiation exposure must be tempered by the need to obtain a complete study. The radiologist plays a vital role in choosing which limited views should be obtained and in ensuring appropriate shielding.

- Many seriously injured patients are rapidly evaluated and taken to surgery or the intensive care unit. Consequently, important injuries can be overlooked. It is important to carefully follow serial examinations and assess radiographs for injuries obscured or overlooked on initial evaluation. This includes not only fractures but other entities such as diaphrag-

matic disruption or the delayed development of thoracic outlet syndrome or clavicular posttraumatic osteolysis.

- **Systematic evaluation, quality imaging, and close cooperation with the trauma team** maximize radiographic impact on the acute trauma patient's care.

10.2 VASCULAR INJURIES

- **Acute traumatic aortic injury (ATAI)** is a common cause of mortality in MVCs. The typical mechanism of injury is rapid deceleration with rotation and torsion of the relatively mobile aortic arch tethered by the ligamentum arteriosum, diaphragm, and aortic root. A direct blow with osseous pinch of mediastinal structures against the spine is another potential mechanism. ATAI can be catastrophic, accounting for 15 percent of all MVC fatalities, 85 percent of patients dying before any intervention. Clinical findings include shock, systolic murmur from disrupted flow, and acute coarctation syndrome with differential upper and lower extremity pressures.

    The **location of ATAI** is predictable because of the mechanism of injury. Greater than 90% of injuries in survivors occur at the aortic isthmus adjacent to the ligamentum arteriosum, and the remainder occur at the ascending aortic root, arch, or rarely, the descending aorta near the diaphragmatic hiatus.

    Patients with complete transection of the aorta generally die. Those with a contained rupture (pseudoaneurysm) or intimal injury of the aorta may survive the "golden hour" following trauma. These patients have small vessel mediastinal bleeding, which accounts for many of the radiographic manifestations. The blood obscures adjacent structures such as the aortic knob, and mass effect from the hematoma causes displacement of anatomic landmarks such as the trachea and left main bronchus.

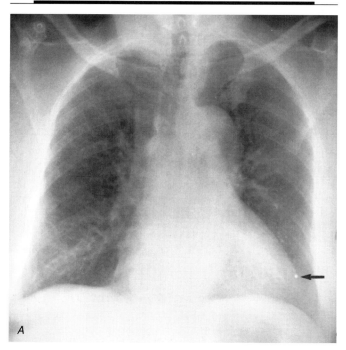

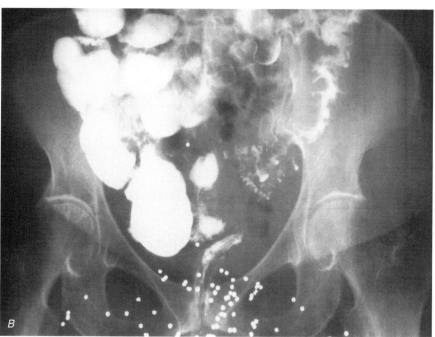

FIGURE 10-2   Pellet embolism. (*A*) Radiograph in a 70-year-old woman who sustained a shotgun injury to the pelvis with a solitary pellet embolized to the left lower lobe (arrow). (*B*) Pelvic film following a barium enema shows the concentrated pellets of the blast.

- **Radiographic findings** vary in their sensitivity and specificity, and a normal frontal chest radiograph has a 98 percent negative predictive value for ATAI. Sensitivity for aortic injury exceeds 85 percent, yet specificity is low at 45 percent. The most discriminating findings include obscuration of aortic contour, a widened right or left paraspinal stripe in the absence of a spinal fracture, rightward displacement of an NG tube and opacification of the aorticopulmonary window (Fig. 10-3).

Other radiographic findings may include rightward tracheal shift, a hemothorax, depression of the left main bronchus (angle >40 degrees below horizontal), a wide mediastinum (>8 cm or a mediastinum/chest ratio >0.25) (**Differential 105***) and a right paratracheal line >5 mm (Fig. 10-4). An apical cap can be seen, although this can be due to other causes including venous bleeding and fractures with a concomitant extrapleural hematoma. Fractures of the first and second ribs can be seen in association with ATAI and imply significant trauma but do not by themselves mandate angiography.

- **Further evaluation with CT** is performed in cases where the chest radiograph is equivocal or perhaps suggestive of ATAI and the patient is hemodynamically stable. The scan should be rapidly performed with intravenous (IV) contrast and without oral contrast. IV contrast enhances evaluation of the vascular structures, definition of the lumen, and detection of wall irregularities. It is also often required for evaluation of other injuries, particularly visceral organ involvement. Spiral technique allows more rapid scanning as well as multiplanar reconstructions. CT angiography may show occlusion or pseudoaneurysm caliber change but generally does not replace aortography. CT angiography has an increasing role and may eventually replace conventional angiography in certain circumstances.

  The purpose of CT is to detect or exclude a mediastinal hematoma apparent as soft tissue density adjacent to the aorta (Fig. 10-5). This finding is usually due to venous bleeding but can also be due to fractures or other mediastinal injuries. Therefore, a hematoma from aortic injury should abut the aorta and, at least partially, encase it. A small amount of fluid in the anterior and posterior aortic pericardial recesses is normal and should not prompt alarm. The thymus may pose a diagnostic challenge in young victims, and symmetry and a preserved aortic fat plane may help in differentiation.

  A negative CT, one that shows no hematoma or mediastinal hematoma but a preserved aortic fat plane, requires no further evaluation. Those that are positive should be followed by angiography along with cases where the radiograph is strongly suggestive of ATAI. By this algorithm, 50 percent or more of patients can be spared angiography. A majority of CT-proven hematomas are due to nonaortic causes such as fractures and small venous bleeds. **Angiography** is the gold standard and is discussed in Section 14.3. It may demonstrate

---

*Please refer to Chapter 2, in which the differential diagnoses are discussed in numerical order.

a contour abnormality, an intimal tear, or an aortic pseudo-aneurysm (Fig. 10-6).

- **Other vessels** may be injured in chest trauma. Almost 20 percent of thoracic arterial injuries from trauma occur in the

great vessels. The left subclavian artery is most commonly injured, followed by the brachiocephalic, right subclavian, left common carotid, and vertebral arteries. Over 70 percent fail to be noted by physical examination. Essentially all these patients have plain radiographic findings of a mediastinal hematoma similar to those seen with ATAI. These injuries are frequently missed on CT examinations, particularly those tailored to evaluate the aorta. Aortography is required.

- The **inferior vena cava** (IVC) is the most frequently injured vein in thoracic trauma. Caval injuries may be difficult to repair and may be fatal. They are manifested as a mediastinal hematoma with widening that may be more prominent on the right. Fractures of the distal third of the clavicle can injure the subclavian or axillary vessels, as can traumatic central line insertion. This injury may be apparent as an extra-pleural density in the subclavicular area and can produce a hemothorax if the pleura is violated. Penetrating trauma can injure vessels directly or as a result of proximity.

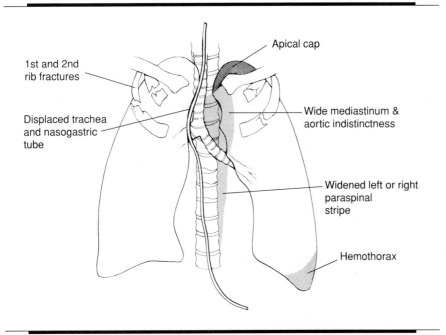

FIGURE 10-3   Radiographic findings of ATAI.

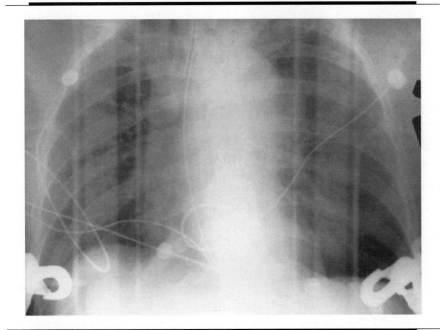

FIGURE 10-4   ATAI, radiographic findings. Supine AP chest radiograph in a 34-year-old trauma victim who is on a backboard. The mediastinum is widened, the aorta indistinct, and the left paraspinal stripe widened. Both the ETT and NG tubes are displaced rightward beyond the thoracic vertebrae. The left main bronchus is depressed.

10.3 PNEUMOTHORAX AND AIRWAY INJURIES

- In all trauma cases, the airway is initially assessed in the field and the patient may be intubated. On arrival at the trauma center, reevaluation of the airway is undertaken. This usually involves auscultation and physical examination. The chest radiograph is essential to confirm appropriate ETT positioning.

  Tracheal intubation is well demonstrated on chest radiographs, and the tip of the ETT should reside below the thoracic inlet, ideally 3 cm proximal to the carina, limiting dead space. Prolonged intubation may lead to tracheomalacia and stenosis.

  A **malpositioned ETT** can be seen within a main bronchus, almost always the right mainstem bronchus because of the bifurcating angle (Fig. 11-2). This limits contralateral lung aeration, and the ETT should be withdrawn appropriately.

  Esophageal intubation is another frequent site of ETT malposition. The

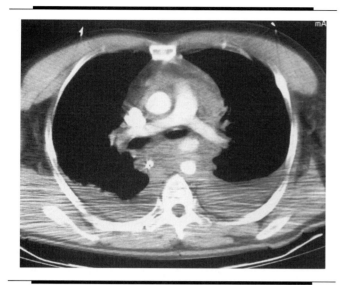

FIGURE 10-5   ATAI, CT findings. Contrast-enhanced CT in a patient following an MVC demonstrates mediastinal hematoma. This is manifest as soft tissue density encircling the ascending and descending aorta as well as the main pulmonary artery. There are bilateral hemothoraces and rightward displacement of the NG tube.

accompanying radiograph will demonstrate bilaterally decreased pulmonary volumes with concomitant gastric distention. The ETT may project over the trachea, although it is frequently advanced within the esophagus past the level of the tracheal carina.

- Likewise, **NG** tubes may be incorrectly placed within the airway and can have deleterious effects including pneumothorax, aspiration, and collapse (Fig. 10-7). Drowned lung and ensuing pneumonia can occur if gastric lavage is attempted.

Air Collections

- A **pneumothorax**, air within the pleural space, is a common sequela of thoracic trauma and is often observed in association with rib fractures (**Differentials 5 and 70**). While apical pneumothoraces are generally seen on upright films, supine radiographs of the traumatized patient may show air collecting adjacent to the mediastinum, anteriorly, and at the lung base. These features may be difficult to detect on plain film, and CT is more sensitive. The radiograph shows a pleural line with absent lung markings peripherally (Fig. 7-5). An air-fluid level on erect positioning indicates a hemopneumothorax.

  Although expiratory radiographs increase pneumothorax conspicuity by increasing their relative size and contrast difference compared to the smaller, more opaque lung, they should not be obtained in the trauma setting. Expiratory films make the mediastinum appear broader, may limit radiographic detail of other structures such as the posterior ribs, and have a similar sensitivity to upright inspiratory radiographs in pneumothorax detection.

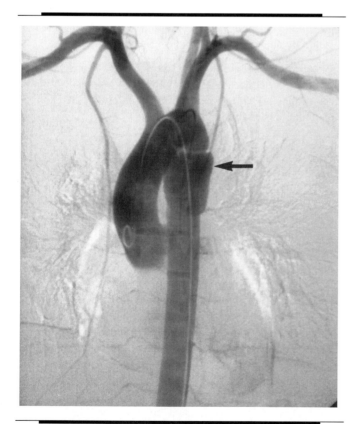

FIGURE 10-6   ATAI, angiographic findings. Aortogram demonstrating a pseudoaneurysm (arrow) at the aortic isthmus following an MVC.

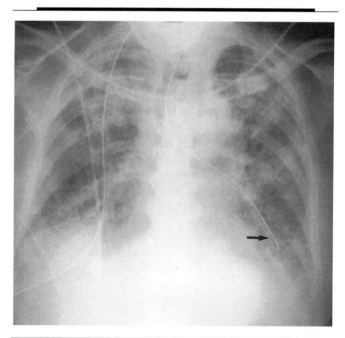

FIGURE 10-7   Pulmonary positioning of NG tube. Frontal chest radiograph demonstrating a NG tube (arrow) in the left lower lobe in a patient with underlying lung disease.

- In a **tension pneumothorax**, positive intrapleural pressure leads to compression of the normal, contralateral lung, creating a ventilation-perfusion mismatch through ventilatory restriction. It may clinically lead to respiratory distress, absent unilateral breath sounds, and distended neck veins. The radiograph demonstrates a large unilateral pneumothorax with partial or total collapse of the ipsilateral lung and mediastinal and tracheal deviation into the contralateral hemithorax (Fig. 10-8). Immediate decompression with a catheter or chest tube is mandated. Reexpansion pulmonary edema is uncommon in acute pneumothoraces.

- **Chest tube placement** should be radiographically confirmed. Generally, the thoracostomy tube is placed in the fourth or fifth intercostal space just anterior to the midaxillary line. It usually immediately decreases pneumothorax size. Malpositioned chest tubes may reside in the chest wall, pulmonary parenchyma, or interlobar fissures, or with the tip against the mediastinum.

- **Subcutaneous emphysema** is often seen in conjunction with a pneumothorax. It may also be the sequela of soft tissue laceration or pneumomediastinum and is generally innocuous but should prompt a search for the etiology. A pneumothorax must be excluded.

- **Pneumomediastinum** can be seen in the setting of barotrauma, penetrating, or blunt injury (**Differential 102**). Airway or esophageal injury must be excluded. Pneumomediastinum may extend cephalad to the aortic knob, decompress into the cervical soft tissues or caudally to yield the

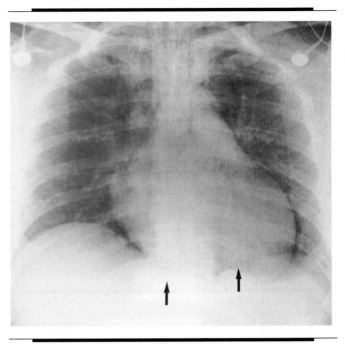

FIGURE 10-9 Pneumomediastinum. Chest radiograph in a patient who was stabbed in the cervical trachea, showing subcutaneous gas extending inferiorly to produce pneumomediastinum. Note the distinct cardiac margins and the so-called continuous diaphragm sign (arrows).

so-called **continuous diaphragm sign**. This distinguishes pneumomediastinum from pneumopericardium, which is generally due to penetrating trauma (Fig. 10-9).

- **Pneumoperitoneum** in the setting of blunt trauma requires further evaluation, generally with CT. It is usually due to abdominal hollow viscus injury or inferior extension of pneumomediastinum.

Airway Injury

- **Tracheobronchial injuries** are rare, yet serious, results of thoracic trauma. They cause 3 percent of blunt trauma deaths and have a 30 percent mortality, perhaps due to associated injuries and delayed detection. They may be intra- or extrathoracic, the latter resulting from direct trauma to the neck. There may be cervical crepitus, hoarseness, and dyspnea, and injuries may be treated conservatively with flexible bronchoscopy and intubation.

   Intrathoracic tracheobronchial fractures occur within 3 cm of the carina in 80 percent of cases. They are difficult to detect radiographically, and delayed diagnosis is common. They may be suspected from a pneumothorax that fails to resolve despite adequate thoracostomy tube decompression.

   Other plain film findings include tracheal or bronchial cutoff, ETT displacement or balloon overdistension, and mediastinal and deep cervical emphysema. The so-called **fallen-lung sign** is an uncommon finding where a bronchial fracture leads to the ipsilateral lung collapsing adjacent to the mediastinum. The chest radiograph is normal in 10 percent of

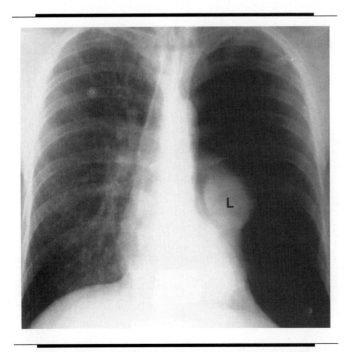

FIGURE 10-8 Tension pneumothorax. Chest radiograph in a 33-year-old victim of an MVC showing a left tension pneumothorax with complete collapse of the left lung (L), contralateral mediastinal shift, and downward displacement of the left hemidiaphragm.

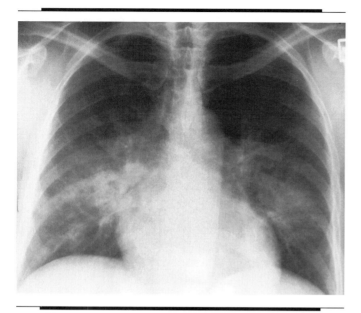

FIGURE 10-10 Toxic inhalation. Chest radiograph showing perihilar infiltrates and peribronchial thickening in a 47-year-old woman following gasoline inhalation.

tracheobronchial injuries. CT may show the airway discontinuity, especially with spiral thin-collimation technique. Airway scarring and stenosis are late complications.

- **Acute inhalational injury** may be due to smoke, chemical, or noxious fume inhalation (Fig. 10-10). While specifics may vary, these events cause injury by surface irritation and variably by allergic response, toxic absorption, and displacement of ambient air, yielding asphyxiation. Fire is the most frequent source of inhalational injury, and its composition may vary. Generally, tracheobronchitis occurs with possible ulceration. Often, there is central pulmonary edema which may progress to pneumonitis. Radiographs are normal with limited exposure. Further exposure to the irritant produces peribronchial thickening, infiltrates, and atelectasis.

- **Esophageal injury** is rarely due to a blunt mechanism; generally, it is the result of penetrating trauma. It can also be iatrogenic or caused by violent retching (Boerhaave disease). Radiographic manifestations include pneumomediastinum, pneumothorax, pleural effusions, and possibly mediastinitis and abscess. A triangular focus of gas is sometimes seen in the left medial cardiophrenic sulcus and is called the **V sign of Naclerio.**

10.4 POSTTRAUMATIC FLUID COLLECTIONS AND CARDIAC INJURIES

- **Hemorrhage** is a common result of thoracic trauma. Blood may collect in any space including the subcutaneous tissues,

pleural or pericardial spaces, mediastinum, or pulmonary parenchyma.

- **Hemothorax** may be due to intercostal, internal mammary, subclavian, or other chest wall vascular injury as well as cardiac, parenchymal, and mediastinal injuries (**Differential 77**). It is considered massive when in excess of 1500 ml. The radiographic appearance of hemothorax is generally indistinguishable from that of other effusions. To prevent fibrothorax, a hemothorax should be evacuated once the bleeding has stopped.

- **Chylothorax** should be differentiated from hemothorax; it represents the accumulation of lymph in the pleural space. While chylothorax does have nontraumatic etiologies, traumatic chylothorax is due to **thoracic duct injury (Differential 78)**. There is a 7- to 10-day latent period following duct disruption. Chylothorax is radiographically indistinguishable from any other pleural fluid collection. A right chylothorax occurs with thoracic duct disruption below T4 to T6 and on the left in more superior injuries. The thoracic duct empties into the venous system at the left jugular and subclavian confluence.

Cardiac Injury

- **Hemopericardium** can result from direct cardiac injury or retrograde dissection from a mediastinal vascular injury. It may be manifested as globular cardiomegaly, perhaps with pericardial fat stripe separation on the lateral radiograph (**Differentials 114 and 116**). CT can demonstrate fluid attenuation broadening the pericardial space. Echocardiography is the study of choice for evaluation. Penetrating trauma may lead to hemopneumopericardium seen as an air-fluid level limited to this space.

- **Cardiac tamponade** may result from hemopericardium, and it must be urgently addressed. Clinically it may demonstrate the triad of muffled heart sounds, pulsus paradoxus, and distended neck veins. It is a clinical diagnosis supported by the previously discussed radiographic findings of hemopericardium.

- **Myocardial injuries** are uncommon and include cardiac contusion, pericardial and myocardial rupture, and valve injuries. The aortic valve is the most frequently injured, leading to aortic insufficiency. Radiographic findings are nonspecific and generally those of hemopericardium. Sternal fracture may be present and directly cause contusions or lacerations. Arrhythmias are a dangerous complicating factor in cardiac contusions.

- **Penetrating cardiac injury** is often lethal. Imaging findings are generally those of hemopericardium. Surgery is required to detect and repair the myocardial defect. A bullet can embolize to the heart from a distant site of vascular injury and is often trapped in the trabeculae of the right ventricle. Assessing the patient for site of injury is critical in making this diagnosis, as a direct cardiac injury can have an identical appearance.

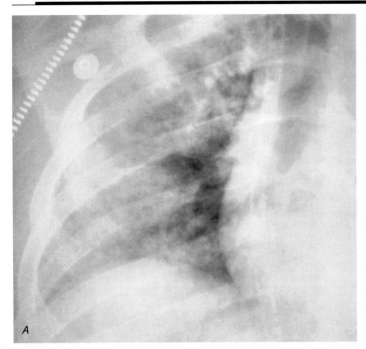

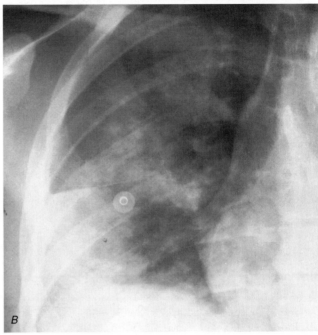

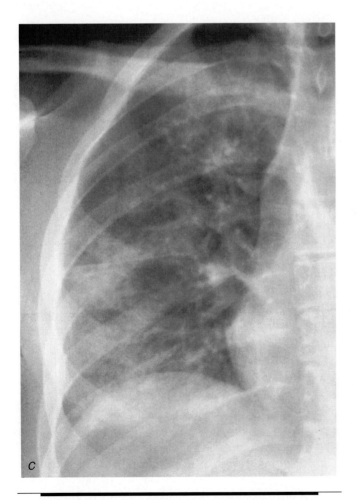

FIGURE 10-11 Pulmonary contusion. (*A*) Initial chest radiograph showing right lower lobe contusion following an MVC. (*B*) A subsequent film 1 day later showing a more defined and smaller infiltrate. (*C*) Final image 2 days after the accident demonstrating substantial clearing.

10.5 PULMONARY INJURIES

- Pulmonary parenchymal injuries are common following blunt and penetrating trauma and should be recognized. Moderate injuries may compromise oxygenation. Failure of these injuries to resolve should suggest superimposed aspiration or infection.

- **Pulmonary contusion** represents a parenchymal bruise and may be deep to the site of trauma or distributed in a contrecoup location. It represents interstitial and alveolar edema and blood, limiting gas exchange and oxygenation. A contusion appears on plain films within 6 hours of injury and resolves within 3 to 6 days. Hence, initial radiographs may be normal (Fig. 10-11).

- A **pulmonary laceration** is generally due to a shearing or penetrating force that leads to cystic spaces which fill with blood and air. They are more common in young patients and pose a risk of air embolism, a frequently fatal complication.

  A laceration may fill with blood, yielding a **pulmonary hematoma** (Fig. 10-12). It is a fairly homogeneous parenchymal mass which becomes apparent as the overlying contusion resolves. Pulmonary hematomas may persist for several months following the acute event. They become smaller and better defined on plain films and CT images within 6 to 8 weeks.

- **Traumatic pneumatoceles** are unilocular or multilocular air cavities within the parenchyma which may appear within the first 2 days following thoracic trauma. They have the radiographic appearance of a bulla or bleb and generally resolve within several weeks (**Differential 23**).

- **Aspiration** is fairly common following trauma because of altered consciousness, alcohol impairment, and increased

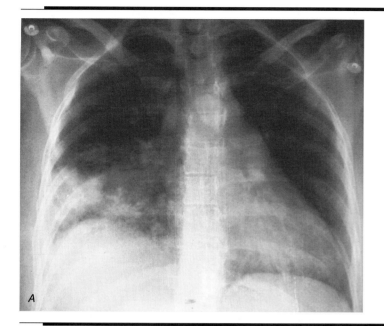
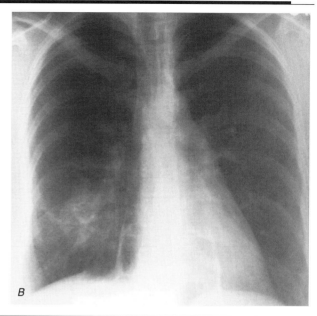

FIGURE 10-12   Pulmonary hematoma. (*A*) Chest radiograph in a 42-year-old woman involved in an MVC with pulmonary contusion in the right base. (*B*) Follow-up film 11 days later showing resolution of the contusion and reveals a persistent, well-defined pulmonary opacity representing a hematoma.

intra-abdominal pressure. Location depends on victim positioning at the time of aspiration. The lower lobes (particularly the right) and middle lobe are common in erect patients, and the posterior segment of the upper lobes and superior segment of the lower lobes in supine victims. This condition may appear similar to a contusion, although it is slower to resolve. Foreign bodies and fractured teeth can be aspirated, leading to postobstructive atelectasis or pneumonia.

- **Fat embolism** occurs commonly on a subclinical level and is generally the result of pelvic or long bone fractures. Fat droplets from bone marrow gain intravascular access and cause injury by thrombosis and vasculitis. The more dramatic "fat embolism syndrome" is distinctly uncommon and affects the lungs, brain, kidneys, and skin. There is a clinical latent period of 12 to 48 hours. Chest radiographs may be normal or show multiple alveolar infiltrates or edema. Pleural effusions are uncommon.

10.6   FRACTURES AND DISLOCATIONS

- **Chest wall injuries** are the most common posttraumatic thoracic injury (Fig. 10-13). Thoracic fractures may be subtle or obvious. Dramatic findings should not be allowed to limit the search for other injuries or the potential complications of various fractures.

- **Rib fractures** are very common and can be the result of even minor trauma, particularly in osteopenic patients. Such fractures may be a source of pain, but dedicated rib films are rarely indicated as it is the complications of these fractures, particularly pneumothorax, that cause significant morbidity and warrant surveillance. Intercostal nerve blocks may pro-

vide substantial pain relief. First and second rib fractures signify significant energy transfer and have been reported in association with ATAI, while posterior lower rib fractures may lead to visceral organ injury. Cortical disruption and potential displacement are demonstrated on radiographs.

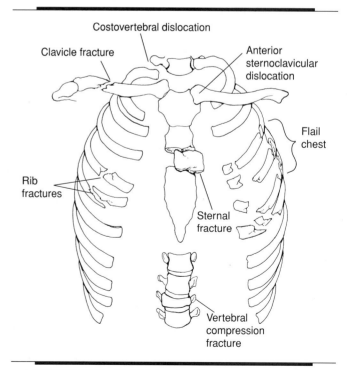

FIGURE 10-13   Skeletal trauma. Demonstrating the various skeletal injuries that follow thoracic trauma. Adapted from Lange S, Walsh G. *Radiology of Chest Disease.* 2nd ed. New York: Thieme; 1998.

- A **flail chest** is paradoxical movement of a thoracic cage segment from multiple rib fractures. Usually this requires segmental rib fractures at three contiguous levels or single fractures at five adjacent levels. There may be significant associated injuries, and a flail chest can be clinically overlooked because an acute hematoma may help stabilize the hypermobile segment. It hinders respiratory mechanics. Mortality exceeds 5 percent.

- **Costal cartilage fractures** are generally occult on plain radiographs but can cause pain and costochondritis (Tietze syndrome).

- **Vertebral fractures** result from hyperflexion in the midthoracic to lower thoracic spine and axial loading at the thoracolumbar junction. They may occur at discontinuous levels, and 10 percent are multiple. Vertebral fractures may be associated with focal pain or cord injury, or be nearly asymptomatic. A hematoma may cause paraspinal widening.

  Plain radiographs may show focal scoliosis, kyphosis, loss of vertebral body height, and a widened interpedicular distance (Fig. 10-14). The so-called ***rule of twos*** states that there should be less than a 2-mm change between interspinous or

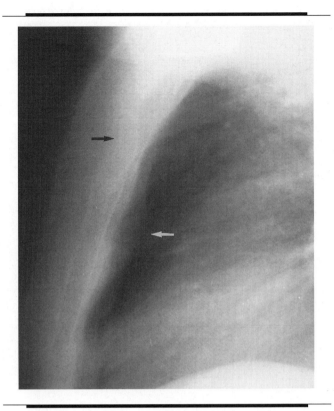

FIGURE 10-15   Sternal fracture. Radiograph in a 34-year-old motorcyclist showing a transverse fracture through the first sternal segment (black arrow) with approximately 50 percent offset. Notice the retrosternal hematoma (white arrow).

interpedicular distance at adjacent levels, facet joints should be no more than 2 mm wide, and anterior vertebral body height should be no more than 2 mm less than posterior height. **CT** can assess for osseous detail and canal encroachment, while **MR** depicts cord, marrow, and soft tissue injuries including traumatic disc herniation.

- **Sternal fractures**, seen in up to 8 percent of blunt thoracic trauma victims, are due to direct blows, often against the steering wheel in a MVC. Their significance is in the 20 percent associated cardiac contusions and potentially fatal arrhythmias. Displaced fractures may rarely cause pericardial or cardiac laceration, and they can heal with a persistent deformity. Lateral chest radiographs are best at demonstrating the fracture line (Fig. 10-15). Axial CT may fail to show the fractures which occur in the plane of imaging.

- **Sternoclavicular dislocations** are rare and frequently occult on radiographs. CT provides a more sensitive examination. Anterior dislocations are more common and easily detected clinically. Posterior dislocations can be associated with severe vascular and airway injury (Fig. 10-16).

- **Clavicular fractures** commonly occur in the middle third, and muscular traction may cause displacement, shortening, and deformity. They are usually readily identified on chest radiographs. Fractures of the distal third can cause vascular injury and persistent pain.

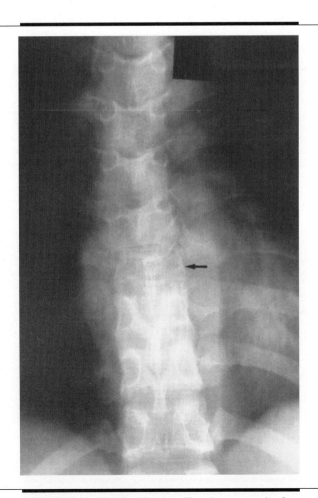

FIGURE 10-14   Vertebral fracture. There is a compression fracture and facetal dislocation of T8 (arrow). This appears as loss of vertebral body height, malalignment, and loss of the pedicles.

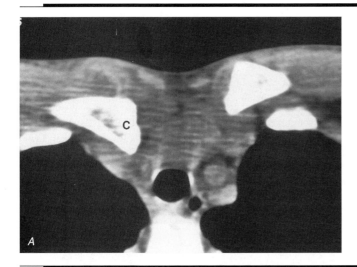
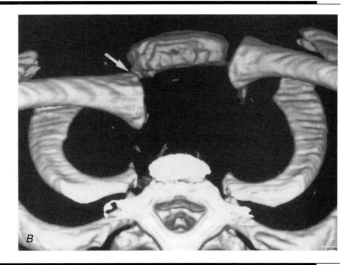

FIGURE 10-16 Posterior sternoclavicular dislocation. (*A*) CT in a 14-year-old boy with a palpable step-off at the sternoclavicular joint, showing a posterior dislocation of the proximal right clavicle (C) compared with the contralateral clavicular head. (*B*) A shaded surface display demonstrating the dislocation (arrow) from a superior projection.

- **Posttraumatic thoracic outlet syndrome** can result from brachial plexus or vascular compression. First rib, clavicular, or soft tissue injury is usually present. Symptoms may include shoulder pain and neurologic findings. First rib resection can be curative in up to 75 percent of patients.

- **Posttraumatic osteolysis** is an infrequent sequela in distal clavicular fractures. It results in osseous resorption weeks to months following fracture, persists for 10 to 18 months, and spontaneously regresses in another 6 months. Radiographs may demonstrate distal clavicular rarefaction, soft tissue swelling, and acromial deformity.

- **Glenohumeral dislocations** are anterior in over 90 percent of cases, with the humeral head in an anterior subcoracoid or subglenoid location. A **Hill-Sachs fracture** of the posterolateral humeral head or a **Bankhart lesion** of the inferior glenoid may be observed (Fig. 10-17). These dislocations may be readily evident on chest radiograph or require additional views such as posterior oblique, axillary, Stryker notch, or scapular Y projections.

  Posterior shoulder dislocations are uncommon and often difficult to identify. Persistent overlap of the glenoid and humeral head is seen on posterior oblique images (half-moon sign). Scapular Y and transthoracic views show a posterior humeral position. The humerus is held in internal rotation and may appear minified as it is closer than

normal to the film. Reverse Hill-Sachs fractures, seen as a "hatchet" deformity in the humeral head anteromedially, and Bankhart lesions may be present. Inferior dislocations are rare.

- **Scapular fractures** generally signify significant trauma but may be subtle on plain films, with greater than 40 percent overlooked on trauma chest radiographs. Dedicated scapular

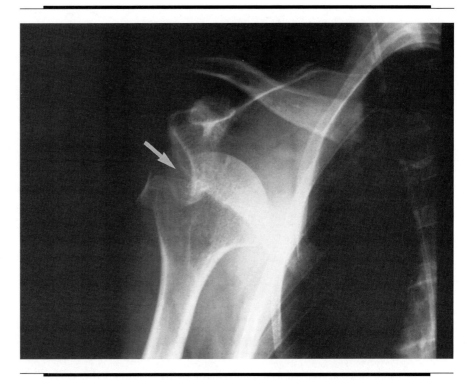

FIGURE 10-17 Glenohumeral dislocation. Radiograph in a patient who sustained a fall and has an anterior glenohumeral dislocation. A large Hill-Sachs deformity (arrow) is noted in the superolateral aspect of the humeral head.

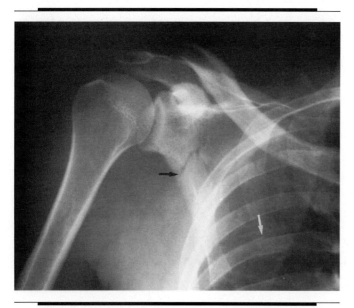

FIGURE 10-18 **Scapular fracture.** Radiograph showing a nondisplaced right scapular neck fracture (black arrow). Also noted is a right sixth-rib fracture (white arrow).

radiographs may be necessary. Fractures often occur at the glenoid and scapular neck (Fig. 10-18).

• **Acromioclavicular separations** result in widening of the joint space beyond the normal 4 to 6 mm. Type I sprains are radiographically occult, type II show acromioclavicular

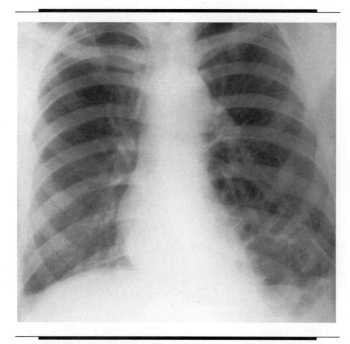

FIGURE 10-19 **Traumatic diaphragmatic rupture.** Chest radiograph demonstrating gas-filled loops of colon in the left hemithorax and an indistinct left hemidiaphragm following blunt thoracoabdominal trauma in a 19-year-old man.

joint widening, and type III have concomitant coracoclavicular widening. Weight-bearing views accentuate subtle joint widening.

10.7 DIAPHRAGM INJURY

• Up to 4 percent of blunt trauma patients have diaphragmatic tears, increasing to 15 percent in victims of penetrating thoracic trauma. This rate approaches 30 percent when the wound is inframammary.

• **Traumatic diaphragmatic rupture** can result from penetrating or blunt injury with elevation of intra-abdominal pressure. This situation accounts for only 5 percent of all diaphragm hernias, but 90 percent of those that are strangulated. The left hemidiaphragm is more often affected and better visualized. Herniation potentially involves the stomach, large or small bowel, omentum, or spleen. Traumatic diaphragmatic rupture can enlarge over time, particularly after cessation of positive pressure ventilation.

Approximately 60 percent of these ruptures are overlooked on initial **chest radiographs**. Consequently, a high index of suspicion must be maintained. There may be an indistinct or elevated hemidiaphragm, often with an associated pleural effusion and basilar consolidation. Intrathoracic bowel or an NG tube above the diaphragm are confirmatory signs (Fig. 10-19).

CT may show discontinuity or lack of visualization of the diaphragm (absent diaphragm sign), abdominal organs or peritoneal fat above the diaphragm, and a gastric narrowing (collar or hourglass sign) at the diaphragmatic defect. Thin-section spiral CT with sagittal reformations can improve depiction of the disruption (Fig. 10-20).

The multiplanar capability of **MR** can be helpful in assessing the diaphragm, as traumatic hernias may be more readily recognized in a coronal or sagittal plane.

10.8 NERVE INJURY

• The **brachial plexus** is formed from roots of C5 through T1 which form trunks, divisions, cords, and branches as they variably join and divide peripherally. They pass between the anterior and middle scalene muscles and then into the axilla.

MR is the modality of choice for imaging of the brachial plexus. The nerves, their relationship to the adjacent scalene musculature, and the surrounding fat can be evaluated. In the case of fractures, CT may show the osseous fragments to better advantage. Both CT and MR may be hindered by artifacts in the case of gunshot wounds.

• Traction can stretch the cervical nerve roots and cause neurologic symptoms. More tension can lead to **nerve root avulsion** and the formation of **pseudomeningoceles**. These features are best demonstrated on coronal MR scans. Distal injury can cause a hematoma, neural edema, or nerve disruption, and potentially formation of a posttraumatic neuroma.

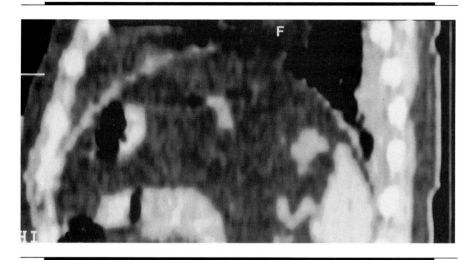

FIGURE 10-20   Traumatic diaphragmatic rupture. Oblique sagittal CT reconstruction showing discontinuity of the left hemidiaphragm with herniation of omental fat (F) in a patient following blunt trauma.

- **Phrenic nerve injury** may occur in the trauma setting. It leads to hemidiaphragm elevation and can mimic traumatic diaphragmatic rupture. Fluoroscopic evaluation with the sniff test is used to diagnose hemidiaphragm paralysis (See Section 8.8).

- **Spinal cord injury** in the thoracic spine can be due to blunt or penetrating trauma. CT may optimally demonstrate osseous fragment retropulsion, but MR can demonstrate intervertebral disks and soft tissues as well as contusion or hemorrhage within the cord.

Bibliography

Creasy JD, Chiles C, Routh WD, Dyer RB. Overview of traumatic injury of the thoracic aorta. *Radiographics.* 1997;17:27–45.

Dee PM. The radiology of chest trauma. *Radiol. Clin. North Am.* 1992; 30(2):291–306.

Graham JM, Beal AC, Mattox KL, Vaughn GD. Systemic air embolism following penetrating trauma to the lung. *Chest.* 1977;72(4):449–454.

Harris JH Jr, Harris WH. Chest. In *The Radiology of Emergency Medicine.* 3rd ed. Baltimore: Williams & Wilkins; 1992, pp. 469–622.

Howell JF, Crawford ES, Jordan GL. The flail chest. *Am. J. Surg.* 1963; 106:628–635.

Israel IS, Mayberry JC, Primack S. Diaphragmatic rupture: Use of helical CT scanning with multiplanar reformations. *Am. J. Roentgenol.* 1996; 167:1201–1203.

Mattox KL. *Complications of Trauma.* New York: Churchill Livingstone; 1994.

Mirvis SE, Bidwell JK, Buddemeyer EU, Diaconis JN, Pais SO, Whitley JE. Imaging diagnosis of traumatic aortic rupture: A review and experience at a major trauma center. *Invest. Radiol.* 1987;22:187–196.

Mueller CF, Hummel MM. Sternal fractures: New perspectives. *Emerg. Radiol.* 1994;1(1):52–55.

Posniak HV, Olson MC, Dudiak CM, Wisniewski R, O'Malley C. MR imaging of the brachial plexus. *Am. J. Roentgenol.* 1993;161:373–379.

Pretre R, Chilcott M. Blunt trauma to the heart and great vessels. *N. Engl. J. Med.* 1997;336:626–632.

Wagner RB, Crawford WO, Schimpf PP. Classification of parenchymal injuries of the lung. *Radiology.* 1988;167:77–82.

Worthy SA, Kang EY, Hartman TE, Kwong JS, Mayo JR, Müller NL. Diaphragmatic rupture: CT findings in 11 patients. *Radiology.* 1995;194: 885–888.

Chapter 11

CHEST DISEASE MANAGEMENT AND POSTTREATMENT IMAGING

Richard M. Slone

11.1 PORTABLE RADIOGRAPHY AND INTENSIVE CARE UNIT IMAGING

- **Portable chest radiographs**, technically termed bedside chest radiographs, account for half of all in-patient chest examinations in most hospitals, particularly in the intensive care unit (ICU). Patients being treated in these units are often very ill, and timely, accurate diagnosis of new or changing conditions, edema (Fig. 11-1) or evolving pneumonia, is important.

  Patient positioning is difficult, and cooperation may be limited. The technologist often requires assistance to position patients and remove overlying devices, minimizing artifacts. Erect positioning is seldom possible, and semierect positioning is the norm.

- **Image quality and interpretation** are limited by several factors. Maximum inspiration is often difficult to achieve, as is timing with mechanical ventilation. Recumbent patients have difficulty taking a deep inspiration, hence there is always some degree of vascular crowding and dependent atelectasis. Typically, only an anteroposterior (AP) examination is obtained.

These factors make assessment of the lung bases, a common site for effusions, atelectasis, and pneumonia, difficult.

An antiscatter grid is seldom used because of the weight and positioning difficulties. Phototiming is not possible, and so the technologist estimates the appropriate exposure. As a result, there are variations in film density, complicating serial film comparisons. The lower power of portable generators often leads to longer exposure times and an increased number of motion artifacts. The radiologist must exercise quality control and should have suboptimal examinations repeated when indicated.

- **Digital imaging techniques**, particularly computed radiography (CR) using photostimulable phosphor plates and digital image processing, has virtually eliminated variations in image density and contrast. Soft-copy display of images on monitors has greatly facilitated the availability of images.

- An important role of portable ICU imaging is to evaluate the location and potential **complications of monitoring and treatment devices**, such as central venous catheters, endotracheal tubes (ETTs), chest tubes, and feeding tubes.

- **Mechanical ventilation** has revolutionized the management of critically ill patients, particularly those at risk for acute respiratory distress syndrome (ARDS). Indications for mechanical ventilation include hypoxemia and hypercarbia unresponsive to conventional therapy. Radiographs are routinely obtained immediately following endotracheal intubation to confirm the position of the tube, and daily thereafter to detect potential complications.

  Most **ETTs** have a radiopaque stripe for identification. Tubes reinforced with a coiled wire are sometimes used intraoperatively to prevent tube compression. Ideally, the ETT tip should be 3 cm above the carina. The exact location of the carina is sometimes difficult to visualize. Comparison with prior radiographs can be helpful, or an estimate can be made based on the location of the fifth thoracic vertebral

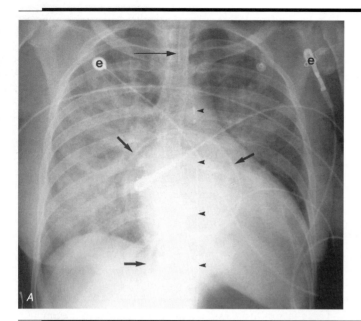
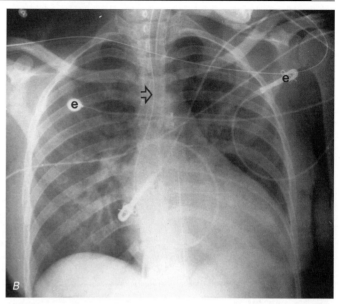

FIGURE 11-1   Congestive heart failure. (*A*) Portable chest radiograph in a patient with cardiomyopathy shows cardiomegaly and diffuse pulmonary infiltrates consistent with pulmonary edema. Note endotracheal tube (long arrow), pulmonary artery catheter (arrows) entering from the inferior vena cava with the tip in the right interlobar pulmonary artery and aortic balloon pump (arrowheads) with the distal marker in the proximal descending thoracic aorta. (*B*) Follow-up radiograph 20 hours later shows substantial interval clearing of the edema and addition of a nasogastric tube (open arrow). Cardiac monitoring leads are common artifacts (e).

body which typically overlies the carina. If positioned too high, the inflatable cuff present on almost all adult ETTs can damage the vocal cords. If positioned too low, selective ventilation of only one lung may occur.

The ETT tip can move several centimeters with flexion or extension of the neck, and this movement should be taken into account. The tip advances distally into the trachea when the patient's head is tilted forward and withdraws when the neck is extended, contrary to intuition.

An ETT advanced too far most frequently enters the right main bronchus because of its oblique course, resulting in airflow obstruction and left pulmonary collapse (Fig. 11-2). Hyperinflation of the intubated lung may cause pneumothorax. **Esophageal intubation** is uncommon but leads to hypoventilation and gastric distention. The ETT may be seen outside the margins of the trachea (Fig. 9-13). Overinflation of the ETT cuff can overdistend the trachea and cause ischemic necrosis and tracheomalacia. The tracheal diameter should not vary. A focal bulge may indicate balloon overinflation.

Barotrauma in mechanically ventilated patients, preferably referred to as **volotrauma**, can lead to pneumomediastinum, pneumothorax, and often substantial subcutaneous emphysema. **Emergent intubation** carries a potential risk of tracheal laceration which may produce similar findings.

Extubation requires alert patients who can generate a moderate inspiratory force. They must have adequate cough and gag reflexes; vital capacity; and cardiac, renal, and nutritional status. Following extubation, lung volumes decrease, with resultant increased vascular crowding, dependent atelectasis, and often increased prominence of pulmonary infiltrates.

• **Nasogastric tubes** are marked with a radiopaque stripe for identification. There is often an interruption in this stripe indicating the location of the most proximal side port, which should be distal to the gastroesophageal junction. Complications include esophageal and airway malposition (Fig. 10-7). Position should be confirmed by radiograph before use.

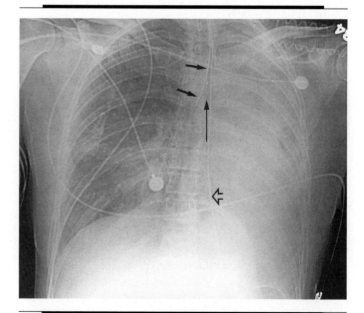

FIGURE 11-2   Right mainstem intubation. Portable chest radiograph showing opacification of the left hemithorax and ipsilateral mediastinal shift due to partial collapse. The ETT (arrows) deviates to the right below the carina (long arrow). Nasogastric tube (open arrow).

- A variety of **feeding tubes** are employed including those with weighted tips. They can be placed at the bedside or under fluoroscopic guidance. A guide wire provides some rigidity during tube placement, and when the appropriate position has been confirmed, this wire is removed. The tip should be in the distal duodenum. The side ports on the weighted tubes are proximal to the weight and not at the tip. Occasionally, feeding tubes are intentionally positioned within the stomach.

  In patients with an intact gag reflex, advancement into the tracheobronchial tree is immediately evident. In some individuals, however, inadvertent placement of tubes into the tracheobronchial tree may occur, with deleterious consequences. Such malposition is readily apparent on the chest radiograph.

- **Central venous catheters or lines (CVLs)** are routinely used for the management of in-patients, particularly those in an ICU. There are a wide variety of catheters, including those with single, double, and triple lumens. Small-caliber catheters are sufficient for fluid infusion, whereas large-caliber catheters are employed for dialysis. Catheters are advanced via the jugular or subclavian vein directly or through a sheath. A femoral approach can be used, although this method carries an increased risk of local infection.

  Catheters are introduced using the Seldinger technique, and malposition and other complications occur with sufficient frequency to warrant imaging following placement. **Pneumothorax** is one of the most common complications (Fig. 11-3). Films should be obtained with the patient in an erect position. Attention should also be given to the contralateral lung, as initial attempts may have been made on that side. Local hematoma is an uncommon complication and seldom demonstrated on radiography.

  Malposition can include intra- or extravascular placement. An unexpected intravascular course such as a subclavian catheter coursing into the jugular vein or a jugular catheter coursing into a subclavian vein may be seen. Advancement into an artery rather than a vein occasionally occurs but is usually clinically evident. A catheter may enter the internal thoracic vein and be seen adjacent to the anterior chest wall on a lateral examination (Fig. 11-4) or follow the left side of the mediastinum in patients with a persistent left superior vena cava (SVC).

  For typical applications, the tip should be within the SVC. Intentional catheter placement within the right atrium for maximum dilution is no longer considered prudent since it can incite arrhythmias and rarely perforation with resultant hemopericardium and tamponade.

  Catheters can inadvertently be withdrawn outside the vessel and into cutaneous tissues. Less commonly, a catheter can perforate venous structures, resulting in hemorrhage and infusion of material into the mediastinum, neck, or supraclavicular regions. Mediastinal widening is a late finding. Treatment is typically conservative, with catheter removal without attempted aspiration of the extravasated fluid. When perforation occurs in the SVC below the azygos vein, hemopericardium and tamponade can occur.

  A catheter directed against the vessel wall should be repositioned. This is most commonly encountered with CVLs entering into the left brachiocephalic vessel. Before turning into the SVC, the catheter tip may be directed against the lateral wall of the SVC (Fig. 11-5). Respiratory motion, cardiac pulsations, and head movements can lead to recurrent impingement of the catheter tip against the SVC wall, increasing the risk of venous perforation.

  For standard chest radiographs, patients are positioned with their arms to the side for the posteroanterior (PA) radiograph, and over their head for the lateral examination. Thus, intravascular distance and the course of the catheter can vary. In particular, the catheter tip often appears lower on the lateral than on the PA examination.

- **Pulmonary artery catheters**, often termed Swan-Ganz catheters and discussed in Section 1.7, are used for pressure, oxygenation, and cardiac output measurements. The catheter tip should be in a lower lobe pulmonary artery, at or below the level of the left atrium, to provide accurate pressure measurements (Fig. 11-6). Complications include malposition (Fig. 11-7) and distal advancement where balloon occlusion can lead to infarction. Balloon overinflation can lead to pulmonary artery rupture or pseudoaneurysm, which may appear as a focal opacity. As with other CVLs, an immediate postplacement radiograph is warranted to evaluate position and complications.

- **Peripherally introduced central catheters (PICCs)** are typically 3 or 4 French in size and are introduced through a brachial or antecubital vein. The catheter should pass into the

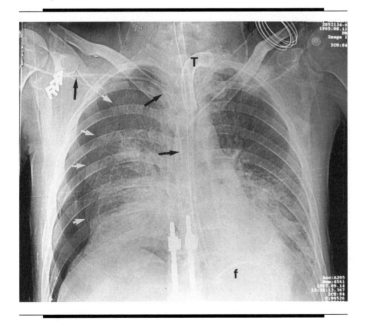

FIGURE 11-3 Pneumothorax following central venous catheter insertion. Portable chest radiograph immediately following placement of a right subclavian central venous catheter (black arrows) showing a large right pneumothorax (white arrows) which was symptomatic requiring thoracostomy tube drainage. Note also tracheotomy (T), nasogastric tube and weighted tip of feeding tube (f) in stomach.

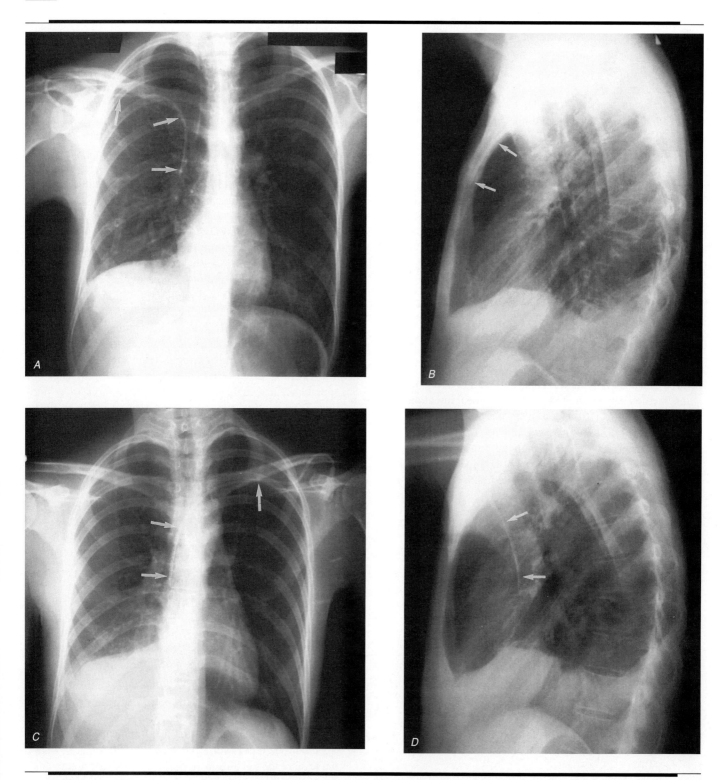

FIGURE 11-4   Central venous catheter entering internal thoracic vein. (*A*) PA chest radiograph showing a central venous catheter (arrows) entering the right subclavian vein. The tip is more lateral than expected for the SVC. (*B*) Lateral chest radiograph showing the catheter adjacent to the anterior chest wall (arrows). (*C* and *D*) Properly positioned central venous catheter entering the left subclavian vein and SVC in the same patient.

subclavian and brachiocephalic veins and subsequently into the SVC. Catheters can be difficult to visualize on conventional chest radiographs. Confident identification is improved by placing the patient in a 15-degree left anterior oblique

(LAO) projection, which moves the SVC off the spine, and using a 70-kVp technique to increase subject contrast. Malposition includes entry into the right heart, coiling or kinking in a vessel, or an aberrant course.

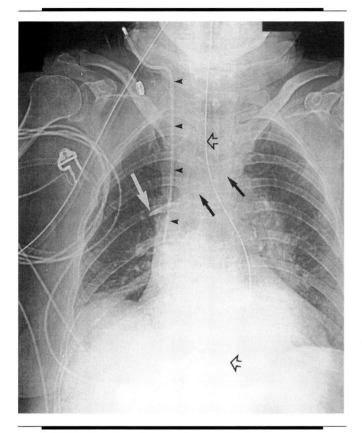

FIGURE 11-5 Poor dialysis catheter positioning. Portable chest radiograph showing a large left subclavian central venous catheter (black arrows) coursing down the left brachiocephalic vein with the tip (white arrow) directed toward the lateral wall of the SVC. This positioning increases the risk of venous perforation. Note the right internal jugular central venous catheter (arrowheads) with the tip in the lower SVC and the nasogastric tube (open arrows).

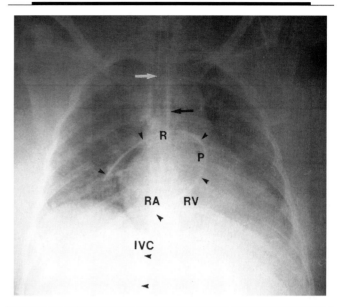

FIGURE 11-6 Pulmonary artery catheter. Portable chest radiograph in a man who sustained severe burns to the torso and left upper extremity. Note staples affixing skin grafts over left hemithorax. There is a pulmonary artery catheter (arrowheads) entering from the inferior vena cava (IVC), passing through the right atrium (RA), right ventricle (RV), pulmonary trunk (P), and right pulmonary artery (R) with the tip in the right interlobar pulmonary artery. Note ETT (white arrow) and feeding tube (black arrow).

of the French size. A 24 French tube is 8 mm in diameter. They have multiple sideholes. A radiopaque stripe with a single interruption indicates the location of the most proximal side port.

- **Subcutaneous reservoir-type catheters**, for example, Port-a-Cath and Infuse-a-Port, are placed in ambulatory patients requiring long-term intermittent infusions, typically chemotherapy. The entire device is internal. The reservoir is placed in subcutaneous tissue, and the catheter enters the central circulation via the subclavian vein or occasionally the jugular vein. These devices can be metallic or plastic and vary in opacity (Fig. 11-8).

  The ports are accessed with a Huber needle with a noncoring tip and a 90-degree bend. The thick membrane overlying the port can be accessed thousands of times, and the port can be used for years. Complications include separation of the catheter and reservoir, catheter fracture (typically between the first rib and clavicle), thrombosis of the reservoir or catheter, venous perforation, and fibrous sheath occlusion. Intravenous contrast injection can be valuable in assessing malfunction.

- **Thoracostomy tubes** (chest tubes) of various sizes are used for drainage of pleural effusions, empyemas, and pneumothoraces. They range from small 9 French angiocath-type devices to larger-bore 30 French standard thoracostomy tubes. The diameter of a tube in millimeters is one-third that

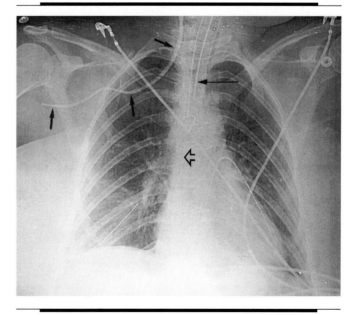

FIGURE 11-7 Pulmonary artery catheter malposition. Portable chest radiograph shows a sheath and aberrantly positioned catheter (arrows) entering the right jugular, subclavian, and then axillary vein. Note also ETT (long arrow), nasogastric tube (open arrow) and bilateral chest tubes.

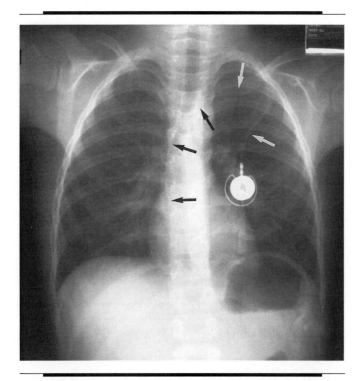

FIGURE 11-8 Subcutaneous reservoir-type catheter. Chest radiograph showing a metallic reservoir implanted in the anterior chest wall and a catheter (arrows) entering the subclavian vein with the tip in the lower SVC.

Tubes are typically directed toward the anterior lung apex for treatment of pneumothorax, and into the posterior costophrenic angle for drainage of effusions. A malpositioned tube can be outside the pleural space, within the chest wall or under the diaphragm, puncture the visceral pleura and enter the lung, lie within a fissure, or push up against mediastinal structures (Figs. 11-9 and 11-10).

A standard examination is required to confidently determine the location of a thoracostomy tube. Computed tomography (CT) is sometimes required in complex cases.

Development of subcutaneous emphysema is frequent, particularly when a persistent air leak or bronchopleural fistula is present. Inadvertent withdrawal of the chest tube ports outside the pleural space can produce significant subcutaneous emphysema and recurrent pneumothorax.

- Most portable examinations have some overlying artifacts, and cardiac monitoring leads are the most common. Other catheters and lines seen on postoperative films include **left atrial lines**, which are small catheters placed in the atria for direct pressure monitoring following surgery (Fig. 11-11). **Temporary pacing leads** are small, thin wires hooked into the epicardial surface to allow pacing of arrhythmias during the immediate postoperative period. They are removed simply by pulling them through the incision site. Complications can include breakage with a fragment remaining and bleeding, but this is rare.

Mediastinal drains are often placed following cardiac surgery. They are simply conventional thoracostomy tubes placed in a mediastinal location and exiting through a subxiphoid incision. **Pericardial drains** are positioned on the

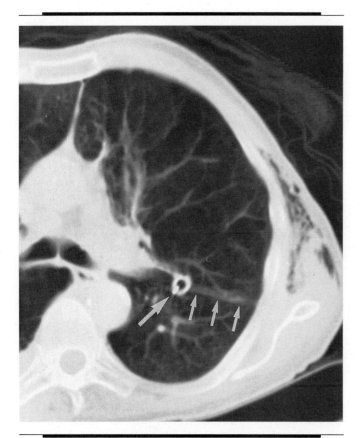

FIGURE 11-9   Chest tube malposition. Chest CT showing a chest tube (large arrow) entering the major fissure (small arrows). Note small amount of subcutaneous emphysema.

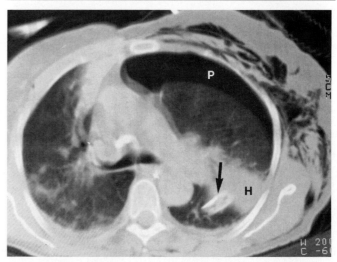

FIGURE 11-10   Chest tube entering lung. Chest CT showing a persistent pneumothorax (P) and subcutaneous emphysema following emergent placement of a thoracostomy tube for a tension pneumothorax caused by mechanical ventilation. Note the chest tube (arrow) entering the lung with a resultant hematoma (H). (With permission from Slone RM, Gierada DS. Pleura, chest wall, and diaphragm. In Lee JKT, Sagel SS, Stanley RJ, Heiken JP, eds. *Computed Body Tomography with MRI Correlation*, 3rd ed. New York: Lippincott-Raven, 1998.)

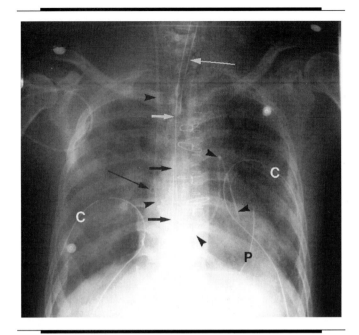

FIGURE 11-11   Catheters following cardiac surgery. Portable chest radiograph showing bilateral chest tubes (C), a pericardial drain (P), a pulmonary artery catheter (arrowheads) in the left lower lobe pulmonary artery, a nasogastric tube (white arrow), an ETT (long white arrow), a mediastinal drain (black arrows), and a left atrial catheter (long black arrow). Note also sternal wires and skin staples in midline.

inferior surface of the heart. **Jackson Pratt (JP) drains** are often used for subcutaneous and intra-abdominal drainage. They are rectangular in cross section with multiple side holes. They connect to a compressed bulb that provides suction. A **Penrose drain** is a thin, flat, latex strap that provides a large potential space for direct drainage to the skin.

- Both transvenous and cutaneous **temporary pacing leads** are available. A temporary transvenous pacer can be differentiated from a catheter by the metallic tip. Ideally they are positioned with the tip in the right ventricular apex, similar to the placement of a conventional pacemaker lead. Zoll transcutaneous pacemaker and defibrillating pads are often seen overlying the chest in patients recently transferred to the cardiac ICU. A metallic lead and wire can be seen attached to the patch. The pads are typically about 10 cm in size and have irregular contours.

- **Extracorporal membrane oxygenation (ECMO),** used most often in infants, is performed to provide gas exchange and allow the lungs to recover in cases of severe pulmonary injury and hypoxemia. Large catheters are placed in central arteries and veins, often the right common carotid artery and SVC in infants, and the blood circulated to an external oxygenation device.

- **Tracheostomy** is often performed in patients requiring prolonged intubation. Dissection is made through the subcutaneous tissues and anterior tracheal wall below the thyroid cartilage. A variety of plastic and metallic tracheostomy

appliances are used. Sometimes a **mini-tracheostomy** is performed between the cricoid and thyroid cartilage and a small lumen device placed to allow suctioning in hospitalized patients.

- **Intra-aortic balloon pumps (IABP)** assist cardiac function in patients with left ventricular failure following cardiac surgery, cardiogenic shock following myocardial infarction, or other low-output cardiac disease. They are inserted via the femoral artery with the tip in the proximal descending thoracic aorta just beyond the left subclavian artery. The catheter tip is radiopaque, although the remainder of the catheter often cannot be visualized (Fig. 11-12). If the IABP is positioned too high, blood flow in the great vessels may be compromised. If it is positioned too low, renal or mesenteric blood flow may be compromised. The tip should be between the aortic arch and carina.

  The balloon inflates during diastole to increase diastolic pressure in the proximal aorta and improve coronary blood flow. The balloon is deflated during systole to reduce afterload. Contraindications include aortic dissection, severe aorto-iliac disease which precludes instrumenting the femoral artery, and aortic insufficiency which would worsen with inflation of the balloon. Complications include lower extremity ischemia, necrosis and perforation.

- A **left ventricular assist device (LVAD)** is a partial bypass circuit which withdraws blood from the left atrium, transfers it to a vortex pump, and returns it to the aorta. The LVAD is positioned with a venous return line in the left atrium via the right superior pulmonary vein and is designed to support a stunned heart which will eventually recover or to provide

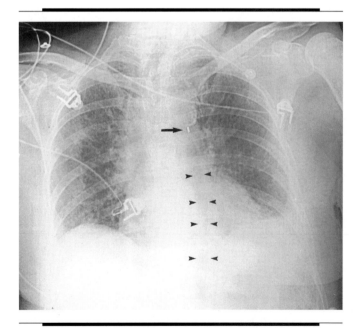

FIGURE 11-12   Aortic balloon pump. Portable chest radiograph showing the radiopaque marker (arrow) at the end of the balloon pump in the proximal descending thoracic aorta just below some atherosclerotic calcifications in the aortic arch. Note the column of gas within the inflated balloon (arrowheads) seen during diastole.

a "bridge" to transplantation. A biventricular assist device (BVAD) provides support to both the right and left heart.

- **Permanently implanted devices**, including cardiac pacemakers, defibrillators, cardiac valves, stents, and orthopedic devices are discussed in Chapter 12.

11.2 SURGICAL INCISIONS AND THORACOSCOPY

- A wide variety of incisions have been developed to gain access to the chest and minimize morbidity. Skin staples are now used almost exclusively in place of sutures. They are typically left in place for 1 to 2 weeks and make the location of the incision readily apparent on postoperative examinations.

- A **median sternotomy** is the most common thoracic incision and is the incision of choice for cardiac operations. It is also used for anterior mediastinal lesions and some bilateral pulmonary procedures. The incision extends from the suprasternal notch to below the xyphoid. The pectoral fascia and interclavicular ligament are divided, and the manubrium is sawed longitudinally.

  Closure is typically performed with four to seven parasternal stainless steel wires. Supplemental wires can be woven between costal cartilage along the side of the sternum if there is significant osteopenia or if sternal fracture develops during surgery. The pectoral fascia and linea alba are sutured. Fluid and inflammatory changes are normally seen in the anterior mediastinum and adjacent soft tissues for several weeks. Air can remain in the mediastinal soft tissues for up to 1 week.

  Wound dehiscence and mediastinitis are uncommon, but carry a high morbidity and mortality. Management includes antibiotics, drainage, and surgical debridement. Chest radiographs are insensitive and nonspecific, and CT is necessary to detect the location of fluid collections and the extent of inflammation. Aspiration may be needed to determine whether collections are infected. Occasionally, months or years after a sternotomy, a patient reports chest pain due to a chronic sternal infection. Fracture of sternal wires can occur years following a sternotomy and is usually inconsequential but may warrant removal of the wires if soft tissue irritation persists.

- A **posterolateral thoracotomy** is the most common incision used for pulmonary surgery. It is performed with the patient in a lateral decubitus position. The incision is typically made through the fifth intercostal space, extending from the anterior axillary line, under the tip of the scapula, and then cephalad between the medial border of the scapula and the spine. The latissimus dorsi muscle is divided, and occasionally portions of the rhomboid, serratus anterior, and trapezius muscles are divided as well. The intercostal muscles and parietal pleura are subsequently incised.

  In the past, long sections of rib were routinely resected, but this is no longer considered necessary in every thoracotomy. The rib is almost always sectioned in patients over 40 years old to decrease the incidence of rib fracture, yet the operation

can be performed through the interspace without transecting a rib. In such cases postoperative films typically show a widened intercostal space.

- An **axillary thoracotomy**, also referred to as a mini thoracotomy, muscle-sparing thoracotomy, or lateral thoracotomy, is performed via dissection between the serratus anterior and latissimus dorsi. The potential benefits of reduced operative time, decreased blood loss from muscle transection, and improved patient comfort postoperatively are balanced with the decreased visibility and maneuverability that this lesser incision allows.

- An **anterior thoracotomy** (Chamberlin procedure) is occasionally used for open lung biopsy, esophageal surgery, and anterior mediastinal and AP window biopsies inaccessible via mediastinoscopy. The incision extends through the fourth or fifth intercostal space from the midaxillary line to a parasternal location.

- A **transverse thoracosternotomy**, sometimes referred to as the "cross-bow" or "clamshell" incision, extends from the left to the right anterior axillary line in the fourth intercostal space. The incision may pass through the sternum or around the sternum through the costal cartilage. It allows access to the heart and hila and is performed primarily for bilateral lung transplantation. It is occasionally used for emergent traumatic cardiac surgery or bilateral thoracic surgical procedures such as resection of pulmonary metastases.

- A **thoracoabdominal incision** is performed to obtain extended exposure for operations in the lower thorax and upper abdomen such as lower esophageal surgery or repair of a thoracoabdominal aneurysm.

- A **cervical** or **suprasternal incision**, running transversely above the manubrium, is used for mediastinoscopy, thymus resections, and occasionally, resection of anterior mediastinal masses and is discussed in Section 1.7.

- **Video-assisted thoracic surgery (VATS)**, sometimes called thoracoscopy, allows less invasive thoracic procedures to be performed. A double-lumen endotracheal tube with single-lung ventilation and ipsilateral lung collapse permit adequate visualization of the lung, pleura, and mediastinum. Three to five small intercostal incisions allow placement of the video camera and instruments. VATS is contraindicated in patients with hilar or deep parenchymal lung lesions, ventilator-dependent, or who have dense pleural adhesions. Disadvantages include difficulty in controlling unexpected major bleeding and the necessity for single-lung ventilation.

  Diagnostic indications include evaluation of indeterminate pleural effusions and biopsy to obtain tissue diagnosis of pleural and peripheral pulmonary lesions. VATS is an alternative to mediastinoscopy for evaluating anterior mediastinal lymph nodes or masses. **Therapeutic** indications include pleural, pulmonary, esophageal, and mediastinal resections; management of pleural effusions; dorsal sympathectomy; apical bleb resection; and pleural abrasion in patients with recurrent spontaneous pneumothoraces.

11.3 THORACIC SURGERY

- **Pulmonary resections** range in extent from wedge resection of small peripheral lesions to complete extrapleural pneumonectomy for mesothelioma. Excisions for malignancy may be extended to include portions of the chest wall, pericardium, diaphragm, or adjacent vascular structures. Postoperative chest radiographs can be confusing, and an accurate interpretation is enhanced by an understanding of the surgical procedure performed.

- **Automated stapling instruments**, which simultaneously deploy several rows of staples, are used to perform partial lung resections as well as to separate incomplete fissures during lobectomy. Stapling instruments are also employed to close bronchial stumps, and to divide and secure blood vessels. Stapling is simpler and faster than manual suturing and produces a symmetric, precise, uniform closure which minimizes inflammation and improves closure strength. There is reduced risk of bronchopleural fistula, aspiration, or contamination of the operative field. Current models deploy titanium staples which minimize artifacts on CT and magnetic resonance imaging (MR) examinations.

- **Hemoclips** are individual metal clips used to control small bleeding vessels such as bronchial branches when dissecting around the hilum.

- A **pneumonectomy** is typically performed through a posterolateral thoracotomy for treatment of bronchogenic carcinoma and occasionally of extensive inflammatory disease such as bronchiectasis or large abscesses. A right pneumonectomy requires separate ligation of the right anterior truncus and descending pulmonary arteries. A single arterial ligature is used on the left. The superior and inferior pulmonary veins are ligated, and the inferior pulmonary ligament is transected. The bronchus is often secured with staples, which are quicker than suturing and may provide more uniform compression and better healing. A tissue flap is frequently placed over the bronchial stump to minimize risk of dehiscence.

  The postpneumonectomy pleural space slowly accumulates serosanguinous fluid, and an air-fluid level may persist for months. The volume of the air component should continually decrease. Any increase in the air volume signals the development of bronchial dehiscence (bronchopleural fistula). Eventually, the space completely fills with fluid and decreases in size as fluid is resorbed. In most patients some fluid remains and becomes organized, but the transverse diameter of the collection is typically less than 5 cm. The hemithorax decreases in size with inward displacement of the chest wall. The remaining volume is filled by the shifted mediastinum and hyperinflated contralateral lung (Fig. 11-13).

- Following **left pneumonectomy**, the mediastinum shifts so that the usual anteroposterior orientation of the aortic arch is maintained. The right lung may herniate posteriorly or anteriorly. Following **right pneumonectomy**, the mediastinum rotates, with a resultant transverse orientation of the aortic arch, and the left lung herniates anteriorly. In general, the smaller the pneumonectomy space, the greater the herniation.

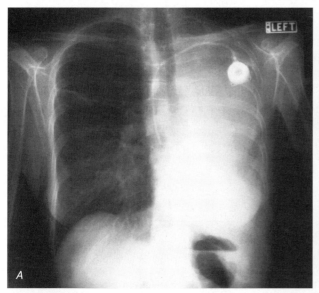 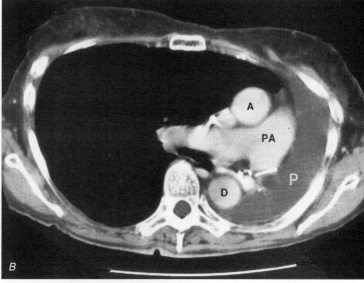

FIGURE 11-13   Left pneumonectomy. (*A*) PA chest radiograph showing complete opacification of the left hemithorax with ipsilateral shift of the mediastinum including the heart and trachea. Note the reservoir port for chemotherapy. (*B*) CT showing a small, normal amount of fluid remaining in the postpneumonectomy space (P). Note staples in the left hilum remaining from the dissection and transection of the left main bronchus and pulmonary veins. The right lung is hyperinflated and herniated anterior to the mediastinum. PA, pulmonary artery; A, ascending aorta; D, descending aorta.

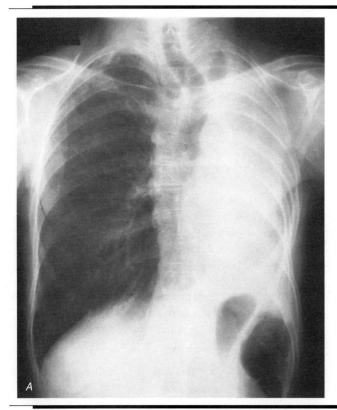
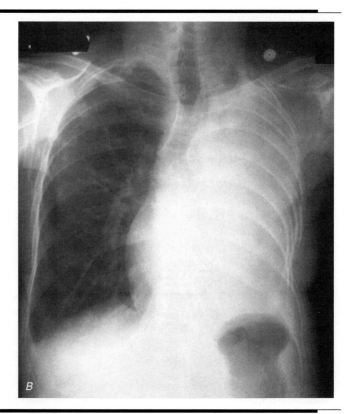

FIGURE 11-14   Recurrent cancer following left pneumonectomy. (*A*) Chest radiograph obtained following a left pneumonectomy for bronchogenic carcinoma. Note normal opacification of the left hemithorax with ipsilateral shift of the heart and trachea. (*B*) Chest radiograph obtained 6 months later showing contralateral shift of the heart and movement of trachea back to the midline with a larger opaque area in the left hemithorax. CT demonstrated recurrent bronchogenic carcinoma within the pneumonectomy space. The patient was subsequently treated with radiation therapy.

Opacification of the hemithorax makes radiographic evaluation of new or recurrent disease in the pneumonectomy space or mediastinum difficult until mediastinal shift occurs (Fig. 11-14). CT is much more sensitive than radiographs for detecting recurrence (Fig. 11-15).

- An **extrapleural pneumonectomy** involves removal of the entire lung, the pleural space, and the parietal pleura and is performed for treatment of mesothelioma and tumors with extensive pleural involvement. **Completion pneumonectomy** refers to removal of remaining lung tissue following prior partial resection. Morbidity approaches 40 percent, and operative mortality is approximately 10 percent compared to 6 percent for a pneumonectomy, 3 percent for a lobectomy, and 1 percent for a wedge resection. Mortality is generally higher for a repeat operation than for the original procedure.

- A **lobectomy** is frequently performed through a posterolateral thoracotomy, with the patient on his or her side. The hilum must be dissected to allow visualization and ligation of the necessary arteries, veins, and bronchus. The artery is ligated, but the vein and bronchus can be stapled. The fissures are often incomplete and must be dissected to allow resection.

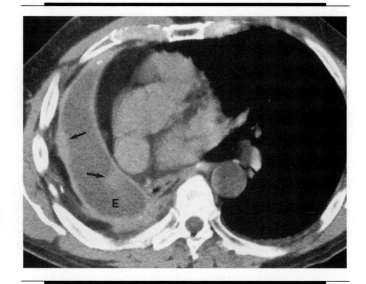

FIGURE 11-15   Recurrent bronchogenic carcinoma. Contrast-enhanced chest CT following right pneumonectomy for bronchogenic carcinoma. There is irregular nodular pleural enhancement (arrows) characteristic of pleural seeding by tumor and a malignant pleural effusion (E).

The fissure is usually completed with a stapler, leaving a chain of staples on the side of the fissure which is to remain in the chest.

The inferior pulmonary ligament is severed during a lower lobectomy to remove the lobe, and during an upper lobectomy to mobilize the lower lobe to fill the pleural space. With expansion of the remaining lung, elevation of the hemidiaphragm, and ipsilateral shift of the mediastinum, the lobectomy space is usually obliterated within 1 week. The radiologic appearance of the various lobectomies is similar to the pattern seen with lobar collapse (Figs. 3-43 to 3-50 and Fig. 11-16).

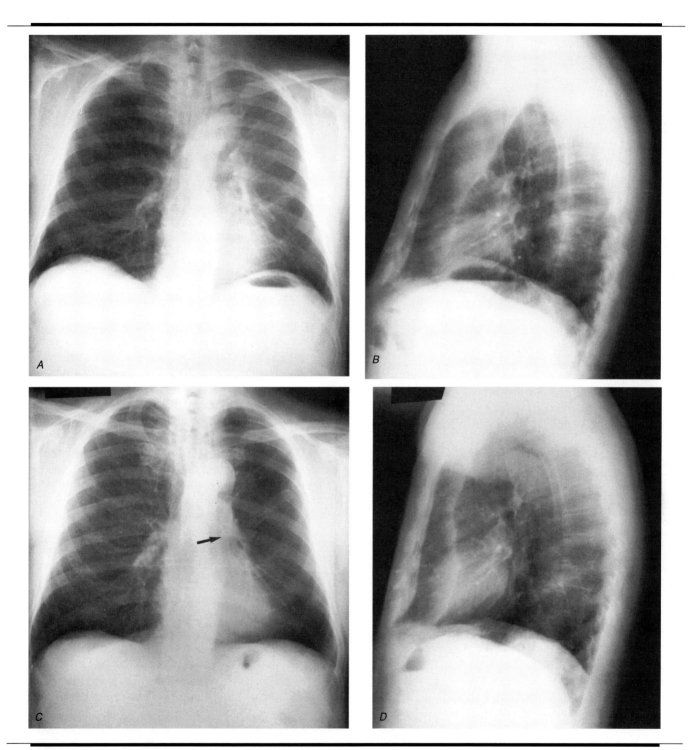

FIGURE 11-16   Cancer causing left upper lobe collapse treated with lobectomy. (*A*) PA chest radiograph showing increased opacity of the left hemithorax with volume loss. (*B*) Lateral radiograph showing a retrosternal opacity characteristic of left upper lobe collapse. (*C* and *D*) PA and lateral examination 6 months following left upper lobectomy showing left hilar staples and hemoclips (arrow) and evidence of a left thoracotomy. Note how similar the findings of lobectomy and collapse are.

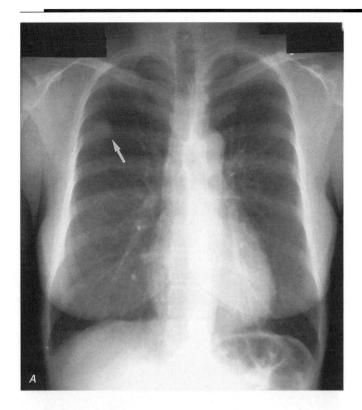

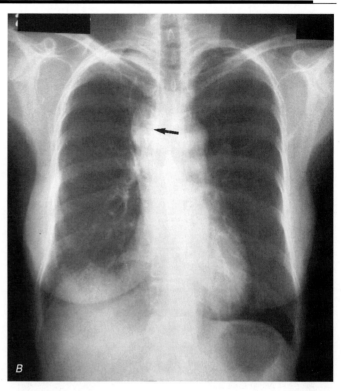

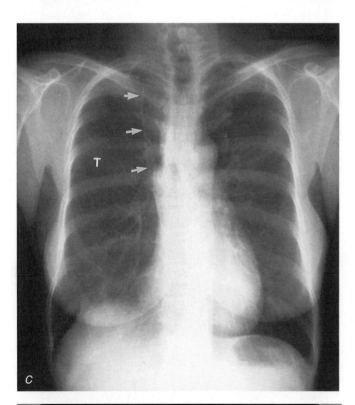

FIGURE 11-17   Right upper lobectomy. (*A*) Preoperative chest radiograph showing a 2-cm bronchoalveolar cell carcinoma in the right upper lobe (arrow). (*B*) Examination 2 weeks following surgery showing a small paramediastinal hematoma (arrow). (*C*) Six months later the hematoma has completely resolved. Note ipsilateral volume loss, widening of the sixth interspace following thoracotomy (T), and a staple line representing completion of the major fissure (arrows).

- **A right upper lobectomy** is typically performed through a posterolateral thoracotomy in the fourth or fifth intercostal space. The hilum is dissected, and the segmental arteries ligated. Hemoclips are often used to secure small vessels. The upper lobe branches of the superior pulmonary vein are divided, taking care not to impinge on the middle lobe branch. The minor fissure and superior portion of the major fissure are divided if they are incomplete, usually with a stapling instrument (Figs. 11.17 and 11.18). If the inferior portion of the major fissure is complete, the lower and middle lobe can be stapled together to prevent middle lobe volvulus. The inferior pulmonary ligament is divided to mobilize the lower lobe. The right upper lobe bronchus is typically divided using a stapling instrument. The right upper lobe has now been completely mobilized and can be removed. The chest is irrigated, chest tubes are placed, and the thoracotomy is closed.

- A **right middle lobectomy** is the lobectomy least commonly performed. The right middle lobe is more often removed along with either the upper or lower lobe because disease has crossed a fissure or involves the hilum. It is carried out through the fifth intercostal space with either a posterolateral or anterolateral thoracotomy. It requires transection of the middle lobe arteries arising from the descending pulmonary artery and the middle lobe veins which join the superior pulmonary vein. These vessels are usually ligated with suture, but the vein is occasionally stapled. The middle lobe bronchus is usually divided with a stapling instrument, taking care not to impinge on the bronchus intermedius. The minor fissure is rarely complete and usually divided using a stapling

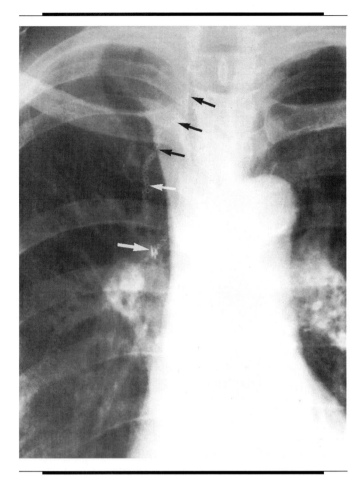

FIGURE 11-18   Right upper lobectomy. Chest radiograph showing a row of surgical staples (small arrows) representing completion of the superior portion of the major fissure. The minor fissure was complete. The upper lobe bronchus was transected (large white arrow) using a stapling instrument. The arteries and veins were ligated with suture.

instrument. If necessary, the major fissure between the middle and lower lobes is also completed with a stapling instrument. Hemoclips are often used to secure small hilar vessels.

- A **right lower lobectomy** is usually performed through a posterolateral thoracotomy in the fifth or sixth intercostal space or through the bed of the sixth rib. The inferior pulmonary vein can be ligated but is more frequently stapled. The lower lobe pulmonary artery branches are ligated, including the superior segment branch. The inferior portion of the major fissure is completed, taking care not to staple the middle lobe vein. The superior portion of the major fissure is divided with a stapling instrument. Stapling the bronchus can be difficult because of the close proximity of the superior segment and middle lobe bronchi, and occasionally both the middle and lower lobes must be taken. The inferior pulmonary ligament is divided, and hemoclips are used for hemostasis. If the minor fissure is complete, the middle lobe can be secured to the upper lobe with staples to prevent volvulus.

- A **left upper lobectomy** is performed through a posterolateral thoracotomy in the fourth or fifth intercostal space.

The left upper lobe pulmonary artery and lingular branches are individually ligated, and the superior pulmonary vein stapled. Both the superior and inferior portions of the major fissure may require completion. The upper lobe bronchus is divided with a stapling instrument and the inferior pulmonary ligament is divided to mobilize the lower lobe. Hemoclips are used to secure small vessels around the hilum and pulmonary ligament (Fig. 11-19).

- A **left lower lobectomy** is usually performed through a posterolateral thoracotomy in the fifth or sixth intercostal space or through the bed of the sixth rib. The superior and basal segmental arteries are individually ligated, and the inferior pulmonary vein ligated or secured with a vascular stapling instrument. The superior and inferior portions of the major fissure usually require completion. The lower lobe bronchus is divided with a stapling instrument and the inferior pulmonary ligament is divided. Hemoclips are often used to secure small vessels around the hilum and in the pulmonary ligament (Fig. 11-20).

- A **segmentectomy** is most frequently performed for removal of the superior segment of the lower lobe or resection of the

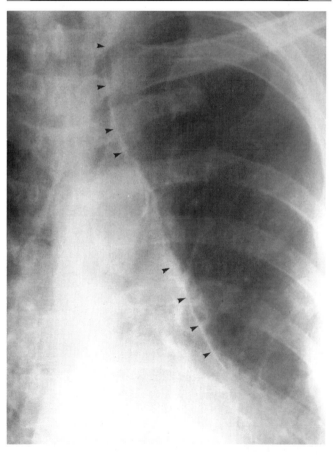

FIGURE 11-19   Left upper lobectomy. Chest radiograph showing a row of surgical staples (arrowheads) representing completion of the major fissure with a stapler. The bronchus and vessels were ligated with suture.

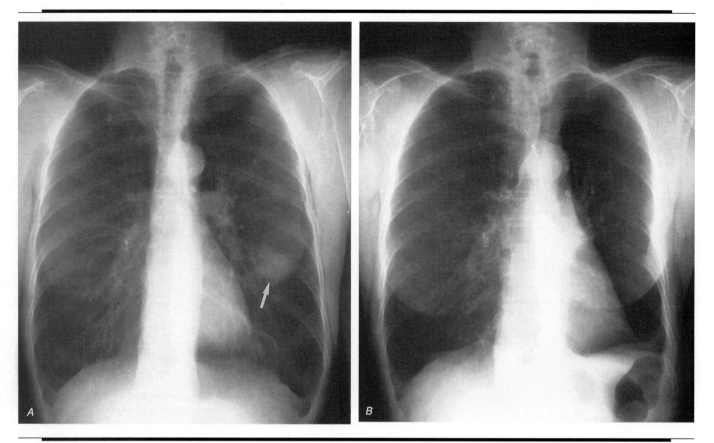

FIGURE 11-20   Left lower lobectomy. (*A*) Preoperative chest radiograph showing a 3-cm squamous cell carcinoma (arrow) in the left lower lobe. (*B*) Follow-up examination 1 year after surgery showing left-sided volume loss with ipsilateral mediastinal shift and upward displacement of the diaphragm. Note hemoclips and downward displacement of left hilum.

lingula. A segmentectomy is seldom performed in the right upper or middle lobe. The basal segments can be resected from either lower lobe. On the left, an apicoposterior segmentectomy can be performed, sparing the anterior and lingular segments of the left upper lobe; likewise, a left anterior segmentectomy or lingular segmentectomy can be performed.

- A **bronchial sleeve resection**, or **bronchoplasty**, is the segmental resection of a bronchial orifice with primary reanastomosis of the transected bronchial segments. This procedure can be considered when tumor involves the junction of the right upper lobe and main bronchus, middle lobe and bronchus intermedius, or left upper and main bronchus. For example, a lesion arising at the orifice of the right upper lobe bronchus can be resected and the bronchus intermedius anastomosed to the right main bronchus, thus obviating a pneumonectomy. Bronchial sleeve resection is an excellent option in patients with T2 and T3 lung cancer and provides superior functional results and survival equivalent to pneumonectomy.

- **Inoperable tumor invasion** obstructing the central tracheobronchial tree is sometimes managed with **laser surgery** or endoluminal **stents**. The yttrium-aluminum-garnet (YAG) laser, in combination with a rigid bronchoscope and general anesthesia, can be used to core out inoperable airway obstruction caused by tumor. A laser can also be used to treat

patients with inflammatory disease such as Wegener granulomatosis producing tracheal, bronchial, or subglottic stenosis. Endobronchial stents, further discussed in Section 12.5, can be used to improve bronchiol patency in malignant and benign conditions including bronchial anastomatic structures following transplantation, Wegeners, primary and secondary tumors, and relapsing polychondritis.

- **Decortication of the lung** consists of removing a restrictive fibrous membrane of tissue from the pleural surface of the lung to treat fibrothorax resulting from an organized hemothorax or empyema. Layers can also be removed from the chest wall and diaphragm. The procedure is designed to free the "trapped" lung, allow reexpansion, obliterate the pleural space, and preserve pulmonary function.

- A **pleural tent** or pleural partition is occasionally indicated to reduce the size of the postlobectomy space when insufficient lung volume remains to fill the pleural space, particularly after an upper lobectomy. The procedure involves dissection of the parietal pleura away from the chest wall to drape over the visceral pleura, creating an extrapleural space and obliterating the pleural space (Fig. 11-21).

  The opposition of the visceral and parietal pleura is felt to reduce the time needed for the sealing of parenchymal air leaks and thus decrease the time to chest tube removal.

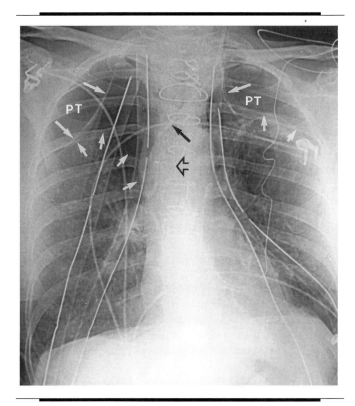

FIGURE 11-21 Bilateral pleural tents following LVRS.
Portable chest radiograph on postoperative day 1 shows dissection of the parietal pleura away from the chest wall (large white arrows) and extrapleural air collections (PT). There are small bilateral pneumothoraces, allowing visualization of the visceral pleura (small arrows). Note chest tubes in the space between the pleural surfaces, central venous catheter (black arrow), and epidural catheter (open arrow) for pain management.

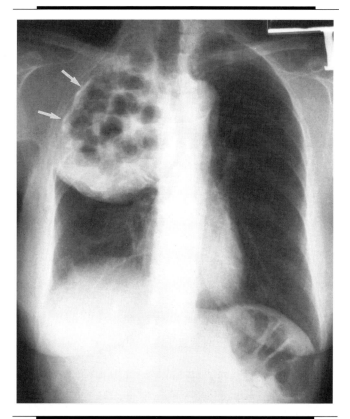

FIGURE 11-22 Plombage. Chest radiograph showing multiple Lucite balls, some with fluid levels, filling the right upper chest. Note thick pleural calcifications (arrows) characteristic of a prior tuberculous empyema.

Although this new extrapleural space is initially air-filled, fluid soon accumulates and then is resorbed, retracting the pleura back toward the chest wall. If the remaining lung is unable to further expand, the extrapleural fluid within the tent organizes, otherwise the fluid is resorbed and only focal pleural thickening remains. Similarly, a therapeutic postoperative pneumoperitoneum to reduce the volume of the ipsilateral hemithorax following lower lobectomy has been advocated.

- **Thoracic outlet syndrome** is the result of compression of the lower nerve roots of the brachial plexus or, less commonly, compression of the subclavian vessels in the thoracic apex. A common cause is a cervical rib, occurring in one-third of patients with the syndrome. A rudimentary, fractured, or bifid first rib, or fusion of the first and second ribs, or a clavicular deformity can also cause symptoms. Surgical management involves resection of the first rib and dissection of the brachial plexus to decompress the soft tissues.

- **Plombage** refers to the placement of oil, wax, Lucite balls, or other space-occupying material in the pleural space to partially collapse the lung. This technique was developed for the treatment of tuberculosis, but its use has largely been abandoned except in rare circumstances (Fig. 11-22).

- **Thoracoplasty** refers to surgical resection or collapse of the skeletal support of the chest wall to reduce the hemithoracic volume and collapse the underlying lung or empty space. This procedure was developed for the treatment of tuberculosis and was based on the premise that collapsing the lung would prevent the growth of infectious organisms. The only current indication is for chronic empyema with excessive dead space (Fig. 8-6).

- Occasionally, in particularly symptomatic patients, a **pectus excavatum** deformity of the chest wall is repaired. The costal cartilages are transected and shortened, and the sternum is lifted and often held in place with a metallic strut. The sternocostal cartilage heals with the sternum in the improved position and the strut is subsequently removed.

- Approximately 20 percent of patients with **myasthenia gravis** present with a thymoma which should be resected. In addition, any myasthenic patient can benefit from a total thymectomy if it is done early in the course of the disease. **Median sternotomy** is the approach of choice when a thymectomy is done for thymoma; however, a **transcervical thymectomy**, performed through a suprasternal transverse incision, is a viable alternative for patients with a tiny thymoma or a nonthymomatous gland. Morbidity is lower, and the hospital stay is shorter for transcervical thymectomy

(Fig. 11-23). It may take up to 18 months before full benefit of the operation is obtained; thus patients are maintained on medical therapy that includes Mestinon and corticosteroids.

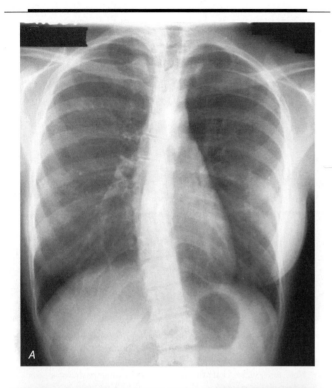

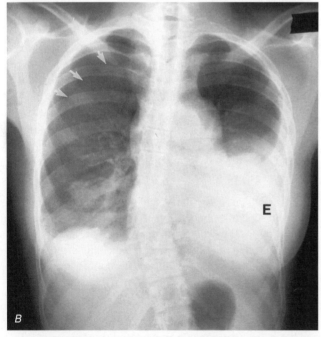

FIGURE 11-23 Transcervical thymectomy. (*A*) Preoperative chest radiograph showing mild thoracic dextroscoliosis. (*B*) Postoperative examination showing widened mediastinum and moderate left pleural effusion (E) secondary to bleeding. Note also right pneumothorax (arrows) and air-fluid level in lung base (hydropneumothorax). Chest radiograph 1 month later showed complete resolution.

- Partial **pericardial resection** is sometimes required to completely remove a lung cancer. Small pericardial defects can be closed by direct suture without causing cardiac compression. Large defects developing after a pneumonectomy pose a danger of cardiac herniation and strangulation at the margin of the defect. This outcome can be prevented on the left by enlarging the defect to the level of the diaphragm, allowing the heart to lie freely within the pleural space without physiologic consequence.

  Following right pneumonectomy, the heart may herniate and rotate, resulting in venous inflow occlusion, engorgement, and rapid death. Right-sided pericardial defects must therefore always be completely repaired. This can be accomplished using bovine pericardium, polypropylene, or a pedicle graft of diaphragm.

- **Complications** of thoracic surgery can be intraoperative or postoperative. The most common **intraoperative** complication is hemorrhage, frequently from the pulmonary artery since it is thin and easily torn. Other intraoperative complications include air embolism, contralateral pneumothorax, and rarely pulmonary embolism, spinal cord injury, or paraplegia.

  Anesthetic complications include arrhythmias, hyper- or hypotension, myocardial infarction, hypoxia, and airway problems. **Postoperative** complications are more common than intraoperative complications. Hemorrhage can be lethal, and bloody chest tube drainage of more than 200 ml/hr for more than 2 hours necessitates reexploration.

  Pulmonary complications include atelectasis, pneumonia, respiratory failure, empyema, bronchopleural fistula, hemothorax, and prolonged air leaks. Atelectasis is most commonly related to retained secretions and poor coughing effort and can lead to hypoxemia and pneumonia. Atelectasis is avoided with excellent pain control (epidural anesthesia) and vigorous respiratory therapy, including chest percussion and drainage. **Pneumonia** occurs in approximately 7 percent of patients and has a 30 percent mortality rate following pneumonectomy. **Empyemas** occur in 3 percent of patients following pneumonectomy and have a 5 percent mortality rate. A bronchopleural fistula may be present. **Chylothorax** occurs in less than 1 percent of patients.

  Cardiac complications are uncommon but are the most likely to cause death. Pulmonary surgery leads to adrenergic activity, increased catecholamines, and hypercoagulability. Hypertension and tachycardia increase the risk of ischemia (4 percent) and myocardial infarction (1 percent). Congestive heart failure (CHF) due to fluid overload is common in the postoperative period. Acute cor pulmonale is very rare. Atrial arrhythmias are quite common (20–30 percent) and more frequent following left-sided surgery.

  Subcutaneous emphysema is commonly present following pulmonary surgery, often secondary to parenchymal air leaks in severely emphysematous lungs. It is usually benign. Sudden massive subcutaneous emphysema suggests a bronchopleural fistula. A **persistent air leak** lasting more than 7 days is more common after upper lobe resections. A pleural tent may help reduce the incidence by apposing visceral and parietal pleura and speeding the closure of visceral leaks.

The left **recurrent laryngeal nerve** can be damaged, leading to aspiration and ineffective cough. This nerve is at highest risk for injury during extrapleural pneumonectomy, esophageal resection, or extensive lymph node dissection. The **phrenic nerve** can also be damaged, more commonly on redo operations. Sometimes the damage is intentional for complete resection of a tumor. In such a case, the diaphragm is often plicated to reduce redundancy.

Esophageal injury is rare and often manifests late as an empyema or a hydropneumothorax on the side of the surgery. Esophageal injuries are more common in cases involving inflammatory disease, extensive lymph node dissections, or resection of a central tumor.

Wound **infections** are rare, although lung surgery is actually a clean/contaminated procedure since the bronchial tree, which is open to the environment, is exposed to the operative field. **Wound dehiscence** is a very rare complication.

- A **bronchopleural fistula** is uncommon now that bronchial closure is routinely performed with stapling devices that provide uniform pressure and closure of the bronchus. The incidence is further reduced when a tissue flap is used. Bronchopleural fistula usually occurs approximately 1 week following surgery. The risk is highest with pneumonectomy, more so on the right side than on the left side. Patients at additional risk include those who receive preoperative radiation therapy, those with diabetes, those with extensive bronchial manipulation during the procedure, or those who require ventilatory assistance postoperatively (Fig. 11-24).

If diagnosed early, reexploration and closing of the stump with pericardial fat, omentum, or intercostal muscle is performed. Delayed detection is often associated with an empyema requiring chest tube drainage followed by an open-window thoracostomy (Clagett window or Eloesser flap) allowing open drainage and irrigation (Fig. 11-25). The window is eventually closed with a muscle flap or omentum.

- **Lobar torsion** with resultant gangrene is the rare complication which is the result of the rotation of a pulmonary lobe on the vascular pedicle. It can occur spontaneously in patients with a freely mobile middle lobe as the result of a complete major and minor fissure but also can occur in the upper or lower lobes. When this condition remains unrecognized, vascular occlusion, infarction, gangrene, and death can occur. To prevent torsion, the middle lobe is sometimes sutured to the remaining lobe following a lobectomy. Suspicion should prompt an immediate bronchoscopy. When confirmed, immediate reexploration is indicated. Lobectomy may be necessary if the lobe is not viable.

- **Complications unique to pneumonectomy** include acute mediastinal shift, postpneumonectomy syndrome, and cardiac herniation. In up to 5 percent of patients, **postpneumonectomy ARDS** may develop 2 to 5 days following pneumonectomy. The cause is unknown but is thought to be related to alterations in the capillary microcirculation and lymphatic drainage. Mortality is 50 percent.

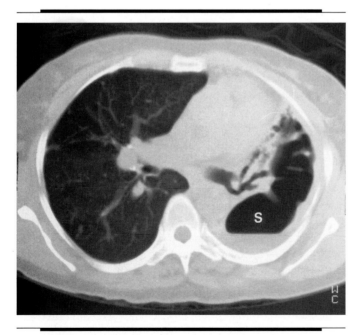

FIGURE 11-24 Bronchopleural fistula with empyema. CT following left upper lobectomy showing bronchi leading to an air-fluid level in the infected postlobectomy space (S). Note volume loss with ipsilateral mediastinal shift following partial pulmonary resection.

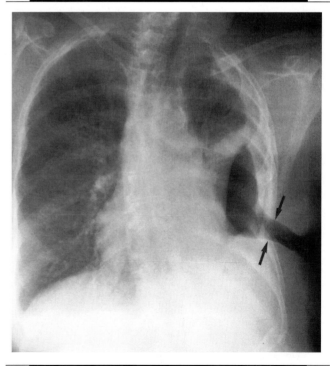

FIGURE 11-25 Claggett window. Chest radiograph demonstrating a surgically created left chest wall defect (arrows) for management of a bronchopleural fistula.

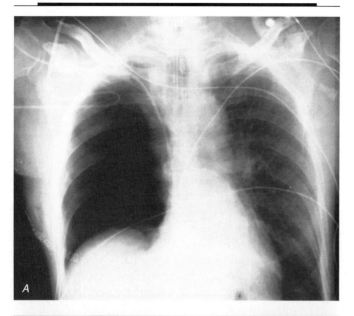

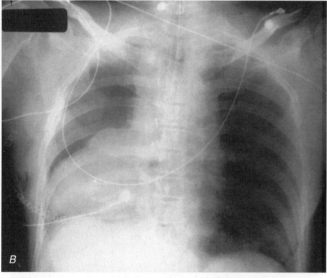

FIGURE 11-26   Cardiac herniation. (*A*) Portable chest radiograph obtained in the recovery room following right pneumonectomy. (*B*) Cardiac arrest occurred when the patient was rolled onto their right side. Radiograph showing heart rotated into the right chest. Immediate median sternotomy and cardiac replacement at the bedside was lifesaving.

Acute mediastinal shift with hypotension, arrhythmias, and respiratory failure following pneumonectomy can be fatal. Mediastinal shift can cause kinking of the SVC, hypotension, and arrhythmias. A tracheal shift impedes respiratory clearance. An inappropriate mediastinal shift following pneumonectomy is typically a self-limited problem and can be controlled with air insufflation into the pneumonectomy space.

Cardiac herniation is a rare, sudden, and frequently fatal complication occurring within 1 day following right pneumonectomy with intrapericardial resection. Herniation into the right chest with the apex of the heart near the right axilla is usually fatal within minutes. Herniation following a left

pneumonectomy is associated with hypotension but is not usually as catastrophic. Emergent reopening of the thoracotomy and repositioning of the heart are required (Fig. 11-26). Prevention includes patching the pericardial defect with pleura, bovine pericardium, diaphragm, or prosthetic material. Enlarging the pericardial opening to avoid cardiac strangulation is an alternative on the left side but not an option on the right side.

Postpneumonectomy syndrome, seen most commonly in children or asthenic adults, refers to dyspnea or recurrent lung infections due to compression of the distal trachea and main bronchus after pneumonectomy. It can occur following a left pneumonectomy in patients with a right-sided aortic arch but is most common after right pneumonectomy. Treatment involves mediastinal repositioning, often with prosthetic spacers such as breast implants.

11.4 TRANSPLANTATION AND EMPHYSEMA SURGERY

- **Pulmonary emphysema** is a severe debilitating disease affecting millions of Americans. Palliative medical management includes bronchodilators, steroids, pulmonary rehabilitation, and supplemental oxygen. A series of surgical procedures have been advocated and subsequently abandoned because of lack of efficacy and risk of an adverse outcome. Procedures currently considered viable options for emphysema management include bullectomy, lung transplantation, and lung volume reduction surgery (LVRS).

- **Radiologic examinations** play an important role in identifying anatomically appropriate candidates. Large bulla, lung compression, and hyperinflation can be evaluated with radiographs. CT demonstrates the severity and distribution of emphysema and may detect unsuspected pleural disease, bronchiectasis, compressed lung simulating a mass, or extensive coronary artery calcification suggesting advanced atherosclerotic disease. CT can also detect small bronchogenic carcinomas seen in 3 to 5 percent of patients. Indeterminate soft tissue nodules can be resected or they can be further evaluated with a transthoracic needle biopsy, positron emission tomography (PET) or serial CT to assess interval growth.

  Nuclear medicine ventilation-perfusion studies provide useful information regarding the relative global and regional distribution of disease. The heterogeneity of perfusion is valuable in selecting the regions for resection in patients selected for LVRS or selecting the less functional lung for single-lung transplantation.

- **Bullectomy** refers to the removal of a large bulla which compresses underlying normal lung. Giant bullae are often well circumscribed and can be removed without destroying nearby normal lung parenchyma. Ventilation-perfusion mismatch, impaired respiratory muscle function due to hyperinflation, and compressed normal lung contribute to pulmonary compromise (Fig. 11-27). Unilateral bullectomy can be per-

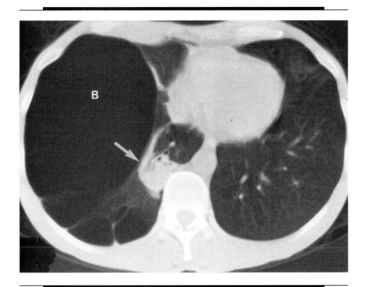

FIGURE 11-27   Bullectomy candidate. CT demonstrating a large bullae (B) compressing adjacent lung and producing a "pseudo-mass" (arrow). Note the relatively normal lung on the left characteristic of paraseptal (distal acinar) emphysema. The mass reexpanded following bullectomy.

formed by limited thoracotomy or VATS while bilateral bullectomy may be done via a median sternotomy. Plication of large bullae or intracavitary suction and drainage are alternative approaches that accomplish similar results with less morbidity.

Unfortunately, isolated large bullae with underlying normal lung parenchyma are an uncommon manifestation of emphysema. Transplantation and LVRS are potential options for critically disabled emphysema patients without giant, discrete bullae suitable for resection.

Lung Volume Reduction Surgery

• **Lung volume reduction surgery (LVRS),** first performed in the 1950s and revived and modified in recent years, involves nonsegmental resection of the most severely emphysematous lung (Fig. 11-28).

Removing lung to improve pulmonary function in a disease characterized by lung destruction seems counterintuitive. Reducing lung volume returns the thorax to a more normal configuration, improves respiratory mechanics, and reduces the work of breathing. Resecting severely emphysematous lung improves $\dot{V}/\dot{Q}$ matching and lung elastic recoil. Patients have improved dyspnea, pulmonary function, gas exchange, and exercise tolerance following surgery. Preoperative pulmonary rehabilitation to improve physical conditioning is an important component of treatment. In some patients, LVRS has palliated patients for years prior to eventual lung transplantation.

Basic clinical indications include severe airflow obstruction due to emphysema, intolerable dyspnea, and exercise intolerance which impairs daily activities despite maximal medical therapy. Testing includes spirometry to measure air

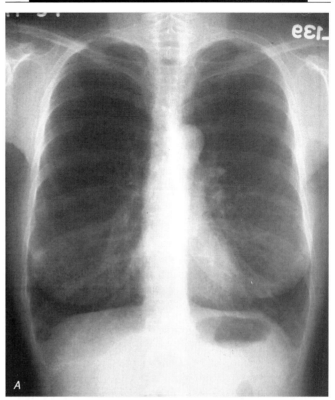

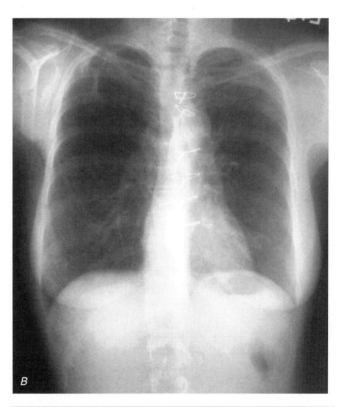

FIGURE 11-28   LVRS. (*A*) Chest radiograph showing advanced pulmonary emphysema with thoracic distention, downward displacement, and flattening of the diaphragm and predominantly upper lobe parenchymal destruction. (*B*) Chest radiograph 6 months following surgery showing return of the chest wall and diaphragm to a more normal configuration. (With permission from Slone RM, Gierada DS. Radiology of emphysema and lung volume reduction surgery. *Semin. Thorac. Cardiovasc. Surg.* 1996;8(1): 61–82.)

flow rates, plethysmography to evaluate lung volumes, arterial blood gas analysis to determine hypoxemia and hypercapnea, and standardized exercise tolerance testing.

- **Radiologic evaluation** including chest radiography, CT, and perfusion scans play a significant role in identifying suitable candidates. Anatomic features associated with the greatest degree of improvement include upper lobe-predominant emphysema, lung compression, regional heterogeneity with "target areas" for surgical resection, hyperinflation, and a satisfactory amount of normal or mildly emphysematous lung. Advanced age, hypercapnea, and lower lobe predominant or severe, diffuse emphysema are poor prognostic factors.

- **Surgical techniques** have included unilateral and bilateral procedures performed by thoracotomy, median sternotomy, and VATS. Staple lines are often buttressed with bovine pericardium to reduce air leaks. A thoracic epidural catheter is placed for pain management. Laser ablation has been shown to be ineffective by comparison, despite similar morbidity and mortality.

- **Postoperative management** is critical because of the patient's depressed pulmonary function and limited reserve. Immediate postoperative examinations typically demonstrate bilateral thoracostomy tubes, a central venous line, and an epidural catheter (Fig. 11-29). Opacities adjacent to the

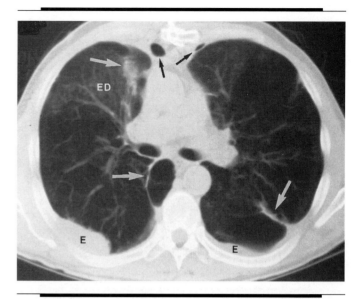

FIGURE 11-30　CT following LVRS. Note significant residual emphysema, small mediastinal air collections (black arrows), loculated pleural effusions (E), staple lines (white arrows), and mild edema (ED) in an area of normal lung parenchyma.

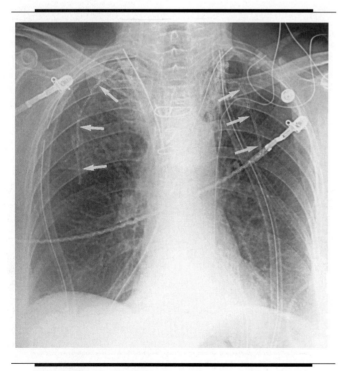

FIGURE 11-29　Normal postoperative examination. Portable chest radiograph immediately following LVRS showing bilateral chest tubes and staple lines (white arrows) indicating the site of resection of a crescent of emphysematous lung from both upper lobes. (With permission from Slone RM, Gierada DS. Exploring imaging options in lung volume reduction surgery. *Diagn. Radiol.* 1996;October:50–56,73).

staple line due to focal hemorrhage, edema, and atelectasis typically decrease or resolve in days to weeks.

The lung tissue is fragile and easily damaged, predisposing the patient to prolonged air leaks and pneumothorax, and so suction is minimized. A basilar component is common. Invagination of the visceral pleura leads to triangular fluid and air collections. Small pleural effusions are common, but empyema is rare. Pulmonary edema may have an atypical distribution and be difficult to differentiate from pneumonia due to persistent regions of emphysema. CT can be used to evaluate complicated cases (Fig. 11-30).

Pleural tents represent separation of the parietal pleural from the chest wall to allow it to drape over the lung. Apposition of the visceral and parietal pleura speed the closing of visceral pleural air leaks. Tents are easily confused with a pneumothorax, particularly when the visceral and parietal pleura are in contact with each other and the pleural tent is air filled. Fluid slowly accumulates over days and then resorbs, drawing the pleura back toward the chest wall. Pleural thickening remains at the site. Extrapleural hemorrhage is a potential complication (Fig. 11-31).

Lung Transplantation

- Approximately 1000 **lung transplantations** are performed throughout the world each year, primarily in the treatment of pulmonary fibrosis, primary pulmonary hypertension, cystic fibrosis, and end-stage emphysema including α_1-antritrypsin deficiency (Fig. 11-32). Donor availability is the major limitation. Approximately 2500 patients are currently awaiting a transplant. The average wait is 12 to 18 months, with 500 patients dying each year awaiting transplantation. Bilateral

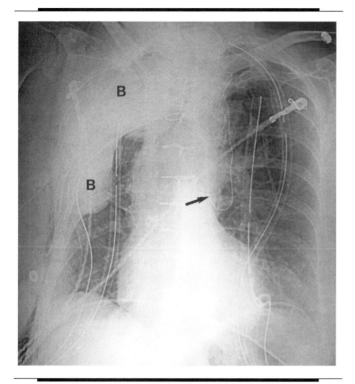

FIGURE 11-31   Hemorrhage into pleural tent following LVRS. Portable chest radiograph on postoperative day 2 showing a large extrapleural fluid collection along the right upper chest representing bleeding (B) into the pleural tent. The previous examination showed a much smaller air collection. Note bilateral chest tubes and a thoracic epidural catheter (arrow). (With permission from Slone RM, Gierada DS, Yusen RD. Preoperative and postoperative imaging in the surgical management of pulmonary emphysema. *Radiol. Clin. North Am.* 1998;36(1):57–89.)

transplantation is preferred in younger patients and required in patients with cystic fibrosis because of the risk of donor lung infection from the native lung.

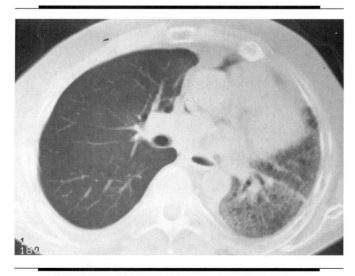

FIGURE 11-32   Right lung transplant. CT showing a small left native lung with coarse interstitial thickening and architectural distortion following unilateral transplant for pulmonary fibrosis.

- **Functional results** after lung transplantation are excellent, and patients reach peak performance within a few months. Transplantation for obstructive disease carries a longer survival than for pulmonary hypertension, fibrosis, or cystic fibrosis. Hospital **survival** is approximately 95 percent, 1-year survival 80 percent, and 5-year survival greater than 50 percent. Causes of late death include bronchiolitis obliterans due to chronic rejection, sepsis, and posttransplant lymphoproliferative disease.

  Lung transplantation is seldom considered in patients older than 65 years of age. Acceptable candidates are ambulatory and without significant systemic disease or recent malignancy. Patients are enrolled in an ongoing program of pulmonary rehabilitation while awaiting transplantation to optimize physical conditioning.

- Preferred **donors** are less than 55 years old, have normal chest radiographic and bronchoscopic exams, negative serologic studies for hepatitis B and HIV, no significant history of smoking or pulmonary disease, and adequate gas exchange. Only blood group typing, rather than tissue cross-matching, is performed. Donor lung extraction requires separation from pleural attachments, division of the pulmonary veins with a left atrial cuff, and division of the pulmonary artery and bronchus. Preservation is maintained with electrolyte solutions and cold storage. Size matching of the donor lung and recipient thorax are important and may be performed using chest radiograph measurements or nomograms based on height and age.

- **Single-lung transplantation** is performed via a posterolateral thoracotomy, and **bilateral lung transplantation** as sequential unilateral transplantation through a transverse thoracosternotomy or clamshell incision. The bronchial anastamosis is covered with peribronchial lymphatic tissue to reduce the risk of dehiscence. The pulmonary artery is anastomosed end to end. The bridge of tissue separating the superior and inferior pulmonary veins is amputated, creating a left atriotomy for anastomosis with the donor. Cardiopulmonary bypass is rarely needed during transplantation for pulmonary emphysema, in contrast to the situation for pulmonary vascular disease. Typical immunosuppressive agents include cyclosporin or tacrolimus, steroids, and azathioprine.

- Recently, **living related lung donors** have been used, primarily for children with cystic fibrosis or bronchopulmonary dysplasia. A right lower lobe harvested from a donor is transplanted into the right hemithorax, and a left lower lobe from a second donor is transplanted into the left hemithorax. The usual indications include a patient likely to die before a donor lung becomes available. Donors are usually family members. Standard immunosuppression is used. Episodes of rejection are usually unilateral, yet both lungs require surveillance. There is a 10 percent complication rate and about a 20 percent reduction in force expiratory volume in 1 second (FEV_1) and forced vital capacity (FVC) in each donor.

- **Postoperative radiologic examinations** demonstrate the location of thoracostomy tubes in the pleural space, usually one in the apex and one near the lung base. The presence of a

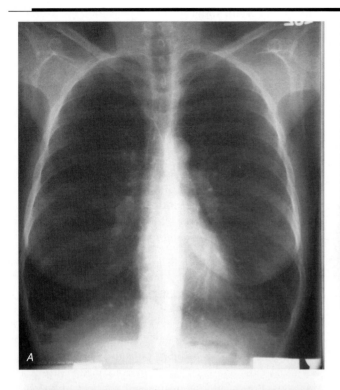

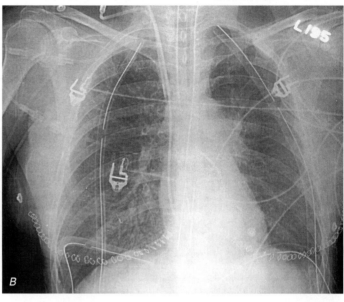

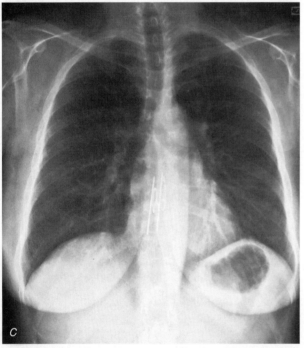

FIGURE 11-33   Bilateral lung transplantation for treatment of emphysema. (*A*) Preoperative chest radiograph showing advanced pulmonary emphysema. (*B*) Portable chest radiograph on postoperative day 1 showing immediate reconfiguration of the thorax. Note skin staples indicating location of transverse thoracosternotomy incision, bilateral chest tubes, pulmonary artery and central venous catheters, and endotracheal and nasogastric tubes. (*C*) Chest radiograph 6 months following surgery showing normal lung and chest wall. Note costochondral circlage wires and Kirshner wires traversing the lower sternum to provide stability. (With permission from: Slone RM, Gierada DS, Yusen RD. Preoperative and postoperative imaging in the surgical management of pulmonary emphysema. *Radiol. Clin. North Am.* 1998;36(1):57–89.)

CVL and an ETT is routine. There are usually small pleural effusions and air collections, but large pneumothoraces are uncommon. Thoracic hyperinflation quickly reverses in patients with emphysema. The lung is generally well expanded, although mild edema and small areas of atelectasis are common (Fig. 11-33).

Routine radiologic examinations serve an important role in surveying for complications, including infection and rejection which can be asymptomatic. However, findings are seldom specific, and regular surveillance, including bronchoscopy with lavage and biopsy, is the mainstay for diagnosis.

- **Bronchoalveolar lavage** involves instillation into and suction removal of aliquots of saline from a segment or subsegment of the lung, usually the middle lobe. Focal or patchy infiltrates usually resolve over days. Four to eight **transbronchial biopsy** specimens are also routinely obtained. Bleeding can produce infiltrates or pulmonary nodules representing small hematomas that may not be evident on immediate postbiopsy radiographs but can persist on CT for 1 month. Nodules can appear solid or cavitary and indistinguishable from infection or rejection.

- **Early complications** following transplantation include pneumothorax, reimplantation edema, acute rejection, infection, airway ischemia and dehiscence, hemorrhage, phrenic nerve paralysis or laryngeal nerve injury, and bronchiolitis obliterans with organizing pneumonia. Graft dysfunction from donor lung injury, ischemia, or vascular stenosis manifests as diffuse alveolar damage. **Late pulmonary complications** include infections, acute and chronic rejection, bronchiectasis, airway stenosis, and posttransplant lymphoproliferative disorders.

- The **reimplantation response** (reperfusion pulmonary edema) in the donor lung is a form of noncardiogenic pulmonary edema, likely a response to lymphatic interruption, pulmonary denervation, surgical trauma, and organ preservation. It occurs in virtually all patients to varying degrees within the first three postoperative days. Management is supportive. Radiographic findings include those of pulmonary edema and typically progress for a few days, peak by day 5, and resolve by day 10 (Fig. 11-34). Infiltrates that continue to worsen beyond 5 days may represent infection or rejection of the allograft.

- **Pleural abnormalities** include pneumothorax, parapneumonic effusions, empyemas, hemothorax, and chylothorax. A single communicating pleural space may result following bilateral lung transplantation, allowing fluid and air to move between the hemithoraces. Ipsilateral pleural effusion occurs in all lung transplant recipients, beginning immediately following transplantation, in part because of severing of the allograft lymphatics. These reconstitute and become functional within a month. Continued increase in size or failure of resolution by day 9, or a new pleural effusion suggests a pathologic process such as infection or rejection and necessitates diagnostic thoracentesis. Empyema occurs in less than 5 percent of patients but may be asymptomatic and can be a serious complication in these immunosuppressed patients.

- **Acute transplant rejection** occurs in almost all patients within the first 3 months after transplantation. Symptoms include cough, fever, dyspnea, and reduced oxygenation. The most common radiologic finding is septal lines and new or increasing pleural effusions, but abnormalities may be subtle or absent. There is significant overlap with reimplantation response, fluid overload, early graft dysfunction, atelectasis, mucous plugging, and pneumonia. CT findings include ground-glass attenuation, septal thickening, nodules, and consolidation. Decreased perfusion on posttransplant scintigraphy suggests acute rejection, and transbronchial biopsy is used to confirm the diagnosis. There is usually rapid clearing of the radiographic abnormalities following initial treatment with high-dose intravenous steroids.

- **Posttransplant infection** is the most common complication and the leading cause of mortality following lung transplantation. Immunosuppression increases the risk of infection.

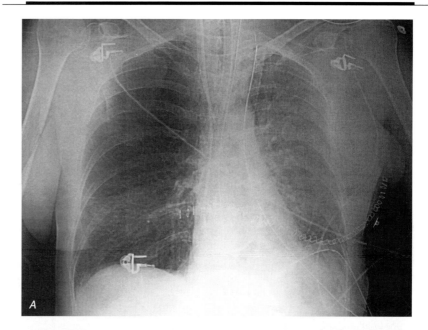

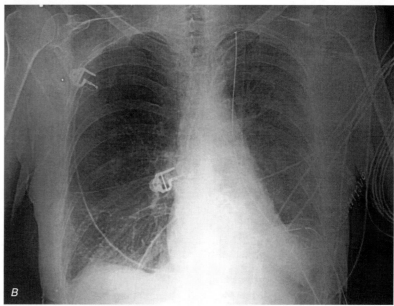

FIGURE 11-34   Reperfusion pulmonary edema. (*A*) Portable chest radiograph 1 day following left lung transplantation for treatment of pulmonary emphysema showing a diffuse left-sided infiltrate. Note chest tubes, central venous and pulmonary artery catheters, and endotracheal and nasogastric tubes. (*B*) Follow-up examination on postoperative day 4 showing interval clearing of the infiltrate. The remaining opacity represents the difference between the emphysematous right and "normal" left lung parenchyma. (With permission from Slone RM, Gierada DS, Yusen RD. Preoperative and postoperative imaging in the surgical management of pulmonary emphysema. *Radiol. Clin. North Am.* 1998;36(1):57–89.)

The transplanted lung is more susceptible than the native lung because of ischemic injury, interrupted lymphatic drainage, impaired mucociliary clearance, and diminished cough reflex because of denervation. Extrapulmonary infections and dissemination are common as a result of immunosuppression. The radiologic appearance of opportunistic pulmonary infections is often nonspecific, and the chest radiograph can be normal. Healing rib fractures, often first visualized 1 month following transplantation, can appear as pulmonary nodules mimicking infection.

- **Bacteria**, particularly *Pseudomonas* and *Staphylococcus*, are the most common infecting organisms, particularly in the first 2 months following transplantation, and prophylactic antibiotics are routinely used. The radiologic appearance is often nonspecific and overlaps with findings seen in rejection, including lobar or diffuse consolidation, cavitation, or nodules. Bacterial bronchitis is also common.

- **Cytomegalovirus (CMV)** is the most common opportunistic infection following transplantation. It occurs most commonly in the first 4 months when immunosuppression is highest. This virus is a ubiquitous organism, with most adults having serologic evidence of prior infection. Infection occurs in the majority of seronegative patients receiving a seropositive lung. When possible, CMV matching is performed between donor and recipient to prevent this occurrence. Although patients are often asymptomatic, symptoms can include fever, nonproductive cough, malaise, leukopenia, dyspnea, and hypoxemia. Diagnosis is made by bronchoscopy with lavage and biopsy. Radiographs may be normal or show interstitial and reticular opacities, small nodules, ground-glass areas, consolidation, or small effusions (Fig. 11-35). Less frequently, viral infections are due to herpes simplex virus, adenovirus, influenza virus, and respiratory syncytial virus.

- Pulmonary **fungal infections** are less common than bacterial and viral infections but are associated with higher mortality. Fungi endemic to the regions of both the recipient and donor must be considered. Invasive pulmonary aspergillosis may progress slowly or rapidly disseminate and has a high mortality. It can manifest as pneumonia, ulcerative tracheobronchitis, or a systemic infection. The most frequent radiographic findings include nodules and focal consolidation. *Candida* colonization of airways is common, but invasive infection is uncommon.

- Potential **airway complications** following transplantation include dehiscence, necrosis, stenosis, or bronchomalacia. The incidence of airway complications is approximately 5 percent per anastomosis, with a 2 to 3 percent mortality. Endoluminal flaps and small perianastomatic air collections can be a normal finding at telescoping anastomoses.

  Bronchial dehiscence is the most common surgical complication. The central bronchi are supplied by bronchial arterioles which are not anastamosed during transplantation, making the bronchial anastomoses susceptible to ischemia, necrosis, and resultant dehiscence. Small defects typically heal without intervention. Some heal with stenosis, but larger ones may be fatal. Management includes bronchoscopic surveillance, stent placement, or even retransplantation. Bronchial dehiscence is well demonstrated on CT by the presence of extraluminal air, although air may normally be seen outside the bronchus several weeks following transplantation.

  Bronchial stenosis occurs in approximately 10 percent of patients. CT with multiplanar reconstructions is generally

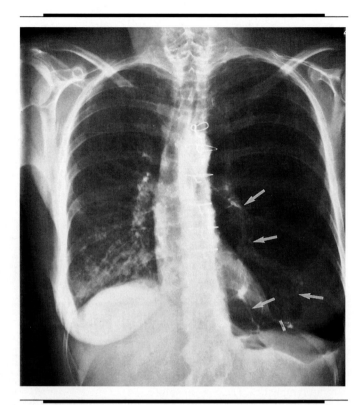

FIGURE 11-35   CMV infection following lung transplantation. Chest radiograph showing a small pleural effusion and new infiltrate in the transplanted right lung. Note advanced emphysema in the native left lung and staples (arrows) from prior LVRS. (With permission from Slone RM, Gierada DS, Yusen RD. Preoperative and postoperative imaging in the surgical management of pulmonary emphysema. *Radiol. Clin. North Am.* 1998;36(1):57–89.)

more accurate than thin-section axial CT alone in demonstrating mild stenoses and the length of stenoses. Bronchoscopic dilatation of strictures and stent placement are sometimes required.

- **Bronchiolitis obliterans** is the pathologic manifestation of **chronic rejection**, a major source of morbidity and the principal cause of late death. It is characterized physiologically by airflow obstruction and is typically associated with multiple episodes of acute rejection and CMV infection. It can begin a few months or years after transplantation and progress rapidly or slowly. Symptoms include worsening dyspnea and nonproductive cough without evidence of infection. The disease may be diffuse or focal and therefore can be overlooked on transbronchial biopsy. Radiologic findings include reduced lung volumes, subsegmental atelectasis, bronchial thickening, decreased peripheral vascular markings, and thin, linear opacities or nodular infiltrates, although a normal chest radiograph is common. High-resolution CT (HRCT) findings include mosaic perfusion, decreased peripheral vascular markings, mild cylindrical bronchiectasis (often worse in the lower lobes), and air trapping on expiration.

- **Posttransplantation lymphoproliferative disease (PTLD)**, which affects 2 percent of all organ transplant recipients, refers to a spectrum of disorders ranging from polyclonal lymphoid hyperplasia to aggressive lymphoma. PTLD rarely occurs before 2 months, but commonly occurs in the first year after transplantation and is a consequence of chronic immunosuppression exacerbated by cyclosporin administration. It may be associated with Epstein-Barr virus-infected lymphocytes in the donor lung. Symptoms include fever, fatigue, and weight loss. Common radiologic findings are pulmonary nodules and mediastinal adenopathy (Fig. 3-14). Pleural effusions and air space consolidation may be seen. Treatment includes antiviral agents and reduced immunosuppression while trying to prevent graft rejection. Untreated PTLD is almost always fatal, and chemotherapy or radiation may be considered.

11.5 ESOPHAGEAL AND GASTRIC SURGERY

- **Gastroesophageal reflux (GER)**, a common disorder accompanied by hiatal hernia, can generally be treated with medication. **Surgical management** is indicated in patients with refractory or recurrent symptoms following a satisfactory duration of adequate medical treatment and in patients with airway or pulmonary complications or advanced esophagitis, especially if associated with peptic stricture or acquired shortening. Evaluation includes an upper gastrointestinal contrast examination, endoscopy, and manometry. The **Angelchik prosthesis** sometimes encountered on radiographs is an obsolete silicone-filled silastic implant that encircles the esophagus below the diaphragm to help reduce GER.

  Antireflux surgical procedures include those performed through the thorax and abdomen and minimally invasive laparoscopic techniques. Surgery involves mobilization of the esophagus and stomach and restoration of a 3-cm segment of abdominal esophagus below the hiatus. The repair is reinforced with a cuff of stomach (fundoplication), and with anatomic reapproximation of the diaphragmatic crura. These procedures are designed to secure the esophageal hiatus below the diaphragm and provide an artificial valvelike mechanism to create a lower esophageal sphincter.

- **Nissen fundoplication** is the most common antireflux operation. It can be performed transabdominally or transthoracically and entails a 360-degree wrap of gastric fundus around the terminal esophagus. It has a 90 percent long-term success rate in controlling reflux symptoms. An excessively long or tight wrap can cause postoperative dysphagia and inability to belch or vomit. A "slipped Nissen" refers to migration of the wrap down along the gastric body.

- A **Belsey fundoplication** (Belsey Mark IV) is performed through a left thoracotomy and involves a 240- to 270-degree fundoplication. It is indicated in obese patients, those with advanced esophagitis, and those with decreased peristaltic motility. The Belsey procedure controls symptoms in more than 85 percent of patients.

  Toupet is a 180-degree posterior fundoplication most similar to the Nissen. The wrapped fundus is sewn to the right and left edges of the esophagus, and the whole repair is then sutured to the diaphragm crura.

- A **Hill fundoplication** involves a crural plication added to a posterior gastropexy. The stomach is attached to the median arcuate ligament, and the crura of the diaphragm approximated over the distal esophagus to increase the resting tone of the lower esophageal sphincter. The goal is the same: the creation of a length of intra-abdominal esophagus exposed to abdominal pressures.

- A **Collis gastroplasty** can be performed in addition to a Nissen or Belsey fundoplication to lengthen the esophagus and reduce tension on the repair. A Collis gastroplasty involves stapling of the gastric cardia parallel to the lesser curvature of the stomach, to lengthen the esophagus by transforming a portion of the gastric cardia into the neoesophagus.

- A laparoscopic Nissen fundoplication is considered **minimally invasive antireflux surgery**. Candidates include both young, healthy and old ill individuals desiring surgical management. The procedure requires five abdominal incisions through which gas insufflation of the peritoneal cavity, retraction, and instrumentation are performed.

  Contraindications include esophageal shortening, prior upper abdominal or antireflux surgery, morbid obesity, a massive left hepatic lobe, a large hiatal hernia, or an intrathoracic stomach. Potential complications include esophageal, gastric, or bowel perforation and distal esophageal ischemia. **Side effects** of fundoplication are more frequent following laparoscopy and include dysphagia, bloating, and inability to belch.

- The **modified Heller esophagomyotomy** for treatment of **achalasia** is performed through a left posterolateral thoracotomy. Starting several centimeters above the gastroesophageal junction and avoiding the vagus nerve, an incision is made through the muscular layer of the esophagus down to but not through the mucosa. The incision is continued through the lower esophageal sphincter 1 cm onto the stomach. Complications can include empyema, atelectasis, pneumonia, wound infection, and phlebitis. Because reflux often develops in these patients, a thorough myotomy is generally paired with a Belsey fundoplication (Fig. 11-36).

- **Esophageal cancer** accounts for 12,000 deaths per year in the United States. Esophagectomy is the treatment of choice for fit patients with localized disease. Tumors that are unresectable and patients who cannot undergo surgery can be treated palliatively with stents, chemotherapy, or radiation. The newer silicone-covered metallic stents are preferred to plastic stents (Fig. 11-37). Preoperative radiation does not improve resectability or survival. Postoperative radiation decreases local recurrence but does not improve survival. Five-year survival following complete resection is approximately 65 percent for stage I disease, 30 percent for stage II disease, and 15 percent for stage III disease, with the vast majority of patients falling into stage III. The technique for esophageal resection

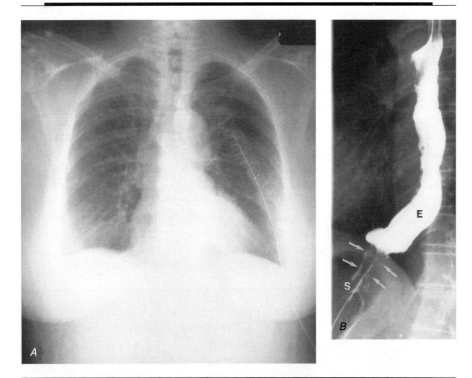

FIGURE 11-36   Heller myotomy and Belsey fundoplication for achalasia. (*A*) Postoperative chest radiograph showing left chest tube and skin staples marking thoracotomy site. Note also partial resection of the seventh rib. (*B*) Esophagram showing evidence of the gastric wrap (arrows) below the diaphragm. E, Esophagus; S, Stomach.

and replacement depends on tumor size, location, and surgeon preference.

- **Transhiatal esophagectomy** and gastric replacement with a cervical anastomosis provide the best functional results for tumors in the distal third of the esophagus, small mobile tumors in the midesophagus, and Barrett esophagus with severe dysplasia or carcinoma in situ. This procedure also works well for esophageal replacement in benign disease, such as peptic or lye stricture, motor disorders such as diffuse spasm, achalasia, and scleroderma.

An upper midline abdominal incision is made, and the esophageal hiatus is dissected and enlarged. The paraesophageal and gastric tissues are dissected, including ligature of the short gastric vessels. The lesser curvature of the stomach is divided with a stapler and oversewn. A left-sided neck incision is made anterior and parallel to the sternocleidomastoid muscle, and the cervical esophagus mobilized. The esophagus is then removed and the stomach is drawn into the neck through the

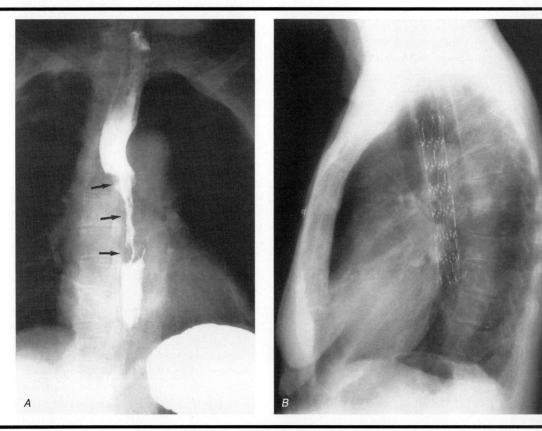

FIGURE 11-37   Esophageal cancer. (*A*) Esophagram showing a large constricting mucosal lesion (arrows) consistent with esophageal carcinoma. (*B*) Lateral chest radiograph showing a silastic coated metal esophageal stent placed for palliative management.

mediastinum. Finally, a cervical esophagogastric anastomosis is performed (Fig. 11-38).

Complications include anastomotic leak, stricture, and recurrent laryngeal nerve palsy. A quarter of patients have an anastomotic leak following transhiatal esophagectomy, although few are of clinical significance.

The stomach is the preferred organ for esophageal replacement, since it is sturdier, has a more reliable blood supply, and only requires one anastomosis. The **colon** or **jejunum** can also be used, but their use requires the creation of three, rather than one anastomosis (Fig. 11-39). The left colon is preferred because of its smaller diameter, more con-

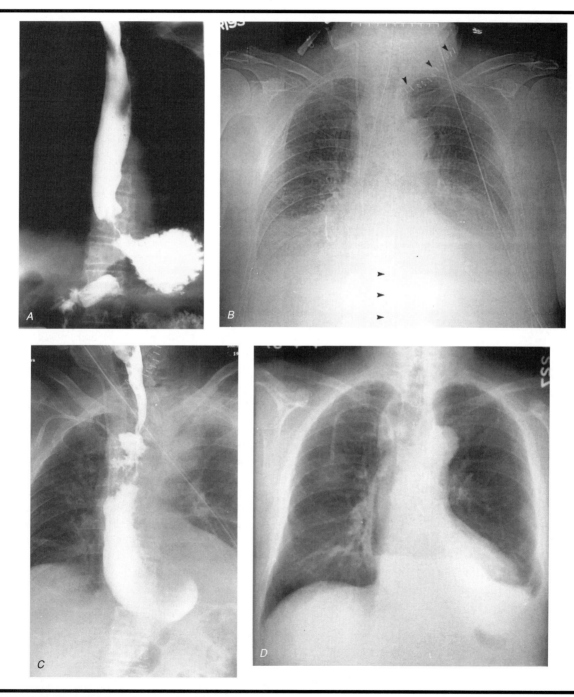

FIGURE 11-38 Transhiatal esophagectomy with gastric replacement. (A) Esophagram showing distal esophageal carcinoma. (B) Postoperative chest radiograph showing skin staples (arrowheads) at the site of the upper abdominal and cervical incisions, bilateral pleural effusions, a nasogastric tube, a central venous catheter, and an infus-a-port for chemotherapy. (C) Postoperative esophagram showing site of cervical anastamosis and intrathoracic stomach. (D) Chest radiograph 2 weeks following surgery showing expected widened mediastinum and air-fluid level in stomach. Note small left pleural effusion.

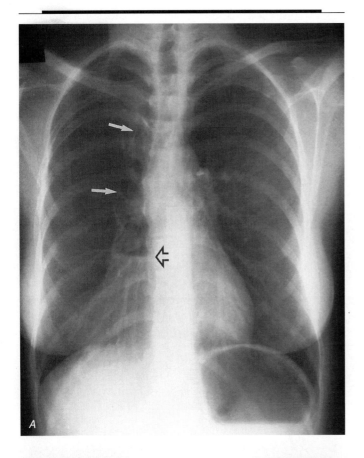

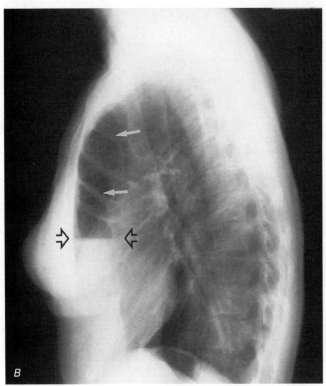

FIGURE 11-39 Esophagectomy with colonic interposition.
(*A* and *B*) PA and lateral chest radiographs showing an air-fluid level (open arrows) in the anterior mediastinum. Note the colonic wall and haustrations seen more superiorly (white arrows).

stant and reliable blood supply, and adequate length for total esophageal replacement.

- An **Ivor-Lewis esophagectomy** is a partial esophagectomy and gastric interposition. First a laparotomy is performed, and the stomach is mobilized and brought up through the diaphragm. The patient is then placed in a lateral decubitus position, and a midthoracic esophagogastric anastomosis is performed through a right thoracotomy.

  A midthoracic anastomotic leak is less common (5 versus 20 percent), but potentially more disastrous than a cervical leak following transhiatal esophagectomy. In contrast to a transhiatal approach in which the stomach is contained in the mediastinum, an Ivor-Lewis esophagectomy leads to displacement of the stomach into the right chest.

11.6 VASCULAR SURGERY

- **Pulmonary thromboendarterectomy** is a viable treatment alternative for select patients with chronic pulmonary embolism. Indications for surgery include significant pulmonary hypertension with progressive exercise impairment or dyspnea at rest. The embolic occlusions must extend sufficiently proximal to permit surgical accessibility. Contraindications include severe coronary artery, renal, or parenchymal lung disease.

  The procedure is performed by median sternotomy during deep hypothermia and circulatory arrest. The main pulmonary arteries are incised, and an eversion endarterectomy carried out into the segmental and subsegmental vessels. Reperfusion edema ranging from mild pulmonary edema to pulmonary hemorrhage is common and may initially appear as late as 3 days following surgery. Patients are often kept intubated for several days in anticipation of this potential complication.

- **Carotid endarterectomy** provides better outcome than nonoperative management of severe carotid stenosis and is indicated in patients with a 60 to 80 percent stenosis depending on symptoms. The incidence of stroke is 0.5 percent, and the risk of death is 2 percent, following endarterectomy. Simultaneous carotid endarterectomy and coronary bypass surgery may be performed without increased risk of stroke or death. The length of hospitalization, anesthesia exposure, and cost are reduced by combining these operations in select patients.

- **Thoracic aortic aneurysms** are generally considered for surgical repair when their diameter exceeds 6 cm or when there is a dramatic increase in size or symptoms over a short time. Significant aortic insufficiency is a reason for aortic replacement even with aneurysms smaller than 6 cm. Descending thoracic aortic aneurysms are repaired through a left thoracotomy. There is a 10 percent mortality rate and a 4 percent incidence of paraplegia.

- **Thoracoabdominal aneurysms** are repaired through a thoracoabdominal incision with the patient in the left lateral decubitus position. Repair is associated with high morbidity and has a 30 percent mortality and a 15 percent rate of paraplegia. The celiac, superior mesenteric, and right renal arteries are often reanastamosed together as one pedicle (Fig. 11-40).

- **Acute traumatic aortic injury (ATAI)** of which transection is the most severe manifestation warrants emergent repair because of the high incidence of rupture and death. The aortic tear typically occurs at the ligamentum arteriosum just distal to the left subclavian artery, and repair involves a left thoracotomy. A median sternotomy is required for ascending aortic injuries (Figs. 10-3 to 10-6 and Fig. 14-9).

- **Type A aortic dissections** are repaired to prevent the complications of aortic regurgitation, coronary occlusion, and pericardial tamponade rather than to "fix" the dissection. Planning the repair includes decisions regarding management of the aortic valve, coronary arteries, and transverse thoracic aortic arch. In patients with aortic insufficiency the aortic valve can be replaced or the native valve resuspended.

  Coronary artery management may include reimplantation or bypass. If the coronaries are spared from involvement, the aortic valve can be repaired or replaced and an ascending aortic tube graft can be placed above the coronary ostia. Dissection involving the arch requires placement of either a beveled anastomosis that extends under the great vessels or an arch graft that is sewn to the distal aorta and the arch vessels separately.

- The **Bentall procedure** involves the placement of a composite valve and tube-graft conduit (valved-conduit) in the ascending aorta with the right and left coronary orifices implanted into the valved-conduit. A valved-conduit repair is generally indicated in patients with Marfan syndrome because of the risk of valvular degeneration and in patients with aneurysmal dilatation of the aortic segment containing the coronary orifices.

11.7 INTERVENTIONAL CARDIOLOGY

- **Percutaneous techniques** applied to the coronary circulation include balloon angioplasty, laser ablation, arthrectomy, and coronary stent placement. Balloon valvuloplasty is sometimes used for management of mitral and aortic stenoses.

- **Percutaneous transluminal coronary angioplasty (PTCA)**, originally proposed in 1979, has become standard therapy for patients with single-vessel and many patients with multivessel coronary artery disease (CAD). Patients are generally also candidates for coronary artery bypass grafting (CABG) since an emergent bypass may be required in the event of complications. PTCA works by fracturing the stenotic plaque and underlying intima and stretching the normal vessel wall. Indications include acute myocardial infarction (PTCA within 3 hours), significant angina, or positive exercise testing in the presence of a 75 percent narrowing with single- or double-vessel CAD refractory to medical treatment.

  Although initially successful in over 90 percent of patients, up to 50 percent restenose after 6 months. Success is lower with severe stenosis, dense arthrosclerotic calcification, intraluminal thrombus, and right coronary lesions. Contraindications include left main and heavily calcified lesions, chronic occlusions, lesions spanning a bifurcation, and long-segment lesions difficult to cross with a balloon catheter.

  Technical failures include inability to reach or traverse the lesion or inability to dilate the lesion despite crossing it. **Restenosis** occurs in over one-third of patients because of a fibroproliferative response to balloon injury, recurrent plaque formation, and accelerated atherosclerosis. **Complications** occur in less than 10 percent of procedures but include definitive myocardial infarction or death in 2 percent. Emergent CABG is required in up to 4 percent of cases.

- Endovascular **coronary stents** deployed immediately following conventional balloon angioplasty reduce the incidence of abrupt closure and late restenosis. They can be placed in vessels as small as 2.5 mm (see Section 12.5). The introduction of antiplatelet agents and platelet receptor blockers has provided a powerful tool against acute thrombotic complications, particularly when combined with stent placement.

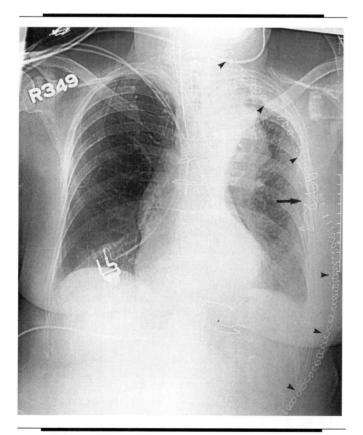

FIGURE 11-40 Thoracoabdominal aortic aneurysm repair. Chest radiograph on postoperative day 5. Note left pleural effusion, skin staples overlying thoracoabdominal incision (arrowheads), and circlage wires approximating fifth through seventh ribs (arrow).

- A number of **mechanical atherectomy devices** have been developed for atherosclerotic CAD but as yet have documented little advantage over PTCA or stents, and the risk of perforation is higher. These include a directional coronary arthrectomy device for excising eccentric plaques, a rotablator with a rotating burr that can emulsify atheromanous plaques, and a transluminal extractor endarterectomy catheter that excises and aspirates athermanous plaque. **Laser recannulation** has been attempted but has shown little advantage over PTCA.

- **Transmyocardial laser revascularization** refers to the creation of ventricular myocardial sinusoidal channels to improve subendocardial perfusion to the myocardium. The procedure results in dramatic improvement in angina scores and scintigraphic perfusion defects in patients with inoperable end-stage ischemic heart disease but does not clearly impact ventricular function or survival. Factors contributing to improvement likely include concomitant angiogenesis and local denervation.

- **Percutaneous mitral balloon valvuloplasty**, introduced in 1985, is an efficacious nonsurgical technique for treating patients with symptomatic mitral stenosis without significant mitral regurgitation, left atrial thrombus, or recent embolic events. The balloon catheter is placed antegrade across the mitral valve and inflated following transseptal left heart catheterization.

  The procedure succeeds by splitting the fused commissures of the valve toward the mitral annulus and may fracture calcified valvular deposits. **Complications** include mitral leaflet, papillary muscle, or chordae tendineae tears; left ventricular or atrial septal perforations; rupture of the mitral annulus; embolic events including stroke; severe mitral regurgitation; and rarely pericardial tamponade and death.

- **Percutaneous aortic valvuloplasty** is a palliative treatment for patients with calcific aortic stenosis at high risk for surgical valve replacement. Restenosis occurs in over one-half of patients within the first year, and it is therefore limited to nonsurgical candidates who have critical aortic stenosis, or as a bridge to aortic valve replacement in patients with cardiogenic shock due to critical aortic stenosis. **Complications** include pericardial tamponade, annular rupture, leaflet damage, and thromboembolic events including stroke and induction of severe aortic regurgitation.

11.8 CARDIAC SURGERY

- **Coronary artery bypass graft (CABG) surgery** may improve patient survival but primarily improves quality of life in terms of pain-free survival. Coronary revascularization has the greatest benefit in patients with reduced ejection fractions and unstable angina. Specific indications include triple-vessel CAD, double-vessel CAD with reduced ejection fraction, angina refractory to medical therapy, and left main and proximal left anterior descending CAD. Survival is increased in patients with triple-vessel and double-vessel CAD, with a reduced ejection fraction as compared to medical management alone.

  At the present time the "gold standard" for coronary revascularization is surgical anastomosis between the left internal mammary (thoracic) artery (LIMA) and left anterior descending (LAD) coronary artery (Fig. 11-41). The 10-year patency of saphenous vein grafts is reduced due to intimal hyperplasia and atherosclerosis. The patency is about 50 percent, compared to 95 percent 10-year patency for internal thoracic grafts.

  One theoretic disadvantage of the LIMA graft is the propensity for spasm during the perioperative period, though this is rarely of clinical significance. While both the right and left IMAs are used for bypass grafts, only one IMA is generally utilized in immunocompromised patients, patients with chronic renal failure, and diabetics because of the risk of suboptimal chest wound healing. Other potential conduits for coronary revascularization include the greater and lesser saphenous vein and the gastroepiploic, inferior epigastric, and radial arteries. Arm veins have extremely poor patency rates and are not routinely used except as a last resort in a patient with no other accessible conduit.

- **Cardiopulmonary bypass** is a process in which systemic venous blood is withdrawn from the patient, transferred to a pump oxygenator, and delivered back to the arterial circulation. It can be performed at 37°C or by cooling the patient to as low as 15°C in preparation for complete circulatory arrest. An aortic cross-clamp is applied, and a high-potassium **cardioplegia** solution is used to cause electromechanical diastolic arrest of the myocardium. This decreases myocardial oxygen utilization substantially and protects the heart from ischemia. Cooling the heart further reduces oxygen consumption.

  Various cannulation sites are used, depending on the procedure and the surgeon's preference. A single two-stage venous cannula is used to remove blood from the IVC and right atrium. If the right atrium must be entered, separate SVC and IVC cannulae are used. A retrograde cardioplegia line is often inserted through the right atrium into the coronary sinus.

  Blood enters a reservoir and subsequently a temperature-regulating device and hollow fiber membrane pump oxygenator where carbon dioxide and oxygen exchange takes place. The blood is filtered and then returned into the arterial circuit of the patient. Two aortic cannula sites are used, one large cannula to perfuse oxygenated blood and one small cathether to administer the cardioplegia solution and to vent the aorta of blood and air.

- **Femorofemoral bypass** refers to full cardiopulmonary bypass established by withdrawing venous blood from a large cannula placed in the femoral vein, transferring it to a pump oxygenator, and returning it through a cannula in the femoral artery. This procedure is most frequently used when the ascending aorta is unsuitable for cannulation or in descending thoracic or thoracoabdominal aortic operations to improve spinal cord protection by perfusing both the ascending aorta and the distal circulation simultaneously.

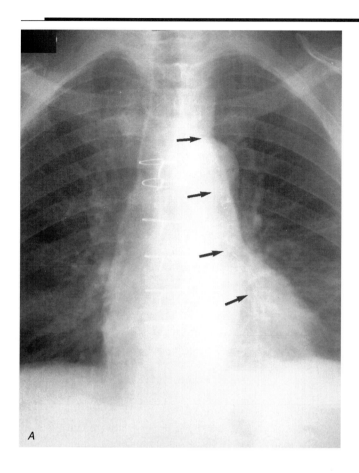
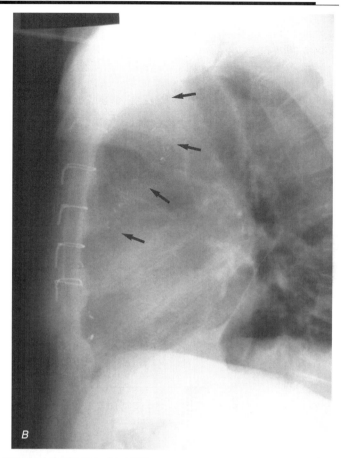

FIGURE 11-41 **Coronary bypass with left internal mammary artery** (LIMA). (*A* and *B*) PA and lateral chest radiographs showing sternal wires from median sternotomy and a series of hemoclips (arrows) along the course of the internal thoracic artery which has been dissected away from the chest wall for anastamosis with the left anterior descending coronary artery.

- A **left atrial-femoral bypass** is a partial bypass in which an oxygenator is not involved. Oxygenated left atrial blood is withdrawn and propelled by a pump to a femoral artery cannula. This technique is employed to provide spinal protection below the level of the cross-clamp, such as in descending thoracic and thoracoabdominal aortic aneurysm repairs.

- A **venovenous bypass** is used in special situations, particularly for IVC procedures including liver transplantation, resection of renal and adrenal tumors with caval involvement, and traumatic injury to the retrohepatic IVC. Blood drained from the lower half of the body from the femoral vein is delivered by centrifuge pump to the right atrium or axillary vein. The portal system can be drained by an inferior mesentery vein. An oxygenator is not used.

- **Mechanical cardiac support devices**, in particular **left ventricular assist devices (LVADs)** which work in conjunction with the patient's native heart, have undergone considerable development and are used primarily as a bridge to transplantation. Third-generation rotary (radial or axial) devices that are small, easily implanted, and durable are being developed and tested in animals. Human trials should begin soon. Research continues on the development of a total artificial heart, with

a device scheduled for human implantation at the turn of the century.

- Extracorporeal membrane oxygenation (**ECMO**) and **aortic balloon pumps** are covered in Section 11.1.

- A **left ventricular aneurysmectomy** can be performed in patients with poor ventricular function due to a dyskinetic or akinetic infarct segment. A dilated ischemic aneurysm causes an increase in wall stress, and dyskinesia sequesters cardiac output, leading to CHF. The aneurysm and scar also cause arrhythmias. Indications include a large aneurysm with decreased cardiac output, CHF, and ventricular arrhythmias. Most aneurysms are anterolateral in position, and organized thrombus is frequently present. This operation is often performed in conjunction with CABG surgery.

- **Left ventricular reduction surgery**, called a *Batiste partial left ventriculectomy* or a *dynamic cardiomyoplasty*, improves left ventricular function by reducing its size. The procedure is gaining acceptance as a viable surgical option in a very select subset of patients with CHF.

- **Cardiac transplantation** has become a standard treatment option for select patients with CHF. The limited supply of donor hearts is the factor determining the number of procedures performed. The dynamic status of heart failure in individual patients necessitates continued reevaluation of recipient criteria.

The three major factors contributing to posttransplant mortality are right ventricular failure, pulmonary artery hypertension, and posttransplant CAD. Long-term immunosupression requires continued radiologic surveillance to detect opportunistic infections. Rejection is monitored by periodic myocardial biopsies performed via right heart catheterization.

- A **commissurotomy** for treatment of mitral stenosis is performed off cardiopulmonary bypass by opening the left atrium and placing a gloved finger or other device through the mitral valve to open the stenotic valve. Valvuloplasty is less effective in aortic stenosis because of the risk of producing severe aortic insufficiency. These are historic procedures rarely performed by surgeons today. Percutaneous equivalent procedures have been developed and are being employed in cardiac catheterization laboratories.

- **Mitral valve repair**, which may include commissurotomy, excision of thickened chordae, and placement of an annuloplasty ring (see Section 12.2), is the procedure of choice for suitable patients with mitral regurgitation. Repair is simple, is typically feasible, and has been so successful that surgery is now recommended for asymptomatic patients with mitral regurgitation. The hemodynamic results of repair may not be as satisfactory as mitral valve replacement, but the elimination of the mechanical valve and its attendant need for anticoagulation makes repair preferable. Prolapse of the anterior leaflet, a bileaflet valve, calcified mitral annulus, and active endocarditis are more difficult to repair, and valve replacement should be considered. The operative mortality for mitral valve repair is about 1 percent. Surgical techniques also exist for repairing incompetent aortic valves. Repair of stenotic aortic valves is less successful.

- **Mitral valve replacement** is more appropriate than repair in patients with mitral regurgitation caused by acute myocardial infarction with ventricular wall and papillary muscle damage. **Mitral stenosis** can often be managed with percutaneous balloon valvuloplasty (see Section 11.7).

- The **Ross procedure** is a technique of aortic valve replacement with a pulmonic valve autograft and reconstruction of the pulmonic valve with a homograft. Advantages include excellent hemodynamics, freedom from anticoagulants, and a potential for growth of the autograft in children. Disadvantages include the fact that this is a complex operation requiring long cardiopulmonary bypass and aortic cross-clamp times. Furthermore, the patient leaves the operating room with two potentially abnormal valves after having arrived there with one. Contraindications include Marfan syndrome, an abnormal pulmonary valve, a dilated aortic annulus, depressed left ventricular function, and three-vessel CAD.

- **Minimally invasive cardiac surgery** techniques are emerging for the treatment of heart disease. CABG can be performed through a small anterior thoracotomy and the assistance of thoracoscopy by mobilizing the internal thoracic artery and grafting it to the LAD coronary artery during isolation and immobilization of the anterior cardiac wall. Catheter systems have also been developed for peripheral cardiopulmonary bypass and "endoaortic cross clamping," facilitating less invasive CABG, mitral valve repair or replacement, and other cardiac procedures.

11.9 LUNG CANCER TREATMENT, RADIATION, AND CHEMOTHERAPY

- **Surgical resection** is the treatment of choice for attempted cure of patients with stage I and II bronchogenic carcinoma (see Section 15.3 for lung cancer staging). The 5-year survival for patients with T1, N0, M0 disease exceeds 70 percent. The lesion itself must be surgically resectable, and the patient a suitable candidate for thoracotomy and pulmonary resection (operability). Unfortunately, less than one-third of patients diagnosed with lung cancer are suitable surgical candidates because advanced disease or medical status renders them inoperable, such as poor pulmonary function or significant cardiac disease. A key test in assessing suitability includes measurement of FEV_1. Patients predicted to be left with less than 0.8 L postoperatively are excluded. A Pa_{CO_2} greater than 45 mmHg is also a contraindication.

- A **lobectomy** is the standard procedure for surgical resection of bronchogenic carcinoma; however, a segmentectomy can be considered in some situations, particularly patients with small tumors and limited pulmonary reserve. However, segmental resections have a higher incidence of local recurrence than lobectomies, and wedge resections a higher incidence of local recurrence than segmentectomies (twice that of a lobectomy). The difference is minimal with squamous cell cancer and greater with adenocarcinomas. Large tumors crossing the fissures or involving the main bronchus usually require a pneumonectomy. Five-year survival following surgery in patients with stage I disease is approximately 60 percent, and with stage II disease, 40 percent.

- **Locally advanced cancer** implies extension outside the lung parenchyma directly or lymph node metastasis. Some patients with **stage IIIa** are candidates for surgery, including those with chest wall invasion. Surgical management usually includes a lobectomy and a full-thickness chest wall resection. Five-year survival is 30 percent when regional nodes are negative. Occasionally an extrapleural dissection is performed in patients with only parietal pleural involvement.

  Ipsilateral mediastinal lymphadenopathy (N2 disease) is typically a contraindication to surgery; however, some studies have shown acceptable survival, particularly with right-sided disease following surgical resection and lymph node dissection. Five-year survival of up to 30 percent has been reported in patients treated with neoadjuvent radiation and chemotherapy followed by surgery. Some surgeons also consider a left upper lobe cancer with isolated subaortic mediastinal adenopathy resectable. In general, the risk of recurrence increases with the number and level of involved lymph nodes.

- **Superior sulcus tumors** are typically low-grade squamous cell carcinomas. They may invade the endothoracic fascia, lower roots of the brachial plexus, sympathetic chain, adjacent ribs, or vertebral body (Fig. 1-20). Management options include surgery, RT, chemotherapy, and often combinations of these treatments. RT alone can relieve pain and prolong survival. Sometimes treatment includes preoperative RT with 30 to 40 Gy (3000 to 4000 rads) followed by surgical resection in 4 weeks. Surgical resection is technically challenging. Both a posterior and, more recently, an anterior cervical thoracic approach allowing en bloc resection of the involved chest wall and underlying lung have been advocated.

- **Chemotherapy** is used for systemic control of tumor, and **radiation therapy (RT)** for local control. Both are key components in the multidisciplinary treatment of bronchogenic carcinoma. Chemotherapy is the primary treatment for small cell lung cancer, and is often supplemented by RT. A number of studies have been conducted evaluating the role of combined RT and chemotherapy for the treatment of non-small-cell cancer. Although surgical resection is clearly the first line of treatment, survival is further increased by chemotherapy in patients with unresectable or incompletely resected lung disease or with mediastinal spread. RT can improve the quality of life and be a component of curative treatment. High-dose chemotherapy and whole-body RT are also an essential final treatment in patients undergoing bone marrow transplantation.

- **Chemotherapy** requires patients with good functional status, including cardiac and renal function and minimal weight loss. Newer chemotherapy agents, including vinorelbine tartrate (Navelbine®), gemcitabine (Gemzar®), and the taxanes, i.e., paclitaxel (Taxol®), and docetaxel (Taxotere®), are more effective than cisplatin, vinblastine, and other first-line agents previously used. Chemotherapy improves survival in patients with N2 disease and is an important adjuvant to radiation therapy in patients with stage III non-small-cell carcinoma. Neoadjuvant chemotherapy generally increases 5-year survival to approximately 20 percent.

- The **side effects of chemotherapy** vary by dose and agent, and the toxic effects are often cumulative. Pulmonary toxicity can lead to capillary leak and interstitial edema, pleural effusions, and pneumonitis. Pulmonary fibrosis often ultimately develops, particularly with busulfan, bleomycin, and cyclophosphamide (Fig. 11-42). Rarely, bleomycin can cause pulmonary nodules indistinguishable from metastases. Chemotherapy may induce hypercalcemia and can also potentiate the effects of radiation-induced pneumonitis.

- **Preoperative RT** in combination with chemotherapy is not advocated for treatment of bronchogenic carcinoma with the exception of superior sulcus tumors; however, the benefits remain controversial. Resection can be difficult following radiation therapy due to fibrosis and impaired wound healing.

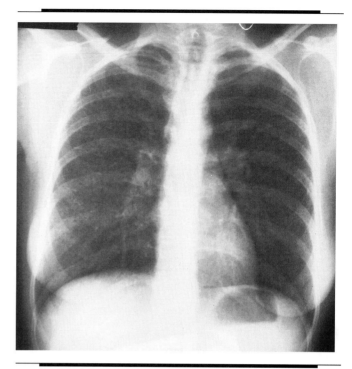

FIGURE 11-42 Chemotherapy toxicity. Chest radiograph showing diffuse interstitial infiltrates following treatment with BCNU.

Postoperative RT may be used in a locally aggressive or marginally resected tumor. Although postoperative RT reduces the incidence of local recurrence of N2 disease, only 5-year disease-free survival is increased. Postoperative RT is clearly not beneficial for increasing survival in patients with stage I or stage II disease. Accurate dose delivery and portal design are crucial for providing adequate coverage while minimizing the dose to critical normal structures such as the heart and spinal cord.

RT also improves the 5-year survival over medical management alone in patients with **inoperable** stage I or II lung cancer. Definitive treatment includes 65 to 75 Gy to the primary site. Five-year survival is approximately 30–40 percent.

- **Complications of thoracic RT** include pneumonitis (5 percent), esophagitis (15–30 percent) particularly when concomitant chemotherapy is given, pericarditis (1–2 percent), esophageal stricture (<1 percent), and myelopathy (<0.5 percent).

Radiation pneumonitis does not always develop following RT, but can occur 1 to 3 months following therapy and is usually self-limited. Symptoms develop in the first 3 months in about 5–10 percent of patients and include dyspnea, nonproductive cough, hypoxemia, a low-grade fever, and mild leukocytosis. Individual susceptibility varies. Risk factors for radiation fibrosis include a higher dose, hypofractionation, a greater volume of lung, and possibly concomitant administration of chemotherapy. Radiologic evidence of injury is rare below 20 Gy (2000 rads).

Typically there is gradual evolution from a homogeneous increase in density to discrete areas of consolidation (Fig. 11-43). Small nodular abnormalities can be confused with

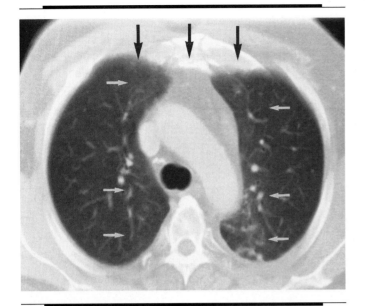

FIGURE 11-43   Radiation pneumonitis. Chest CT in a 68-year-old man following mediastinal radiation, showing evidence of radiation pneumonitis in the medial aspects of the lung (white arrows) contained within the radiation port (black arrows). (With permission from Slone RM, Gierada DS. Pleura, chest wall, and diaphragm. In Lee JKT, Sagel SS, Stanley RJ, Heiken JP, eds. *Computed Body Tomography with MRI Correlation*, 3rd ed. New York: Lippincott-Raven, 1998.)

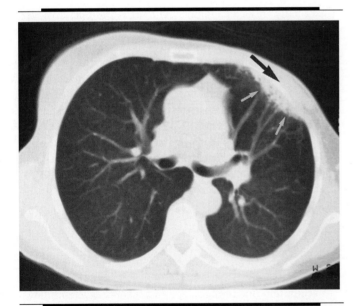

FIGURE 11-44   Radiation fibrosis. Chest CT in a 52-year-old woman who had undergone a left mastectomy and radiation therapy for treatment of breast cancer. The fibrosis adjacent to the anterior lateral chest wall (white arrows) was contained within the radiation port which passed tangential to the chest wall (black arrow). Note associated volume loss. (With permission from Slone RM, Gierada DS. Pleura, chest wall, and diaphragm. In Lee JKT, Sagel SS, Stanley RJ, Heiken JP, eds. *Computed Body Tomography with MRI Correlation*, 3rd ed. New York: Lippincott-Raven, 1998.)

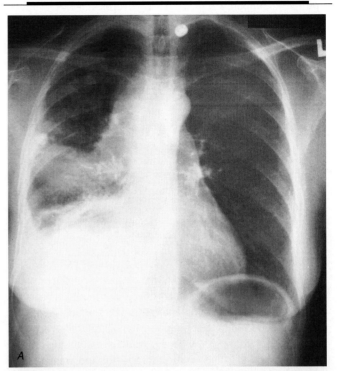

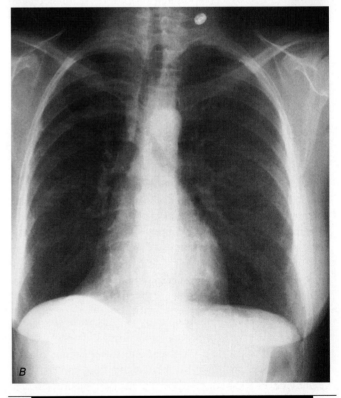

FIGURE 11-45   Small cell carcinoma treated with chemotherapy. (*A*) Chest radiograph at the time of diagnosis in a 50-year-old woman with small cell carcinoma, showing postobstructive pneumonia and mediastinal adenopathy. (*B*) Chest radiograph obtained following 2 months of treatment showing dramatic interval resolution of the adenopathy and associated parenchymal lung disease.

pulmonary metastases. PET can be useful in differentiating radiation fibrosis from recurrent tumor. Pneumonitis gradually transforms to radiation fibrosis, which usually stabilizes 9 to 12 months following treatment. The chest radiograph and CT show infiltrates that increase in density and decrease in volume. Traction bronchiolectasis and volume loss also occur, producing honeycombing. The findings cross anatomic boundaries and conform to the radiation port shape. This is more apparent on CT than on radiography (Fig. 11-44).

- Few patients with **stage IV** lung cancer live beyond 1 year (median survival <6 months). Treatment is palliative. RT in the range of 40 to 50 Gy often relieves chest pain, cough, and dyspnea. Chemotherapy can increase survival for several months and has been reported to improve quality of life and decrease hospitalizations.

- **Small cell carcinoma** accounts for about 20 percent of primary lung cancer. It is often diagnosed in an advanced form and results in earlier death than other lung cancers. Two-thirds of patients have metastases at diagnosis, and those that do not are presumed to have micrometastases that are not detectable. Stage is classified simply as limited or extensive (Section 15.3). Untreated small cell cancer is rapidly fatal, with a mean survival of less than 3 months. A peripheral small cell cancer without mediastinal involvement is the only indication for resection, but this is limited to a small fraction of patients.

  Small cell cancer is very sensitive to chemotherapy (Fig. 11-45). Regimens typically include a combination of agents delivered over a 6-month period. Over 50 percent of limited disease and 20 percent of extensive disease go into complete remission. Combined RT and chemotherapy reduces local recurrence and further increases survival. Prophylactic cranial irradiation reduces central nervous system involvement and increases survival.

- **Endobronchial RT** is palliative for treatment of patients with symptomatic obstructive tumor. Iridium is placed endobronchially near the obstruction. The most common severe complications are bronchial stricture and hemoptysis. **Endobronchial stents** available for management of airway narrowing are discussed in Section 12.5. Other techniques for treatment of endobronchial obstruction include cryotherapy and laser oblation of the tumor.

- **Gene therapy for thoracic malignancies** is now feasible given our ability to transfer novel genetic material to tumor cells. Gene replacement therapy has proven difficult in practice because of the inability of current vectors to provide sufficient levels of gene product for a long enough period of time. Gene therapy for malignant mesothelioma is being studied.

Bibliography

Carter AR, Sostman HD, Curtis AM, Swett HA. Thoracic alterations after cardiac surgery. *Am. J. Roentgenol.* 1983;140:475–483.

Edmonds LH, Norwood WI, Low DW. *Atlas of Cardiothoracic Surgery.* Philadelphia: Lea and Febiger, 1990.

Fishman AP, Elias JA, Fishman JA, Grippi MA, Kaiser LR, Senior RM. *Fishman's Pulmonary Diseases and Disorders.* 3rd ed. New York: McGraw-Hill; 1998; vol 1–2.

Libshitz HI, Shuman LS. Radiation-induced pulmonary change: CT findings. *JCAT* 1984;8:15–19.

Murphy GP, Lawrence W, Lenhard RE. *Clinical Oncology.* 2nd ed. Atlanta: American Cancer Society; 1995.

Murray JF, Nadel JA. *Textbook of Respiratory Medicine.* 2nd ed. Philadelphia: WB Saunders; 1994, vol 1–2.

O'Meara JB, Slade PR. Disappearance of fluid from the postpneumonectomy space. *J. Thorac. Cardiovasc. Surg.* 1974;67:621–628.

Pearson FG, Deslauriers J, Ginsberg RJ, Hiebert CA, McKneally MF, Urschel HC. *Thoracic Surgery.* New York: Churchill Livingstone; 1995.

Randall PA, Trasolini NC, Kohman LJ, et al. MR imaging evaluation of the chest after uncomplicated median sternotomy. *Radiographics.* 1993;13: 329–340.

Ravitch MM, Steichen FM, Schlossberg L. *Atlas of General Thoracic Surgery.* Philadelphia: WB Saunders; 1988.

Ravitch MM, Steichen FM, Welter R, eds. *Current Practice of Surgical Stapling.* Philadelphia: Lea and Febiger; 1991.

Roth JA, Ruckdeschel JC, Weisenburger TH. *Thoracic Oncology.* 2nd ed. Philadelphia: WB Saunders; 1995.

Sabiston DC, Spencer FC. *Surgery of the Chest.* 6th ed. Philadelphia: WB Saunders; 1996; vol 1–2.

Slone RM, Gierada DS, Yusen RD. Preoperative and postoperative imaging in the surgical management of pulmonary emphysema. *Radiol. Clin. North Am.* 1998;36(1):57–89.

Yamashita H. *Roentgenologic Anatomy of the Lung.* Tokyo:Igaku-Shoin, 1978.

Chapter 12

THORACIC IMPLANTS AND DEVICES

Andrew J. Fisher and Matthew J. Fleishman

12.1 INTRODUCTION

• Thoracic implants and devices are becoming increasingly utilized in the management and treatment of both cardiac and pulmonary pathology. As endoluminal techniques and technology continue to advance, this trend will continue.

   In addition to prosthetic valves, pacemakers, and defibrillators, coronary stents are now available. Noncardiac appliances are also frequently encountered on chest examinations. These include tracheal, esophageal, and vascular stents and orthopedic hardware. Thoracostomy tubes, pulmonary embolization coils, and interventional procedures are described in Chapter 14. Temporary devices such as nasogastric tubes and Swan-Ganz catheters are discussed in Chapter 11.

12.2 CARDIAC VALVES

• Cardiac valve repair and replacement is a common and accepted mode of treatment for valvular heart disease. Currently, millions of prosthetic valves are in place in patients worldwide; however, early valve surgery was much less successful than current techniques.

   Valve surgery began in the 1920s and consisted primarily of closed heart procedures for attempted treatment of mitral and aortic stenosis. These procedures were complicated by a high mortality rate. Patients who survived often rapidly progressed to valvular restenosis. In 1954, Charles Hufnagel implanted the first prosthetic valve, adapting a bottle-stopper design initially patented in the 1800s. This ball valve was inserted into the descending aorta for the treatment of aortic insufficiency. Although the procedure improved lower extremity perfusion, it did little to improve blood flow to the head, heart, and upper extremities.

• **Advances** critical to the progression of cardiac valve replacement included **cardiopulmonary bypass**, opening up the possibility for complex intracardiac surgery. Also in the 1950s, systemic **anticoagulation therapy**, necessary for maintaining mechanical prosthetic valves, evolved. While heparin, a product of bovine lung, gained popularity in the 1940s, it was not until the 1950s that coumadin was found to be effective in the human population. Before this time, it had served as a rat poison and was felt to be too toxic for human administration.

• **Albert Starr**, a cardiothoracic surgeon, and **Lowell Edwards**, an engineer, were the first to successfully devise and implant a prosthetic cardiac valve. Their mechanical valve, based on a ball-in-cage technology, was implanted in the mitral position as the first long-term prosthetic valve implant in 1960 and became commercially available in 1965. Complications, partly related to its high profile, included obstruction of the left ventricular outflow tract and injury to aortic valve leaflets. These valves were also predisposed to thrombus formation, particularly models with a metallic ball.

   These problems subsequently led to development of the **Björk-Shiley** valve. This device was based on a low-profile design with a tilting stainless steel disk contained by a pair of small, welded metal struts which improved flow characteristics and lessened complications.

Types of Valves

• Numerous valves have since been devised, and over 40 models are currently in use worldwide. Prosthetic valves can be classified as **mechanical**, **bioprosthetic**, or **human homograft** (Fig. 12-1).

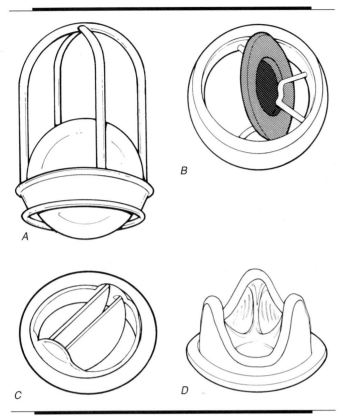

FIGURE 12-1   Types of valves. Illustrating four common valve types: *(A)* Ball-in-cage, *(B)* tilting disk, *(C)* bileaflet, and *(D)* bioprosthetic.

- **Mechanical valves** are based on three distinct designs. One is a ball-in-cage construction similar to the original Starr-Edwards valve. Another is a tilting disk configuration similar to the Björk-Shiley valve, and the third is a bileaflet valve of which the **St. Jude valve** is the most prevalent example.

- **The ball-in-cage valve** is used much more rarely than in the early era of valve replacement. Current examples are the modified **Starr-Edwards valve** (Fig. 12-2A) and the **Smeloff-Cutter valve** (Fig. 12-2B). The main disadvantages are their bulky size and thrombogenicity. They are the most obstructive type of prosthetic valve, causing disruption of flow in the left ventricular outflow tract. They are advantageous in that they have limited regurgitation compared to other designs. Starr-Edwards valves placed in the mitral position typically have four struts, whereas those placed in the aortic position have three struts.

- **Tilting disk valves** have increased in popularity since their initial introduction by Björk and Shiley (Fig. 12-3). They have a lower profile than ball-in-cage valves and are less disruptive of flow. These valves are prone to more significant regurgitation than ball-in-cage valves; however, this backwash of blood across the disk can be beneficial as it decreases thrombus formation.

    The tilting disk is set on several struts and a supporting annulus. During their evolution, the metallic struts were prone

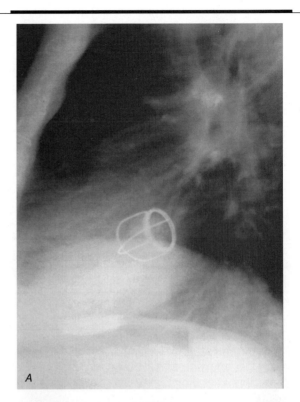

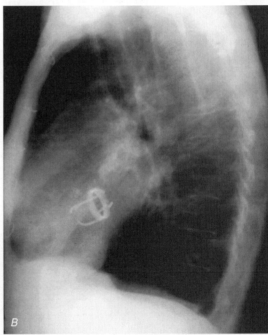

FIGURE 12-2   Ball-in-cage valve. (A) Lateral chest radiograph showing a Starr-Edwards valve in the mitral position. This can lead to left ventricular outflow obstruction. (B) Smeloff-Cutter valve in the mitral position. The struts on this type of ball-in-cage valve are normally discontinuous as shown. The ball in both valves is radiolucent.

to weakening and potentially fracture, resulting in abrupt, severe regurgitation and malfunction. This problem has been largely circumvented by constructing the valve from a single piece of metal alloy. The **Medtronic Hall valve** is a similar and commonly used tilting disk valve.

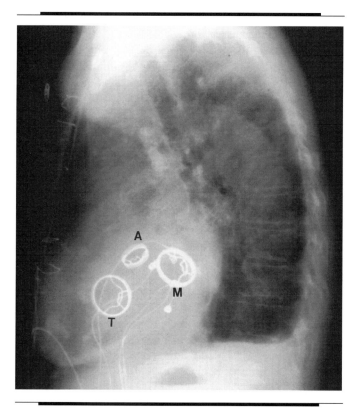

FIGURE 12-3 Tilting disk valves. Lateral chest radiograph showing aortic (A), mitral (M), and tricuspid (T) Björk-Shiley valves.

- **Bileaflet valves** have the lowest profile of all cardiac valves and are made of pyrolitic carbon, making them difficult to detect on radiographs unless they are perfectly profiled. The **St. Jude medical valve** is the prototype of this group (Fig. 12-4). Valve leaflets pivot within grooves, and each opens to approximately an 85-degree angle and closes at 30–35 degrees with respect to the base (Fig. 12-10, *C–D*). Valve function can be assessed fluoroscopically.

- **Bioprosthetic valves** include preserved porcine valves and those constructed of harvested bovine pericardium. The **Carpentier-Edwards valve** is an example of a porcine aortic valve (Fig. 12-5). This harvested material is tanned with gluteraldehyde and stretched over an annulus with several supporting struts which add stability and internal structure. The supporting frame is an undulating wire which typically has three prongs attached to a ring, allowing for ease in suturing the valve to the supporting cardiac annulus. The first porcine valve was inserted in 1965.

  Another type of bioprosthetic valve, the **Hancock porcine valve**, is seen as an uninterrupted circular ring without the

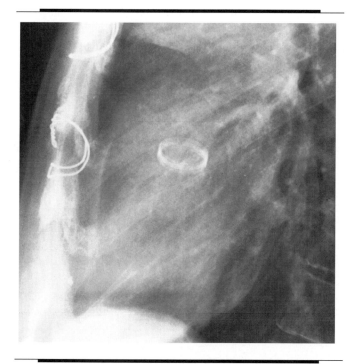

FIGURE 12-4 Bileaflet valve. Lateral chest radiograph showing an aortic St. Jude valve with a metal annulus which makes the valve radiographically evident. Most housings are made of pyrolitic carbon, making them very difficult to visualize (see Fig. 12-10).

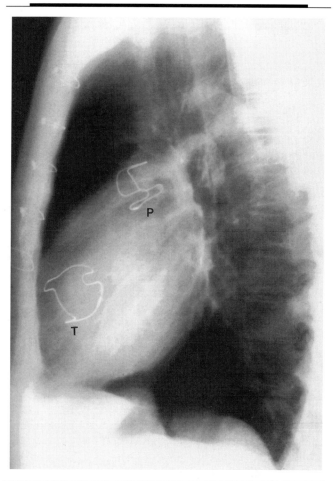

FIGURE 12-5 Bioprosthetic valve. Lateral chest radiograph showing right heart Carpentier-Edwards valves in a patient with carcinoid. Pulmonic (P) and tricuspid (T).

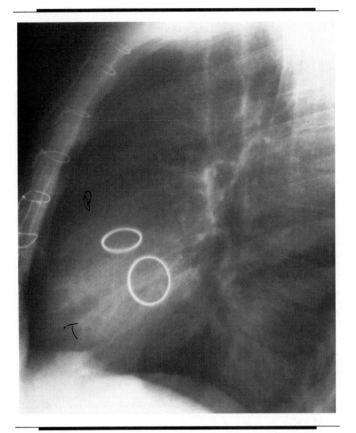

FIGURE 12-6   Bioprosthetic valve. Lateral chest radiograph showing the smaller aortic and larger mitral Hancock bioprosthetic valves. The complete metal annulus distinguishes this valve from an annuloplasty.

three prongs (Fig. 12-6). The interrupted ring seen typically in the mitral or tricuspid position is not a bioprosthetic valve but an annuloplasty, generally used to prevent regurgitation (Fig. 12-11).

- **Human homograft valves** are harvested from a donor heart and inserted into the recipient valve annulus. They are ideal for small aortic roots and are particularly beneficial in that anticoagulation is not required because of the very low rate of thromboembolism. The surgery is technically difficult because of the lack of a supporting frame, which lends structure and facilitates operative insertion. Also, these valves are more difficult to acquire.

Valve Positions and Indications

- Prosthetic valve location on a chest radiograph can usually confidently confirm which valve has been replaced. On a **frontal chest radiograph** (Fig. 12-7A), the most cephalad valve is the pulmonic valve, followed by the aortic valve slightly to the right. Slightly more inferior and to the left is the mitral valve, and the most inferior and right lateral is the tricuspid valve.

On the **lateral chest radiograph** (Fig. 12-7B), the aortic valve is the smallest valve and resides in the middle of the heart. If a line is drawn from the pulmonary hila through the cardiac apex, the mitral valve lies immediately posterior to the aortic valve in the center of the line. The pulmonic valve is the most superior and anterior of the valves. The tricuspid valve is located along the bisecting line anteriorly. Valves are typically better demonstrated and more easily visualized on a lateral radiograph because of the absence of overlapping structures.

Indications for valve replacement have been discussed in Section 6.11. Patient functional status as classified by the New York Heart Association (Section 15.10) is a primary criterion. The most severe debility is class IV in which patients are symptomatic at rest. Typical causes of both stenotic and regurgitant lesions include rheumatic heart disease, acute bacterial endocarditis, trauma, connective tissue disease, and congenital abnormalities such as a bicuspid aortic valve. The mitral and aortic valves are more commonly affected in these diseases and consequently are more frequently replaced in comparison with right-sided valves.

Complications

- The mortality rate from cardiac valve replacement is not trivial. Mortality rates for aortic and mitral valve replacement range from 3 to 7 percent. If multiple valves are replaced, mortality rates double. Reoperation likewise raises the mortality rate to between 9 and 14 percent, with a third aortic operation having a perioperative mortality of up to one-third of patients, and third mitral operation, approximately 65 percent mortality. Numerous potential complications can develop if patients survive the perioperative period.

- **Thromboembolism** is the most important problem facing patients with valve replacement. The risk of thromboembolic disease is 8 percent per year for mechanical valves, which have a higher thromboembolic rate than bioprosthetic valves.

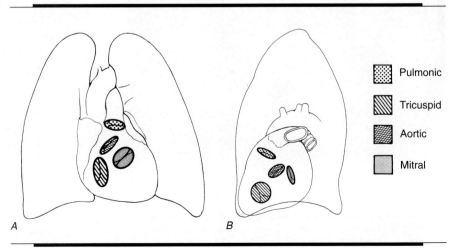

FIGURE 12-7   Valve position. Indicating the relative positions of the cardiac valves. *(A)* Frontal and *(B)* lateral.

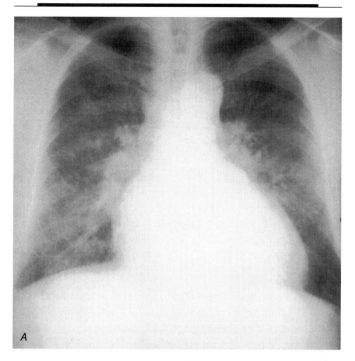

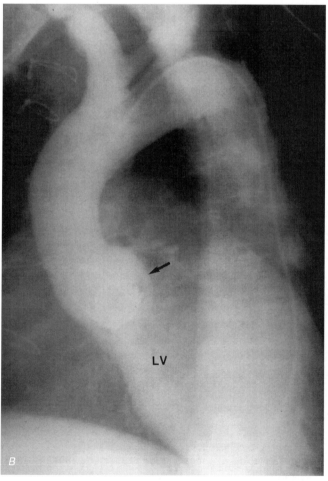

FIGURE 12-8   Periprosthetic leak. (*A*) Chest radiograph showing pulmonary edema and cardiomegaly. (*B*) Aortogram showing periprosthetic leak of contrast (arrow) around the Starr-Edwards valve and into the left ventricle (LV). There is infraprosthetic aortic regurgitation as well.

The risk is increased during the first year. The risk of thromboembolism is aggravated by conditions that lower cardiac output, including left atrial enlargement, poor left ventricular function, atrial fibrillation, and conditions such as endocarditis and multiple valves. Thromboembolism accounts for 18 percent of minor complications in patients with prosthetic valves and carries a 1 percent mortality risk per patient per year.

- **Long-term anticoagulation** is required for patients with mechanical valves. Patients are placed on prolonged coumadin therapy which adds the risk of hemorrhage. This treatment has a 5 to 15 percent yearly morbidity rate and a 1 percent yearly mortality rate. Hemorrhage may be spontaneous or the result of trivial or overt trauma. Additionally, coumadin has multiple documented adverse drug reactions and can be teratogenic. Usually bioprosthetic valves require only short-term post-operative anticoagulation.

- **Infection** is a dreaded complication. It may occur early in the postoperative period or as a delayed complication. The infection rate is about 1 percent per year, with a mortality rate exceedingly high. The rate of infection is similar for both mechanical and bioprosthetic valves. Common infectious agents include *Staphylococcus*, gram-negative bacilli, and *Candida* species. This potential complication mandates antibiotic prophylaxis during dental or other procedures associated with bacteremia.

  Valve infection has several potentially lethal complications including septic emboli to both the pulmonary parenchymal and systemic circulations. Within the lungs this infection is generally manifested as cavitary pulmonary nodules. The other complication is valve dehiscence and consequent periprosthetic leak (Fig. 12-8).

- **Other potential complications** include hemolytic anemia, which is present in the overwhelming majority of patients as a result of mechanical factors and is usually subclinical. Severe anemia may herald significant valve dysfunction and disruption of normal laminar flow. Other potential complications include obstruction, as can be seen with ball-in-cage valves; mechanical failure, such as a strut fracture in some Björk-Shiley valve models; and operative complications including pseudoaneurysm formation at the cannula sites of a cardiac bypass (Fig. 12-9). An often overlooked problem with the St. Jude valve is an audible mechanical click which can be unsettling to the patient.

- **Valve fluoroscopy** can be used to assess function. C-arm fluoroscopy allows optimal positioning to view the valve on edge and en face, allowing both subjective and quantitative assessment of symmetry and arc of excursion (Fig. 12-10). Thrombus formation and tissue ingrowth can limit excursion. As bileaflet valves have the lowest profile, they are the most difficult to visualize radiographically.

- **Valve selection** is based on several factors. The clinical goal is to relieve symptoms and minimize morbidity, mortality, and reoperation rates. Mechanical valves are durable but

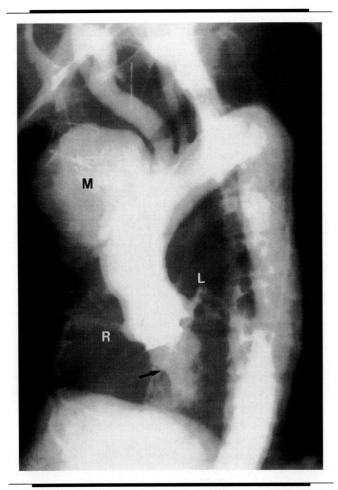

FIGURE 12-9 Mycotic pseudoaneurysm. Aortogram demonstrating a large pseudoaneurysm (M) arising from the ascending aorta and aortic insufficiency (arrow). An aortic Björk-Shiley valve is present. Also note filling of the right (R) and left (L) coronary arteries.

require long-term anticoagulation. Consequently, these valves are generally reserved for young patients (less than 65 years old) and patients with no known bleeding problems or risks for anticoagulation. Coumadin is teratogenic, making its use with mechanical valves inappropriate for women who wish to conceive.

Biological valves require only short-term anticoagulation and have less risk of thromboembolism and hemolysis, but they are less durable, having up to a 65 percent failure rate at 15 years. Consequently, bioprosthetic valves are reserved for older patients with a shorter life expectancy and for women of childbearing age. Also, bioprosthetic valves are placed in patients with contraindications to coumadin therapy such as a history of medical noncompliance or a known anticoagulation risk factor.

Other Procedures

- **Valve annuloplasty** refers to placement of an interrupted ring into the soft tissues of the valve ring in an effort to reform the annulus to the appropriate size and shape

(Fig. 12-11). The small gap is present to accommodate the bundle of His. This annuloplasty ring should not be confused with the complete ring of a bioprosthetic Hancock valve. Valve annuloplasty is typically performed in the treatment of mitral regurgitation.

- Thousands of patients undergo **coronary artery bypass grafting** each year. These procedures may involve internal mammary artery vein grafts or saphenous grafts from the leg. The origin of the graft from the anterior margin of the aorta is often marked with metallic rings for identification if subsequent coronary angiography is required (Fig. 12-12). The vertical median sternotomy approach is used for the vast majority of cardiac surgery. Multiple **sternal wires** are radiographically identified. It is important to evaluate these wires for disruption and possible sternal dehiscence. Late fractures are typically of no significance, although the broken end may cause pain, warranting removal.

- **Transcatheter closure** of a **patent ductus arteriosus (PDA)** is becoming more common (Fig. 12-13). Although surgical occlusion of a PDA is a safe, reliable procedure in infants and young patients, adult patients with brittle PDAs are at risk of hemorrhage and increased morbidity. This technique also obviates the need for general anesthesia. Coil occlusion with detachable Gianturco coils has safely been performed without a need for general anesthesia on an outpatient basis. Flow through the PDA is interrupted immediately in most cases, but it may take as long as several months before complete obliteration is achieved in a small percentage of patients. A Rashkind occluder or a buttoned device is accompanied by a less than 40 percent incidence of residual shunt.

12.3 PACEMAKERS

- As early as the 1700s it was recognized that electric shock could revive patients who had suffered acute cardiac arrhythmia and death. Consequently, devices that applied external electric shock were developed but were rarely successful. Attempts to construct pacemakers in the 1800s included the use of a metronome to provide alternating current to pace the heart. The first true cardiac pacemaker was developed in 1952 by Paul Zoll. No implantable wires were placed, but a belt was strapped across the chest, the patient was sedated, and current was applied across the chest wall. This procedure provided short-term therapy.

- In 1958 **C. Walton Lillehei** placed the first transthoracic epicardial leads. Initially, the external units were large, but as technology evolved, they became smaller and transvenous pacers were connected to external power sources. These early systems were plagued by skin entrance site infections and perforations at the site of cardiac insertion.

  As technology improved, power sources were made small enough to be implanted into subcutaneous tissues. The earliest power sources were implanted in the anterior abdominal wall. These pacemakers required a thoracotomy, as leads had to be sewn or screwed into the myocardium.

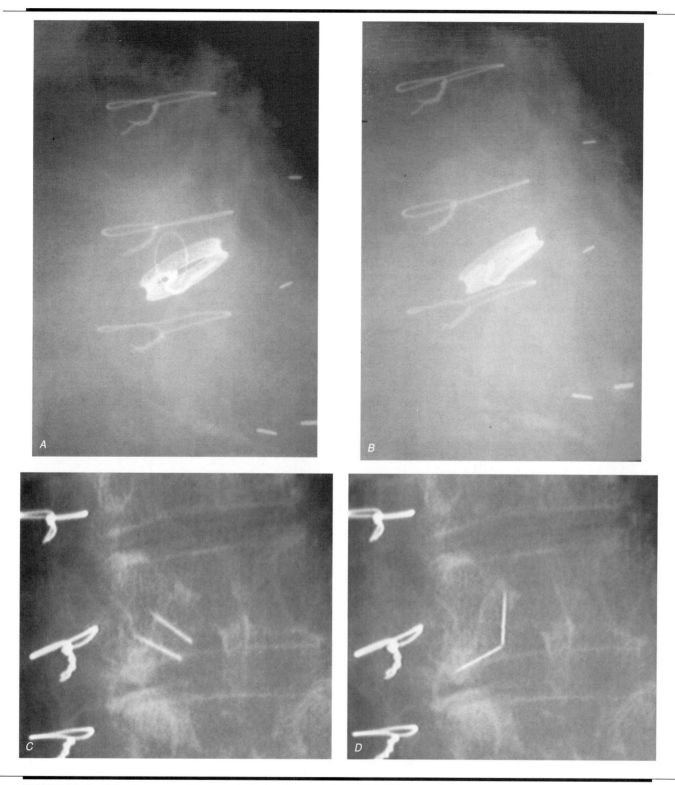

FIGURE 12-10   Valve fluoroscopy. Fluoroscopic images demonstrating a Björk-Shiley valve in the open (*A*) and closed (*B*) positions and a St. Jude valve in the open (*C*) and closed (*D*) positions. Only the St. Jude valve hemileaflets are seen in this profile view.

- **Terminology:** Pacemakers consist of a **power generator** and **sensing and pacing leads**. They may sense arrhythmias, pace the heart, and even cardiovert. A **unipolar** lead has only a cathode, with the pacing pulse transmitted back to the gen-erator through the body, whereas a **bipolar** lead contains both a cathode and an anode, with the second lead transmit-ting the pulse back to the generator. Pacemakers can function at a **fixed rate** or on **demand**. A **single lead** or **dual leads**

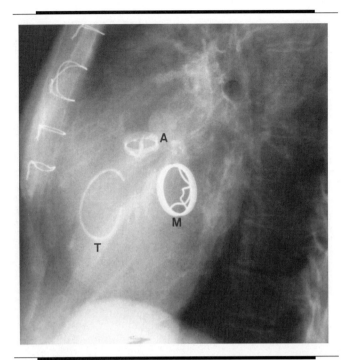

FIGURE 12-11   Annuloplasty. Lateral chest radiograph showing a tricuspid annuloplasty (T), a Björk-Shiley mitral (M) and a Medtronic-Hall aortic (A) valve.

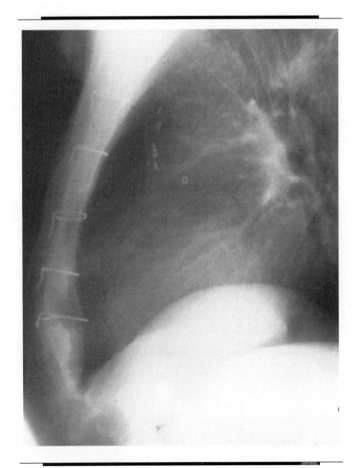

FIGURE 12-12   Coronary artery bypass graft markers. Six circular coronary bypass graft markers identify the saphenous vein grafts.

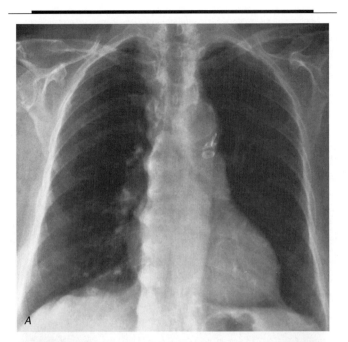

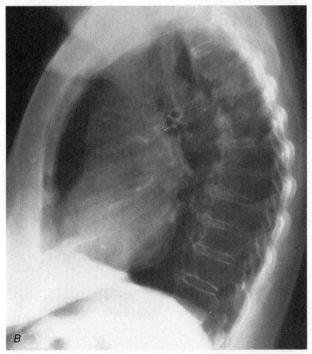

FIGURE 12-13   Patent ductus arteriosus occlusion. (*A* and *B*) PA and lateral chest radiographs demonstrating a percutaneously placed occlusion device seen between the aorta and pulmonary artery. Subtle calcification of the ductus is present.

may be present, with the latter firing sequentially in the atrium and then in the ventricle.

- **Indications for placement** of a transvenous pacer include two primary problems. The first is abnormalities of impulse formation, with typical etiologies including sick sinus syndrome, asystole, sinus tachycardia, atrial fibrillation, and atrial flutter. The other indication is defects in electrical conduction, predominantly complete heart block.

Unipolar Versus Bipolar Pacemakers

- Early pacemaker units tended to have a single **unipolar** lead. The implanted generator was the positive anode, while the lead within the right ventricle was the negatively charged cathode. A unipolar pacemaker was highly functional, although its sensing capabilities were poor because of the large distance between the anode and cathode and interference from muscular electrical potentials in both the chest wall and the arm.

- A **bipolar design** is found in most modern pacemakers. Bipolar pacemakers contain a double wire leading from the pacemaker which can be insulated within one lead (Fig. 12-14). The cathode and anode are separated at the distal tip within the right ventricle, which has improved sensing capabilities over the unipolar pacer and is not affected by chest wall musculature.

    Electrodes are secured to the right ventricular endocardium by one of two means. In most cases there is a screw along the distal aspect that is directly secured to the myocardium. Less commonly there is a tine adjacent to the terminal tip of the pacemaker, which becomes entangled within the trabeculae of the right ventricular wall. Both become more secure with time as local scar tissue develops.

- Patients with a **sequential pacemaker** have two separate leads. One is within the right atrium, and the other within the right ventricle (Fig. 12-15). The atrial lead is secured by a preshaped "J wire." This wire is straightened by a stylet, and during placement a formed J loop is secured within the right

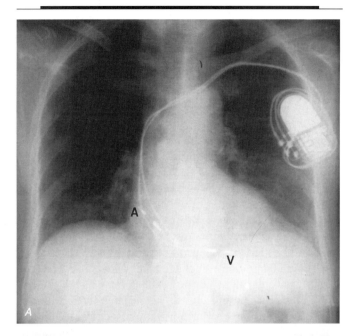

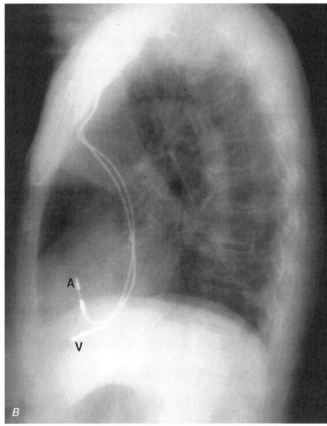

FIGURE 12-15 Sequential pacemaker. Frontal (*A*) and lateral (*B*) radiographs demonstrating the normal position of the right atrial (A) and ventricular (V) leads.

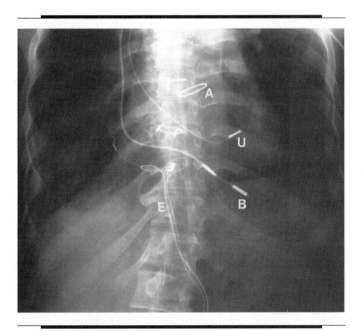

FIGURE 12-14 Pacing leads. Bipolar (B), unipolar (U), aortic bioprosthetic valve (A), and epicardial (E) leads.

atrial appendage, allowing sequential pacing of the atria followed by ventricular contraction.

- **Battery systems** have also undergone significant evolutionary change. The earliest pacemaker was charged by a mercury zinc battery, and five circular batteries were evident on radiographs as concentric disks within the transistor itself. The life span of these batteries was only 2 to 3 years. They emitted hydrogen gas and sodium hydroxide during the decay process and consequently had to be embedded in a resin to prevent patient exposure. Furthermore, the mercury oxide was converted to metallic mercury.

In an effort to prolong the life of a given generator implant, rechargeable **nickel cadmium batteries** were introduced. These batteries required weekly recharging and had a unit life of up to 30 years. An additional alternative power source was a nuclear pacemaker, which involved plutonium-238 as a power source. Thirty-five hundred batteries were implanted, yet problems with patient tracking, plutonium disposal, and public relations led to their quick demise. The radiation risk to the patient was essentially theoretical, with no proven malignancies found. Public risk was real when the fuel capsule was exposed during either trauma or cremation.

Current pacemaker technology is centered about a **lithium iodide power source**, which was introduced in 1971 and is able to generate more energy per unit weight. The lifetime of the lithium iodide power source is 15 years, and new units have a 7- to 9-year life span.

- A **letter system** for designating **pacemaker mode and function** is commonly employed. The first letter indicates the chamber that is paced, with V representing ventricle, A representing atrium, and D representing double or both chambers. The second letter indicates the chamber assessed and includes the previous designations plus an O indicating that no chamber is assessed. This example represents a fixed-rate pacemaker. Finally, the third letter represents the response mode. Here, I represents inhibited mode, which is blocked by a sensed signal, while T represents triggered mode, where the pacemaker is just charged by a sensed signal.

- **Monitoring of pacemakers** can be accomplished in several ways. Typically, outpatient monitoring is done electronically over the telephone on a regular basis, perhaps every 2 months. Patients can be seen in a clinic on a longer-term basis, typically annually, where more sophisticated monitoring can be performed.

Placement Complications

- Radiology plays a role in monitoring complications following transvenous pacemaker insertion, including detection of pneumothorax, hemothorax, lead malposition, and fracture. Tricuspid valve damage during placement can lead to tricuspid regurgitation.

- **Lead malposition** occurs in roughly 6 percent of cases, and 50 percent of lead dislodgements occur in the first 2 weeks following placement. Lead malposition should be detected before fibrous ingrowth occurs at the site of myocardial implantation. Locations of lead malposition include the right atrium, the pulmonary outflow tract, the hepatic veins, and the coronary sinus.

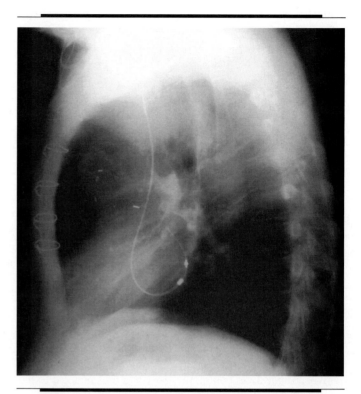

FIGURE 12-16   Coronary sinus malposition. Lateral chest radiograph showing the posterior position of a pacemaker lead in the coronary sinus.

Coronary sinus malposition is somewhat common. The coronary sinus drains the myocardium and empties into the right atrium between the inferior vena cava and the tricuspid valve. It is guarded by an incompetent semilunar valve. Placement here is usually inadvertent, although it is occasionally used for intentional atrial pacing. The key to radiographic detection is a lateral radiograph demonstrating posterior positioning of the lead with its tip directed cephalad (Fig. 12-16).

Left ventricular malposition is a serious problem and may occur through a patent foramen ovale, intraventricular septum, fossa ovalis, or sinus venosus defect or via an inadvertent transatrial placement. Clinically, this situation is manifested as a right bundle branch block on electrocardiography, whereas a normal right ventricular lead produces a left bundle branch pattern. Plain radiographs demonstrate the pacer lead within the left ventricle (Fig. 12-17). Management is controversial, with surgical removal versus anticoagulation therapy employed to prevent thromboembolism.

- An additional complication is **perforation**, which occurs in less than 3 percent of patients. It is manifested by failure to pace the myocardium or pacing of the heart with an increased threshold. Rarely, a perforation can present as cardiac tamponade because of hemopericardium and bleeding. A perforation through the inferior wall may lead to pacing of the diaphragm and compromise normal respiration. It may also

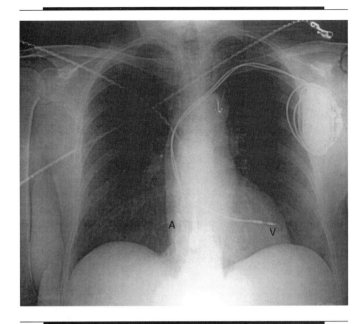

FIGURE 12-17   Left ventricular malposition. Frontal chest radi-ograph showing a pacemaker lead (V) more superior and lateral in position than expected. Lateral chest radiograph confirmed the malposition. The right atrial lead (A) is in a normal position.

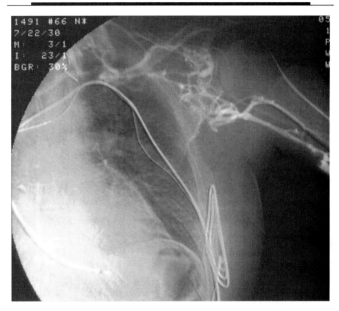

FIGURE 12-19   Lead-induced thrombophlebitis. Venogram showing thrombosis of the left subclavian and axillary veins with collateral vessel filling in a patient with a transvenous cardiac lead.

penetrate into the pulmonary parenchyma of pleural space (Fig. 12-18).

- **Thrombophlebitis** can occur early following insertion but is relatively uncommon (Fig. 12-19). Pulmonary emboli as well as septic emboli may occur as a result.

- **Lead fracture** is an additional complication that can be demonstrated radiographically (Fig. 12-20). Although a lead is fractured, it may continue to function intermittently and be difficult to detect radiographically if the wire is not dis-placed. This complication generally results from a lead being either too taut or too slack. It can also be due to excessive

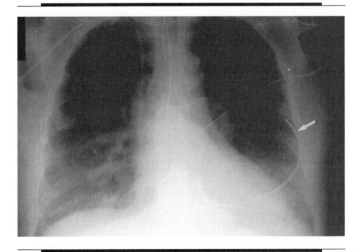

FIGURE 12-18   Pleural malposition. The pacemaker lead has perforated the heart and entered the pleural space (arrow).

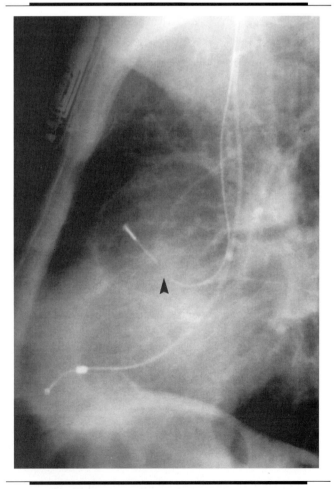

FIGURE 12-20   Pacemaker lead fracture. Lateral chest radio-graph demonstrating a fracture (arrowhead) of the atrial lead in a sequential pacemaker.

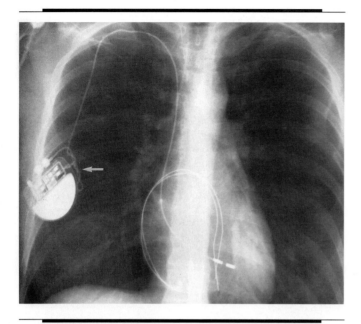

FIGURE 12-21　Twiddler syndrome. Radiograph showing a single-lead bipolar pacemaker in place and retained epicardial pacing wires. Note entanglement of the pacing wire (arrow) produced by excessive patient manipulation. The baseline chest radiograph 1 month earlier was normal.

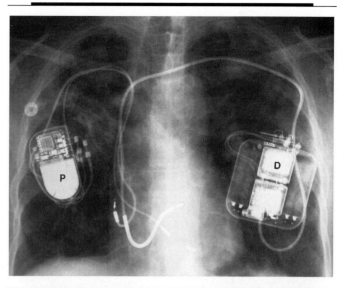

FIGURE 12-22　Pacemaker and defibrillator. Frontal chest radiograph showing a sequential bipolar pacemaker (P) entering from a right subclavian approach. There is also a transvenous defibrillator (D) entering from the left. The ventricular lead is intentionally directed away from the pacer lead to prevent interaction.

shoulder motion, kinking, or direct trauma. Atrial J-wire disruption can be determined with high-resolution fluoroscopy.

- **Twiddler syndrome** is caused by excessive patient manipulation of the implanted generator, which can progress to lead dislodgment, fracture, or detachment with ineffective pacing and sensing capacities (Fig. 12-21).

12.4　CARDIAC DEFIBRILLATORS

- Approximately 500,000 sudden deaths attributable to cardiac arrythmias occur annually in the United States. Individuals who are successfully resuscitated have a significant risk of recurrence. Few patients are candidates for surgical cure for their arrhythmias, and medical treatment may be limited by lack of efficacy as well as by proarrhythmic and intolerable side effects.

- **Implantable cardiac defibrillators** have significantly altered the treatment of cardiac arrhythmias. These devices function as cardioverters and can terminate both tachy- and bradyarrhythmias, although they were initially used only for ventricular arrythmias. They have been highly successful, with a less than 5 percent arrhythmia mortality rate over 5 years compared to a 40 percent annual mortality rate for untreated tachyarrhythmias. These devices continue to evolve as technology improves (Fig. 12-22).

- **Implantable cardiac defibrillators (ICDs)** are the classic example. They contain sensing leads, a shock generator, and cardioverting patches. The sensing apparatus consists of

epicardial screw-in or trabecular hook leads. The shock pads are titanium mesh within silicone elastic placed in the pericardial space. A radiodense wire within the mesh is present solely for radiographic delineation. The lithium silver vanadium oxide batteries last 3 to 5 years.

The radiographic appearance can vary greatly. Anywhere between one and four patches are placed depending on electrophysiologic pathology and thresholds. They appear on plain film as rectangular or concentric oval wire patches (Fig. 12-21). The pacing leads appear as conventional epicardial leads with terminal screws and may be intra- or extrapericardial. The shock generator is a square device implanted in the subcutaneous tissues.

- More recently, **ICDs** have been developed with additional capabilities. They have antitachycardia pacing algorithms that can terminate ventricular tachycardia without shocks, and they can serve as single- or dual-chamber bradycardia pacemakers.

Transvenous leads have been developed that do not require thoracotomy and thus are minimally invasive. The lead has proximal and distal coils for shock delivery, and has sensing and pacing capabilities (Fig. 12-23).

- **Complications** include malfunction if the leads fracture, typically as they penetrate the chest wall (Fig. 12-24). Fractures result from mechanical stress and probable compression between the clavicle and anterior first rib.

The lead may migrate, as it is not mechanically secured in position, perhaps resulting in inadequate defibrillation, sensing, or pacing which would render it ineffective. Patch distortion is common and often of no clinical significance, although it may cause lead fractures or signify infection or

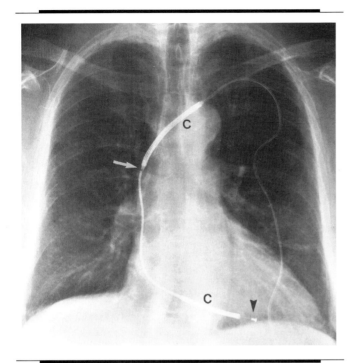

FIGURE 12-23   ICD. An ICD in place with the shock generator implanted in the anterior abdominal wall. The apparent disruption seen in the lead (arrow) is normal, although it is commonly mistaken for a fracture in this CPI brand lead. Note the sensing lead (arrowhead) in the right ventricular apex and the two defibrillator coils (C).

adjacent fluid collection (Fig. 12-25). Distorted patches are also common following cardiac transplantation. Finally, lead disconnection from the pulse generator is uncommon.

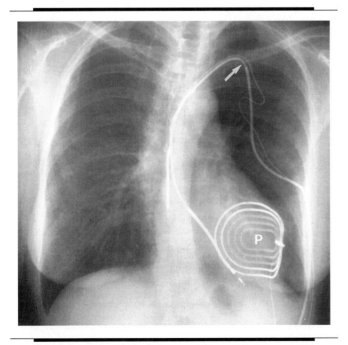

FIGURE 12-24   ICD lead fracture. ICD malfunction caused by disruption of the outer coil of the sensor, pacer, defibrillator lead as it passes through the chest wall (arrow). The replacement lead fractured at the same site 6 months later. Note the single pericardial patch (P).

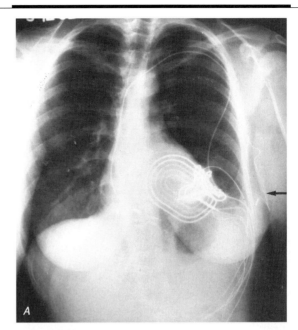

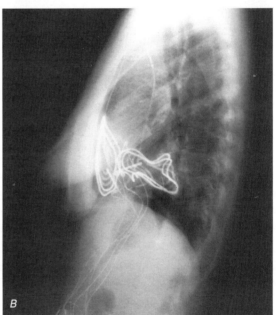

FIGURE 12-25   ICD malfunction caused by patch distortion. Frontal (*A*) and lateral (*B*) chest radiographs demonstrating distortion of one of the pericardial patches and a replacement subcutaneous patch in the left lateral chest wall (arrow).

- **External defibrillators,** such as the Zoll patch, may be temporarily employed. These devices have a characteristic "cobra head" or a pentagon shape.

12.5 ESOPHAGEAL, AIRWAY, VASCULAR, AND CORONARY STENTS

- **Endoluminal stents** are gaining in popularity for the treatment of many intrathoracic diseases. They are often palliative but can also be therapeutic, such as radioactive stents placed

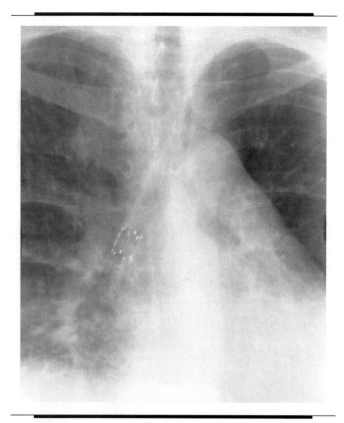

FIGURE 12-26 Bronchial stent. Gianturco stent placed in the right mainstem bronchus across an anastomotic stricture in a patient who has undergone a lung transplant.

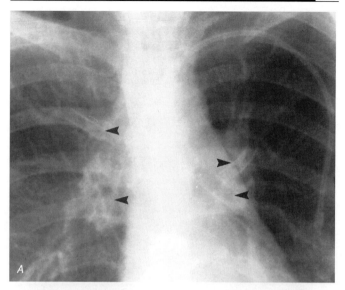
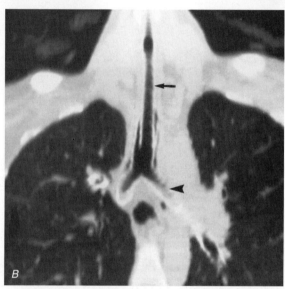

FIGURE 12-27 Airway stents. (*A*) Radiograph and (*B*) coronal reformatted CT in a 26-year-old woman with relapsing polychondritis. She has had both expandable metallic stents (arrowheads) placed in the bronchi and plastic stents placed in the trachea (arrow).

within the coronary arteries. While in their infancy, these stents and other devices are becoming more prevalent in the treatment of malignant esophageal fistulae and perforations, coronary artery disease, and vascular and airway stenoses.

- **Esophageal stents** are more commonly being employed in the treatment of esophageal perforations and fistulae. They are often reserved for palliation of dysphagia related to unresectable cancer which, unfortunately, is a rather common occurrence. Over 60 percent of esophageal cancer patients have incurable disease at the time of initial diagnosis. Earlier therapy centered around palliative surgery or radiation therapy. Unfortunately, these interventions have inherent risks, and recurrent dysphagia occurs in approximately 20 percent of cases.

  The original rigid plastic stents were plagued by perforation, dislodgment, and occlusion (Section 11.5). They have generally been replaced by expandable metallic stents which have lower complication and mortality rates. The Ultraflex Nitinol® stent, the Gianturco Z® stent, the Wallstent®, and the Esophacoil® are several of the stents currently used. They are either stainless steel or a metal alloy. Self-expanding stents may take several weeks to obtain maximal dilatation.

  Expandable metallic stents also can have multiple potential complications including perforation, aspiration, and incomplete expansion during the periprocedural period. Later

complications include stent occlusion or migration, tumor ingrowth or overgrowth, erosions, and bleeding. Tumor overgrowth is reduced in metal stents (6 to 9 percent) as compared with plastic stents (5 to 22 percent).

The radiographic appearance is similar to that of metallic stents elsewhere. Paying particular attention to position on serial examinations should allow early detection of migration. An esophagram can be obtained in cases where tumor overgrowth or stent occlusion is suspected clinically.

- **Tracheobronchial stents** have been employed for the treatment of airway stenoses, particularly those due to compression or cicatrix. More recently, self-expanding Nitinol stents have been successfully used in cases of intraluminal nonoperative tumor.

Tracheobronchial stents have several benefits. They avoid having the device exit the neck like a tracheostomy, and they maintain airway patency without necessarily requiring repeated procedures as intraluminal laser therapy generally does; however, there are multiple potential complications including migration, wall erosions and tracheoesophageal fistulae, reocclusion, and hemoptysis.

Plastic stents were associated with infection, granulation tissue formation, tumor overgrowth, and obstruction. These complications may be reduced with the use of expandable metallic stents (Fig. 12-26). Besides extrinsic compression from lymphadenopathy and mediastinal tumor, conditions such as primary tracheobronchial tumor, relapsing polychondritis, and endobronchial non-Hodgkin lymphoma have been treated with stenting (Fig. 12-27).

- **Coronary stenting** began a decade ago, but early stents had thrombosis rates approaching 20 percent. Improved antiplatelet therapy and new techniques in deployment such as intravascular ultrasound have led to improved results. Coronary stenting has been shown to be an effective adjuvant to angioplasty in treating new focal stenoses and flow-limiting dissections.

  While initially contraindicated in acute myocardial infarction, more recent work has been encouraging in this setting. Angioplasty has better than a 30-day benefit, but there may be better long-term preservation of vessel caliber with stenting, as angioplasty has rates of restenosis between 30 and 60 percent. Consequently, stents may reduce the restenosis rate by 30 percent compared with angioplasty. Restenotic narrowings generally have a worse outcome after stenting than de novo lesions.

  Potential disadvantages include lack of flexibility, limiting deployment in tortuous vessels, and low axial strength. The advantages are several, namely, lower restenosis rates and general avoidance of potential intimal dissection and subsequent complications. Also, catheter-based radiotherapy with iridium 192 in conjunction with stenting has been preliminarily shown to result in a substantially reduced restenosis rate.

- The Palmaz-Schatz stent, a 15-mm device consisting of two 7-mm slotted stainless steel tubes connected by a 1-mm bridging strut, is commonly used. A Gianturco-Roubin stent is also used. Stents can be deployed alone or in tandem (Fig. 12-28).

- While **vascular stents** are not yet approved by the U.S. Food and Drug Administration (FDA) for use in the chest other than the heart, there are numerous roles for arterial, venous, and even aortic stenting in both experimental and routine clinical settings. The origins of the great arteries can be stented for arm claudication, transient ischemic attacks, and stroke prevention. Stenting can be performed from a trans-femoral approach or via a surgical cut-down in the carotid artery. Palmaz stents and Wallstents have been used in this role, but the newer Nitinol stents have not yet been extensively tested.

  Venous stenting is generally reserved for the subclavian vein in hemodialysis patients with flow-limiting stenosis resulting in refractory arm swelling (Fig. 12-29). Wallstents are currently preferred for this indication. Other less common roles involve treatment of venous stenosis resulting from iatrogenic stenosis (a pacemaker or a central line) in the subclavian vein and superior vena cava occlusion resulting in superior vena cava syndrome. The Wallstent is the stent of choice, but the long-term patency of venous stenting has been questioned and remains controversial.

  Advances in covered stents may revolutionize the treatment of atheroscelrotic and traumatic aortic pathology, as well as expand applications for stenting the great vessels. Early reports suggest that percutaneously placed stent-grafts can be used to successfully treat traumatic injuries of the aorta and atherosclerotic aneurysms. Much additional work and improvement in the existing technology needs to take place in this area before covered stents can be commonly employed, particularly in the treatment of thoracic vascular disease.

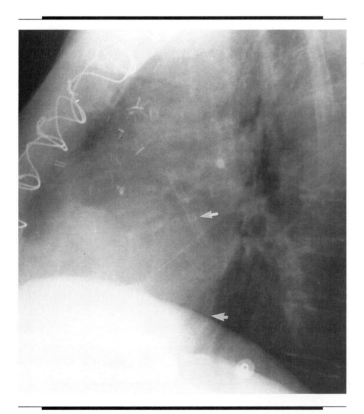

FIGURE 12-28 Coronary artery stents. Lateral chest radiograph showing metallic stents (arrows) in the marginal branch of the circumflex artery.

12.6 ORTHOPEDIC DEVICES

- The chest radiograph often bears evidence of prior orthopedic or neurosurgical intervention. Although spinal surgery may involve only a laminectomy to gain access to the spinal canal

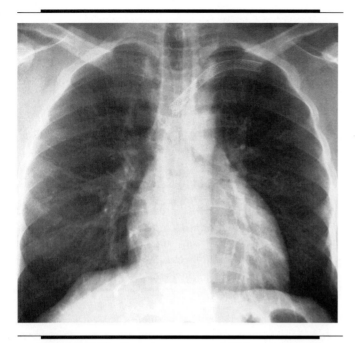

FIGURE 12-29 Central venous stent. A Wallstent stent in the left subclavian and brachiocephalic veins in a 33-year-old dialysis patient.

or intervertebral disks, multilevel fusion is usually accompanied by fixation. Entities that may require fixation include traumatic burst fractures, degenerative disk disease, scoliosis, congenital deformities, and occasionally tumors causing mechanical instability.

- **Spinal fixation** includes rods, plates, screws, and wires placed anteriorly or posteriorly to provide stability and maintain alignment during osseous fusion. **Osseous fusion** is facilitated by the placement of bone graft in the form of morselized bone within the facet joints, between transverse processes, or in intervertebral disk spaces. Structural allografts or metallic cages packed with morselized bone are also used following corpectomy (vertebral body removal) (Fig. 12-30). These cages can also be placed in disk spaces for fusion between vertebrae. Methylmethacrylate is occasionally used following corpectomy for a tumor when palliation rather than long-term correction is the goal.

    Harrington compression and distraction rods were introduced in the 1960s. They apply corrective forces at the end of the rod via **laminar hooks** (Fig. 12-31). Paired rod systems have since become the most common posterior instrumentation. **Luque rods**, introduced in the 1970s, are smooth rods, often contoured and attached with segmental wiring, allowing corrective force to be applied at multiple levels (Fig. 12-32).

    More recently Cotrel-Dubousset (CD), Texas Scottish Rite Hospital (TSRH) and other paired rod systems have been utilized in combination with both laminar hooks and **pedicle screws** which pass through the pedicle into the vertebral body, providing three-dimensional segmental control to maximize correction and stability. **Plates and rods** are sometimes placed along the vertebral bodies for anterior fix-

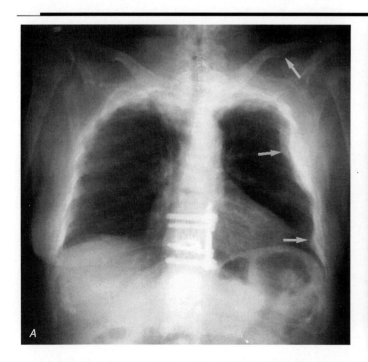

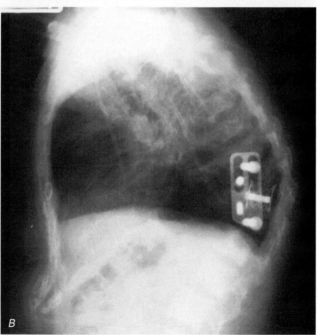

FIGURE 12-30 Anterior spinal fusion. Chest radiograph in a woman with metastatic breast cancer with an unstable spine. There has been resection of the eighth thoracic vertebral body and an anterior plate and vertebral body screws have been placed in the seventh and ninth thoracic vertebrae. The titanium cage filling the corpectomy space is typically filled with morselized bone to promote fusion. Note the destructive osseous metastases in the left clavicle and lateral ribs (arrows).

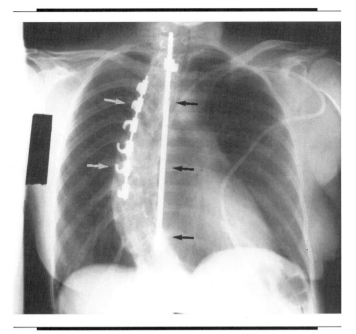

FIGURE 12-31   Harrington rods. PA chest radiograph following a posterior spinal fusion for management of scoliosis showing both Harrington compression rods (white arrows) and Harrington distraction rods (black arrows).

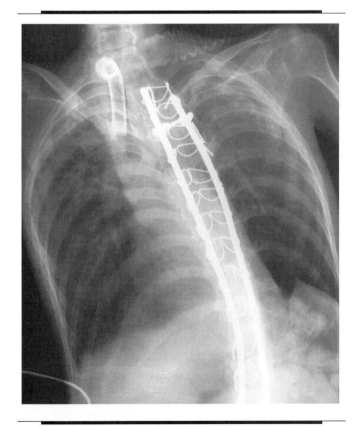

FIGURE 12-32   Luque rods. PA chest radiograph showing paired Luque rods with segmental sublaminar wiring following posterior thoracolumbar fusion for treatment of neuromuscular scoliosis. Note metallic tracheotomy tube and ventilator tubing.

ation. In some settings, both anterior and posterior fixation are used in combination.

- **Other orthopedic instrumentation** seen on chest radiographs may include shoulder arthroplasties. Reconstructive surgery of the shoulder may utilize **sutural anchors** which are small screws threaded into the bone cortex that have suture attached to the screws for reattaching tendons and ligaments. Screws and other wires are occasionally used to attach the clavicle to the acromion or the coracoid to the clavicle in shoulder separation injuries.

- **Instrumentation is generally not removed** but left in place after fusion has occurred because of the morbidity associated with removal. In the absence of a successful osseous fusion, recurrent stresses can lead to metal fatigue and fracture of the instrumentation. Other **complications** include dislodgment of laminar hooks, fracture of wires, osseous resorption around screws due to loosening or infection, and migration of the hardware which may encroach on critical structures.

Bibliography

Akagi T, Hashino K, Sugimura T, Ishii M, Eto G, Kato H. Coil occlusion of patent ductus arteriosus with detachable coils. *Am. Heart J.* 1997; 134:538–543.

Almagor Y, Feld S, Kiemeneij F, Serruys PW, Morice MC, Colombo A, Macaya C, Guermonprez JL, Marco J, Erbel R, Penn IM, Bonan R, Leon MB. First international new intravascular rigid-flex endovascular stent study (FINESS): Clinical and angiographic results after elective and urgent stent implantation—The FINESS trial investigators. *J. Am. Coll. Cardiol.* 1997; 30:847–854.

Bejvan SM, Ephron JH, Takasugi JE, Godwin JD, Bardy GH. Imaging of cardiac pacemakers. *Am. J. Roentgenol.* 1997;169:1371–1379.

Eagar G, Gutierrez FR, Gamache MC. Radiologic appearance of implantable cardiac defibrillators. *Am. J. Roentgenol.* 1994;162:25–29.

Fischman DL, Leon MB, Baim DS, Schatz RA, Savage MP, Penn IM, Detre K, Veltri L, Ricci D, Nobuyoshi M, Cleman M, Heuser R, Almond D, Teirstein PS, Fish RD, Colombo A, Brinker J, Moses J, Shaknovich A, Hirshfeld J, Bailey S, Ellis S, Rake R, Goldberg S. A randomized comparison of coronary stent placement and balloon angioplasty in the treatment of coronary artery disease. *N. Engl. J. Med.* 1994;331:496–501.

Gollub MJ, Gerdes H, Bains MS. Radiographic appearances of esophageal stents. *Radiographics* 1997;17:1169–1182.

Mittal S, Weiss DL, Hirshfeld JW Jr, Kolansky DM, Herrmann HC. Comparison of outcome after stenting for de novo versus restenotic narrowings in native coronary arteries. *Am. J. Cardiol.* 1997;80:711–715.

Morgan RA, Ellul JP, Denton ER, Glynos M, Mason RC, Adam A. Malignant esophageal fistulas and perforations: Management with plastic-covered metallic endoprostheses. *Radiology* 1997;204:527–532.

Morse D, Steiner RM, Fernandez F. *Guide to Prosthetic Cardiac Valves.* New York: Springer-Verlag; 1985.

Shah R, Sabanathan S, Mearns AJ, Featherstone H. Self-expanding tracheobronchial stents in the management of major airway problems. *J. Cardiovasc. Surg.* 1995;36:343–348.

Slone RM, McEnery KW. Principles, imaging, and complications of spinal instrumentation: Radiologist's perspective. In: Jenkins RJ, ed. *Post-therapeutic Neorodiagnostic Imaging.* Philadelphia: Lippincott-Raven; 1997: 245–266.

Takasugi JE, Godwin JD II, Bardy GH. The implantable pacemaker-cardioverter-defibrillator: Radiographic aspects. *Radiographics.* 1994;14: 1275–1290.

Teirstein PS, Massullo V, Jani S, Popma JJ, Mintz GS, Russo RJ, Schatz RA, Guarneri EM, Steuterman S, Morris NB, Leon MB, Tripuraneni P. Catheter-based radiotherapy to inhibit restenosis after coronary stenting. *N. Engl. J. Med.* 1997;336:1697–1703.

Vesely TM, Hovsepian DM, Pilgram TK, Coyne DW, Shenoy S. Upper extremity central venous obstruction in hemodialysis patients: Treatment with Wallstents. *Radiology.* 1997; 204:343–348.

Wagner HJ, Stinner B, Schwerk WB, Hoppe M, Klose KJ. Nitinol prostheses for the treatment of inoperable malignant esophageal obstruction. *J. Vasc. Interv. Radiol.* 1994;5:899–904.

Wallace MJ, Charnsangavej C, Ogawa K, Carrasco CH, Wright KC, McKenna R, McMurtrey M, Gianturco C. Tracheobronchial tree: Expandable metallic stents used in experimental and clinical applications. *Radiology.* 1986;158:309–312.

Chapter 13

UPPER ABDOMEN

Andrew J. Fisher

13.1 UPPER ABDOMEN
13.2 STOMACH
13.3 LIVER
13.4 GALLBLADDER AND BILIARY TREE
13.5 PANCREAS
13.6 ADRENAL GLANDS
13.7 KIDNEYS
13.8 SPLEEN

13.1 UPPER ABDOMEN

• The upper abdomen is visualized on almost all standard chest radiographs. The similarity of various tissue densities and relative underexposure to optimize pulmonary visualization limit, but do not preclude, display of abdominal pathology. For these reasons, it is important to be familiar with the normal anatomy, variants, and common pathologic entities of the upper abdomen.

Patients may have upper abdominal disease thought to be chest-related, such as a subphrenic abscess or pancreatitis. Chest disease may extend into the abdomen, although abdominal disease more frequently involves the thorax, particularly sympathetic effusions from pancreatitis or pulmonary metastases from abdominal malignancies. Systemic disease processes may involve both compartments.

Similarly, chest computed tomography (CT) and magnetic resonance imaging (MR) examinations include portions of the abdomen, both as a consequence of including the posterior sulcus of the lung in the examination and intentionally to visualize the adrenal glands and liver in patients being staged for lung cancer.

Fluid and Air

• **Pneumoperitoneum**, abdominal free air, is always abnormal. It is best identified on an upright chest radiograph, where it is evident as lucency below a hemidiaphragm or between the liver and abdominal wall on a left lateral decubitus view (Fig. 13-1). CT imaging, particularly with lung windows, is very sensitive for free air. It can be the result of bowel perforation, peritoneal dialysis, abdominal surgery, or percutaneous

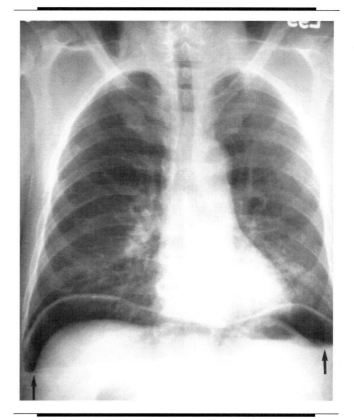

FIGURE 13-1   Pneumoperitoneum. Radiograph showing free air underneath both hemidiaphragms resulting from recent surgery in a 66-year-old woman. There is an air-fluid level in the subphrenic space (arrows).

tube placement. The rate of absorption is variable, but post-procedural air generally resolves within the first week.

• **Pneumatosis**, air in the bowel wall, can be a harbinger of bowel ischemia or infarction. Less ominous causes include overuse of steroids, bowel obstruction, and chronic obstructive pulmonary disease. Repeat CT imaging with the patient in the decubitus position may help differentiate intraluminal air from pneumatosis.

• **Ascites** is a common finding in abdominal pathology. It can be malignant or infectious or related to cirrhosis, local inflamma-

283

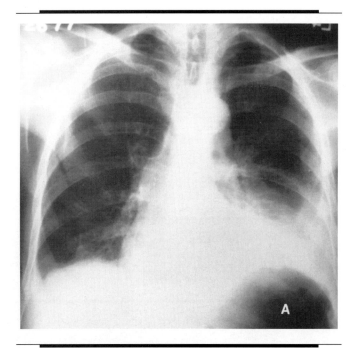

FIGURE 13-2   Subphrenic abscess. There is elevation of the left hemidiaphragm with associated atelectasis and pleural effusion. The gas collection in the left upper abdomen was a subphrenic abscess (A) from prior splenectomy.

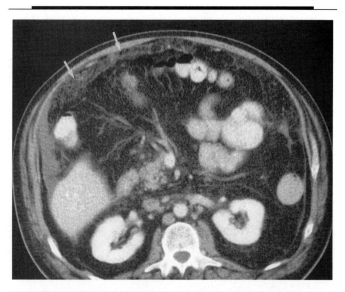

FIGURE 13-3   Carcinomatosis. There is an "omental cake" (arrows) of soft tissue stranding within the omentum representing peritoneal carcinomatosis. Also note a small amount of malignant ascites. This patient had a large distal esophageal cancer.

tion, or peritoneal dialysis. Enhancement of the peritoneum suggests peritonitis or malignant ascites with studding of the peritoneal surface.

- A **subphrenic abscess** may result from abdominal surgery, penetrating trauma, or bowel perforation. On plain radiographs the hemidiaphragm may be elevated, there may be basilar atelectasis or an effusion, and gas bubbles or an air-fluid level may be seen in the subdiaphragmatic space (Fig. 13-2). CT shows a fluid attenuation lesion with an enhancing rim and internal air or debris.

Omentum and Mesentery

- The **omentum** has been called "the policeman of the abdomen," as it can compartmentalize pathologic processes including infection and neoplasm. It is draped over the anterior aspect of the viscera. The abdominal **mesentery** contains numerous upper abdominal ligaments including the gastrocolic, gastrosplenic, gastrohepatic, phrenicocolic, and splenorenal ligaments. The lesser sac is located posterior to the stomach, anterior to the pancreas, and medial to the gastrosplenic ligament with access via the foramen of Winslow.

- **Carcinomatosis** is seeding of the abdominal mesentery and omentum with tumor (Fig. 13-3). This condition is classically seen in ovarian cancer, although it can be observed in numerous other tumors, including esophageal, gastrointestinal, pancreatic, and renal primaries, as well as lymphoma and cholangiocarcinoma. Small nodules and soft tissue stranding are present, and there may be malignant ascites and an enhancing peritoneum.

- **Lymphadenopathy** can be present in both infectious and neoplastic processes. Lymphoma is common, although a specific distribution, such as gastrohepatic ligament lymphadenopathy in esophageal cancer, or **low-density adenopathy** as seen in tuberculosis (TB), *Mycoplasma avium-intracellulare* (MAI), Whipple disease, seminoma, and treated lymphoma may provide differential clues.

- There are many types of hernias, including **ventral hernias** due to diastasis of the midline rectus fascia. **Incisional hernias** are the most common type and occur adjacent to laparotomy or stoma sites. **Spigelian hernias** occur at the fascial aponeurosis between the rectus and lateral abdominal musculature. They can be difficult to identify clinically, as they remain covered by the external oblique muscle. **Internal hernias** such as paraduodenal and foramen of Winslow types are uncommon but often lead to obstruction caused by a narrow hernia opening.

- **Bowel dilatation** can be seen in conjunction with an ileus or mechanical obstruction. A transition point and an obstructing lesion such as a tumor should be sought.

13.2   STOMACH

- The **stomach** is a distensible, muscular structure divided anatomically into the cardia, fundus, antrum, and pylorus. Normal rugal folds can be seen on both plain films and CT. The stomach is best examined when distended with fluid or gas. Water has recently gained popularity over conventional oral contrast as a luminal contrast agent in the CT evaluation of gastric cancer.

- **Gastric overdistention** can be seen in gastroparesis resulting from diabetes or secondary to mechanical obstruction caused by ulcer disease, duodenal or pancreatic tumors, duodenal webs and diaphragms, and superior mesenteric artery syndrome.

- A **nondistensible stomach**, termed *linitis plastica*, suggests fibrosis or tumor. Considerations for linitis plastica include infiltrating adenocarcinoma, lymphoma, gastritis, granulomatous conditions, and Ménétièr disease (Fig. 13-4). Tuberculosis, histoplasmosis, sarcoidosis, and syphilis can all involve the stomach and be manifested as thickening and indistensibility.

- **Rugal fold thickening** can be seen with tumor and inflammatory conditions. Gastritis can be due to alcohol abuse or nonsteroidal antiinflammatory agents, Ménétièr disease, Zollinger-Ellison disease, eosinophilic gastritis, or granulomatous infections. **Ménétièr disease** is a hypertrophic gastritis characterized by pain, hypochlorhydria, and hypoproteinemia. It typically spares the antrum.

Benign Disease

- **Ulcers** are difficult to appreciate on CT but may cause local wall thickening or be evident as a focal defect within the gastric wall. Perforation leads to adjacent inflammation and pneumoperitoneum. Ulcers are best evaluated with a barium study.

- Gastric **varices** are seen as densely enhancing tubular structures in the setting of portal hypertension. They often extend to surround the distal esophagus.

- Gastric **diverticula** are outpouchings of the muscular wall. Unopacified diverticula may simulate a mass.

- A **bezoar** is an intraluminal concretion composed of hair, inorganic substances, or indigestible vegetable matter. It is seen as an intraluminal solid mass in a distended stomach, possibly causing obstruction.

- A **Billroth I** is an end-to-end gastroduodenostomy now rarely performed, and a **Billroth II** is an end-to-side gastrojejunostomy. An unopacified afferent loop can simulate a mass lesion, but its characteristic position and fluid contents should allow differentiation from pathologic processes.

Gastric Tumors

- **Benign gastric tumors** include leiomyomas, fibromas, hemangiomas, and lipomas. A lipoma can be distinguished by its fatty attenuation.

- **Gastric cancer** is the third most common gastrointestinal malignancy, with an increased incidence in Asia. Predisposing factors include pernicious anemia, chronic atrophic gastritis, adenomatous polyps, and prior gastric surgery. Adenocarcinomas may be polypoid, ulcerating, or infiltrating. Ulceration can lead to perforation. CT may show focal masses or diffuse gastric wall thickening and indistensibility (Fig. 13-5). Tumor may spread locally, hematogenously to the liver, within the peritoneum, or to Virchow's node in the left supraclavicular fossa.

- The stomach is the most common site of gastrointestinal involvement in **non-Hodgkin lymphoma**. It too can demon-

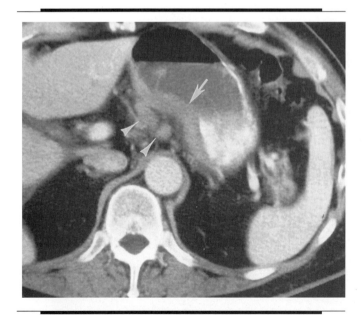

FIGURE 13-4   Nondistensible stomach (linitis plastica). A rind of soft tissue (arrow) is thickening the lesser curve of the stomach in a 72-year-old man with non-Hodgkin lymphoma. Enlarged lymph nodes (arrowheads) are present in the gastrohepatic ligament.

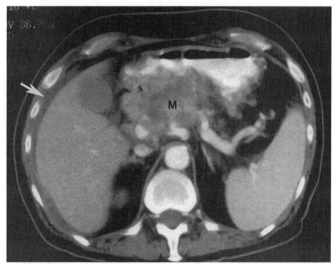

FIGURE 13-5   Gastric cancer. Large, heterogeneous mass (M) arising from the posterior wall of the stomach and extending posteriorly is adenocarcinoma of the stomach, not pancreas. Necrotic regions are present centrally, and there is perihepatic fluid (arrow). The patient had a periumbilical (Sister Mary Joseph) node of identical histology.

strate focal or diffuse wall thickening and lack of distention and favors the antrum. Intra-abdominal lymphadenopathy may suggest the diagnosis.

- **Gastric leiomyosarcomas** are often large gastric masses with both intra- and extramural components. They frequently ulcerate and can show central necrosis and low attenuation. Rarely, they occur in conjunction with pulmonary chondromas and extra-adrenal paragangliomas, which constitute the **Carney triad**.

- **Metastatic disease** is most commonly from breast cancer and is seen as infiltrative wall thickening. Other primaries include melanoma, Kaposi's sarcoma, lung cancer, and intestinal tumors.

13.3 LIVER

- The **liver** is the largest abdominal parenchymal organ. Its functions include filtering toxins from the blood, storing glycogen, secreting bile salts, and synthesizing many substances, including coagulation factors and complement.

  The liver receives a dual blood supply, approximately 25 percent from the hepatic artery, which delivers only oxygen, and 75 percent from the portal vein, which delivers oxygen and nutrients from the splanchnic bed. Venous outflow is via the right, middle, and left hepatic veins into the inferior vena cava (IVC) near the hepatic dome.

  These hepatic veins divide the liver into **lobes and segments** that are both surgically and structurally important. The right and left hepatic lobes are separated by a vertical plane through the middle hepatic vein and the gallbladder fossa. The left hepatic lobe has medial (closer to the hilum) and lateral segments separated by the left hepatic vein and falciform ligament. The right lobe consists of anterior and posterior segments separated by the right hepatic vein. The caudate lobe encompasses the anterior IVC margin. **Couinaud** has numbered the segments, further subdividing them into superior and inferior portions by an axial plane at the level of the portal vein (Fig. 13-6). The bare area of the liver lacks a visceral peritoneal covering and is surrounded by leaves of the coronary ligament.

Diffuse Disease

- Normal **hepatic attenuation** is roughly the same as that of the spleen, measuring 30 to 70 HU on unenhanced CT. A number of conditions increase hepatic density relative to the spleen, including amiodarone, glycogen storage diseases, Wilson disease, gold therapy, and Thorotrast. Hemochromatosis increases

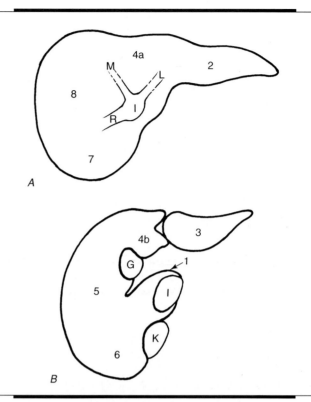

FIGURE 13-6   Couinaud segments. I, IVC; L, left hepatic vein; M, middle hepatic vein; R, right hepatic vein; G, gallbladder; K, right kidney. Numbers represent Couinaud segments.

the density of both the liver and spleen. Basilar fibrosis supports the diagnosis of amiodarone toxicity (Fig. 13-7).

- The liver may undergo **fatty infiltration**, particularly in the setting of obesity, steroid use, ethanol abuse, Cushing

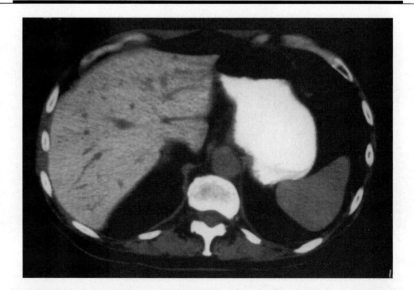

FIGURE 13-7   Increased hepatic density. The liver is diffusely increased in attenuation on this non-contrast-enhanced CT with the hepatic vasculature seen as very prominent low attenuation. The patient had been on prolonged amiodarone therapy.

disease, and chemotherapy with agents such as Taxol. It can be patchy, geographic, diffuse, or even micronodular, mimicking other pathology such as microabscesses. Preferential sites include adjacent to the gallbladder fossa and along the falciform ligament. Focal sparing in a diffusely fatty infiltrated liver can simulate an enhancing mass (Fig. 13-8).

• **Cirrhosis**, a chronic fibrotic disease characterized by volume loss, scarring, and nodular regeneration, is frequently due to alcohol abuse, hepatitis, or biliary origins, but it can also be cryptogenic. In advanced cirrhosis, the liver has a bumpy, nodular surface, often along with left lobe and caudate hypertrophy (Fig. 13-9).

• **Hepatitis**, typically of viral etiology, may produce nonspecific enlargement and has very limited CT findings; diagnosis is based on serologic titers.

• **Hepatic trauma** is the second most common parenchymal abdominal injury after splenic trauma. **Hepatic lacerations** are manifested as a low-attenuation thrombus, typically in the right lobe, which may extend to the hilum. If intrahepatic vessels are transected, the peripheral parenchyma may not enhance. **Subcapsular hematomas** can be seen as peripheral lenticular low-density collections (Fig. 13-10).

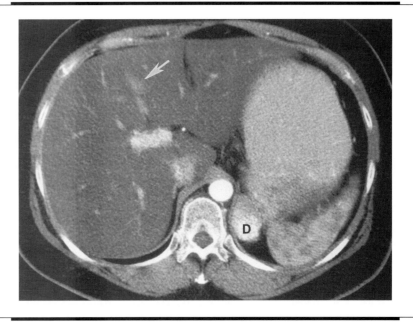

FIGURE 13-8 Hepatic fatty infiltration. Radiograph showing diffuse low attenuation of the hepatic parenchyma with a minimal amount of focal sparing (arrow) in a 46-year-old woman. The high attenuation in the region of the left adrenal gland is a gastric diverticulum (D).

Vascular Abnormalities

• **Budd-Chiari syndrome** or hepatic vein thrombosis is often (>60 percent) idiopathic, although hypercoaguable states such as pregnancy, polycythemia vera, and trauma are potential causes. CT may demonstrate a thrombus or failure of the hepatic veins to enhance with intravenous (IV) contrast, while the caudate may show dense enhancement because of its

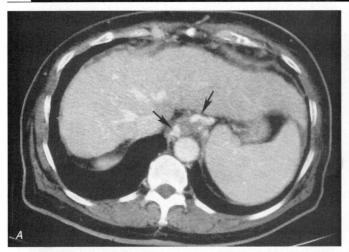
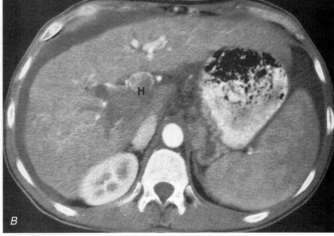

FIGURE 13-9 Cirrhosis. (A) CT in a 73-year-old alcoholic with a nodular hepatic surface, left lobe hypertrophy, and esophageal varices (arrows). (B) CT in a 36-year-old with hemochromatosis and a cirrhotic morphology with surface nodularity, left lobe enlargement, and ascites. A hepatoma can be seen invading the hepatic portal vein (H).

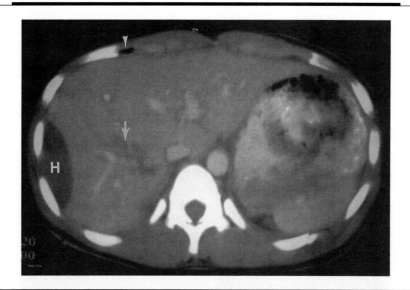

FIGURE 13-10 Intrahepatic laceration and subcapsular hematoma. Linear, low-attenuation laceration traverses the right hepatic lobe (arrow), and a crescentic, well-marginated subcapsular hematoma indents the hepatic margin (H). The tiny focus of air anteriorly (arrowhead) is the anterior pulmonary sulcus.

small penetrating veins draining into the IVC directly. The hepatic parenchyma may show mosaic enhancement.

- **Congestive heart failure** can also produce a mosaic enhancement pattern caused by passive congestion (nutmeg liver), with dilatation of the IVC and hepatic veins. Diffuse metastases from breast cancer can have a similar appearance following treatment and therapeutic response.

- **Portal vein thrombosis** may be due to portal hypertension, sepsis, dehydration, or tumor or be idiopathic. It is seen as low-attenuation thrombus within the portal vein or its segmental branches. Enhancing hilar collaterals may be evident. Thrombus enhancement suggests tumor extension and warrants further work-up (Fig. 13-9*B*).

    Portal venous hypertension occurs in the setting of cirrhosis. Portal vein pressures increase as a result of elevated flow resistance, and the main portal vein may enlarge or undergo thrombosis, giving rise to numerous hilar collaterals. This condition is termed **cavernous transformation of the portal vein**, a misnomer as it is actually collateral vessel formation. Portal hypertension leads to splenomegaly, ascites and formation of collaterals, including gastric and esophageal varices, a recanalized umbilical vein, and the formation of retroperitoneal collaterals,

most notably a spontaneous splenorenal shunt.

- **Superior vena cava (SVC) obstruction** from thrombus, tumor, or nodal compression may produce "downhill varices" as well as medial segment left hepatic lobe enhancement caused by umbilical pathway drainage.

- **Transient hepatic attenuation difference (THAD)** is a phenomenon related to the liver's dual blood supply, which is evidenced by segmental hyperdensity when images are obtained during the hepatic artery dominant phase. It is related to portal shunting from the hyperenhanced segment and may be caused by segmental tumor, portal vein occlusion, or arteriovenous shunting.

Benign Lesions

- Benign tumors of the liver are common and include cysts, focal fat, hemangiomas, adenomas, and focal nodular hyperplasia. Imaging features and demographics may suggest a diagnosis, although biopsy or excision is often required for definitive diagnosis.

- **Hepatic cysts** are common and occur as sporadic findings or in other processes, including autosomal dominant polycystic kidney disease (ADPCKD) and von Hippel-Lindau syndrome. Imaging features are identical to those of cysts elsewhere, including uniform water attenuation, single or thin

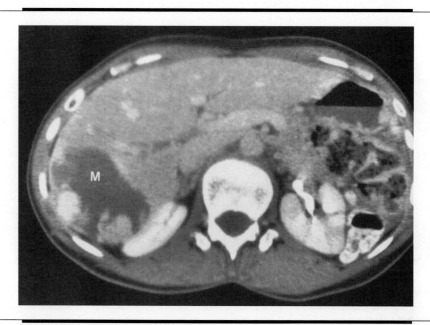

FIGURE 13-11 Cavernous hemangioma. There is a large, predominantly low-attenuation mass (M) in the posterior segment of the right hepatic lobe with peripheral, "puddling" of contrast characteristic of a cavernous hemangioma. The lesion filled with contrast on delayed images.

septations, an imperceptible wall, and lack of enhancement with IV contrast. They may rupture, become infected, or bleed, altering their appearance. Posttraumatic and echinococcal cysts may also occur.

- **Cavernous hemangioma**, the most common benign hepatic tumor, is typically small and asymptomatic, although giant cavernous hemangiomas (over 4 cm) are at an increased risk for hemorrhage. Hemangiomas seen in conjunction with thrombocytopenia represent the **Kasabach-Merritt phenomenon**. The classic CT appearance is a low-density mass demonstrating dense, nodular, and peripheral enhancement which gradually fills in with contrast (Fig. 13-11). Atypical lesions can be confirmed on MR or tagged red blood cell scans.

- **Hepatic adenomas** are benign tumors seen in young women. Patients with long-term oral contraceptive use or glycogen storage disease have an increased risk of developing adenomas. They are hypervascular lesions with a discernible capsule and low T1 and increased T2 signals on MR. Adenomas do not contain bile ducts on biopsy, distinguishing them from focal nodular hyperplasia, and they do not accumulate sulfur colloid, appearing as cold defects on liver-spleen scintigraphy. Excision is often required because of the propensity for hemorrhage with increasing size.

- **Focal nodular hyperplasia (FNH)** is a hypervascular encapsulated hepatic tumor which contains a central scar in 60 percent of cases. It is usually peripheral and can be multiple. The tumor is well demonstrated on arterial phase CT. On MR, the scar may be high signal on T2-weighted images, whereas that of a hepatoma may be low signal. FNH accumulates sulfur colloid levels equal to or greater than that in the hepatic parenchyma in most cases.

- **Regenerating nodules** of cirrhosis are typically dark on both T1- and T2-weighted MR sequences, while hepatomas show an increased T2 signal and are enhancing. They may appear hyperdense on noncontrast CT. **Adenomatous hyperplastic nodules**, intermediate lesions, are bright on T1-weighted images. Distinction and hepatoma exclusion often mandate biopsy. **Confluent hepatic fibrosis** may result in focal capsular retraction.

- **Hepatic abscesses** are usually pyogenic but may be amebic or echinococcal. Amebic abscesses are caused by *Entamoeba histolytica*. Patients with pyogenic abscesses are typically very ill with fever, pain, sweating, emesis, and even jaundice. CT shows a hypodense lesion with an irregularly and densely enhancing margin. While up to one-quarter of these nodules are multiple, isolated lesions are seen predominately within the right lobe (Fig. 13-12). There may be evidence of an adjacent inflammatory process such as cholecystitis serving as the infectious source. Patients usually require aggressive antibiotic therapy and drainage.

- **Calcified hepatic granulomas** are the result of prior exposure to histoplasmosis or other granulomatous organisms.

Malignant Hepatic Tumors

- **Metastatic disease** is the most common hepatic neoplasm. While it can appear as an isolated lesion on CT, multiple low-density masses of varying size and scattered distribution are the hallmarks. Specific imaging features may limit the differential.

  Hypervascular metastases include melanoma, islet cell tumors, and carcinoid along with more common primaries such as breast cancer (Fig. 13-13). Hepatic arterial imaging may demonstrate additional lesions that are occult on conventional CT. Multiple calcium-containing lesions suggest a primary tumor of mucinous origin, usually colon or ovarian cancer. Sarcomas, such as osteosarcomas, are an additional etiology. Infiltrating hepatic metastatic disease is commonly due to breast cancer.

- **Hepatocellular carcinoma** (hepatoma) is more frequently seen in Asian and African patients. Clinical features include pain, mass, weight loss, and elevated α-fetoprotein levels. Imaging features overlap with those of adenomas and FNH, and this tumor appears as an enhancing, often irregular mass. Clues to its malignant nature include lymphadenopathy, portal vein invasion, and satellite lesions. Predisposing conditions include hemochromatosis, cirrhosis, glycogen storage diseases, and aflatoxin exposure (Fig. 13-9*B*).

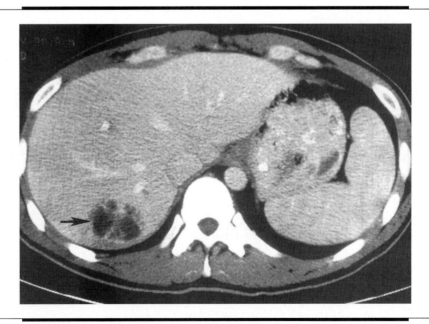

FIGURE 13-12   Hepatic abscess. CT showing a complex, partially cystic right hepatic lobe lesion (arrow) representing a hepatic abscess from appendicitis in a 38-year-old male with shaking chills and diffuse abdominal pain.

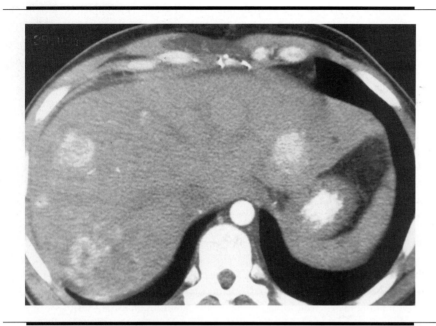

FIGURE 13-13 Hypervascular metastases. CT showing numerous densely enhanced hepatic masses during arterial phase imaging in 26-year-old man with tricuspid valve replacement associated with endocardial fibroelastosis. These were carcinoid metastases.

childbearing age. Predisposing factors include hemolytic states such as sickle cell disease, cholestasis, strictures, parasites, inflammatory bowel disease, and genetic predilection. Stones are of varied composition, the most common consisting of cholesterol alone or combined with calcium carbonate or bilirubinate. Pigmented stones are soft and frequently intrahepatic.

About 15 percent of gallstones can be seen on plain films and 65 percent on CT, depending on their calcium content. They may contain nitrogen gas from negative internal pressure, demonstrable as the "Mercedes Benz sign." These densities are typically seen within the gallbladder on CT, although **choledocholithiasis** with an obstructing distal common bile duct stone can be demonstrated and can be a source of biliary obstruction and pain. Ultrasound is the modality of choice for detecting cholelithiasis.

The **fibrolamellar variant**, seen in younger patients (<35 years old), has a better prognosis. This tumor is low density, shows variable enhancement, and, in up to 60 percent of cases, has a central fibrous scar with low T2 signal.

- **Angiosarcomas** are rare, occurring after exposure to arsenic, polyvinyl chloride, or **Thorotrast**, an alpha-emitting angiographic contrast agent used until the mid-1950s. Thorotrast persists in the reticuloendothelial system and can be seen radiographically as increased density, particularly in the spleen, hepatic periphery, and lymph nodes. An angiosarcoma is a densely enhancing, infiltrative tumor often with central necrosis. It carries a grim prognosis.

13.4 GALLBLADDER AND BILIARY TREE

- The **gallbladder** serves as a reservoir for bile awaiting transport to the duodenum to aid digestion. It has a muscular wall which contracts on stimulation by cholecystokinin. The cystic artery possesses few anastamoses, predisposing the gallbladder to ischemia.

  Bile is formed in the liver at a rate of 1.5 L/day. The dominant conjugated form aids in lipid metabolism. The intrahepatic biliary radicles form right and left hepatic ducts which have a confluence near the hilum, forming the common hepatic duct. The cystic duct joins the common bile duct which traverses the pancreatic head to empty into the duodenum at the ampulla of Vater with its sphincter of Oddi.

Cholelithiasis and Gallbladder Pathology

- **Cholelithiasis** (gallstones) is a very common cause of abdominal discomfort typically seen in obese women of

- **Biliary sludge** represents calcium bilirubinate granules or cholesterol crystals and may increase bile attenuation on CT. Hemobilia, mucus, parasitic infestations, and tumors may have a similar appearance.

- **Cholecystitis** is typically the result of cystic duct obstruction from an impacted stone. Symptoms include pain, fever, and right upper quadrant tenderness with leukocytosis and a **Murphy sign** of inspiratory arrest on gallbladder fossa palpation. The gallbladder is usually distended, with a thick wall, cholelithiasis, pericholecystic fluid, and soft tissue stranding. A perforation or hepatic abscess may be evident. **Acalculous cholecystitis** is seen in debilitated, postoperative, and posttraumatic patients and in those receiving total parenteral nutrition.

- **Chronic cholecystitis** is characterized by cholelithiasis and gallbladder wall thickening. It is best diagnosed with hepatobiliary scintigraphy with delayed visualization of the gallbladder.

- **Emphysematous cholecystitis** is seen in elderly patients and in diabetics, with *Clostridium perfringens* as the primary infectious agent. Patients may have a normal white blood cell (WBC) count and lack focal tenderness. Gas can be seen within both the gallbladder wall and the lumen (Fig. 13-14). Treatment is surgical.

- **Adenomyomatosis** is a hyperplastic cholecystosis causing segmental or diffuse gallbladder wall thickening. A localized form may simulate gallbladder cancer. It is best diagnosed sonographically.

- **Mirrizi syndrome** is an uncommon cause of biliary obstruction in which a stone impacted in the gallbladder or cystic duct compresses the adjacent common bile duct.

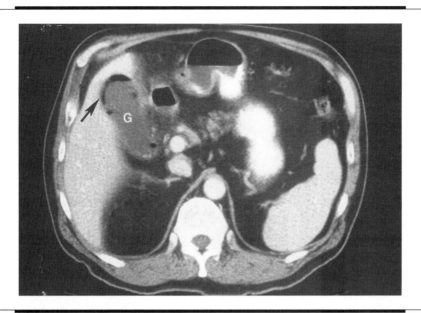

FIGURE 13-14　Emphysematous cholecystitis in a 68-year-old diabetic male with gas in both the gallbladder wall (arrow) and lumen. There is inflammation in the pericholecystic fat. G, Gallbladder.

Bile Duct Disease

- **Biliary dilatation** appears as linear, fluid-attenuating structures tracking adjacent to the portal veins on CT (Fig. 13-15). They are generally observed on only one side of the vessel and are seen out to the hepatic periphery. This is in contradistinction to periportal edema, which surrounds the portal structures. Causes of dilatation include choledocholithiasis, cholangitis, benign strictures, cholangiocarcinoma, pancreatic head masses, and ampullary stenosis.

- **Pneumobilia**, or air within the biliary tree, can be caused by surgery, instrumentation including endoscopic sphincterotomy, fistulae (gallstone ileus), and infection. Surgery is the most common cause, and clinical history can confirm this etiology. Biliary air may be more central and confluent than portal venous gas, although these conditions can be difficult to differentiate (Fig. 13-16). **Portal venous gas** is an ominous finding suggesting bowel ischemia.

- **Bilomas** are the sequelae of iatrogenic or traumatic biliary injury. They may be free-flowing or loculated portal or perihepatic collections. Image-guided drainage is indicated for infected or symptomatic bilomas.

- **Sclerosing cholangitis** is a chronic inflammatory condition of the biliary

tree characterized by jaundice, pain, pruritis, and occasionally fever. It has an association with inflammatory bowel disease. Segmental stricturing and dilatation of both intra- and extrahepatic ducts is seen, having a "pruned tree" appearance. Ductal wall thickening may be indistinguishable from **acquired immunodeficiency syndrome (AIDS) cholangitis** due to infection by cryptosporidium, CMV, or human immunodeficiency virus (HIV).

- **Recurrent pyogenic (Oriental) cholangiohepatitis** is a common disease in Asia caused by *Clonorchis sinesans* infestation. It is manifested as intermittent bouts of fever, abdominal pain, and jaundice. Dilated intrahepatic ducts contain sludge or pigment stones. Hepatic abscesses are a relatively common complication, and pancreatitis occurs less commonly.

- **Choledochal cysts** are dilatations of the extrahepatic biliary tree and are manifested as cystic lesions along the portal vein. They may arise from reflux of pancreatic enzymes into the distal duct. Choledochal cysts are infrequently asociated with the classic triad of right upper quadrant pain, jaundice, and a palpable mass. It can be difficult to determine the origin, gastrointestinal duplication cysts being the primary differential consideration in the pediatric population.

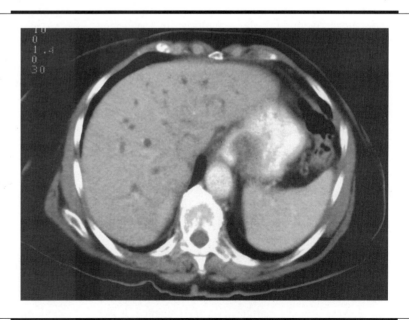

FIGURE 13-15　Biliary dilatation. Dilated intrahepatic biliary ducts are noted adjacent to accompanying portal venous branches in a patient with pancreatic adenocarcinoma.

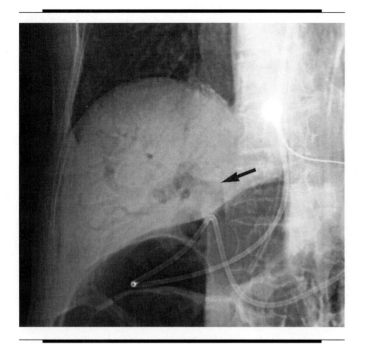

FIGURE 13-16   **Portal venous gas.** There is air throughout the portal venous system including the main portal vein (arrow). This patient had pneumatosis and a colonic infarct. An enteral feeding tube is in place. (Figure courtesy of Harold F. Bennett, M.D. Mallinckradt Institute of Radiology.)

Choledochoceles are a type of choledochal cyst and represent dilatations of the terminal portion of the common bile duct, often herniating into the duodenum and causing pancreatitis or stone formation.

- **Caroli disease** is the rare entity of saccular intrahepatic biliary dilatation often associated with medullary sponge kidney, congenital hepatic fibrosis, and infantile polycystic kidney disease. Patients may develop cholangitis, intrahepatic stones or cholangiocarcinoma. CT shows multiple interconnected hepatic cystic lesions which may exhibit the "central dot sign" of the cysts encasing portal triads, although this feature is better demonstrated on sonography.

Malignant Tumors

- **Cholangiocarcinoma** is a tumor of the bile ducts which invades hepatic parenchyma, metastasizes to local lymph nodes, and may cause proximal biliary obstruction. These tumors are usually adenocarcinomas and carry the eponym of **Klatskin tumor** when they occur at the bifurcation of the common hepatic duct. They appear as an infiltrating, enhancing mass usually near the hepatic hilum, although they can be more peripheral. Delayed enhancement may be demonstrated on delayed CT in about 40 percent of cases if the diagnosis is considered (Fig. 13-17).

- **Gallbladder cancer** follows colorectal, pancreatic, gastric, and esophageal primary malignancies in frequency. It is a disease of the elderly. Predisposing factors include cholelithiasis, porcelain gallbladder, and chronic cholecystitis. A thick-

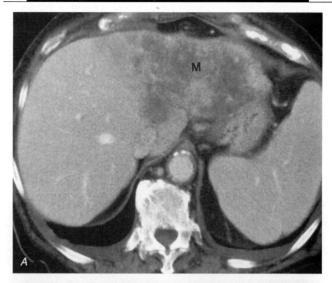

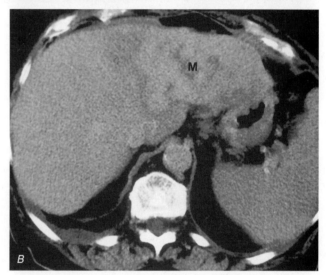

FIGURE 13-17   **Cholangiocarcinoma.** (*A*) A heterogeneous, partially necrotic hepatic mass (M) replacing the lateral segment of the left hepatic lobe as shown by contrast-enhanced CT in a 78-year-old woman. (*B*) CT image obtained 20 minutes later demonstrating delayed enhancement of the majority of the tumor, characteristic of cholangiocarcinoma.

ened or irregular gallbladder wall, polypoid mass, or replacement of the lumen may be a sign of malignancy, with hepatic invasion and lymphadenopathy present in up to 75 percent of cases at diagnosis. Peritoneal spread and omental disease are common. Metastases to the gallbladder do occur but are uncommon.

- **Porcelain gallbladder** refers to dystrophic calcification of the gallbladder wall or within dilated Rokitansky-Aschoff sinuses (Fig. 13-18). Patients are usually asymptomatic unless there is associated cholelithiasis, and most cases are identified incidentally. Elective cholecystectomy is performed because of the strong predisposition for malignancy.

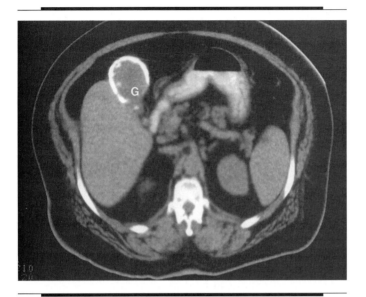

FIGURE 13-18   Porcelain gallbladder. Non-contrast-enhanced CT demonstrating a calcific rim encasing the gallbladder (G) in an elderly patient. The gallbladder did not contain cancer at surgical resection.

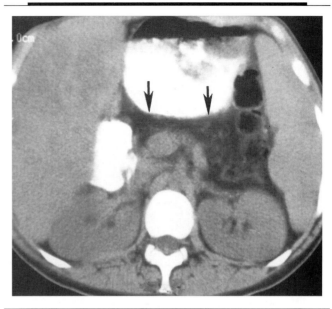

FIGURE 13-19   Fatty replacement of the pancreas in a 22-year-old woman with cystic fibrosis and elevated liver enzyme levels. Near total fatty replacement of the pancreatic parenchyma is seen as fat attenuation in the pancreatic bed (arrows).

13.5 PANCREAS

- The pancreas, both an **endocrine** and **exocrine gland**, produces insulin and glucagon for glucose control, and trypsin, chymotrypsin, amylase, and lipase for enteric digestion. Ventral and dorsal anlages rotate and fuse during embryogenesis, leaving a main ventral duct of Wirsung draining through the major papilla at the ampulla of Vater. An accessory dorsal duct of Santorini exits at the minor papilla.

  The gland is retroperitoneal in position and is contained within the anterior pararenal space. It shows soft tissue attenuation and a lobular contour and is less than 3 cm thick. The main pancreatic duct should be less than 2 mm in diameter. The head and uncinate process partially encompass the superior mesenteric vein, with the neck, body, and tail residing immediately anterior to the splenic vein.

- **Pancreas divisum**, caused by failure of fusion of the anlage, is seen in less than 8 percent of the population. It may be incidentally detected or seen as a source of recurrent pancreatitis from presumed impaired drainage.

- The pancreas normally undergoes fatty atrophy with aging. Extensive or premature **fatty replacement** is also seen in cystic fibrosis, Cushing syndrome, obesity, exogenous steroid use, and Schwachman-Diamond syndrome, congenital absence of pancreatic exocrine tissue (Fig. 13-19).

Pancreatitis and Sequelae

- **Acute pancreatitis** is a common source of abdominal pain. Etiologies include alcohol abuse, cholelithiasis, and idiopathic causes, with trauma, drugs, infection (including mumps), pancreas divisum, and metabolic factors less frequently implicated. Patients have pain, emesis, and elevated levels of pancreatic enzymes. Leukocytosis, hypocalcemia, and hyperglycemia occur with necrotizing pancreatitis.

  Plain film findings can include a left pleural effusion, atelectasis, and an elevated hemidiaphragm. In the abdomen, there may be a "sentinel loop" of dilated duodenum resulting from local ileus or "colon cutoff" caused by phrenicocolic ligament edema, spasm, or neural inflammation causing a transverse colon ileus and decompressed descending colon. On CT, the pancreas may be normal or enlarged, indistinct, hypoattenuating, and surrounded by fluid and mesenteric infiltration (Fig. 13-20). There may be areas of hyperattenuation caused by hemorrhage, or failure to show enhancement caused by necrotizing pancreatitis. Emphysematous changes can be seen.

  In addition to hemorrhage and necrosis, pancreatitis can cause a phlegmon (an inflammatory mass), pseudocyst, or pseudoaneurysm of the gastroduodenal or hepatic arteries seen as a hyperdense enhancing lesion. Biliary obstruction, abscess, or splenic vein thrombosis may also occur.

- **Chronic pancreatitis** is typically seen in alcoholics. The gland may be somewhat enlarged, with numerous intraductal calcifications (present in up to 50 percent of cases due to alcohol) evident on both plain films and CT. These patients are at risk for pancreatic carcinoma.

- Pancreatic **pseudocysts** are sequelae of pancreatitis and may prevent clinical resolution. They are encapsulated collections of pancreatic fluid usually seen in conjunction with other imaging findings of pancreatitis, although the acute findings

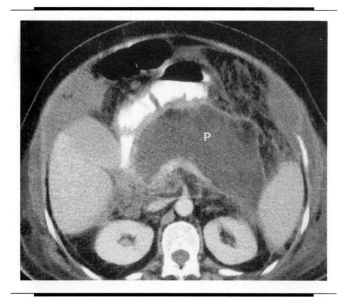

FIGURE 13-20 Ischemic pancreatitis. 53-year-old alcoholic with failure of the parenchyma (P) to show contrast enhancement, representing necrotic pancreatitis. Adjacent stranding and inflammation are present.

may have resolved. The majority are located within the pancreas, and half of them communicate with the pancreatic duct; however, pseudocysts can dissect along fascial planes and be found in the retroperitoneum, intraperitoneal space, and even the mediastinum after dissecting through the esophageal hiatus (Fig. 13-21).

- **Pancreatic trauma** is usually caused by a blunt mechanism of injury, such as a motor vehicle accident, with the gland compressed between the steering wheel and the spine. Signs of injury include adjacent soft tissue stranding, linear low attenuation within the gland, or areas of parenchyma that are not enhancing. Fluid between the pancreas and splenic vein posteriorly is a specific sign of a pancreatic laceration.

Cystic Tumors

- Isolated **pancreatic cysts** are uncommon. Multiple cysts can be seen in association with von Hippel-Lindau syndrome and ADPCKD.

- **Microcystic cystadenoma**, or serous cystadenoma, is a benign neoplasm of centroacinar cell origin observed typically in older women. While it can arise anywhere within the gland, there may be a predilection for the pancreatic head. These tumors are well-marginated aggregates of numerous (less than 2 cm) cysts with a characteristic central scar demonstrating sunburst calcification in 30 percent of cases. These are glycogen-rich tumors with no malignant potential.

- **Macrocystic cystadenomas**, or mucinous cystadenomas, occur in a similar patient group yet have a high rate of transformation to **mucinous cystadenocarcinoma**, necessitating surgical intervention. They stain densely for mucin (periodic acid-Schiff [PAS]-positive) and appear on CT as thick-walled lesions containing one or more cysts often greater than 2 cm in size. Mural calcifications are infrequent. Vascular encasement and local invasion support a diagnosis of malignant change.

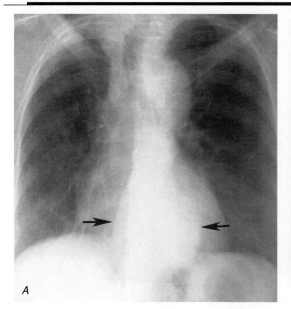

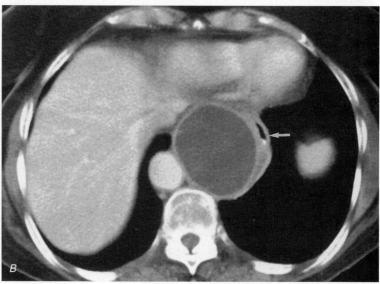

FIGURE 13-21 Mediastinal pancreatic pseudocyst. (*A*) A pancreatic pseudocyst has dissected through the esophageal hiatus and can be seen as a retrocardiac density (arrows). (*B*) CT demonstrates its cystic nature. The esophagus is displaced (arrow). (With permission from Glazer HS, Semenkovich JW, Gutierrez FR. Mediastinum. In Lee JKT, Sagel SS, Stanley RJ, Heiken JP, eds. *Computed Body Tomography with MRI Correlation*, 3rd ed. New York: Lippincott-Raven; 1998.)

- **Solid and papillary neoplasms** are rare, low-grade malignancies found in women under 30 years old. They contain variable amounts of cystic and solid components and are typically large and low density at presentation.

Islet Cell Tumors

- Islet cell tumors are neuroectodermal in origin and may be hormonally hyperfunctioning. When the tumor is a **non-hyperfunctioning islet cell tumor**, it appears later because of lack of symptomatology and is larger than those that are hyperfunctioning. These tumors have a greater than 80 percent rate of malignant transformation. They are large, hypervascular pancreatic masses with regions of necrosis and possible nodal and hepatic metastases.

- **Insulinomas** are the most common variety of islet cell tumor and develop early as a result of insulin secretion and symptoms of the Whipple triad, including hypoglycemia, starvation attacks, and obtaining relief with IV dextrose. These tumors are small (<1.5 cm), low-density masses which are often difficult to detect, are densely enhancing, and are optimally depicted on arterial phase CT imaging. They have a low (<10 percent) rate of malignant transformation.

- **Gastrinomas**, the second most common type of islet cell tumor, are responsible for the **Zollinger-Ellison syndrome** of gastric hypersecretion, recurrent peptic ulcer disease, malabsorption, and gastrointestinal bleeding. Imaging features are similar to those of insulinomas, although they may be slightly larger and demonstrate concomitant rugal fold thickening. Up to one-third may be ectopic and located near the portal vein and duodenum. Most (60 percent) are malignant.

- **VIPomas** are tumors that secrete **vasoactive intestinal peptide** and cause the **WDHA (Verner-Morrison) syndrome** of watery diarrhea, hypokalemia, and achlorhydria. Most (60 percent) are malignant. **Somatostatinomas** and **glucagonomas** are very uncommon islet cell tumors which have a high rate of malignancy and similar imaging features. Glucagonomas are characterized by a characteristic rash, necrolytic erythema migrans.

Malignant Tumors

- **Pancreatic adenocarcinoma** is of ductal origin and is the fourth most common cause of cancer deaths. These tumors are seen in older patients, and predisposing factors include alcohol abuse and hereditary pancreatitis. The majority of patients have advanced local or metastatic disease at diagnosis. Symptoms include abdominal pain, weight loss, fatigue, painless jaundice, new-onset diabetes, and thrombophlebitis (Trousseau syndrome). This disease carries a dismal prognosis, with <1 percent survival at 5 years.

  Pancreatic adenocarcinoma is the primary differential consideration when confronted with a solid pancreatic mass in an older patient. The mass may require dual-phase, small-field-of-view CT imaging for accurate evaluation. It may be small and show enhancement with low central attenuation, proximal gland atrophy, and biliary obstruction, depending on the location. Invasive tumor may demonstrate local spread, superior mesenteric vasculature and celiac artery encasement, splenic vein thrombosis, and regional lymphadenopathy (Fig. 13-22).

- Other epithelial tumors include **ductectatic mucinous tumors**, which cause dilatation of the pancreatic duct and branches by producing copious mucin, and **acinar cell tumors**, which may result in systemic fat necrosis caused by lipase production.

- **Primary lymphoma** of the pancreas is rare and usually of the non-Hodgkin type, although tumor within local lymph nodes can spread to the pancreas. **Metastases** to the pancreas are uncommon but are sometimes seen, particularly in association with melanoma.

- A **Whipple procedure** is a pancreaticoduodenectomy with choledochojejunostomy and gastrojejunostomy and is typically performed for tumor in the pancreatic head. A **Peustow procedure** involves a lateral side-to-side pancreaticojejunostomy, and a Roux-en-Y operation is performed in treating ductal decompression in chronic pancreatitis.

13.6 ADRENAL GLANDS

- The **adrenal glands** lie along the anterosuperior renal margin. On CT, they appear as thin, inverted Y- or V-shaped structures with smooth medial and lateral limbs. The limbs should be at least as thin as the adjacent diaphragmatic crura.

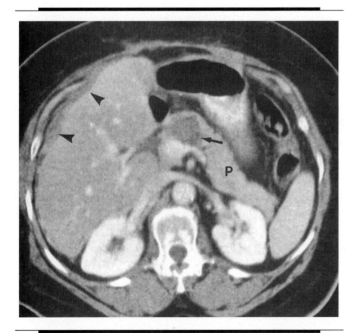

FIGURE 13-22 Pancreatic adenocarcinoma. CT demonstrates a focal, low-attenuation mass (arrow) in the body of the pancreas (P), which was pancreatic adenocarcinoma on biopsy. This 71-year-old man also has omental metastases (arrowheads).

They are encompassed in the perinephric fat and are consequently contained within Gerota fascia.

The adrenal cortex has three layers, the zonae glomerulosa, fasiculata, and reticulosa, which produce aldosterone, cortisol, and testosterone, respectively. The adrenal medulla synthesizes epinephrine and norepinephrine. Arterial supply is via the superior, middle, and inferior adrenal arteries arising from the inferior phrenic artery, aorta, and renal arteries, respectively. Venous drainage is usually through a single central vein.

An incidental adrenal lesion can be seen in up to 1 percent of all CTs, with at least half representing adenomas, even in oncologic patients.

Benign Lesions

• **Adrenal adenomas** are common benign tumors of the adrenal cortex which produce variable amounts of gluco- or mineralocorticoids. Clinical appearance depends on the type and amount of hormone production, with the majority incidentally identified. Only 10 to 20 percent of Cushing syndrome patients have adrenal cortisol-producing adenomas, and the rest are mostly secondary to pituitary adenomas. **Conn syndrome**, which includes hypokalemia, hypernatremia, and hypertension, is generally due to small (typically less than 2 cm) aldosterone-producing adenomas.

Adenomas are seen as nodules of varying size and enhancement. They are often of low attenuation because of intracellular fat from steroid synthesis. Thus, an attenuation <10 HU on noncontrast CT confirms this diagnosis. They may be densely enhancing, similar to metastases, yet show lower HU values on delayed images, with less than 24 or 37 HU at 15 minutes and less than 37 HU at 30 minutes as proposed cutoff levels. **MR** may confirm an adrenal adenoma if there is signal dropout on opposed-phase imaging (Fig. 13-23) caused by intravoxel cancelation of fat and water.

• **Adrenal hyperplasia** is generally a bilateral process of adrenal enlargement producing **Cushing syndrome**. Cushing syndrome is manifested by hypertension, buffalo hump fat deposition, striae, and glucose intolerance. In 85 percent of patients an adrenocorticotropic hormone (ACTH)-producing pituitary adenoma is the cause, although exogenous steroids and paraneoplastic syndromes, especially those associated with oat cell carcinoma of the lung, can produce this clinical scenario of increased levels of plasma cortisol and urinary 17-hydroxy catecholamines. The adrenal glands may be normal, may be smoothly thickened, or less commonly demonstrate nodular thickening (Fig. 13-24).

• **Pheochromocytomas**, or paragangliomas, are neuroendocrine tumors of chromaffin cell origin which produce catecholamines leading to symptoms of headache, flushing, hypertension, and palpitations. Urinary catecholamine and vanillylmandelic acid (VMA) levels are elevated, and IV contrast is avoided to prevent precipitation of a hypertensive crisis requiring alpha-adrenergic blockade with phentolamine. The "rule of tens" states that 10 percent of pheochromocytomas are extra-adrenal, 10 percent are malignant, 10

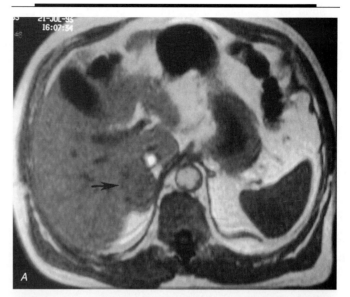

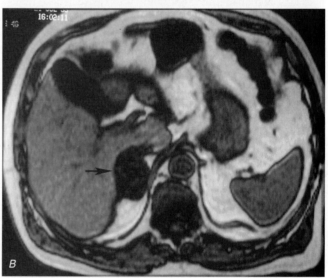

FIGURE 13-23   Adrenal adenoma. (*A*) In-phase MR demonstrating a right adrenal mass (arrow) nearly isointense to hepatic parenchyma. (*B*) Out-of-phase MR showing that the signal intensity drops out, confirming an adrenal adenoma (arrow).

percent are familial, and 10 percent are bilateral. They are associated with multiple endocrine neoplasia (MEN) types 2a and 2b, as well as with von-Hippel Lindau syndrome.

Pheochromocytomas are apparent as soft tissue adrenal lesions which are densely enhancing if IV contrast is administered. Limited noncontrast thin sections through the adrenal fossa can be obtained if a pheochromocytoma is suspected. This is both to avoid IV contrast administration and to diagnose the lesion in the appropriate clinical setting. These tumors are generally "light-bulb" bright on T2-weighted MR. Ectopic lesions can be localized with In-111 octreotide or iodine-131 methyliodobenzylguanidine (MIBG) scintigraphy.

• **Myelolipomas** are uncommon, benign adrenal tumors containing bone marrow and fatty elements. Consequently, CT

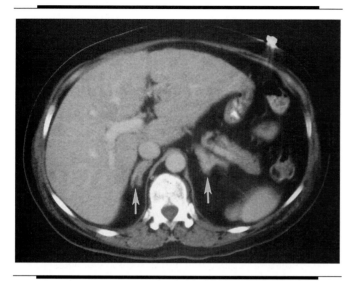

FIGURE 13-24   Adrenal hyperplasia. Bilateral adrenal thickening (arrows) due to an ACTH-secreting bronchogenic tumor in a 68-year-old woman.

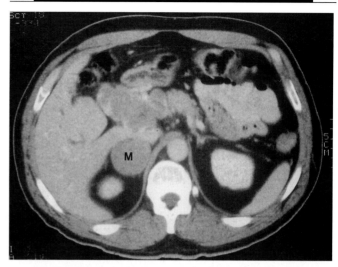

FIGURE 13-26   Adrenal metastasis. A circumscribed homogeneous adrenal mass (M) displacing the liver and IVC anteriorly represents metastatic melanoma in a young man.

demonstrates macroscopic fat, obviating biopsy. However, soft tissue elements may predominate, and calcification is seen in about 20 percent of patients (Fig. 13-25).

- Adrenal **cysts** are rare and possess imaging characteristics of similar cysts located elsewhere. Adrenal **hemorrhage** may lead to a mass lesion, often precipitated by sepsis, birth trauma, or hypoxia in newborns, and anticoagulation, trauma, surgery, or meningococcal sepsis (**Waterhouse-Friderichsen syndrome**) in other patients. Diagnosis is based on clinical presentation and decreased size or attenuation on short-interval follow-up. Calcification is common as a late sequela.

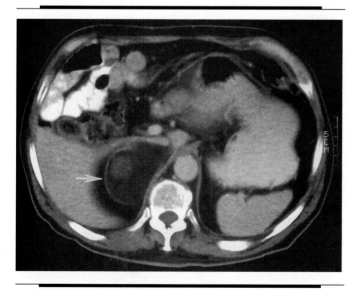

FIGURE 13-25   Myelolipoma. A large, predominantly fat attenuation mass replacing the right adrenal gland (arrow). The macroscopic fat confirms the diagnosis of adrenal myelolipoma.

Malignant Tumors

- Chest CT scans traditionally extend through the adrenal glands to exclude **metastatic disease** in patients with bronchogenic cancer. Metastases commonly occur in the adrenal gland and arise from bronchogenic cancer, renal cell cancer, breast carcinoma, melanoma, and gastrointestinal malignancies. Some metastases may spontaneously hemorrhage and produce stranding in the adjacent fat.

  The imaging characteristics of metastatic deposits are not conclusive. Typically, an adrenal metastasis appears as a nodule of variable size which enhances with IV contrast (Fig. 13-26). Unless noncontrast CT demonstrates a density of less than 10 HU (a conservative value, with values up to 18 HU cited in the literature) characteristic of benign adenomas, the lesion remains indeterminate.

  MR may confirm an adrenal adenoma if there is signal dropout on opposed-phase imaging. Lack of a signal dropout does not exclude an adenoma, and the lesion remains indeterminate. The multiplanar capabilities of MR may prove beneficial in determining from which organ a lesion near the adrenal arises. Definitive diagnosis may require biopsy.

- **Adrenocortical carcinomas** are typically large (>5 cm), heterogeneous, and partially necrotic tumors arising from the adrenal cortex in older patients. They are enhancing and infrequently calcify. They spread by local extension to involve the kidney, liver, or IVC or by hematogenous dissemination to lung and lymph nodes (Fig. 13-27). These tumors are discovered incidentally or are manifested as abdominal fullness or tenderness. Approximately 40 to 50 percent are mildly hyperfunctioning.

- **Neuroblastoma** is a primary adrenal malignancy arising from neural crest cells. It is the most common solid abdominal mass in infancy and the second most common tumor in chil-

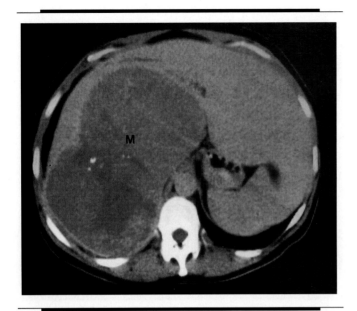

FIGURE 13-27   Adrenocortical carcinoma. CT showing a large suprarenal mass (M) displacing the liver in a patient complaining of abdominal distension. The mass shows necrosis and central calcifications.

dren. In addition to abdominal pain and mass, symptoms can include diarrhea from VIP secretion, paroxysmal flushing from catecholamines, and myoclonus or opsoclonus. Early diagnosis, at less than 1 year of age, is correlated with decreased mortality, and 1 percent of these tumors spontaneously convert to benign ganglioneuromas.

Neuroblastoma can arise anywhere along the sympathetic chain. Adrenal lesions are large, heterogeneous, and irregularly marginated soft tissue masses with frequent necrosis. The majority contain stippled calcifications. Regional spread is common, as are nodal, hepatic, osseous, and pulmonary metastases. Most patients have a positive marrow aspirate at diagnosis.

13.7   KIDNEYS

- The paired kidneys reside in the retroperitoneum encompassed by Gerota fascia and perinephric fat and encased within the renal capsule. They receive a disproportionate amount of cardiac output, filtering the blood as well as regulating arterial pressure and secreting vital substances such as erythropoetin. The cortex contains glomeruli, and the medulla is predominantly composed of tubules.

Arterial supply is by a main renal artery usually originating off the aorta at the L2 level. Accessory renal arteries can be present, and there is a solitary main renal vein. Corticomedullary differentiation can be demonstrated on CT imaging at 30 seconds following IV contrast administration with a nephrographic phase at 70 to 100 seconds.

- When there is an **empty renal fossa**, several possibilities should be considered. The kidney may have been excised, may be atrophic, or may be ectopic. Renal ectopia includes

horseshoe kidney, where there is an isthmus of renal parenchyma joining low-lying kidneys across the midline. These kidneys are prone to reflux, hydronephrosis, calculi, Wilm tumor, and trauma. In **crossed-fused ectopia**, the left kidney is usually fused with the inferior pole of the right kidney. In cases of collecting system duplication, the upper pole tends to obstruct and the lower pole refluxes (Weigert-Meyer rule).

Calculi and Infection

- **Hydronephrosis** is dilatation of the renal collecting system. It is most commonly caused by obstructing calculi, although it can be due to transitional cell carcinoma or pelvic malignancies, sloughed papillae, blood clots, retroperitoneal fibrosis, aortic aneurysms, or reflux disease. Delayed contrast excretion or a persistent nephrogram may be evident.

- **Renal calculi** are well demonstrated on noncontrast CT, and this modality is rapidly becoming the technique of choice in evaluating emergency room patients with suspected urolithiasis. Hydronephrosis is easily demonstrated on CT. In about 85 percent of cases, renal calculi are visible on plain films.

- **Medullary nephrocalcinosis** is commonly seen in renal tubular acidosis (type 4, distal), medullary sponge kidney, and hyperparathyroidism. **Cortical nephrocalcinosis** is associated with chronic glomerulonephritis, oxalosis, cortical necrosis, and Alport syndrome of hereditary deafness and nephritis. **Acute cortical necrosis** is a sequela involving shock, sepsis, and obstetric complications such as abruption and previa. In the acute stage, diminished cortical enhancement is evident.

- **Pyelonephritis** is a common cause of flank pain and is often associated with fever, pyuria, and leukocytosis. Offending organisms include *Escherichia coli, Proteus,* and *Klebsiella.* The involved kidney may be focally or diffusely enlarged, perhaps with delayed excretion, perinephric stranding, and focal regions of low attenuation. Perinephric abscesses can be seen, as can pyonephrosis and collecting system debris.

- **Emphysematous pyelonephritis** is a more fulminant renal infection seen in immunocompromised patients and diabetics. Gas bubbles can be seen in the parenchyma, collecting system, and perinephric tissues. Surgical intervention is warranted.

- **Xanthogranulomatous pyelonephritis (XGP)** is an infection characterized by infiltration of lipid-laden macrophages due to a large, staghorn calculus in 75 percent of cases. *Proteus mirabilis* is the usual infecting organism. CT shows the obstructing stone, renal enlargement, low-attenuation infiltration, obstruction, and associated inflammation which can be extensive (Fig. 13-28).

- **Renal trauma** is common and can be manifested as a subcapsular hematoma, a contusion with focal low density, a laceration that may extend to the collecting system, or a shattered kidney with vascular pedicle disruption and failure to enhance with IV contrast.

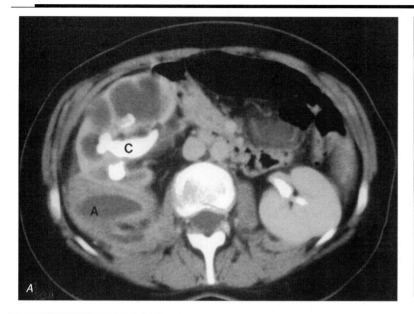
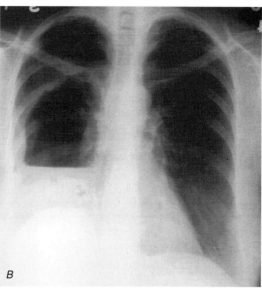

FIGURE 13-28   Xanthogranulomatous pyelonephritis. (*A*) Staghorn calculus (C) is present within an infiltrated, low-attenuation kidney displaced anteriorly by an associated abscess (A). (*B*) The inflammatory process has spread across the diaphragm, causing an empyema in the right hemithorax.

Benign Lesions

- **Renal cysts** are very common and are seen in approximately half of patients over 50 years old. They do not cause symptoms unless they hemorrhage, become infected, or grow to a very large size. Bosniak has divided these cysts into four categories based on risk of associated malignancy:

Category I: simple cyst (water attenuation without enhancement; imperceptible, smooth wall)

Category II: minimally complicated cysts (thin septations or calcifications; may be hyperdense; no enhancement)

Category III: complex cysts (thick, irregular, multiple septations or calcifications; thick or nodular wall; no enhancement)

Category IV: cystic neoplasm (irregular, thickened, or enhancing wall or septae or a solid component)

Simple or minimally complicated cysts do not warrant follow-up, although category III and IV cystic lesions should be excised as they have a high likelihood of representing neoplasm. The Bosniak system is a useful guideline but significant interobserver variability exists.

- **Autosomal dominant polycystic kidney disease (ADPCKD)** is a relatively common inherited disorder which generally progresses to renal insufficiency. The hallmark is numerous simple renal cysts which may hemorrhage or rupture. There is no increased risk of renal cell carcinoma unless the patient is on prolonged dialysis. Associations include hepatic (>25 percent) and pancreatic (10 percent) cysts, intracranial berry aneurysms (approximately 10 percent), and mitral valve prolapse (Fig. 13-29).

- **Angiomyolipomas (AMLs)** are benign renal tumors which are sometimes resected because of their potential for catastrophic hemorrhage. They are variably composed of vascular, fatty, and solid elements. Hence, macroscopic fat on CT

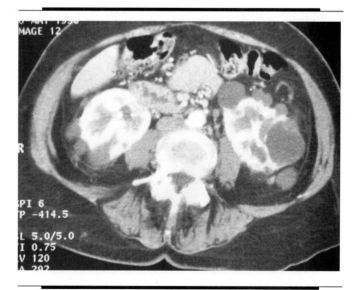

FIGURE 13-29   Autosomal dominant polycystic kidney disease (ADPCKD). There are numerous, bilateral, simple renal cysts demonstrated on this arterial phase abdominal CT. Several of these cysts are hyperdense.

is nearly pathognomonic, since renal cell carcinomas very rarely show macroscopic fat, usually as a result of fat necrosis or encasement of adjacent tissue. Multiple AMLs are seen in association with tuberous sclerosis (Fig. 13-30).

• **Oncocytomas** are uncommon benign renal adenomas seen in older patients. They are usually large (>5 cm) at diagnosis and are often discovered incidentally. They are homogeneous, low-density, enhanced masses, and one-third may have a central scar. Oncocytomas are excised to exclude malignancy; however, preoperative consideration of an oncocytoma may permit wedge resection.

Malignant Tumors

• **Renal cell carcinoma** is a common malignancy and is associated with von Hippel-Lindau syndrome and acquired cystic disease. Patients may develop fever, weight loss, hematuria, and anemia. The tumor ranges from a complex renal cyst to a large, heterogeneous, densely enhancing mass often with central necrosis (Fig. 13-31). It invades the renal vein and IVC, as well as causing local, mediastinal and bilateral hilar lymphadenopathy; lytic bone metastases; and adrenal, pulmonary, hepatic, and contralateral renal metastases. The Robson staging system is as follows:

Stage I: contained within the renal capsule; treated with a parenchyma-sparing procedure or nephrectomy

Stage II: contained within Gerota fascia, including ipsilateral adrenal metastases; treated with nephrectomy

Stage IIIA: renal vein or IVC invasion; may be amenable to resection

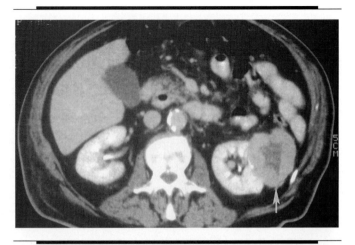

FIGURE 13-31   Renal cell carcinoma. CT showing a soft tissue mass (arrow) emanating from the left renal midpole, with central low attenuation representing necrosis. Pulmonary and osseous metastases were also present.

Stage IIIB: local lymphadenopathy

Stage IIIC: both vascular invasion and local lymphadenopathy

Stage IV: distant metastases

• **Transitional cell carcinoma** arises from the urothelium of the renal pelvis and also occurs in the bladder or ureter. It is seen as an enhancing mass within the collecting system. It can be large or obstructing, or it can produce a "faceless" kidney with an absence of normal hilar morphology.

• **Lymphoma** can appear as a primary tumor within the kidney or result from direct extension and is usually of the non-Hodgkin type. It can diffusely enlarge the kidney or occur as single or multiple low-density parenchymal lesions. More commonly, the kidney is involved secondarily, with associated retroperitoneal lymphadenopathy present.

• **Metastases** to the kidney are common at autopsy yet infrequently seen on imaging studies. They originate from the contralateral kidney, the adrenal gland, or melanoma most frequently. Lung cancer also metastasizes to the kidneys but is infrequently imaged.

13.8 SPLEEN

• The **spleen** is part of the reticuloendothelial system, filtering blood-borne cellular elements and serving an important immunologic function. It is composed of red, white, and marginal pulp, and differential flow through the parenchyma can yield bizarre and heterogeneous enhancement patterns during the arterial phase of CT imaging. Splenic enhancement should be homogeneous when scanning in the portal venous phase.

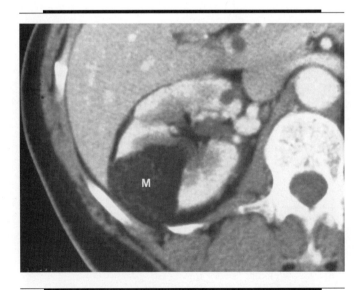

FIGURE 13-30   Angiomyolipoma in a 55-year-old woman being evaluated for newly diagnosed colon cancer has a wedge-shaped 4 cm fatty attenuation renal mass (M) with minimal stranding in soft tissue. A "beak" of parenchyma is seen adjacent to the lesion, indicating its intrarenal nature.

There may be prominent splenic clefts and lobulations. Failure of several mesodermal buds to coalesce can yield **splenules**, round foci of soft tissue density near the splenic hilum and of similar attenuation and enhancement. **Spleno-sis**, with multiple deposits of splenic tissue in the left upper quadrant or at distant sites including the chest, can be seen following trauma and diaphragm rupture.

- The spleen normally weighs 150 g and has a maximum cephalocaudal span of 13 cm. **Splenomegaly** can be seen with lymphoma and leukemia, mononucleosis, cirrhosis and portal hypertension, splenic vein thrombosis, glycogen storage diseases, sarcoid, and hemolytic anemias.

- The spleen may be **small** or **absent** in asplenia and polysplenia syndromes or following surgery, trauma, infarction, or irradiation. **Sickle cell disease** leads to splenic infarction and "autoamputation." The spleen is small and often calcified. Plain radiographic findings may include a small, calcified spleen, cardiomegaly from high cardiac output, osseous changes, and cholecystectomy due to hemolysis with sludge formation.

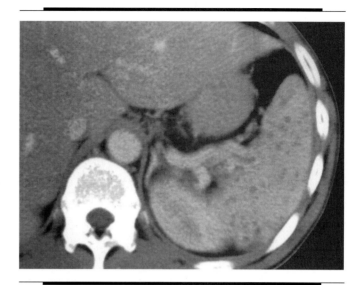

FIGURE 13-32 Candida microabscesses. Contrast-enhanced CT showing multiple foci of splenic low attenuation in the spleen without a dominant lesion or lymphadenopathy in an HIV-positive patient.

Benign Lesions

- **Splenic cysts** are uncommon and are typically due to prior trauma. Other etiologies include echinococcal cysts, dissecting pancreatic pseudocysts, and epithelial cysts. **Echinococcal cysts** (hydatid disease) are asymptomatic or can cause pain, eosinophilia, or urticaria and anaphylaxis with rupture. Humans are accidental intermediate hosts, acquiring the parasite (*Echinococcus granulosus* more commonly than *multilocularis*) from contaminated food. They appear as large cysts with crescentic or circumferential calcification and internal septations.

- **Hemangiomas** are the most common benign splenic lesion. They show low attenuation with enhancement, often peripheral or heterogeneous, on CT following IV contrast administration.

- **Splenic abscesses** can be pyogenic; however, **fungal microabscesses** are becoming more common with an enlarging AIDS population (Fig. 13-32). *Candida* and *Pneumocystis carinii* are the most common infectious agents. Numerous tiny, low-attenuation foci are apparent following IV contrast enhancement of the normal parenchyma. Liver abscesses may also be present. Treatment is systemic.

- **Calcified splenic granulomas** are the result of prior exposure to histoplasmosis or other granulomatous organisms. They generally do not have any findings in the acute phase.

- **Sarcoidosis** can also lead to splenic granulomas. Splenic involvement in sarcoidosis is present in over one-third of patients. Abdominal imaging findings include hepatosplenomegaly, low-attenuation splenic nodules, and lymphadenopathy. Pulmonary disease is present in the vast majority of cases.

- The spleen is the most common abdominal parenchymal organ injured in **trauma**. While partially protected by the ribs, almost half of splenic injuries are associated with fractures of the lower left thoracic cage. It can be lacerated, fractured with devascularized and nonenhancing parenchymal portions, or completely avulsed from its vascular pedicle. Subcapsular hematomas appear as a crescentic, low-density region. A high-density (approximately 60 HU) "sentinel clot" may show splenic injury as the source of hemoperitoneum. The spleen can rupture spontaneously or with very minimal trauma (coughing) in patients with mononucleosis or lymphomatous splenomegaly.

Malignant Tumors

- Primary neoplasms of the spleen are predominately **lymphoma** and leukemia. The organ may be diffusely enlarged or contain multiple low-attenuation foci. Concomitant lymphadenopathy is a diagnostic clue. **Angiosarcoma** is a very uncommon malignancy. It appears as a heterogeneous, densely enhancing tumor. **Metastases** arise most commonly from lung cancer, breast cancer, or melanoma.

Bibliography

Balthazar EJ, Birnbaum BA, Naidich M. Acute cholangitis: CT evaluation. *J. Comput. Assist. Tomogr.* 1993;17(2):283–289.

Bosniak MA. The current radiological approach to renal cysts. *Radiology.* 1986;158:1–10.

Davidson AJ, Hartman DS, Choyke PL, Wagner BJ. Radiologic assessment of renal masses: Implications for patient care. *Radiology.* 1997;202(2): 297–305.

Dunnick NR, Sandler CM, Amos S, Newhouse J. *Textbook of Uroradiology,* 2nd ed. Baltimore: Williams and Wilkins; 1997.

Itai Y, Ohhashi K, Furui S, Araki T, Murakami Y, Ohtomo K, Atomi Y. Microcystic adenoma of the pancreas: Spectrum of computed tomographic findings. *J. Comput. Assist. Tomogr.* 1988;12(5):797–803.

Korobkin M, Brodeur FJ, Francis IR, Quint LE, Dunnick NR, Goodsitt M. Delayed enhanced CT for differentiation of benign from malignant adrenal masses. *Radiology.* 1996;200(3):737–742.

Korobkin M, Francis IR, Kloos RT, Dunnick NR. The incidental adrenal mass. *Radiol. Clin. North Am.* 1996;34(5):1037–1054.

Lee JKT, Sagel SS, Stanley RJ, Heiken JP. *Computed Body Tomography with MRI Correlation*, 3rd ed. New York: Lippincott-Raven; 1998.

Radin R. HIV infection: Analysis in 259 consecutive patients with abnormal abdominal CT findings. *Radiology.* 1995;197(3):712–722.

Soyer P, Gouhiri MH, Boudiaf M, Brocheriou-Spelle I, Kardache M, Fishman EK, Rymer R. Carcinoma of the gallbladder: Imaging features with surgical correlation. *Am. J. Roentgenol.* 1997;169:781–785.

Taylor AJ, Carmody TJ, Quiroz FA, Erickson SJ, Varma RR, Komorowski RA, Foley WD. Focal masses in cirrhotic liver: CT and MR imaging features. *Am. J. Roentgenol.* 1994;163(4):857–862.

Chapter 14

INTERVENTIONAL RADIOLOGY OF THE CHEST

Robert Y. Kanterman

14.1 PULMONARY ANGIOGRAPHY

• **Pulmonary angiography** is most commonly performed in the setting of suspected acute pulmonary embolism (PE). It is estimated that there are more than 600,000 cases of PE each year in the United States, resulting in a significant number of deaths. The radiologic work-up usually begins with a chest radiograph and ventilation-perfusion scintigraphy. When there is high clinical suspicion and discordant or indeterminate results at scintigraphy, especially when a lower extremity Doppler examination is negative, pulmonary arteriography is warranted.

Technique: A 7 French catheter is inserted via the femoral or jugular vein, through the right heart, and into the pulmonary arteries. Pressure measurements within the right heart and pulmonary arteries give ancillary physiologic information and help to guide the subsequent contrast injections. Nonionic contrast is preferred to minimize coughing, patient discomfort, and the risk of side effects. Contrast is then injected at a relatively high rate and volume (20 to 25 ml/s for 2 seconds) into the main or, preferably, selective pulmonary arteries. If initial pulmonary artery pressure exceeds 70 mmHg or right ventricular end-diastolic pressure is >20 mmHg, subselective angiography should be performed with a lower volume of contrast, and frequent monitoring of pulmonary artery pressures is warranted to prevent acute cor pulmonale.

Interpretation: Traditionally, screen-film angiography was performed, but more recently, digital subtraction angiography has become a competitive technique for displaying pulmonary arterial pathology. An acute thrombus is most often visualized as an intravascular filling defect or a vascular cutoff (Fig. 14-1). Because of the overlapping of

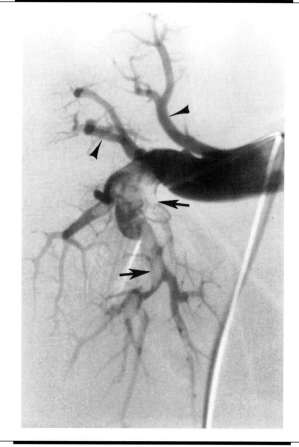

FIGURE 14-1 Pulmonary emboli. Digital subtraction angiogram of the right pulmonary artery from a femoral approach demonstrating extensive embolus in lower lobe branches (arrows). In contrast, there is normal opacification of middle and upper lobe branches (arrowheads).

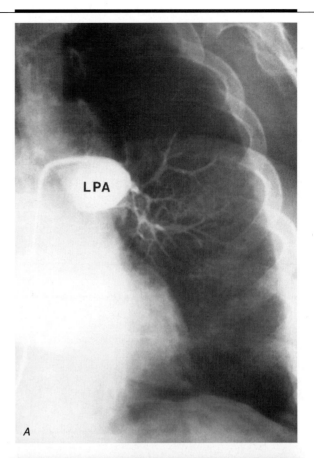
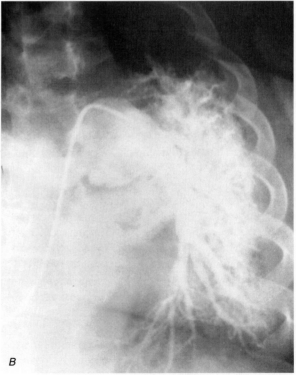

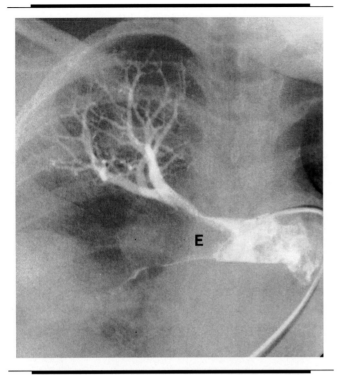

FIGURE 14-2 Pulmonary emboli. Large saddle embolus (E) in the right main pulmonary artery. The patient was treated with intravenous urokinase.

vessels, interpretation of the angiogram can be the most challenging part of the procedure, requiring multiple orthogonal views.

In the setting of PE, percutaneous interventions are not yet widely accepted. Therapeutic techniques used with some success, particularly with larger (saddle) emboli (Fig. 14-2), include pulmonary artery thrombolysis and mechanical thrombectomy. **Pulmonary artery thrombolysis** with urokinase can be achieved via intravenous or intra-arterial infusion through the catheter used to perform the diagnostic examination.

• Pulmonary angiography can also be performed in the setting of **pulmonary artery hypertension** to evaluate for possible chronic thromboembolic disease or to plan treatment. This examination must be made with utmost caution, as the contrast-induced elevation of pulmonary artery pressure may exacerbate underlying pulmonary hypertension and contribute to acute right heart failure and cardiopulmonary decompensation. Oxygen should be administered to reduce pulmonary artery pressure, right ventricular end-diastolic pressure should be monitored and subselective injections of nonionic contrast used.

The angiographic hallmarks of **chronic pulmonary embolism** are pruned vessels with webs and strictures and generally poor opacification of the pulmonary parenchyma during the capillary phase (Fig. 14-3A). At a few centers, patients undergo pulmonary artery endarterectomy, the only successful therapeutic procedure for this condition, and they can demonstrate substantial angiographic improvement (Fig.

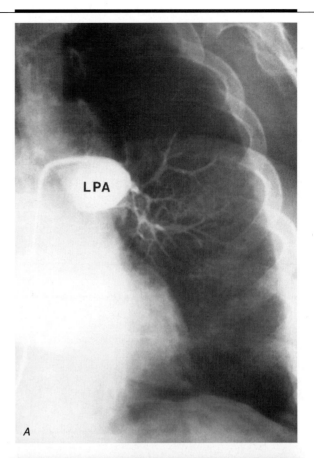

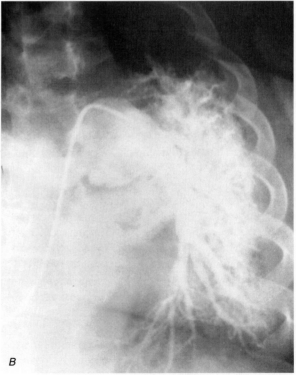

FIGURE 14-3 Thromboendarterectomy. (*A*) Left pulmonary arteriogram in a patient with pulmonary arterial hypertension demonstrates abrupt tapering of the left main pulmonary artery (LPA) and pruning and diminished arborization of the branch vessels. (*B*) After pulmonary artery thromboendarterectomy, there is marked improvement in the pulmonary blood flow.

14-3*B*) after surgery. The presence of acute pulmonary embolism superimposed on chronic pulmonary embolism can be very difficult to diagnose. **Inferior vena cava filters** are indicated to prevent additional pulmonary emboli in many patients afflicted with chronic pulmonary embolism.

- A third role for pulmonary angiography is for the diagnosis and therapy of **pulmonary arteriovenous malformations (PAVMs)**. More than half occur in association with hereditary hemorrhagic telangiectasia, also known as Osler-Weber-Rendu syndrome, an autosomal dominant genetic disorder characterized by abnormalities of vascular structures. Telangiectasias, PAVMs, and vascular abnormalities of the nose, skin, brain, and gastrointestinal tract are characteristic.

  Epistaxis is the most common manifestation and results from spontaneous hemorrhage from mucosal telangiectasias. Symptoms attributable to PAVMs include dyspnea, cyanosis, and polycythemia as a result of right-to-left shunting. Patients also may experience a cerebrovascular accident or develop a brain abscess.

  While angiography is rarely necessary to establish the diagnosis of PAVM (computed tomography [CT] is usually adequate), angiography is necessary for therapeutic planning, particularly when percutaneous embolization is considered. There are two general types of PAVMs. The simple type (80 percent) involves a single feeding artery and a single draining vein. The complex type (20 percent) may involve multiple feeding arteries, a septated aneurysm, and multiple draining veins. Efforts should be made to embolize the feeding arteries when possible.

  Embolization should be considered in patients who have exercise intolerance, to prevent strokes and cerebral abscess and to prevent bleeding. Embolization has been successfully performed with both detachable balloons and coils (Fig. 14-4). Since smaller remaining PAVMs can grow over time, long-term follow-up is essential in these cases. Chest radiographs, determination of arterial blood gases, and bubble echocardiography are effective tools in screening for recurrent or enlarging PAVMs.

- Pulmonary arteriography can also be used in the diagnosis of anatomic variations, pulmonary artery pseudoaneurysm, type IV Takayasu disease, and hepatopulmonary syndrome.

- **Complications** of pulmonary angiography include arrhythmia, worsening pulmonary hypertension, and general com-

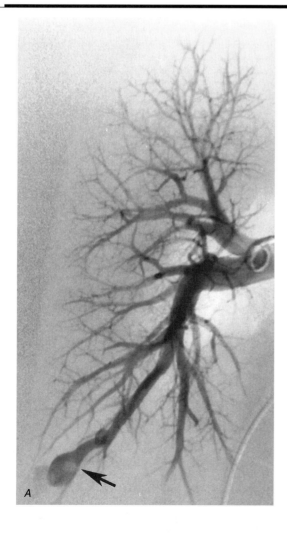

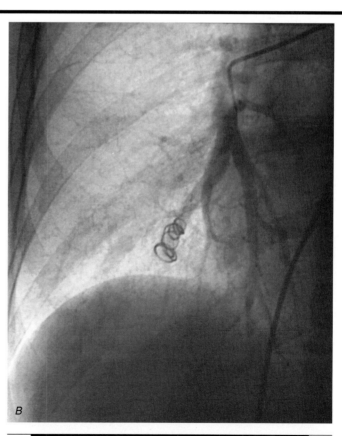

FIGURE 14-4 PAVM embolization. (*A*) Digital subtraction angiogram of the right pulmonary artery demonstrating a large, simple right lower lobe PAVM (arrow). (*B*) After coil embolization of the feeding artery, this PAVM no longer fills with contrast.

plications of bleeding, infection, and contrast toxicity. The major complication rate is approximately 1 percent. Patients with a left bundle branch block should be closely monitored, as right heart catheterization may invoke right bundle branch block leading to a complete heart block. Temporary pacing should be readily available when performing pulmonary angiography in the setting of left bundle branch block. Supraventricular tachycardias are common and usually self-limited or respond to catheter withdrawal or medical therapy. Arrhythmias are felt to result from contact between the bare wire and right atrium, interatrial septum, tricuspid valve, or right ventricle, and this contact should be minimized.

14.2 BRONCHIAL ARTERIOGRAPHY AND EMBOLIZATION

- **Bronchial angiography** is performed in the setting of intractable hemoptysis, particularly in patients with a chronic inflammatory pulmonary condition prone to bleeding, such as tuberculosis, cystic fibrosis, or bronchiectasis. Bronchoscopy is helpful in localizing the side of bleeding (left or right) prior to angiography.

    Technique: A transfemoral artery approach is used to catheterize the bronchial arteries. Bronchial artery anatomy is extremely variable (Fig. 14-5), with the arteries generally arising from the anterolateral thoracic aorta between T3 and T8, most often two from the left side and one from the right side. Coaxial microcatheters are often necessary to engage and deploy embolic materials in these vessels.

    Embolic agents most commonly used in bronchial arteries include gel foam and polyvinyl alcohol (PVA).

Embolotherapy is successful in 75 percent of patients for long-term bleeding control. Bronchial artery embolization using coils should be discouraged as they may limit or prevent access to the source of bleeding if hemoptysis recurs.

Complications of bronchial artery embolization include spinal cord infarction (very rare) and bronchial infarction (two reported cases), as well as the usual complications of angiography. The artery of Adamkiewicz, a large tributary to the anterior spinal artery, may arise with or near a bronchial artery, and this should be recognized prior to embolization. Accidental embolization of this important artery could result in permanent spinal cord injury and paralysis. Chest pain and dysphagia are common postprocedure symptoms and are usually self-limited.

14.3 THORACIC AORTOGRAPHY

- **Indications** for thoracic aortography include atherosclerotic disease as well as blunt and penetrating chest trauma. Aneurysm, dissection (Fig. 14-6), penetrating ulceration (Fig. 14-7), and great vessel origin stenosis or occlusion (Fig. 14-8) are final pathways of atherosclerosis that may warrant angiographic evaluation. While diagnosis of carotid or subclavian origin narrowing is best accomplished with angiography, CT and magnetic resonance imaging (MR) are often employed for evaluation of uncomplicated aneurysms and dissections.

    Thoracic aortography remains the gold standard for the diagnosis of blunt and penetrating chest trauma, despite continued improvement in the competing modalities. As discussed in Section 10.4, CT has a role in screening some trauma patients for arteriography. Thoracic aortography can

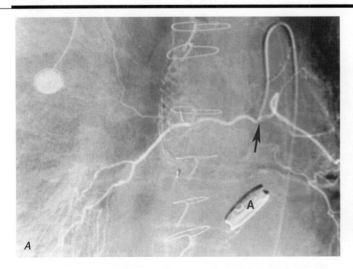 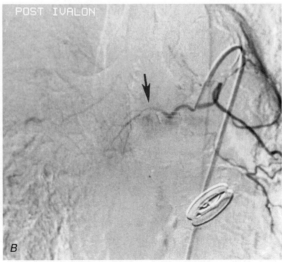

FIGURE 14-5   Bronchial artery embolization. (A) The catheter tip (arrow) is in a common trunk supplying both the right and left bronchial arteries. Incidentally seen is a Bjork-Shiley aortic valve (A). (B) After embolization of the right bronchial artery (arrow) with polyvinyl alcohol, there is stasis of contrast but normal filling of the untreated left bronchial artery.

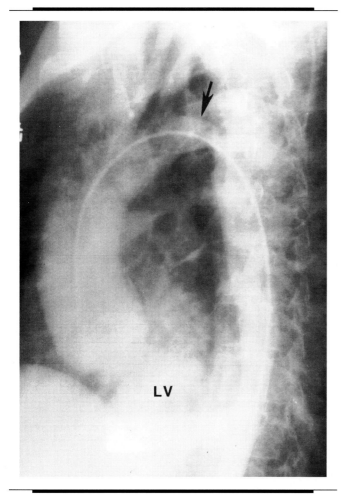

FIGURE 14-6   Type A aortic dissection. Cut-film thoracic aortogram showing the intimal flap (arrow) and evidence of ascending aortic involvement with displacement of the catheter away from the vessel wall and aortic insufficiency with regurgitation of contrast into the left ventricle (LV).

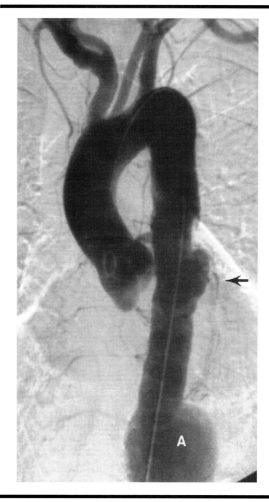

FIGURE 14-7   Penetrating ulcer. A penetrating atherosclerotic ulcer of the aorta (arrow) is several centimeters above a fusiform thoracoabdominal aortic aneurysm (A).

also be useful in the diagnosis of subclavian steal and thoracic outlet syndrome.

   Technique: A transfemoral approach is used in most cases. Thoracic aortography in trauma often requires large volumes of contrast at high injection rates with large catheters (6 French) because of the hyperdynamic physiologic state of the traumatized patient. At least two orthogonal views should be obtained in all cases. Left anterior oblique (LAO) is the single preferred view.

• **Acute traumatic aortic injury (ATAI).** Intimal tears and pseudoaneurysms (Fig. 14-9) are the hallmark signs of **blunt aortic injury** and commonly occur at or near the ligamentum arteriosum. It is important to evaluate all of the visible branch vessels of the aortic arch because these too may be injured (Fig. 14-10). In penetrating trauma to the chest, the angiographic examination should be focused on the region of concern, realizing that gunshot injuries in particular may have harmful effects distant from obvious entry or exit sites.

• Thoracic **aortic aneurysms** are most often atherosclerotic. Postoperative and posttraumatic pseudoaneurysms are so

named because they do not involve all three layers of the vessel. While mycotic aneurysms of the aorta are unusual, they most commonly occur in the descending thoracic aorta. Congenital aneurysms usually involve the sinuses of Valsalva. Syphilis and Ehlers-Danlos syndrome are rare causes of thoracic aortic aneurysms.

• **Marfan syndrome** is an autosomal dominant connective tissue disorder that has cardiovascular manifestations in a majority of those afflicted. Aortic aneurysms due to cystic medial necrosis are a frequent cause of death. Aneurysms of the sinuses of Valsalva, aortic dissection, and aortic regurgitation are also seen.

• **William syndrome**, also called idiopathic hypercalcemia (Fig. 14-11), is a rare disorder characterized by unusual elfin facies, hypercalcemia, mental retardation, and skeletal malformation. A supravalvular aortic stenosis can be seen in these patients, as well as peripheral pulmonary artery stenosis, valvular stenosis, and stenosis of more peripheral arteries.

• **Takayasu arteritis** (Fig. 14-12) is an inflammatory disease of unknown origin that classically occurs in adolescents and

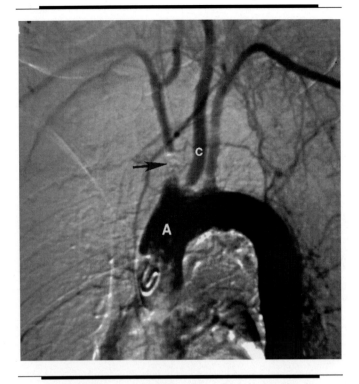

FIGURE 14-8   Atherosclerotic disease. Digital subtraction thoracic aortogram showing complete occlusion of the proximal right brachiocephalic artery (arrow) and narrowing of the left common carotid artery (c) at its origin. There is collateral filling of the right subclavian artery. This may be considered a "right subclavian steal." A, ascending aorta.

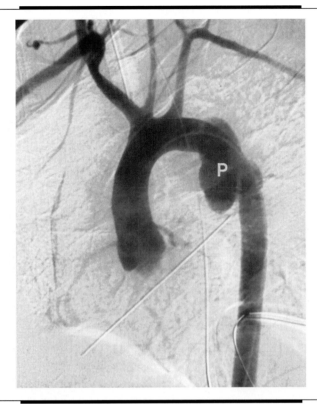

FIGURE 14-9   Pseudoaneurysm. A large, acute posttraumatic pseudoaneurysm (P) of the aorta is found at its most common location at the ligamentum arteriosum. The patient expired during surgery.

young adults and causes diffuse long-segment stenosis and short narrowing and occlusion of the aorta and its major branches. These lesions, particularly in the renal and subclavian arteries, may be amenable to percutaneous angioplasty.

14.4 PERCUTANEOUS BIOPSY

• **Percutaneous chest biopsies** of the lung, pleura, or mediastinum can be performed with either CT, fluoroscopic, or ultrasound guidance. The advantage of CT is that fairly small and deep lesions can be sampled with very little risk to the patient, and the ideal path to the lesion can be defined (Fig. 14-13). Needle placement within the lesion can be made with confidence and appropriately documented. CT is also very sensitive for the diagnosis of postbiopsy bleeding and pneumothorax.

   Fluoroscopically guided biopsy has the advantage of being faster to per-

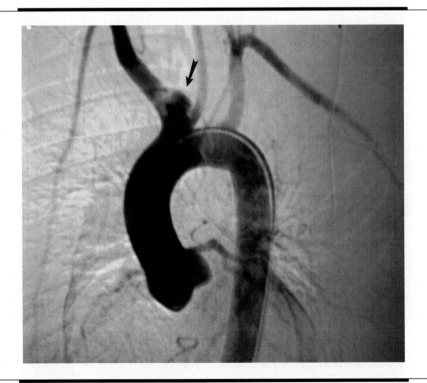

FIGURE 14-10   Penetrating arterial trauma. An acute posttraumatic injury of the brachiocephalic artery (arrow) in a patient whose left common carotid and right brachiocephalic arteries arise from a common trunk.

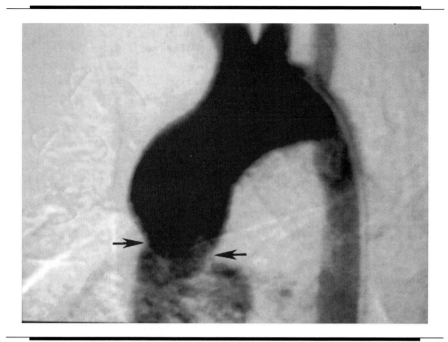

FIGURE 14-11 Aortic stenosis. Supravalvular aortic stenosis (arrows) in a patient with William syndrome.

form, and since one need not seat the needle in the lesion and leave it unattended, there is less chance a needle will be displaced, particularly with peripheral lesions. Should a

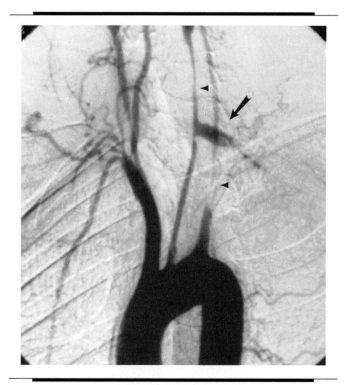

FIGURE 14-12 Takayasu arteritis. Angiogram demonstrating long, tapered stenosis of the left vertebral and common carotid arteries (arrowheads) and occlusion of the left subclavian artery, requiring a carotid-subclavian bypass (arrow).

pneumothorax occur requiring immediate treatment, a fluoroscopy room is the ideal location to place a chest tube, as the catheter can be manipulated under fluoroscopic control to the desired location.

Some physicians even advocate using sonography for lung biopsy, and no doubt, when interventional MR units become more commonplace, there will be proponents for it as well. In most practices, CT remains the modality of choice for percutaneous lung biopsy.

• **Lesion selection:** Much controversy exists about which indeterminate focal lung lesions are appropriate for biopsy. In a smoker with a solitary lung lesion (suspicious for bronchogenic carcinoma) without hilar or mediastinal adenopathy who is a candidate for pulmonary resection, many argue that the lesion should be resected without biopsy. The logic follows that since the clinical suspicion for bronchogenic carcinoma is sufficiently high, a negative (or nondiagnostic) biopsy result would not curtail the workup, and therefore the lesion is destined to be resected no matter what the result of the biopsy.

• **Sampling** can be performed for cytology with an aspirating needle (Chiba) or for histopathology with one of many different types of cutting needles. Some radiologists prefer a coaxial technique with a 22-gauge aspirating needle through a larger 18- or 19-gauge introducer needle. By first advancing the introducer needle into the lesion, multiple samplings can then be performed with the guiding needle without losing access to the lesion (Fig. 14-13). Spring-loaded biopsy guns are favored by some physicians.

• The strength and preference of the hospital pathology department often influence the type of tissue one attempts to acquire during a percutaneous biopsy and the diagnostic success of the procedure. The success of needle biopsy also depends on the technique, the size of the lesion, the experience of the operator, and the lesion location. For focal lung lesions, a percutaneous needle biopsy has a sensitivity of about 90 percent, slightly higher for a cutting needle specimen than for a cytology specimen. When mediastinal masses are biopsied, the sensitivity drops somewhat because of the difficulty in establishing the diagnosis of lymphoma on the basis of needle biopsy specimens.

• **Complications** of lung biopsy include bleeding, air embolism via pulmonary veins, and pneumothorax. Since the latter often necessitates chest tube placement, the physician performing the procedure should be familiar with this technique or should have access to a backup physician who can accomplish it on short notice. To prevent air embolism, the

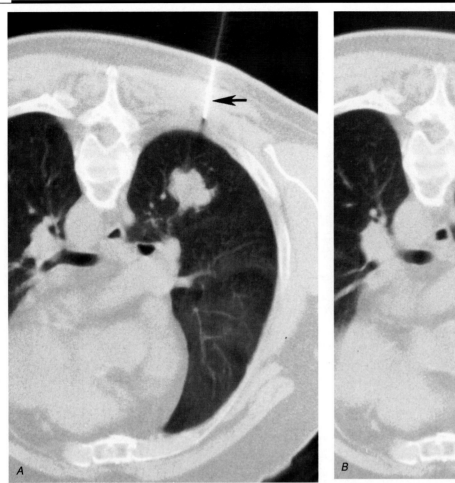
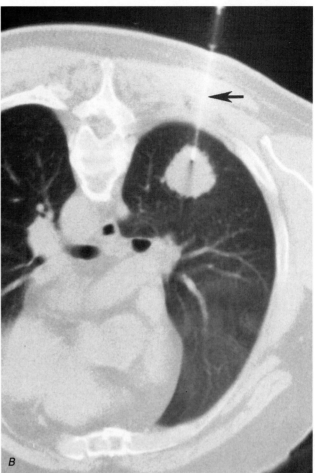

FIGURE 14-13   CT-guided lung biopsy. (*A*) The patient is positioned prone, the lesion is localized under CT, and a 19-gauge "guiding" needle is advanced into the chest wall (black arrow). Note black streak originating at the needle tip, a useful landmark. (*B*) The needle is advanced to the edge of the lesion, allowing multiple aspirations with a 22-gauge Chiba needle which passes through the guiding needle (arrow).

needle should be covered whenever possible. Bleeding is usually self-limited but can result in hemoptysis and obscuration of the lesion during the procedure. Seeding of tumor cells along the needle track is rare.

- **Needle localization** is an extension of the percutaneous lung nodule needle biopsy. This is ideal for small, peripheral lesions which are challenging to biopsy and will likely be resected anyway. The radiologist localizes the lesion in question under imaging guidance (usually CT) with a mammography hookwire, so that the thoracic surgeon can easily locate and resect the lesion at thoracoscopy (Fig. 14-14).

At our hospital, the needle is advanced into the lesion under CT guidance, 1 ml of methylene blue is injected, the appropriate length of hookwire is deployed, and the guiding needle removed. The methylene blue is injected as a safety precaution in the event that the wire is displaced between the time the patient leaves the radiology department and thoracoscopic surgery commences. An evolving pneumothorax is one potential mechanism by which the needle can become displaced.

The surgeon immediately proceeds with thoracoscopic resection of the lesion. This procedure obviously requires tight coordination among the radiologist, thoracic surgeon, and supporting facilities of both. While this procedure has received increasing acceptance for appropriate lesions, some physicians argue that the radiologic technique is so similar to a lung biopsy that a biopsy should indeed be performed prior to thoracoscopic resection, a fairly invasive procedure requiring general anesthesia and hospitalization. Proponents of the needle localization procedure counter that when the lesion is removed, the issue is settled, and there is no consternation as is seen with a negative or nondiagnostic lung biopsy.

14.5 PLEURAL DRAINAGE AND PLEURODESIS

- The simplest pleural drainage procedure is **thoracentesis**, often performed in radiology departments under ultrasound guidance. In most cases, it is adequate to simply localize the fluid with sonography, mark the skin, and proceed with

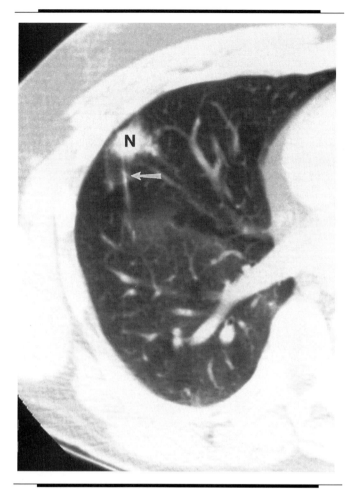

FIGURE 14-14 Localization for thoracoscopy. A hookwire (arrow) is faintly seen passing through a right upper lobe noncalcified nodule (N) which was found to be a granuloma on thoracoscopic resection.

pleural puncture and fluid aspiration at the bedside. For smaller or loculated effusions, a needle guide or dedicated biopsy probe can be used for real-time visualization of the needle passing into the pleural fluid collection. Thoracentesis is ideally performed with the patient sitting upright but can be performed in the supine position if necessary.

- **Recurrent effusions**, particularly when due to malignancy, and complicated pleural effusions (empyema and hemothorax) often require **chest tube drainage**. Chest tubes come in many shapes and sizes and can be inserted with fluoroscopy, ultrasound, or CT guidance (or blindly, under favorable conditions). Tubes appropriate for interventional radiology procedures may use a trocar or an over-the-wire technique and are typically in the 8- to 24-French range with either a Cope loop or a J-tip and multiple side holes.

- Patients with **recurrent, symptomatic malignant effusions** are often treated with **pleurodesis**. The initial step is to insert a pleural drain and remove as much fluid as possible. When fluid output drops to 100 to 150 ml/day, the patient is ready for pleurodesis (Fig. 14-15). Recent literature suggests this can be accomplished on an outpatient basis.

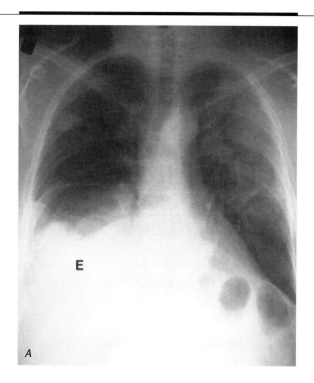

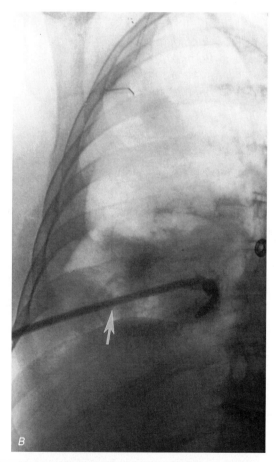

FIGURE 14-15 Pleurodesis. (*A*) Radiograph in a woman with recurrent right pleural effusion (E) as a result of metastatic breast carcinoma who was incapacitated by dyspnea. (*B*) A 12 French pleural drain (arrow) was placed followed by pleurodesis with talc slurry on the following day, resulting in significant symptomatic improvement.

Common **sclerosing agents** include talc slurry, doxycycline, and bleomycin. While there are a number of series that tout the advantage of one agent over another, there is no clear winner. Since talc is by far the least expensive and has had the most clinical use over the years, it remains the preferred agent for many. Lidocaine can be injected into the pleural space with the sclerosing agent to reduce the pain that often accompanies this therapy. The success rate for pleurodesis varies widely, but initial clinical improvement is seen in about 75 percent of patients although it drops to about 60 percent at 90 days.

- **Complications** of pleural drainage include bleeding (from intercostal vessels), pneumothorax, and tube migration. Complications and side effects of pleurodesis include pain, fever, empyema, and respiratory failure, the latter two being fairly unusual. Because of the potential for infection in the pleural space during pleurodesis, some physicians advocate intracavitary administration of antibiotics with the sclerosing agent.

14.6 PNEUMOTHORAX MANAGEMENT

- **Pneumothoraces** can arise spontaneously, but most result as a consequence of trauma or a medical procedure. In the radiology department, one common cause of pneumothorax is percutaneous lung biopsy (Section 14.4). Chest tube placement can be performed by the interventional radiologist with technical considerations as noted previously (Section 14.5).

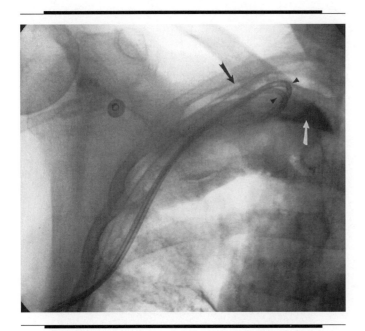

FIGURE 14-16   Air leak management with fibrin glue. Patient who experienced a prolonged, refractory air leak after a right upper lobectomy, despite appropriate positioning of a surgical chest tube in the right apex (black arrow). Two catheters (black arrowheads) were placed side by side, and cryoprecipitate and calcium-thrombin were infused to create fibrin glue to seal the source of the air leak. Contrast (white arrow) has also been injected into the pleural space.

Not all pneumothoraces require drainage. Patients with small, stable, asymptomatic pneumothoraces can be managed conservatively with observation. Larger, increasing, or symptomatic pneumothoraces, including those causing chest pain, dyspnea, or hypoxia, should be evacuated.

One difference in the approach to draining a pneumothorax compared to fluid collection is that, in general, smaller catheters can be used since the viscosity of air is so much less than that of fluid (particularly blood or pus). Smaller drains are more likely to become plugged with mucus, though, and tube patency should therefore be monitored regularly. Patency can be tested and restored with saline injection.

- Patients who sustain a pneumothorax without an ongoing air leak can be managed with a **Heimlich valve**, a one-way valve that allows air to leave the pleural space but not return. Patients can be sent home with the Heimlich valve and further observed on an outpatient basis. When there is evidence or concern of an active air leak, the chest tube should be placed to suction.

   The presence of an **air leak** should be closely monitored by the person managing the pneumothorax drainage. Resolution of the air leak can signal sealing of the violated visceral pleural but also can be seen when the tube is occluded. A chest radiograph obtained with the chest tube on water seal can help determine when the air leak has resolved and the tube is ready for removal. Pneumothoraces that occur with persistent air leaks can be difficult to manage and may require multiple pleural drains and a considerable amount of time for resolution.

- We use a **fibrin glue** to help seal persistent air leaks in patients who have undergone pulmonary resection. Under CT or fluoroscopic guidance, we place two 8 French drainage catheters adjacent to one another and near the expected location of the leak (Fig. 14-16). Cryoprecipitate is infused in one tube and a calcium-thrombin mixture in the other to create a fibrin glue. In our initial set of patients, we have been 70 percent successful at reducing or eliminating the air leak with this fibrin glue procedure, with no complications.

14.7 EMPYEMA MANAGEMENT

- An **empyema** is an infection of the pleural space that is most commonly a complication of an infected perapneumonic effusion. Historically, drainage was performed with a surgically placed chest tube, but despite this, many patients ultimately required a thoracotomy and decortication. Drainage catheters can also be placed by the interventional radiologist (as described in Section 14.5). Empyemas differ from uncomplicated effusions in that larger-bore catheters are required for drainage because of the increased viscosity of the fluid and debris. Usually 20 to 30 French catheters are recommended.

- **CT** or **sonography** is often required to best localize and access empyemas, as they are likely to be loculated, occasionally requiring more than one chest tube.

- **Urokinase** is a useful adjuvant for chest tube drainage because it helps to break up loculations and improve drainage of the infected material. Dosing regimens are variable and can be repeated until the patient is clinically and radiologically improved or until no additional progress is made. Surgical decortication may then be warranted. The clinical success for radiologic treatment of empyemas is about 75 percent and compares favorably to surgical treatment.

- An **empyema** must always be distinguished from a **pulmonary abscess**, which occurs in the lung parenchyma. Tube drainage of pulmonary abscesses should be reserved for patients who are not improving with antibiotics and conservative measures, particularly those who have larger abscesses. The potential creation of a bronchopleural fistula is a feared complication of percutaneous drainage of a pulmonary abscess. The amount of normal lung tissue traversed by the drain should be minimized to reduce the risk of creating a fistula. Other potential complications of lung abscess drainage include pneumothorax, empyema, and bleeding.

14.8 CENTRAL VENOUS CATHETERS

- A modern interventional radiology practice is increasingly involved in **venous access** procedures. From peripherally inserted central catheters (PICCs) to ports, a whole host of central access procedures can be placed by radiology department personnel. Sterile conditions are mandatory for these procedures.

- The choice of which device to place depends on the purpose, length of time it will be in place, patient preference and lifestyle, and available venous access. For short-term access, a PICC line or nontunneled central line is appropriate. Dialysis generally requires large-bore, high-flow catheters. Ports are appropriate for long-term intermittent access requirements and patients with an active lifestyle.

- **Fluoroscopic guidance** is useful for placement, and venography or sonography can be used to aid in venous access. Both tunneled and nontunneled central catheters can be placed, primarily via subclavian or internal jugular vein access. Rarely, patients have occluded subclavian and internal jugular veins, requiring a more creative approach. Using venographic and percutaneous transhepatic techniques, the interventional radiologist is best suited to place direct translumbar inferior vena cava catheters and percutaneous hepatic vein catheters, respectively.

- Procedural **complications** accompanying central access procedures include bleeding, pneumothorax, and air embolism. The major complication rate is well under 5 percent. Catheter fracture can also occur, particularly when a catheter is compressed between the first rib and clavicle, the so-called

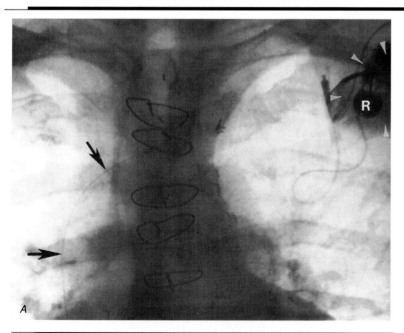
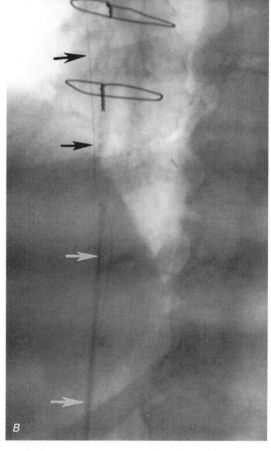

FIGURE 14-17 Catheter fragment retrieval. (*A*) Radiograph showing a catheter (arrows) that has become dissociated from the port reservoir (R) in a patient with lymphoma. Note the free extravasation of contrast (white arrowheads) injected into the port and the gap between the reservoir and catheter. (*B*) A snare (white arrows) is used to retrieve the catheter fragment (black arrows) via the right femoral vein. The snare can be seen pulling the catheter fragment caudally into the inferior vena cava.

"pinch-off" syndrome. Catheter-related thrombosis occurs in up to 10 percent of patients.

Catheter-related **infection** is seen in up to one-fifth of patients because of the relative sterility of conditions during placement and routine use and the immunosuppressed state of many patients who receive these catheters. While permanent catheters should not be placed in patients who are known to be bacteremic, the use of prophylactic antibiotics during catheter placement is controversial. Known or suspected catheter infection almost always necessitates removal.

Interventional radiologists are often called on to aid in treating various complications of central venous access. Migrated or dissociated catheter fragments can be snared by a transvenous approach (Fig. 14-17). While snares are also employed to strip the fibrin sheath from an occluded central catheter, urokinase can be used effectively for this purpose in most cases.

Bibliography

Denny DF. Placement and management of long-term central venous access catheters and ports. *Am. J. Roentgenol.* 1993;161:385–393.

Fisher RG, Chasen MH, Lamki N. Diagnosis of injuries of the aorta and brachiocephalic arteries caused by blunt chest trauma: CT vs aortography. *Am. J. Roentgenol.* 1994;162:1047–1052.

Kadir S. Arteriography of the thoracic aorta. In: *Diagnostic Angiography*, Kadir S, ed. Philadelphia: WB Saunders; 1986.

Klein JS, Schultz S, Heffner JE. Interventional radiology of the chest: Image-guided percutaneous drainage of pleural effusions, lung abscess, and pneumothorax. *Am. J. Roentgenol.* 1995;164:581–588.

Mauro MA, Jaques PF. Transcatheter bronchial artery embolization for inflammation (hemoptysis). In: *Abrams Angiography*, Vol. III, Baum S, Pentecost MJ, eds. Philadelphia: Little Brown; 1997.

Patz EF, McAdams HP, Goodman PC, Blackwell S, Crawford J. Ambulatory sclerotherapy for malignant pleural effusions. *Radiology* 1996;199: 133–135.

Shah RM, Spirn PW, Salazar AM, Steiner RM, Cohn HE, Wechsler RJ. Role of thoracoscopy and preoperative localization procedures in the diagnosis and management of pulmonary pathology. *Semin Ultrasound CT MR.* 1995; 16:371–378.

Westcott JL, Rao, N, Colley DP. Transthoracic needle biopsy of small pulmonary nodules. *Radiology.* 1997;202:97–103.

White RI, Pollak JS, Wirth JA. Pulmonary arteriovenous malformations: diagnosis and embolotherapy. *J. Vasc. Interv. Radiol.* 1996;7:787–804.

Yankelevitz DF, Davis SA, Chiarella DA, Henschke CI. Pitfalls in CT-guided transthoracic needle biopsy of pulmonary nodules. *Radiographics.* 1996; 16:1073–1084.

Zuckerman DA, Sterling KM, Oser RF. Safety of pulmonary angiography in the 1990s. *J. Vasc. Interv. Radiol.* 1996;7:199–205.

APPENDIX

APPENDIX

Richard M. Slone

A.1 NORMAL LABORATORY VALUES AND PRESSURE MEASUREMENTS

Serum chemistry	
Albumin	3.6–5.0 g/dl
Calcium (total)	8.9–10.3 mg/dl
Chloride	97–110 mmol/L
Creatinine	0.5–1.7 mg/dl
Potassium	3.3–4.9 mmol/L
Protein (total)	6.2–8.2 g/dl
Sodium	135–145 mmol/L
Urea nitrogen	8–25 mg/dl

Serum enzymes	
Alkaline phosphatase	38–126 IU/L
Amylase	35–118 IU/L
Lipase	2.3–20 IU/dl
SGOT (AST)	11–47 IU/L
SGPT	7–53 IU/L

Serum hormone levels	
ACTH (fasting)	< 60 pg/ml
Aldosterone	10–160 ng/L
Cortisol	8–25 μg/dl
Parathyroid	10–55 pg/ml
Thyroxin (total T4)	4.5–12 μg/dl
TSH	0.35–6.2 μU/ml

Hematologic values	
Bleeding time	2.5–9.5 min
Erythrocyte sedimentation rate	0–30 mm/h
Fibrinogen	150–360 mg/dl
Hematocrit (men)	41–50
Hematocrit (women)	36–44
Partial thromboplastin time (PTT)	25–33 s
Platelet count	140–440 $10^3/\mu l$
Prothrombin time (PT)	10.7–13 s
Thrombin time	11.3–18.5 s
White blood cells (total)	3.8–9.8 $10^3/\mu l$

Arterial blood gas analysis	
Pa_{O_2}	80–105 mmHg
Pa_{CO_2}	35–45 mmHg
pH	7.35–7.45

Blood pressure measurements	
Left atrium	0–5 mmHg
Left ventricle	120/5 mmHg
Aorta	120/80 mmHg
Right atrium	0–5 mmHg
Right ventricle	30/5–8 mmHg
Pulmonary artery pressure	30/12 mmHg
Pulmonary capillary wedge pressure	5–12 mmHg

Source: Ewald GA, McKenzie CR. *The Washington Manual of Medical Therapeutics.* 28th ed. St Louis: Lippincott-Raven; 1995.

A.2   NORMAL SIZE OF THORACIC STRUCTURES

Vessels	
Aortic root	3.0 to 4.2 cm
Ascending aorta	2.4 to 3.6 cm
Descending thoracic aorta	2.0 to 2.8 cm
Main pulmonary artery	2 cm
Right interlobar pulmonary artery	< 16 mm in men; < 15 mm in women
Superior vena cava	1.4 to 2.6 cm
Inferior vena cava	1.8 to 3.6 cm
Pulmonary artery to bronchus ratio, erect	0.6 to 1.1, upper lobe; 1.0 to 1.7, lower lobe
Pulmonary artery to bronchus ratio, supine	0.8 to 1.2, upper and lower lobe

Cardiac	
Left atrium on PA radiograph	< 7 cm diagonally from left main bronchus to right inferolateral left atrium
Left atrium on lateral radiograph	< 4 cm from posterior wall to a line dropped from anterior right main PA
Left ventricle on lateral radiograph (Hoffman-Rigler sign)	< 1.8 cm between posterior wall and IVC, measured 2 cm above crossing
LV thickness (diastole)	< 15 mm
RV thickness	< 6 mm
Pericardial thickness	< 4 mm
Cardiothoracic ratio	< 0.55 (ratio of maximum cardiac width to maximum interthoracic width)

Lymph nodes	
Axillary lymph nodes	Up to 1 cm, larger if center is fatty
Retrocrural	≤ 0.6 cm
Supraclavicular lymph nodes	≤ 0.5 cm short axis
Subcarinal lymph nodes	≤ 1.5 cm
Mediastinal lymph nodes	≤ 1 cm short axis
Prevascular lymph nodes	≤ 0.5 cm short axis
Pericardial lymph nodes	No more than two 0.5 cm nodes

Airway	
Trachea, mean transverse diameter	16 to 21 mm in men; 12 to 18 mm in women (10% smaller on expiration)
Right paratracheal stripe	< 4 mm
Right main bronchus	12 to 20 mm
Left main bronchus	10 to 17 mm
Subcarinal angle	40 to 80°
Posterior tracheal band on lateral radiograph (tracheoesophogeal stripe)	< 5 mm
Posterior wall of bronchus intermedius on lateral radiograph	< 3 mm
Bronchiectasis suggested when bronchioles seen	< 3 cm of pleura on CXR, < 2 cm by CT, < 1/cm HRCT

Thymus	
Visible on CT	100% age < 30, 70% age 30 to 50, 15% age > 50
Maximum thickness	7 mm age > 50, 13 mm age > 20 years (measured perpendicular to lobe)

A.3   COMMON ABBREVIATIONS USED IN CHEST DISEASE

AAA	Abdominal aortic aneurysm
ABG	Arterial blood gas analysis
ABPA	Allergic bronchopulmonary aspergillosis
ACE	Angiotensin-converting enzyme
ACTH	Adrenocorticotropic hormone (corticotropin)
AFP	Alpha fetoprotein
AI	Aortic insufficiency
AIDS	Acquired immunodeficiency syndrome
ALL	Acute lymphocytic leukemia
AMBER	Advanced multiple beam equalization radiography
AML	Acute myeloblastic leukemia (or angiomyolipoma)
ANA	Antinuclear antibodies
APUD	Amino precursor uptake decarboxylation cell
APVR	Anomalous pulmonary venous return
ARDS	Adult respiratory distress syndrome
AS	Aortic stenosis (or ankylosing spondylitis)
ASD	Atrial septal defect
AVM	Arteriovenous malformation
AVR	Aortic valve replacement
BAC	Bronchoalveolar carcinoma
BALT	Bronchial-associated lymphoid tissue
BOOP	Bronchiolitis obliterans with organizing pneumonia

Source: Rosenberg RD. *Radiographic Measurements.* Philadelphia: JB Lippincott;1989. Bouchard L, Cordeau MP, Samson LM. Pictorial essay of normal reference values in thoracic x-ray, CT and MR imaging. *Chest.* 112(3):51S;1997.

BPD	Bronchopulmonary dysplasia	LVE	Left ventricular enlargement
CABG	Coronary artery bypass graft	LVH	Left ventricular hypertrophy
CAD	Coronary artery disease	LVOT	Left ventricular outflow track
CAM	Cystic adenomatoid malformation	LVRS	Lung volume reduction surgery
CF	Cystic fibrosis	MAC	*Mycobacterium avium* complex
CFA	Cryptogenic fibrosing alveolitis (IPF)	MAI	*Mycobacterium avium* intracellulaire
CHF	Congestive heart failure	MFH	Malignant fibrous histiocytoma
CIP	Chronic interstitial pneumonia	MIBG	Metaiodobenzylguanidine (radiopharmaceutical)
CLL	Chronic lymphocytic leukemia	MPA	Main pulmonary artery
CM	Cardiomegaly	MR	Mitral regurgitation
CML	Chronic myelogenous leukemia	MS	Mitral stenosis
CMV	Cytomegalovirus	MVR	Mitral valve replacement
COP	Cryptogenic organizing pneumonia	N/V	Nausea and vomiting
COPD	Chronic obstructive pulmonary disease	NG	Nasogastric
CP	Chest pain	NHL	Non-Hodgkin lymphoma
CR	Computed radiography	PA	Pulmonary artery
CT	Computed tomography	PAP	Pulmonary alveolar proteinosis
CWP	Coal worker's pneumoconiosis	PAPVR	Partial anomalous pulmonary venous return
CXR	Chest radiograph	PCP	*Pneumocystis carinii* pneumonia
DDx	Differential diagnosis	PCWP	Pulmonary capillary wedge pressure
DIC	Disseminated intravascular coagulation	PCXR	Portable chest radiograph
DIP	Desquamative interstitial pneumonitis	PDA	Patent ductus arteriosis or posterior descending coronary artery
DISH	Diffuse idiopathic skeletal hyperostosis		
DOLV	Double-outlet left ventricle	PE	Pulmonary embolism (also physical examination)
DORV	Double-outlet right ventricle	PEEP	Positive end expiratory pressure
DVT	Deep venous thrombosis	PET	Positron emission tomography
Dx	Diagnosis	PFO	Patent foramen ovale
ECD	Endocardial cushion defect	PG_1	Prostaglandin 1
ECG	Electrocardiogram	PIE	Pulmonary interstitial emphysema
EF	Ejection fraction	PMF	Progressive massive fibrosis
EG	Eosinophilic granuloma	PPD	Purified protein derivative (typically referring to TB)
ERCP	Extracorporeal shock wave lithotrypsy		
ESR	Erythrocyte sedimentation rate	PT	Prothrombin time
FA	Free air	PTLD	Posttransplant lymphoproliferative disease
FEV_1	Forced expiratory volume in 1 second	PTT	Partial thromboplastin time
FVC	Forced vital capacity	PTX	Pneumothorax
GER	Gastroesophageal reflux	PVH	Pulmonary venous hypertension
GVH	Graft vs. host disease	RA	Right atrium
HH	Hiatal hernia	RAA	Right atrial appendage
HRCT	High-resolution CT	RAD	Right axis deviation on ECG
IHSS	Idiopathic hypertrophic subaortic stenosis	RAE	Right atrial enlargement
IPF	Idiopathic pulmonary fibrosis	RAO	Right anterior oblique projection
IV	Intravenous	RBC	Red blood cell
IVC	Inferior vena cava	RLL	Right lower lobe
LA	Left atrium	RML	Right middle lobe
LAA	Left atrial appendage	ROI	Region of interest
LAD	Left anterior descending coronary artery or left axis deviation on an ECG	RPA	Right pulmonary artery
		RSV	Respiratory syncytial virus
LAE	Left atrial enlargement	RUL	Right upper lobe
LAM	Lymphangioleiomyomatosis	RV	Right ventricle (or residual volume)
LAO	Left anterior oblique projection	RVE	Right ventricular enlargement
LCx	Left circumflex coronary artery	RVH	Right ventricular hypertrophy
LIP	Lymphocytic interstitial pneumonitis	Rx	Therapy
LLL	Left lower lobe	SBE	Subacute bacterial endocarditis
LPA	Left pulmonary artery	SPECT	Single photon emission computed tomography
LUL	Left upper lobe	SVC	Superior vena cava
LV	Left ventricle	SVT	Supraventricular tachycardia

TA	Tricuspid atresia or truncus arteriosis
TAPVR	Total anomalous pulmonary venous return
TB	Tuberculosis
TCC	Transitional cell carcinoma
TGA	Transposition of the great arteries
TLC	Total lung capacity
TOF	Tetralogy of Fallot
TV	Tidal volume
UIP	Usual interstitial pneumonia
VATS	Video-assisted thoracoscopic surgery
VC	Vital capacity
VSD	Ventricular septal defect
WBC	White blood cell
XGP	Xanthogranulomatous pyelonephritis

A.4 SURGICAL EPONYMS

- **Belsey fundoplication** is a treatment for gastroesophageal reflux in which a double telescoping of the distal esophagus onto the cardia of the stomach and 270-degree gastric wrap are performed along with tightening of the esophageal hiatus. The procedure is performed via a left thoracostomy.

- **Bentall procedure**, performed for treatment of a type A aortic dissection or ascending aortic aneurysm. It involves replacement of the native valve and proximal aortic root with a composite aortic valved-conduit graft and reimplantation of the coronary arteries. The *Cabrol procedure* is a modification in which the coronaries are sewn to a separate tube graft which is then attached to the composite valved-conduit.

- **Blalock-Hanlon procedure** refers to resection of a portion of the atrial septum to create a large atrial septal defect for the palliative treatment of transposition of the great arteries in patients with an intact atrial septum.

- **Blalock-Taussig shunt** is an anastomosis of the subclavian artery to the ipsilateral pulmonary artery to increase blood flow to the lungs in cyanotic patients with tetrology of Fallot or other right-sided obstructive lesions. In the classic procedure (1949) performed via thoracotomy, the subclavian artery on the side opposite the aortic arch is anastomosed to the ipsilateral pulmonary artery. The procedure can also be performed on the side of the arch with the use of prosthetic graft material to create a conduit between the subclavian and pulmonary arteries. The ideal operation is total open correction on cardiopulmonary bypass.

- **Eloesser flap** (1935) or *open-window thoracostomy* refers to an open pleural drainage for treatment of a postpneumonectomy empyema or bronchopleural fistula that has failed thoracostomy tube management. The opening is created by dissecting through the chest wall and resecting 5–10 cm of one or two ribs. A skin flap is marsupialized into the wound

to optimize drainage and prevent closing by healing. The cavity is packed with dressing and, when fully healed, closed with a soft tissue and skin graft. Clagett described a three-step treatment for empyema in 1963, the first step being an Eloesser flap.

- **Fontan procedure** (1971) is a right atrium-to-pulmonary artery anastomosis, usually performed for tricuspid atresia. The original procedure involved a superior vena cava to right pulmonary artery anastomosis, a homograft valve in the inferior vena cava–right atrial junction, and a valved conduit between the right atrium and left pulmonary artery.

- **Glenn shunt** (1954) is a surgical shunt between the superior vena cava and right pulmonary artery for palliation of cyanotic patients, usually those with tetralogy of Fallot. A *bidirectional Glenn* procedure creates a bidirectional superior cavopulmonary anastomosis.

- **Jatene operation** (1975), also called the *arterial switch procedure*, is the procedure of choice and the definitive treatment of transposition of the great vessels. The procedure involves switching the ascending aorta and pulmonary artery attachments and reimplanting the coronary arteries.

- **Mustard procedure** (1964) is an atrial switching operation for the repair of complete transposition of the great vessels. The procedure is performed via a median sternotomy incision. The atrial septum is removed, and an atrial baffle is made with autologous pericardium to reroute the blood in the atria.

- **Nissen fundoplication** is an antireflux procedure in which the fundus of the stomach is mobilized and wrapped 360 degrees around the distal intra-abdominal esophagus. The procedure can be performed laparoscopically or via a standard upper abdominal midline incision.

- **Norwood procedure** is a three-staged operation for treatment of hypoplastic left heart consisting of an initial palliation, a hemi fontan, and a completion fontan. Mortality can be high. Cardiac transplantation has been proposed as an acceptable alternative though long-term results in neonates remain unclear.

- **Potts procedure** (1946) is the creation of a shunt between the descending aorta and left pulmonary artery formerly used to increase pulmonary blood flow in cyanotic patients with tetralogy of Fallot or tricuspid atresia.

- **Rashkind procedure** (1966) refers to a percutaneous balloon atrial septostomy for palliation of cyanotic patients with transposition of the great arteries. It used to be performed at initial catheterization in almost all infants with transposition of the great arteries to improve mixing between the pulmonary and systemic circulations and thus improve systemic oxygen delivery until formal correction could be performed.

- **Rastelli procedure** (1969) is an operation that creates a conduit between the right ventricle and pulmonary artery in patients with right-sided obstructions.

Source: Pearson FG, Deslauriers J, Ginsberg RJ, Hiebert CA, McKneally MF, Urschel HC. *Thoracic Surgery.* New York: Churchill Livingstone; 1995.

- **Ross procedure** is replacement of the aortic valve with the patient's own pulmonic valve (autograft) and reconstruction of the pulmonic valve with a homograft (allograft).

- **Senning procedure** (1959) is a technique formerly used for repairing transposition of the great vessels by creating intra-atrial transposition of venous return. In this procedure, performed via median sternotomy, the atrial walls and septum are used to form a baffle to redirect blood from the vena cava into the left ventricle, and pulmonary venous blood into the right ventricle. The procedure avoids the use of any type of prosthetic material and thus increases the potential for future growth.

- **Waterson-Cooley procedure** (1962) refers to creation of an anastomosis between the ascending aorta and right pulmonary artery formerly used in the treatment of tetralogy of Fallot and tricuspid atresia.

A.5   SYNDROMES WITH THORACIC MANIFESTATIONS

- A **syndrome** refers to a specific collection of signs and symptoms forming a recognizable pattern repeated in other individuals. Over 2000 syndromes have been recorded. Following are some syndromes associated with thoracic manifestations. An **association** is a grouping of abnormalities that arise together more frequently than they would by chance alone.

- **Achondroplasia** is an autosomal dominant disease often occurring as a sporadic mutation that results in defective endochondral bone formation. It is characterized by rhizomelic dwarfism with short limbs, normal trunk size, square chest, and protuberant abdomen and buttocks. Thoracic skeletal manifestation includes square inferior scapular angles, wedged vertebrae with posterior scalloping, narrow interpedicular spaces, wide neural foramina, and accentuated lumbar kyphoses. Restriction of the thoracic cage can produce pulmonary hypoplasia. Patients have normal intelligence and life expectancy.

- **Behçet disease**, also called *Hughes-Stovin syndrome*, is a rare vasculitis. Primary manifestations include uveitis and skin involvement, but systemic and pulmonary thromboembolism, pulmonary aneurysms, massive pulmonary hemorrhage, and vena cava thrombosis can occur.

- **Buerger disease**, also called *thromboangitis obliterans*, is an idiopathic vascular disease characterized by recurrent seg-

mental obliterative vasculitis of small and medium-sized arteries and veins, particularly in the lower extremities. It is more common in the Eastern Hemisphere and is strongly associated with cigarette smoking.

- **Caplan syndrome** is a rare association, originally referring to pulmonary nodules in coal miners with rheumatoid arthritis. Coal worker's pneumoconiosis need not be present. The term is sometimes used for a condition involving pulmonary nodules, serologic evidence of rheumatoid arthritis, and exposure to some other inorganic dust such as asbestos.

- **Castleman disease**, also called *giant lymph node hyperplasia, angiofolicular lymph node hyperplasia,* or *angiomatous lymphoid hamartoma,* is a rare cause of benign mediastinal adenopathy. Large size and dramatic contrast enhancement on computed tomography are characteristic. No specific cause has been identified, and patients can be symptomatic if the nodes compress adjacent structures. (See Section 5.4.)

- **Churg-Strauss syndrome** is a necrotizing vasculitis occurring in patients with asthma variably associated with pulmonary consolidation (50 percent), neuropathy, and eosinophilia in the blood, lung, and gastrointestinal tract. Sinusitis, myocarditis, and pericarditis can occur. Treatment involves the use of corticosteroids.

- **Cooley anemia,** more commonly called *thalassemia major*, *beta thalassemia*, or *Mediterranean anemia*, is a homozygous hemogammaglobulinopathy that occurs primarily in tropical and subtropical portions of Europe, Africa, and Asia. The incidence is 1 percent in African Americans, 7 percent in the Greek population, and up to 10 percent in some Italian populations. Both sexes are affected. Patients have hypochromic microcytic anemia, bleeding due to thrombocytopenia, and infection due to leukopenia. Patients also have cardiomegaly, expanded ribs, and paraspinal masses due to extramedullary hematopoesis and hepatosplenomegaly. Patients may develop arrhythmias, cirrhosis of the liver, jaundice, or diabetes. Thalassemia minor refers to the condition as it occurs in heterozygous individuals.

- **CREST syndrome** refers to the combined findings of **C**alcinosis, **R**aynaud phenomena, **E**sophageal dysmotility, **S**clerodactyly, and **T**elangectasia present in some patients with systemic sclerosis. Most patients have some degree of pulmonary involvement, with about one-third having apparent fibrosis. About one in ten patients develops pulmonary hypertension predisposing them to death from cor pulmonale.

- **Cri-du-chat syndrome** is characterized by a weak, high-pitched cry due to a hypoplastic larynx, short stature, and microcephaly with wide-set eyes. Patients have profound mental retardation, and one-fourth have congenital heart disease, most commonly a patent ductus arteriosus.

- **DiGeorge syndrome** refers to hypoplasia or aplasia of the thymus and parathyroids with associated facial malformations. Patients have an increased incidence of interruption of the aortic arch and truncus arteriosis.

Sources: Armstrong P, Wilson AG, Dee P, Hansell DM. *Imaging of Diseases of the Chest.* 2nd ed. St. Louis: Mosby-Year Book Inc.; 1995.

Fraser RG, Paré JAP, Paré PD, Fraser RS, Genereux GP. *Diagnosis of Diseases of the Chest.* Vol. II. 3rd ed. Philadelphia: W B Saunders; 1989.

Gilbert P. *The A-Z Reference Book of Syndromes and Inherited Disorders.* 2nd ed. London: Chapman & Hall; 1996.

Taybi H, Lachman RS. *Radiology of Syndromes, Metabolic Disorders, and Skeletal Dysplasias.* Chicago: Year Book Medical Publishers; 1990.

- **Down syndrome** due to trisomy 21, or occasionally to the presence of an extra portion of chromosome 21 on another chromosome (translocation), affects both sexes equally and occurs in 1 in 800 live births. Risk depends on the mother's age. Approximately 40 percent of patients have congenital heart disease, most commonly endocardial cushion defects, patent ductus arteriosus, and mitral prolapse. Upper respiratory tract infections are common in childhood, and recurring ear infections can lead to deafness. Thoracic skeletal abnormalities can include anterior scalloping of the vertebral bodies, hypersegmentation of the manubrium, and only 11 rib pairs. Acute lymphocytic leukemia occurs with a higher incidence than the normal population.

- **Dressler syndrome** is a postcardiac injury syndrome, specifically occurring following myocardial infarction, and is characterized by fever, pneumonitis, and pleural and pericardial inflammation and effusion.

- **Duchenne muscular dystrophy** is an X-linked neuromuscular disorder characterized by infiltration of muscle by fibrous and fatty tissue. Chest deformities, scoliosis, and weakness of the intercostal muscles predispose patients to bronchitis and pneumonia. Cardiac muscle involvement can lead to congestive heart failure.

- **Eaton-Lambert disease** is a myasthenia gravis–like neuromuscular syndrome associated with malignancies including small cell bronchogenic carcinoma.

- **Ehlers-Danlos syndrome**, also called *chondroectodermal dysplasia*, is a very rare inherited connective tissue disorder causing skin, joint, blood vessel, and internal organ problems. Half of patients have congenital heart disease, commonly a single atrium or septal defects. Valvular stenosis and regurgitation often develop. The laxity of ligaments results in hypermobility and common dislocation. Scoliosis, pectus deformities, thin ribs, and spondylolisthesis are common. Subcutaneous calcifications and ectopic bone occur. Skin is especially fragile, and bruising is common. Arterial walls may be thin, predisposing patients to aortic aneurysm, dissection, and rupture. Angiography is contraindicated. Pulmonary involvement can lead to obstructive lung disease with pneumothorax, pneumonia, tracheobronchomegaly, and bronchiectasis.

- **Eisenmenger syndrome** is the progressive development of a right-to-left cardiac shunt and right heart failure from increasing pulmonary vascular resistance induced by a long-standing left-to-right shunt such as a septal defect or patent ductus arteriosus. There are findings of pulmonary artery hypertension, with enlargement of the right heart, pulmonary trunk, and central pulmonary arteries and pruning of peripheral vessels.

- **Ellis-van Creveld syndrome** is an exceedingly rare autosomal recessive form of dwarfism. Half of patients have congenital heart disease, often a single atrium or a septal defect. Patients have accelerated skeletal maturation, with a tall, thin thorax, horizontally oriented ribs, and elevated clavicles. Restrictive thoracic cage abnormalities can lead to pulmonary hypoplasia.

- **Ebstein anomaly** is a congenital cardiac anomaly characterized by displaced, dysplastic tricuspid valve leaflets. There is usually an atrial septal defect or patent foramen ovale. (See Section 6.9.)

- **Farmer's lung** is an extrinsic allergic alveolitis that develops as a result of exposure to fungal antigens present in moldy hay. (See Section 4.7.)

- **Gaucher disease** is a rare autosomal recessive lysosomal storage disease caused by a deficiency of glucosyl-ceramide β-glucosidase. Features include reticulonodular pulmonary opacities, hepatosplenomegaly, anemia, bruising, bone pain, and fractures.

- **Goodpasture syndrome** is a combination of glomerulonephritis and alveolar hemorrhage in patients with basement membrane antibodies. It is seen almost exclusively in young Caucasian men. The typical presentation is cough, dyspnea, and hemoptysis. Blood serum analysis and renal biopsy can confirm the diagnosis. Lung biopsy is seldom performed. Patients may develop hepatospenomegaly, anemia, pulmonary hemosiderosis, and fibrosis.

- **Gorham disease** (destructive lymphangioma-hemangioendothelioma) is a very rare disorder in which intraosseous proliferation of vascular and lymphatic channels infiltrates the chest wall, causing soft tissue swelling, bone destruction, and pleural effusion.

- **Grave disease** is an autoimmune disease in which thyroid-stimulating antibodies lead to hyperplasia and hypertrophy of the thyroid gland, hyperthyroidism, periorbital edema, and proptosis.

- **Guillain-Barré syndrome** is an acute inflammatory demyelinating condition thought to be related to a hypersensitivity reaction to or reactivation of a latent virus. It frequently follows an infection, often beginning with tingling in the hands and feet and shortly thereafter progressing to generalized weakness eventually involving muscles of respiration. The acute period can last for weeks, with inability to breath or swallow requiring hospitalization and intubation. Atelectasis, aspiration, and pneumonia are common. Recovery is usually complete, with little if any residual weakness.

- **Hammond-Rich syndrome**, also called *acute interstitial pneumonia* or *acute diffuse interstitial fibrosis*, is a rapidly progressive disease of unknown etiology that produces diffuse alveolar damage leading to fibrosis, respiratory failure, and often death.

- **Hand-Schüller-Christian disease** is the disseminated form of *histiocytosis–X* characterized by exopthalmus, diabetes, and lytic skull lesions. Pulmonary involvement can include reticulonodular infiltrates and blebs leading to pneumothorax and fibrosis.

- **Henoch-Schönlein purpura** is a diffuse vasculitis caused by IgA immune complex deposition in cutaneous blood vessels and usually follows a respiratory infection. It is much more common in children, but adults are more likely to have pulmonary involvement (<10 percent), particularly pulmonary hemorrhage. Manifestations include lower extremity purpura, abdominal pain, gastrointestinal bleeding, arthralgia, and sometimes glomerulonephritis.

- **Heyde syndrome**, characterized by aortic stenosis and gastrointestinal bleeding, is thought to be due to angiodysplasia of the colon.

- **Holt-Oram syndrome**, also called *heart-hand syndrome*, is an autosomal dominant condition more common in females than in males. The primary manifestations are upper extremity radial ray defects, but cervical scoliosis, pectus excavatum, or hypoplasia of the clavicle may also be seen. Half of patients have congenital heart disease, often septal defects or pulmonary stenosis.

- **Horner syndrome** is the combination of miosis, ptosis, enopthalmus, and anhidrosis due to sympathetic chain or stellate ganglion involvement, classically in patients with a superior sulcus (Pancoast) tumor.

- **Hurler syndrome** is an autosomal recessive mucopolysaccharidosis in which a deficiency in α-L-iduronidase results in a characteristic accumulation of mucopolysaccharides in body tissues. Hepatosplenomegaly, mental deterioration, and characteristic "gargoyle" features develop. Mucopolysaccharide deposition in the heart and coronaries can lead to heart failure.

- **Ivemark syndrome**, also called *asplenia* or *bilateral right-sidedness*, is more common in males than in females. Almost all patients have congenital heart disease, including endocardial cushion defects, total anomalous venous return, duplication of the superior vena cava, transposition, single ventricle, and septal defects. Patients have bilateral trilobed lungs with both major and minor fissures, bilateral eparterial bronchi, no spleen, a centrally located liver, and high infant mortality.

- **Job syndrome** is a rare primary immunodeficiency characterized by elevated levels of IgE. Patients have recurrent bacterial infections of the skin, sinuses, and lung. Pulmonary infections include bronchitis and pneumonia leading to bronchiectasis, multiple cysts, and occasionally empyema, pneumothorax, and bronchopleural fistula. Most patients have eosinophilia.

- **Kartagener syndrome**, also called *primary ciliary dyskinesia* or *immotile or dysmotile cilia syndrome*, is autosomal recessive and affects both sexes. Patients have abnormal mucociliary function due to deficient dynein arms in cilia, resulting in recurrent sinus and chest infections and eventual bronchiectasis. Ear infections and deafness occur, and patients are infertile because of sperm dysfunction. Half of patients have situs inversus. Congenital heart disease, particularly transposition, is common.

- **Klippel-Feil syndrome** patients have restricted cervical motion due to fusion of multiple vertebra. Genitourinary and ear abnormalities are often associated with this condition. A Sprengel deformity with elevation and rotation of the scapula due to an omovertebral bone is present in one-third of patients. Scoliosis and fusion of ribs is also common, and 5 percent of patients have congenital heart defects, most commonly atrial septal defects or coarctation of the aorta.

- **Langerhan cell granulomatosis**, also called histiocytosis–X, is a group of disorders characterized by granulomatous infiltration of bone, skin, lymph node, lung, and exocrine gland tissues. Although it may involve multiple organ systems, limited bone disease is common. Pulmonary involvement is primarily seen in young female smokers. Findings include upper lobe–predominant nodules and small cysts. Fibrosis can develop. Bone lesions are manifested as focal lytic defects.

- **Legionnaire disease** is pneumonia caused by *Legionella pneumophilia*, first recognized in an outbreak that occurred at an American Legion convention in which many of the attendees died. The infection arises from contaminated water sources and can be manifested as local epidemics. Patients have cough and dyspnea, fever, chest and abdominal pain, nausea, and vomiting. Pneumonia appears as a rapidly progressive consolidation, and pleural effusion is common.

- **Letterer-Siwe disease** is the lethal, systemic form of *histiocytosis–X* seen in infancy. It is associated with hemorrhage, anemia, adenopathy, hepatosplenomegaly, and lytic bone lesions in one-half of patients.

- **Löffler syndrome**, also called *acute eosinophilic pneumonia*, refers to acute transient pulmonary infiltrates and consolidation with peripheral blood and pulmonary eosinophilia that can be idiopathic or from an allergic reaction to parasitic infections such as strongyloidiasis or schistosomiasis. Symptoms are absent or minimal, such as a nonproductive cough, dyspnea, or low fever. Underlying asthma is common. Imaging studies show focal nonsegmental peripheral infiltrates which are migratory, changing over days and clearing within a month.

- **Löfgren syndrome** is a constellation of acute clinical symptoms in patients with sarcoid, including fever, erythema nodosum, arthralgias, and hilar adenopathy with focal pulmonary infiltrates.

- **Louis-Bar syndrome**, more often called *ataxia telangiectasia*, is an autosomal recessive disorder characterized by telangiectasis, ataxia, and immunodeficiency, with sinus and pulmonary infections leading to bronchiectasis and often eventually to respiratory failure. Patients have an increased risk of leukemia, lymphoma, and carcinoma.

- **Lutembacher syndrome** refers to the combination of an atrial septal defect and rheumatic mitral valve stenosis. Patients have cardiomegaly with right atrial and pulmonary vascular enlargement.

- **Marfan syndrome** is an autosomal dominant connective tissue disorder affecting both sexes. Some cases arise sporadically. Patients are tall and thin, with limbs disproportionately long relative to trunk size, generalized osteopenia, and long, slender fingers and toes. Joints are generally very mobile, predisposing them to dislocation. Chest deformities including scoliosis, pectus carinatum, and excavatum are common, as is pneumothorax. Cardiovascular abnormalities are present in most individuals, with aortic disease leading to death in over one-half of patients. The ascending aorta is often dilated and predisposed to aneurysmal dilatation and aortic valvular insufficiency. Myxomatous degeneration leads to mitral and tricuspid valve prolapse and regurgitation. Pulmonary aneurysms can develop, and patients are at increased risk for endocarditis. Myopia and lens dislocation are common eye manifestations.

- **Meigs syndrome** as originally described referred to the combination of ascites and pleural effusion that resolves after resection of a benign ovarian fibroma. The terminology has been extended to include other benign pelvic neoplasms. The effusions are more often right-sided.

- **Mounier-Kuhn syndrome**, also called *tracheobronchomegaly*, is a rare disorder affecting primarily men and may be autosomal recessive. Likely due to insufficiency of the supporting structure, it is manifested as tracheal and central bronchial enlargement, often with bronchiectasis and sometimes in association with anatomic variants of the trachea. Patients have recurrent pulmonary infections, increased sputum production, and dyspnea.

- **Noonan syndrome**, sometimes called "male Turner syndrome," occurs in both sexes and is transmitted as an autosomal dominant trait but can occur sporadically. Congenital heart defects, particularly pulmonary stenosis, septal defects, hypertrophic cardiomyopathy, and patent ductus arteriosis, as well as pectus carinatum or excavatum are common. Patients are short in stature and have distinctive facial characteristics including widely spaced slanted eyes, a short neck, a low hair line, a flat nose bridge, and low-set ears.

- **Osler-Weber-Rendu syndrome**, also called *hereditary hemorrhagic telangiectasis*, is characterized by epistaxis, telangiectasis of the skin and mucus membranes, gastrointestinal bleeding, and multiple pulmonary anteriovenous malformations in about 15 percent of patients.

- **Osteogenesis imperfecta** is an autosomal recessive connective tissue disorder causing micromelic dwarfism, blue sclera, lax joints, poor dentition, thin, loose skin, diffuse bone demineralization, and defective cortical bone leading to multiple fractures and often pseudoarthrosis. Congenital cardiac lesions can include aortic, mitral, or pulmonic valve insufficiency. Aortic aneurysm can develop. A restrictive thorax can lead to pulmonary hypoplasia, and patients also have an increased incidence of pulmonary emphysema.

- **Pancoast tumor** was a term originally used to describe a superior sulcus bronchogenic carcinoma invading bone and the sympathetic chain causing ipsilateral Horner syndrome. The term is used more generally to refer to patients with shoulder or arm pain due to invasion of the brachial plexus or sympathetic chain. These are typically squamous cell carcinoma. (See Section 3.3.)

- **Pickwickian syndrome**, also called *alveolar hypoventilation syndrome*, is the result of obstructive sleep apnea and hypoventilation causing hypoxemia and hypercapnea in obese individuals. The heart and central pulmonary arteries may be enlarged.

- **Poland syndrome** is an autosomal recessive condition characterized by variable unilateral absence of the pectoralis muscles (typically the sternocostal head of the pectoralis major). Associated abnormalities can include syndactyly or polydactyly, scoliosis or vertebral body anomalies, scapular hypoplasia, rib or sternal abnormalities, and ipsilateral breast aplasia (Fig. 8-14).

- **Potter syndrome** is one of several syndromes combining pulmonary hypoplasia and gastrointestinal-genitourinary abnormalities. In Potter syndrome there is renal agenesis, abnormal facies, and limb abnormalities.

- **Q fever** refers to a rickettsial pneumonia caused by *Coxiella burnetti*. It is most commonly contracted from tick bites, cattle, or sheep products. Patients have fever, cough, myalgias, headache, and arthralgias. About one-half develop pneumonia, sometimes with a rounded appearance (round pneumonia).

- **Raynaud disease** refers to episodic ischemia in the hands associated with pain, numbness, and cyanosis. It is the result of arterial vasoconstriction induced by cold temperature or emotional upset. Raynaud phenomenon refers to digital ischemia due to occlusion from vascular disease.

- **Rocky Mountain spotted fever** is caused by *Rickettsia rickettsiae* and is transmitted to humans by tick bite. The associated systemic vasculitis often leads to pulmonary edema and hemorrhage.

- **Shone complex** refers to a form of hypoplastic left heart syndrome with subaortic stenosis, coarctation of the aorta, supravalvular left atrial ring, and "parachute mitral valve" in which all chordae arise from a single papillary muscle, thus restricting valve leaflet motion.

- **Silo filler's disease** is a result of nitrous oxide inhalation. Death may occur. Patients have cough, dyspnea, and radiographic findings of pulmonary edema. Untreated bronchiolitis obliterans may develop and manifest as tiny pulmonary nodules. Treatment involves steroids.

- **Sjögren syndrome** is an autoimmune collagen vascular disorder affecting exocrine glands and is characterized by a dry mouth and dry eyes. It is often seen in association with other connective tissue disorders, particularly rheumatoid arthritis, scleroderma, polymyositis, or lupus and termed secondary Sjögrens. Patients have chronic bronchitis, recurrent pneumonia, and a higher incidence of chronic active hepatitis, cirrhosis, thyroiditis, bronchiectasis, and lymphoproliferative disorders such as pseudolymphoma. Patients may have pleural effusions and develop lipoid interstitial pneumonia or pulmonary fibrosis.

- **Sturge-Weber syndrome** is a neurocutaneous syndrome (phakomatosis) characterized by seizures and capillary venous angiomas, classically a unilateral facial port wine stain in the distribution of cranial nerve V. Angiomatous malformations can also occur in the lungs and abdominal organs.

- **Swyer-James syndrome**, also called *MacLeod syndrome*, is a form of bronchiolitis obliterans that occurs in developing lungs (during the first 8 years of life) following a pulmonary insult such as a viral or mycoplasma infection. It is typically unilateral, affecting a single lobe or entire lung which appears smaller and radiolucent compared to the contralateral normal lung. Pathologically it is hypoplastic, with underdeveloped pulmonary vessels, bronchitis, bronchiolitis, and emphysema present. (See Section 9.2.)

- **Takayasu arteritis** (pulseless disease) is a vasculitis of medium and large vessels that commonly affects the aorta and its major branches and pulmonary arteries. Granulomatous inflammation in the media lead to thickening of the vessel wall, eventual fibrosis, and stenosis. It is more common in women than in men and frequently appears in the second decade. Significant ischemia and pulmonary artery hypertension can develop.

- **Taussig-Bing heart** is a form of double-outlet right ventricle with malposition of the great vessels and the pulmonary artery is above the ventricular septal defect.

- **Tetralogy of Fallot** accounts for about 10 percent of congenital heart disease. The four principal components are right ventricular outflow track obstruction, a ventricular septal defect, right ventricular hypertrophy, and an overriding aorta. A bicuspid pulmonic valve, left pulmonary artery stenosis, and right aortic arch are common. Pentalogy includes an atrial septal defect. (See Section 6.9.)

- **Trousseau syndrome** is a hypercoagulable state producing recurrent migratory thrombophlebitis in patients with neoplastic disease, particularly pancreatic carcinoma.

- **Tuberous sclerosis** is a rare autosomal dominant neurocutaneous syndrome with a low penetrance. Over one-half of cases are sporadic. Features include mental retardation and seizures, café-au-lait spots, adenoma sebaceum around the nose and cheeks (dermal angiofibromas), and tumors including subependymal hamartomas, giant cell astrocytomas, cortical hamartomas, and heterotopic islands of white matter. Renal cysts and angiomyolipomas are common, and renal cell carcinoma occurs at an increased rate. Lung involvement is rare but similar to lymphangioleiomyomatosis with small pulmonary cysts, chylothorax, and pneumothorax, but also small nodules. Cardiomyopathy and cardiac rhabdomyoma can occur. Most patients die by early adulthood.

- **Turner syndrome** occurs only in females. An X chromosome is missing. Characteristics include short stature, webbed neck, and infertility. General heart disease, particularly coarctation and aortic stenosis, are common. Atrial septal defects, pulmonic stenosis, and aortic dissection can also occur. The ribs and clavicles may be thin and narrow. A horseshoe kidney is common.

- **VATER association** consists of vertebral anomalies, anal malformations, tracheal and esophageal defects including tracheoesophageal fistulas, renal problems, and radial limb defects. Congenital heart disease is more common than in the general population.

- **Von Recklinghausen disease** is the most common form of neurofibromatosis (type I) and is autosomal dominant. Spontaneous mutations account for half of cases and the severity is variable. Café-au-lait spots, representing increased melanin deposition, and neurofibromas in the subcutaneous tissues and cranial nerve schwannomas are the principal manifestations. Skin nodules can mimic pulmonary nodules on chest radiographs. Neurofibrosarcomas can develop and metastasize to the lung. Skeletal findings include scoliosis, thin, twisted ribs, and rib notching from neurofibromas of the intercostal nerves. About one-fifth of adult patients have fibrosing alveolitis, typically with a basal predominance. Upper lobe bullae are also common. Cardiac manifestations can include aortic and pulmonic stenosis, coarctation, and aortic aneurysms. Pheochromocytoma, medullary thyroid carcinoma, and congenital heart disease including pulmonary stenosis, septal defects, and idiopathic hypertrophic subaortic stenosis occur at a higher incidence than in the general population. Plexiform neurofibromatosis is an exceedingly rare variant in which complex overgrowths of nervous and fibrous tissue occur throughout the body and can be of great size.

- **Waldenström macroglobulinemia** is a rare lymphoproliferative disease characterized by a malignant production of IgM, similar to multiple myeloma. This produces lymphadenopathy, anemia, hepatosplenomegaly, and osteopenia. Lung involvement is uncommon and includes reticulonodular infiltration and pleural effusion.

- **Wegener granulomatosis** is an immunologic reaction with necrotizing vasculitis causing sinusitis and necrotizing glomerulonephritis. Both sexes are affected, typically during middle age. Almost all patients develop lung disease at some time, typically nodules or focal areas of consolidation, often with cavitation. Tracheal involvement can cause thickening and narrowing.

- **Weil disease**, or *leptospirosis*, occurs in the tropics and is caused by the spirochete *Leptospira*. Patients develop fever, jaundice, hemorrhage, nephritis, and meningitis. Hemorrhagic pneumonia with nodules or bronchopneumonia occurs in one-third of patients, often with a peripheral distribution. Pleural effusion is common; adenopathy is rare.

- **White-Bland-Garland syndrome** is a congenital anomaly with the left coronary artery originating from the pulmonary artery. There is usually sufficient myocardial perfusion until shortly after birth when pulmonary artery resistance drops and ischemia ensues. Infants develop congestive heart failure and Q waves are observed on the electrocardiogram.

- **William syndrome** is neonatal hypercalcemia with osteosclerosis, dense vertebral endplates, and metastatic calcification. Congenital heart defects include supravalvular aortic stenosis, septal defects, and peripheral pulmonary stenosis. Patients are mentally retarded and have elfin faces.

- **William-Campbell syndrome** is a result of a diffuse or focal congenital bronchial cartilage deficiency in the fourth to eighth bronchial generations. Affected bronchi collapse during expiration, producing air trapping. Patients develop cystic bronchiectasis and distal emphysema.

- **Wilson disease** is an autosomal recessive disorder characterized by excessive copper retention. Skeletal manifestations include osteopenia, chondrocalcinosis, and premature osteoarthritis.

- **Wiskott-Aldrich syndrome** is an X-linked autosomal recessive disorder characterized by thrombocytopenic purpura, eczema, immunodeficiency, and infection. Hemorrhage and bronchiectasis are common.

- **Wolf-Parkinson-White** is a reentry-type supraventricular tachycardia resulting from an accessory pathway, termed bundle of Kent. The electrocardiogram shows a short PR interval and a widened QRS complex.

A.6 CANCER STAGING

- The TNM system is widely used for describing and recording the stage of various cancers.

  T (primary tumor size and location)

  T1, T2, T3, and **T4** by tumor type, location, and size

  TX Primary not visualized or cannot be assessed

  T0 No evidence of primary tumor

  Tis Carcinoma in situ.

  N (Lymph node involvement)

  N1, N2, and sometimes **N3** by location and size of lymph node involvement

  NX Cannot be assessed.

  M (Distant metastases)

  M0 No distant metastases

  M1 Distant metastases

  MX Cannot be assessed.

TNM Staging of Non-Small Cell Bronchogenic Carcinoma

Tumor size and location		Lymph nodes			
		N0	N1	N2	N3
		No positive nodes	Ipsilateral peribronchial or hilar	Subcarinal or ipsilateral mediastinal	Supraclavicular, scalene, contralateral mediastinal or hilar
T1	≤ 3 cm in diameter surrounded by lung or visceral pleura without invasion proximal to lobar bronchus.	I	II	IIIA	IIIB
T2	> 2 cm distal to carina and > 3 cm or visceral pleural invasion, associated atelectasis or pneumonia extending to hilum.	I	II	IIIA	IIIB
T3	< 2 cm from carina, total lung collapse or consolidation, parietal or mediastinal pleura, chest wall, diaphragm or parietal pericardial invasion.	IIIA	IIIA	IIIA	IIIB
T4	Invasion of the heart, great vessels, trachea, carina, esophagus, spine or malignant pleural effusion.	IIIB	IIIB	IIIB	IIIB

Metachronous primaries increase T by one

Stage IV—Any T, Any N, M1.

Stages IIIB and IV are unresectable

Five Year Survival Following Surgery: Stage I—65%, Stage II—40%, Stage IIIA—20%.

Staging Small Cell Bronchogenic Carcinoma

• Small cell carcinoma is almost always metastatic when diagnosed. Staging is confined to the following two categories.

Limited   Disease limited to one hemithorax with regional hilar and mediastinal adenopathy amenable to a single radiation therapy portal.

Extensive   Disease beyond the boundaries of a single radiation therapy portal.

TNM Staging of Esophageal Cancer

Tumor size and location		Lymph nodes	
		N0	N1
		No positive nodes	Regional lymph node metastases
T1	Invades lamia propria or submucosa	I	IIB
T2	Invades muscularis propria	IIA	IIB
T3	Invades adventitia	IIA	III
T4	Invades adjacent structures (trachea, bronchi, vessels, heart)	III	III

Stage IV—Any T, Any N, M1.

M1 distant metastases; cervical, supraclavicular, or abdominal nodes with thoracic esophageal cancer; any node other than cervical or supraclavicular with a cervical primary.

TNM Staging of Breast Cancer

Tumor size and location		Lymph nodes			
		N0	N1	N2	N3
		No positive nodes	Mobile, ipsilateral axillary	Fixed ipsilateral axillary	Ipsilateral internal mammary
T1	< 2 cm in diameter	I	IIA	IIIA	IIIB
T2	< 5 cm in diameter	IIA	IIB	IIIA	IIIB
T3	> 5 cm in diameter	IIB	IIIA	IIIA	IIIB
T4	Invasion of skin or chest wall	IIIB	IIIB	IIIB	IIIB

M1—Distant metastases including ipsilateral supraclavicular nodes.

Stage IV— Any T, Any N, M1.

TNM Staging of Head and Neck Cancers

Tumor	Lymph nodes			
	N0	N1	N2	N3
Varies by location. See list below.	No clinically positive nodes	Single clinically positive ipsilateral < 3 cm	Single ipsilateral > 3 cm, contralateral or multiple ipsilateral < 6 cm	Metastases > 6 cm
T1	I	III	IV	IV
T2	II	III	IV	IV
T3	III	III	IV	IV
T4	IV	IV	IV	IV

Stage IV— Any T, Any N, M1.

NASOPHARYNX

T1 Tumor not visible or confined to one site
T2 Involving two sites
T3 Extension into nasal cavity or oropharynx
T4 Invasion of skull or cranial nerves

OROPHARYNX

T1 Less than 2 cm in greatest dimension
T2 Less than 4 cm
T3 Greater than 4 cm
T4 Greater than 4 cm with bone, neck, or deep tongue involvement

SUPRAGLOTTIS

T1 Tumor confined to site of origin with normal vocal cord mobility
T2 Involving glottis or adjacent supraglottic sites with normal vocal cord mobility

T3 Limited to larynx with fixation or extension to postcricoid, medial wall of pyriform sinus or preepiglottic space
T4 Extending beyond larynx to oropharynx, neck soft tissues, or thyroid cartilage destruction

GLOTTIS OR SUBGLOTTIS (HYPOPHARYNX)

T1 Tumor confined to subglottic region or vocal cords with normal mobility
T2 Local extension to cords, supraglottis, or subglottic region
T3 Confined to larynx with vocal cord fixation
T4 Thyroid cartilage destruction or extension beyond larynx to oropharynx or neck soft tissues

A.7   LYMPHOMA

Comparison of Hodgkin and Non-Hodgkin Lymphoma

	Hodgkin	Non-Hodgkin
Frequency	12% of lymphoma	
Age peak	20 to 30, 65 to 85	Increases with age
Stage I or II at presentation	45%	10%
Pattern of spread	Contiguous	Noncontiguous
Neck or chest involvement	95% young adults 75% elderly	50%
Retroperitoneal adenopathy	25%	50%
Extranodal sites	Uncommon	Common
Lung involvement	10%, most commonly by bronchovascular spread but can be subpleural, pneumonic, or nodular	< 5%
Prognosis	Stage dependent	Histology dependent

Lymphoma Staging

Stage I   Single lymph node region, contiguous extralymphatic site or organ

Stage II   Two or more regions on the same side of the diaphragm

Stage III   Node regions, extralymphatic sites, or organs on both sides of the diaphragm

Stage IV   Diffuse involvement of extralymphatic site, organs, or node regions

A   No systemic symptoms (important for treatment planning in Hodgkin)

B   Weight loss >10 percent, fever, pruritis, or night sweats

E   Extranodal involvement (important for treatment planning in non-Hodgkin)

S   Spleen involved

Source: Roth JA, Ruckdeschel JC, Weisenburger TH. *Thoracic Oncology.* 2nd ed. Philadelphia: WB Saunders; 1995; and Murphy GP, Lawrence W, Lenhard RE. *Clinical Oncology.* 2nd ed. Atlanta: American Cancer Society; 1995.

Classification of Hodgkin Lymphoma

- **Nodular sclerosis** (50 percent) predominates in young women and is characterized by collagen bands dividing islands of cellular infiltrate in lymph nodes. It is often localized to the neck or chest at diagnosis. Five-year survival is about 70%.

- **Mixed cellularity** (30 percent) predominates in older adults. Five-year survival exceeds 50 percent.

- **Lymphocyte-predominant** (10 percent) is characterized by abundant mature lymphocytes. Five-year survival is 90 percent.

- **Lymphocyte-depleted** (<10 percent) occurs primarily in older adults and has a poor prognosis.

Classification of Non-Hodgkin Lymphoma

- **Low grade** includes (1) small lymphocytic, (2) follicular, small cleaved cell, and (3) follicular, mixed.

- **Intermediate grade** includes (1) follicular, predominantly large cell, (2) diffuse small cleaved cell, (3) diffuse large cell, cleaved or noncleaved.

- **High grade** includes (1) diffuse large cell immunoblastic, (2) small noncleaved cell, and (3) lymphoblastic.

Lymphoma Treatment

- **Hodgkin** Stages I and II are treated with intensive radiotherapy. Stage III is treated with radiation, chemotherapy, or both. Stage IV is treated with chemotherapy alone.

- **Non-Hodgkin lymphoma** of intermediate and high grade are treated primarily with chemotherapy. Radiation is occasionally used to treat localized residual disease.

A.8 PATHOLOGIC CLASSIFICATION OF LUNG AND PLEURAL TUMORS

- Proposed revisions to the World Health Organization (WHO) and International Association for the Study of Lung Cancer (IASLC) Pathology Panel classification system are based primarily on light microscopy to maximize generalizability with a goal toward establishing meaningful, reproducible classifications related to survival differences.

- **Benign epithelial tumors** include squamous, glandular, and mixed-type papillomas and alveolar, papillary, and salivary gland–type adenomas such as pleomorphic adenomas and mucinous cystadenomas.

- **Preinvasive lesions** include squamous dysplasia and carcinoma in situ, precursors of squamous cell carcinoma, atypical adenomatous hyperplasia (which is similar to noninvasive bronchoalveolar carcinoma, possibly a precursor of adenocar-

cinoma), and diffuse idiopathic pulmonary neuroendocrine cell hyperplasia (possibly a precursor of carcinoid).

- **Malignant epithelial tumors** include squamous cell (epidermoid carcinoma), adeno, large cell, adenosquamous, carcinoid, small cell, and salivary gland–type carcinomas, cancer with pleomorphic, sarcomatoid or sarcomatous elements, and unclassified carcinoma.

  Squamous cell carcinoma is characterized by pink keratin pearls in a whirled arrangement and intracellular bridges (prominent tonofilaments by electron microscopy). Variants include papillary, clear cell, small cell, and basaloid subtypes.

  Adenocarcinoma is a histologically heterogeneous mixture of tumors showing glandular differentiation which is divided into acinar, papillary, bronchoalveolar, solid adenocarcinoma with mucin formation, and mixed subtypes. Variants include signet ring, clear cell, mucinous and colloid (which produces significant mucin), mucinous cyst adenocarcinoma, and well-differentiated fetal adenocarcinoma (previously considered a variant of pulmonary blastoma).

  Bronchoalveolar cell carcinoma is a proliferation along preexisting alveolar structures without invasive growth. It is a frequent component of bronchogenic carcinomas but is uncommon in a pure form. It is frequently multicentric. It is classified as mucinous (containing goblet cells, shown well with a mucicarmine stain), nonmucinous (containing Clara cells and type 2 pneumocytes), and mixed mucinous-nonmucinous variants.

  Adenosquamous is a continuum of mixed tumors having both glandular and squamous differentiation and containing more than 10 percent adeno or squamous features.

  Large cell tumors are diagnosed by light microscopy based on the absence of squamous, adeno, or small cell characteristics. Variants include large cell neuroendocrine, basaloid, clear cell, lymphoepithelioma-like cancers and very rare rhabdoid phenotypes. Large cell tumors are larger than three resting lymphocytes and have abundant cytoplasm with a low nuclear/cytoplasm ratio, frequent nucleoli, and coarse chromatin.

  Carcinomas with **pleomorphic, sarcomatoid**, or **sarcomatous elements** are relatively rare tumors that show heterogeneity in their histologic differentiation and have a poor prognosis. They include carcinosarcoma, pulmonary blastoma, and pleomorphic carcinoma with spindle and/or giant cells, which are typically large and peripheral and often invade the chest wall.

- **Neuroendocrine tumors** of the lung are divided into three grades based on prognosis. Low grade includes typical carcinoids, which have a 90 percent 10-year survival rate. Intermediate grade includes atypical carcinoids, which have 60 percent 5-year and 40 percent 10-year survival rates. High grade includes large cell neuroendocrine tumors, which have 30 percent 5-year and 10 percent 10-year survival rates, and small cell carcinoma, which has a 10 percent 5-year and almost no 10-year survival rate.

  Neuroendocrine morphology is defined by immunohistochemistry demonstration of neuroendocrine markers (granules) or by electron microscopy characteristics including

Presented by William D. Travis at the 1997 meeting of the American College of Chest Physicians.

neuroendocrine granules, organoid nesting, and trabecular, palisading, or rosettelike patterns.

Small cell carcinoma is classified based partly on a cell size less than the diameter of three small resting lymphocytes and also on the presence of scant cytoplasm, finely granular nuclear chromatin, inconspicuous nucleoli, extensive necrosis, and a high mitotic rate. The single variant category is termed ***combined small cell carcinoma*** and includes, for example, combinations of small cell with large cell, squamous cell, or adenocarcinoma.

Carcinoid tumors include typical and atypical varieties. **Typical** features include uniform cell size, finely granular nuclear chromatin, a moderate amount of eosinophilic cytoplasm, and organoid nesting. Features of **atypical** carcinoid include a greater number of mitoses or foci of necrosis. All carcinoid tumors are malignant and have the potential to metastasize.

- **Carcinomas** of the **salivary gland type** include mucoepidermoid and adenoid cystic.

- **Mesothelial tumors** include malignant mesothelioma of epithelioid, sarcomatoid, and biphasic subtypes. Immunohistochemistry or electron microscopy may be needed to distinguish mesothelioma from adenocarcinoma. ***Adenomatoid mesothelioma*** is a very rare benign mesothelioma. Tumors invading the lung are by definition adenocarcinomas of the lung.

- **Lymphoproliferative disease** includes lipoid interstitial pneumonia (LIP), nodular lymphoid hyperplasia, low-grade marginal zone B-cell lymphoma of the mucosa-associated lymphoid tissue (MALT), lymphoid granulomatosis, and lymphoma.

- **Secondary tumors** include a wide range of pulmonary metastases.

- **Miscellaneous tumors** include hamartoma (a benign neoplasm), sclerosing hemangioma, clear cell tumor, germ cell tumors such as teratomas, thymomas, and melanomas. Some tumors remain unclassified.

A.9 LEADING CAUSES OF DEATH IN THE UNITED STATES

- Chest-related disease accounts for over one-half of all deaths in the United States.

Cause		Deaths per Year
1	Heart Disease	750,000 (33%)
2	Cancer	530,000 (23%)
	Bronchogenic	(160,000)
	Breast (#2 in women)	(44,000)
	Prostate (#2 in men)	(39,000)
	Colon (#3 in both sexes)	(56,000)
	Lymphoma and leukemia	(48,000)
	Pancreas	(29,000)
3	Stroke	150,000 (7%)
4	COPD	100,000 (5%)
5	Accidents	90,000 (4%)
6	Pneumonia	80,000 (4%)
7–10	Diabetes, HIV, suicide and homicide	200,000 (10%)
All others		400,000 (17%)
Total		2,300,000

Trauma, including accidents, homicide, and suicide, accounts for over 100,000 deaths annually.

A.10 NEW YORK HEART ASSOCIATION CLASSIFICATION OF CONGESTIVE HEART FAILURE

Class I No limitation; ordinary activity does not cause undue fatigue, dyspnea, or palpitations.

Class II Slight limitation; comfortable at rest; ordinary activity results in fatigue, dyspnea, palpitations, or angina.

Class III Marked limitation; comfortable at rest; less than ordinary activity results in symptoms.

Class IV Inability to carry on any activity without discomfort; symptoms of congestion are present at rest and worsen with activity.

Source: Landis SH, Murray T, Bolden S, Wingo PA. *Cancer Statistics*, 1998. *CA Cancer J. Clin.* 1998;48(1):6–29.

INDEX

INDEX

Note: The letter *f* following a page number indicates that a figure is being referenced.

Congenital pulmonary disease and
    pediatrics *(cont'd)*
    cystic fibrosis (CF), 208, 209*f*
    cytomegalovirus (CMV), 212
    histoplasmosis, 212
    human immunodeficiency virus (HIV),
        211–213
    lung abscess, 210–211
    lymphocytic interstitial pneumonitis
        (LIP), 212, 212*f*
    mucormycosis, 212–213
    mycobacterial infection, 213, 213*f*
    obliterative bronchiolitis (OB), 209
    pertussis, 210
    pneumatoceles, 210
    Pneumocystis carinii pneumonia
        (PCP), 211–212
    round pneumonia, 210, 210*f*
    varicella-zoster virus, 212
    viral infection, 211–213
    neonatal chest
        bronchopulmonary dysplasia, 205–206
        chest radiographs, 203
        hyaline membrane disease (HMD),
            203–205, 205*f*
        meconium aspiration, 206
        neonatal pneumonia, 206, 206*f*
        transient tachypnea of the newborn,
            206
        Wilson-Mikity syndrome, 206
    parenchymal lung neoplasms, 213
    pediatric chest imaging, 195
Congestive heart failure, 38, 40, 45–47, 52,
        57–59, 62–63, 207, 230*f*, 288
    neonates, 150
    differential diagnosis, 58–59
Connective tissue disease, 35, 41–43, 51
    ankylosing spondylitis, 28, 41–42, 111
    collagen vascular disease. *See* Collagen
        vascular disease
    dermatomyositis, 28, 41–42, 50, 111
    rheumatoid arthritis, 28, 35, 43, 46,
        51–52, 110
    scleroderma, 27–28, 35, 41–43, 50,
        56–57, 110, 110*f*
    Sjögren syndrome, 42, 110, 324–325
    systemic lupus erythematosus, 110, 110*f*
Conn syndrome, 296
Consolidation, differential diagnosis of. *See*
        Differential diagnosis for the
        chest, consolidation and airspace
        disease
Constrictive bronchiolitis, 102
Constrictive pericarditis, 47, 57, 62–63,
        162, 162*f*
Continuous diaphragm sign, 220
Contralateral mediastinal shift, differential
        diagnosis of, 53
Contrast reaction, 40
Conventional tomography, 11
Cooley anemia, definition of, 321
COPD (chronic obstructive pulmonary
        disease), 61

Coronary arteries, 149, 149*f*
    aneurysms, 160
        differential diagnosis, 62
        arteriography, 160
        calcification, 159–160
        coronary artery bypass graft (CABG)
            surgery, 258, 259*f*, 270, 272*f*
Coronary dominance, 149
Coronary heart disease
    atherosclerosis, 59–60, 62, 159, 308*f*
    coronary arteriography, 160
    coronary artery aneurysms, 62, 160
    coronary artery calcification, 59, 160
    left ventricular aneurysms, 159–160
    overview, 159, 159*f*
    percutaneous transluminal coronary
        angioplasty (PTCA), 160
Coronary sinus, 149–150
Coronary stents, 257, 279
Cor pulmonale, 59
Cortical nephrocalcinosis, 298
Cortriatrium, 62
Costal cartilate fractures, 224
Costochondritis, 64, 181
Costovertebral articulations, 179
Coughing, 5, 5*f*, 6
Couinaud segments, 286, 286*f*
Coxsackie infection, 64
CR (computed radiography), 9–10, 229
CREST (calcification in soft tissues, Raynaud
        disease, esophageal dysmotility,
        sclerodactaly, and telangectasias)
        syndrome, 50, 110, 321
Cri-du-chat syndrome, definition of, 321
Cronchogenic cyst, 52
Crossed-fused ectopia, 298
Croup (acute laryngotracheobronchitis),
        196
Cryptococcosis, 29–30, 33, 80
Cryptococcus infection, 64–65
    gallium 67 scanning, 16
CT. *See* Computed tomography
Cushing syndrome, 57, 296
CVLs (central venous lines), 231,
        231*f*–233*f*, 313*f*, 313–314
Cyanosis, 150
    differential diagnosis, 61
    with increased pulmonary vascularity,
        155–157, 157*f*
    with normal or decreased pulmonary vas-
        cularity, 153–155, 153*f*–155*f*
Cylindrical bronchiectasis, 100, 100*f*
Cyst, 95
Cystadenomas, 294
Cystic adenomatoid malformation, 32–33
Cystic airspace, 61
Cystic bronchiectasis, 32, 100*f*, 100–101
Cystic fibrosis (CF), 25–29, 34–35, 38, 40,
        45, 49, 52, 55, 101–102, 208,
        209*f*
Cystic hygroma, 54–55, 57
    pediatric patients, 199
Cystic lesions

ISBN 0-07-058223-8

90000

9 780070 582231

SLONE: THORACIC IMAGING